Manual
PHYSICAL
THERAPY
OF THE SPINE

THIRD EDITION

To my wife, Janet, and children, Will and Emma,
for their love and support, and for bringing joy to my life

To my parents, John and Anna Mae, for providing a solid foundation to grow and learn

To my grandmother, Miriam, for instilling a passion for helping and teaching

THIRD EDITION

MANUAL
PHYSICAL
THERAPY
OF THE SPINE

Kenneth A. Olson

PT, DHSc, OCS, FAAOMPT
Private Practitioner
Northern Rehab Physical Therapy Specialists
DeKalb, Illinois, USA

Adjunct Faculty
Physical Therapy Program
Northern Illinois University
DeKalb, Illinois, USA

ELSEVIER

Elsevier
3251 Riverport Lane
St. Louis, Missouri 63043

MANUAL PHYSICAL THERAPY OF THE SPINE, THIRD EDITION ISBN: 9780323673396

ISBN: 9780323673396

Previous editions copyrighted 2016, 2009.

Senior Content Strategist: Lauren Willis
Director, Content Development: Ellen Wurm-Cutter
Content Development Specialist: Sara Watkins
Publishing Services Manager: Shereen Jameel
Project Manager: Nadhiya Sekar
Design Direction: Ryan Cook

Printed in India

Last digit is the print number: 9 8 7 6 5 4 3 2

FOREWORD

Dr. Ken Olson's textbook, *Manual Physical Therapy of the Spine*, has evolved over three editions and eleven years. Since the original publication in 2009, we have used this textbook and have found it to be an invaluable manual physical therapy resource for physical therapy students and clinicians. It provides an excellent foundation for a comprehensive examination and clinical management of the spine for an orthopedic manual physical therapist. As President of the International Federation of Orthopaedic Manipulative Physical Therapists (IFOMPT), Dr. Olson leads a multinational organization of physiotherapists who specialize in manual therapy. The IFOMPT defines Orthopedic Manual Therapy as "a specialized area of physical therapy for the management of neuromusculoskeletal conditions, based on clinical reasoning, using highly specific treatment approaches including manual techniques and therapeutic exercises." While lending clarity to the techniques of orthopedic manual physical therapy, Dr. Olson also provides a wealth of patient case examples. This textbook connects all the aspects of the description of orthopedic manual physical therapy and is much more than a book of techniques. These cases demonstrate how to use advanced clinical reasoning to determine the most effective management approach that integrates hands-on skilled manual techniques, targeted exercises, and education to optimize outcomes, including a reduction in pain and improvement in function. Manual physical therapy has been historically viewed as soft tissue or segmental mobilization/manipulation techniques. This textbook provides the reader with a foundation of all aspects of orthopedic manual physical therapy.

We welcome this new edition as it builds on the relevant and practical information in previous versions with clarity and support from the literature. Dr. Olson presents a well-informed approach to evidence-based principles in each chapter. Recognizing the traditions of the past and embracing the need for refinement and support of the evidence, he blends the art, skill, and knowledge to create a foundation for new students and advanced information for skilled clinicians. One hallmark of an expert in OMPT is exceptional education and communication. Readers will find pain science education and psychologically informed communication strategies to describe impairments and the effects of manual therapy. Dr. Olson highlights physical therapy interventions with known effectiveness and recommends that clinicians avoid using language that may induce fear and lead individuals to seek high-risk procedures and medication.

This edition also includes the revision of the IFOMPT Clinical Reasoning Framework for Cervical Arterial Dysfunction, as well as a comprehensive section on red flags. This textbook is a tremendous teaching resource for physical therapy students, academic faculty, and residency/fellowship instructors. Readers will find it an invaluable resource for best practice evaluation and treatment techniques to confidently care for the client at hand and prepare orthopedic manual physical therapists to be frontline providers for patients with spinal pain.

Elaine and Paul Lonnemann

PREFACE

The third edition of this textbook has maintained the format and organization established in the first and second editions but has updated and expanded the research evidence presented to support an impairment-based manual physical therapy approach to evaluate and treat spinal and temporomandibular conditions.

Nearly 200 video clips of the vast majority of examination and manual therapy treatment procedures are available in the eBook. For the third edition, an enhanced eBook version is included *with print purchase*. Those who purchase the print book will be able to access the eBook (for free) on Student Consult via the scratch-off pin code on the inside front cover of the book. Customers will also be able to purchase this enhanced eBook directly on Student Consult if they do not care to purchase the print book. The video clips were filmed at Marquette University with the technical support of the Marquette University Instructional Media Center, where multiple camera angles are used to assure excellent visualization of each procedure.

Each chapter has areas that have been updated and expanded. The primary addition of Chapter 1 involves adding further details related to the history of manipulation and expanded explanation of clinical reasoning associated with biopsychosocial approach to spinal and temporomandibular conditions musculoskeletal. Chapter 2 includes updates and additions to the red flag screening and assessment of central sensitization, pressure pain thresholds, and impaired sleep for the clinical reasoning in musculoskeletal physical therapy practice. Chapter 3 includes an expanded and updated explanation of the effects of manipulation based on new evidence of the mechanical, neurophysiologic, and psychologic effects of manipulation, and expands on the impact of use of language and pain science education in the management of complex musculoskeletal pain conditions. The Chapter 3 section on the safety of manipulation expands on the potential risk factors for vascular pathology of the neck and on safety issues specific to the thoracic spine manipulation.

Chapters 4 through 7 have maintained the same formatting structure for each region of the spine and the temporomandibular joint (TMJ), with updates and expansion on the diagnostic accuracy information and evidence to support the therapeutic exercise and mobilization/manipulation interventions in each region. Chapter 4 expands on the use of psychologically informed management strategies for chronic low back pain. Chapter 5 has updates on the evidence to support the use of thoracic manipulation, especially for shoulder and neck pain conditions. Chapter 6 has updates on the evidence to support classification, manual therapy, and therapeutic exercise for the management of cervical spinal conditions with information added on whiplash associated disorders and headaches. Chapter 7 includes enhanced research evidence to support the examination/classification and treatment of temporomandibular disorders.

This textbook provides the necessary background information and detailed instructional materials to allow full integration of manipulation and manual physical therapy examination and treatment procedures of the spine and TMJ into physical therapist professional education and clinical practice. This textbook combined with the video clips provides the necessary background and instructional information to assist in skill development to effectively implement contemporary evidence-informed treatment recommendations related to manual therapy, manipulation, and therapeutic exercise.

The primary audience for this textbook is physical therapy students and faculty in professional physical therapist education programs. The secondary audience for this textbook is practicing physical therapists and other clinicians who wish to keep up with what is being taught in professional physical therapist education programs. Additionally, persons in manual physical therapy residency, fellowship, and postprofessional degree programs in musculoskeletal and manual physical therapy will find this textbook to be a useful adjunct to other instructional materials.

The textbook and video clips will be very useful additions to the permanent library of clinicians who practice manual therapy techniques to manage spinal disorders. Although the body of research evidence will continue to evolve over time, the technique descriptions and presentations will remain as valuable resources to reference when practitioners are presented with various spinal and TMJ disorders in the future.

Kenneth A. Olson

Acknowledgments

Professionally, I am indebted to the influence and mentorship of Stanley Paris and the faculty and staff of the University of St. Augustine for Health Sciences, who guided my graduate education. Other professional mentors include Annalie Basson, Bill Boissonnault, Tim Dunlop, Laurie Hartman, Mary Jane Harris, Trish King, David Lamb, Steve McDavitt, Catherine Patla, Duncan Reid, Mariano Rocabodo, Bob Rowe, and Guy Simoneau. I am grateful to Jason Beneciuk, Josh Cleland, Elaine Lonnemann, Paul Lonnemann, Louie Puentedura, Ron Schenk, and Guy Simoneau for reviewing chapters of various editions of this textbook and providing useful feedback to improve the quality of the project.

I want to acknowledge the many colleagues I have served with during my 12 years on the International Federation of Orthopaedic Manipulative Physical Therapists (IFOMPT) Executive Committee, and in particular, Laura Finucane and Ali Rushton, who have each led work groups that produced impactful IFOMPT clinical documents on screening red flags and vascular pathology of the neck that have enhanced this textbook and our ability to practice safely and effectively. I also acknowledge my colleagues in private practice, especially physical therapists Aaron Nevdal and Todd Vanatta, and my current and past students who have contributed to my journey and challenged me to find better ways to teach and practice manual physical therapy.

Lauren Willis and Sara Watkins at Elsevier have been helpful and efficient in helping to move this book along in a timely manner. Jim Womack took the photographs used in the textbook, and the video clips were filmed in a professional manner by the Marquette University Instructional Media Center.

Kenneth A. Olson

CONTENTS

VIDEO TABLE OF CONTENTS

Introduction

OVERVIEW

This chapter introduces the purpose of the textbook, describes the history of manipulation, defines common terminology used in the textbook, introduces evidence-based principles, and provides an explanation for use of the textbook and the accompanying video clips.

OBJECTIVES

- Describe the purpose of the textbook.
- Explain the philosophy of treatment used in orthopaedic manual physical therapy.
- Describe the history of manipulation.
- Define common terminology used in orthopaedic manual physical therapy.
- Explain evidence-based principles for assessment of the reliability and validity of clinical examination procedures and clinical trials.
- Explain how to use this textbook and video clips.

PURPOSE

The purpose of this textbook is to provide the necessary background information and detailed instructional materials to allow full integration of manipulation and manual physical therapy examination and treatment procedures of the spine into physical therapist professional education and clinical practice.

Physical therapy students and faculty in professional physical therapist education programs are the primary audience for this textbook. The secondary audience includes practicing physical therapists, chiropractors, and osteopathic physicians who want to keep current with professional physical therapist education programs. In addition, this textbook is a useful adjunct to other instructional materials for manual physical therapy residency, fellowship, and postprofessional degree programs in musculoskeletal and manual physical therapy.

Physical therapists have been practicing manipulation since the inception of the profession, and all physical therapist professional degree programs must demonstrate full integration of both thrust and nonthrust joint manipulation in the curriculum to maintain accreditation in the United States.[1,2]

The intent of this textbook is to provide physical therapist programs detailed instructional materials for the most effective instruction of manipulation.

Prerequisites in the curriculum should include clinical tests and measures for musculoskeletal conditions, including manual muscle testing, muscle length testing, and goniometry. Knowledge of therapeutic exercise, anatomy, physiology, and functional anatomy and biomechanics should also precede instruction in manipulation. Each chapter provides a review of the evidence to support the examination and treatment techniques presented in the chapter and the kinematics and functional anatomy of the anatomic areas covered in the chapter. An impairment-based classification of common conditions treated by physical therapists is presented in each chapter to assist with clinical reasoning, and patient management principles are addressed for each condition. A biopsychosocial approach to spinal and temporomandibular conditions is presented in this textbook with integration of a psychologically informed management principles combined with specific exercise and manual therapy interventions. Detailed descriptions of examination and manual therapy treatment procedures are covered in each chapter and in the video clips. Common exercises to address each diagnostic classification are also included in each chapter.

HISTORY OF MANIPULATION

The utilization of manipulative treatments to address human ailments extends at least 2500 years in Europe and up to 5000 years worldwide with evidence for the use of manipulative therapy provided in the ancient times by Chinese and Egyptian practitioners, Hippocrates (Greek) and Galen (Roman), and then in Europe by bonesetters from the 11th through the 19th century.[3] Manipulation in recorded history can be traced to the days of Hippocrates, the father of medicine (460–370 BC). Evidence is seen in ancient writings that Hippocrates used spinal traction methods. In the paper "On Setting Joints by Leverage," Hippocrates describes the techniques used to manipulate a dislocated shoulder of a wrestler.[4] Succussion was also practiced in the time of Hippocrates. The patient was strapped in an inverted position to a rack that was attached to ropes and pulleys along the side of a building. The ropes were pulled to elevate the patient and the rack as much as 75 feet, at which time the ropes were released, and the patient crashed to the ground to receive a distractive thrust as the rack hit the ground[5] (Fig. 1.1). Some 600 years later, Galen (130–200 AD) wrote extensively on exercise and manipulation procedures in medicine.[4]

Both Greek and Roman medical practitioners used manipulation for hundreds of years starting around 500 BC.[3] When the Roman Empire fell and Europe divided into Western and Eastern realms with fracturing along religious lines, hands-on manipulative interventions continued in the Byzantine East but were removed from the hands of the lay practitioners and medical providers in the West (France/Germany/England) by church restrictions on providing medical interventions outside of religion.[3] With the enlightenment of the 16th and 17th centuries, the pressures restricting the use of hands-on approaches in healing were slowly lifted in Europe (MacDonald).[3] Ambroise Paré (1510–1590) emerged as a famous French physician and surgeon[4] who used armor to stabilize the spine in patients with tuberculosis[5] (Fig. 1.2). His manipulation and traction techniques were similar to those of Hippocrates, but he opposed the use of succussion.[5]

The bonesetters flourished in Europe from the 1600s through the late 1800s. In 1656, Friar Moulton published *The Complete Bone-Setter*. The book was later revised by Robert Turner.[5] The bonesetters where nonmedical lay practitioners of spinal manipulation who learned their skills primarily through apprenticeship and observation.[6] No formal training was required for bonesetters; the techniques were often learned from family members and passed down from one generation to the next. The clicking sounds that occurred with manipulation were thought to be the result of bones moving back into place.[5]

In 1871, Wharton Hood published *On Bone-Setting*, the first such book by an orthodox medical practitioner.[7] Hood learned about bonesetting after his father had treated a bonesetter, Richard Hutton. Hutton was grateful for the medical care and offered to teach his practitioner about bonesetting. Instead, it was the practitioner's son, Wharton Hood, who accepted the offer. Hood thought that the snapping sound with manipulation was the result of breaking joint adhesions.[7] Paget[8] believed that orthodox medicine should consider the adoption of what was good and useful about bonesetting but should avoid what was potentially dangerous and useless.

Osteopathy, like physical therapy, manual medicine, and chiropractic, was founded as an alternative to opium-, cocaine-, morphine-, and alcohol-based approaches to medicine in the 1800s in response to the demands of a growing middle class in Europe and the Unites States seeking better health and quality

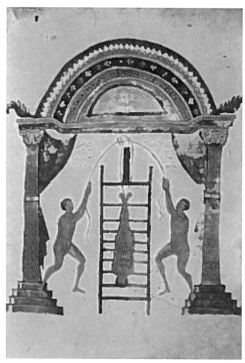

FIG. 1.1 Falling ladder (also known as succussion). (From Schoitz.)

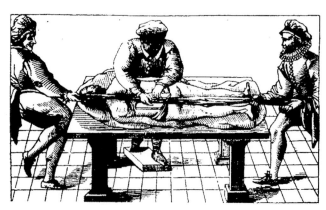

FIG. 1.2 Ambroise Paré applied manual therapy to the spine in conjunction with spinal traction, similar to Hippocrates' methods described over 1000 years earlier. (From Paré, Ambroise. Opera. Liber XV, Cap. XVI. Paris; 1582: p. 440-441.)

of life.[3,9] Andrew Still (1826–1917) explored alternative forms of treatment, such as bonesetting, and founded Osteopathy in 1874 while practicing as a physician in Baldwin City, Kansas.[9] In 1896, Still formed the first school of osteopathy in Kirksville, Missouri.[5] Still developed osteopathy based on the "rule of the artery," with the premise that the body has an innate ability to heal and that with spinal manipulation to correct the structural alignment of the spine, the blood can flow to various regions of the body to restore the body's homeostasis and natural healing abilities. Still's philosophy placed an emphasis on the relationship of structure to function and used manipulation to improve the spinal structure to promote optimal health.[10] The osteopathic profession continues to include manipulation in the course curriculum but does not adhere to Still's original treatment philosophy. Many osteopathic physicians in the United States do not practice manipulation regularly because they are focused on other specialty areas, such as internal medicine or emergency medicine. Osteopathy in many European countries remains primarily a manual therapy profession. In Spain and many South American countries, Osteopathy is not regulated as a profession but has become a postprofessional training program for physical therapist interested in specializing in manual therapy.

Chiropractic was founded in 1895 by Daniel David Palmer (1845–1913). One of the first graduates of the Palmer School of Chiropractic in Davenport, Iowa, was Palmer's son Bartlett Joshua Palmer (1882–1961), who later ran the school and promoted the growth of the profession. D. D. Palmer was a storekeeper and a "magnetic healer,"[6] and there is historical speculation that Palmer may have interacted with Still before the formation of Chiropractic.[11] According to legend, in 1895, Palmer used a manual adjustment directed to the fourth thoracic vertebra that resulted in the restoration of a man's hearing.[12] Palmer integrated popular natural health and scientific models of the day to develop the theory of chiropractic by incorporating the concept of an inherent healing ability of the body that he named "innate intelligence" into concepts drawn from contemporary knowledge about anatomy and physiology.[6] The original chiropractic philosophy is based on the "law of the nerve," which states that adjustment of a subluxed vertebra removes impingement on the nerve and restores innervation and promotes healing processes.[4] Palmer criticized the use of drugs and surgery as unnatural invasions to the body and focused on what he perceived as normalizing the function of the nervous system as the key to health.[6] The "straight" chiropractors continue to adhere to Palmer's original subluxation theories and use spinal adjustments as the primary means of treatment. The "mixers" incorporate other rehabilitative interventions into the treatment options, including physical modalities, such as therapeutic ultrasound and exercise.

The origins of physical therapy can be traced to the Royal Central Institute of Gymnastics (RCIG), founded in 1813 by Pehr Henrik Ling (1776–1839) in Stockholm, Sweden[13,14] (Figs. 1.3 and 1.4). Ling's educational system included four branches: pedagogic gymnastics (physical education), military gymnastics (mostly fencing), medical gymnastics (physical

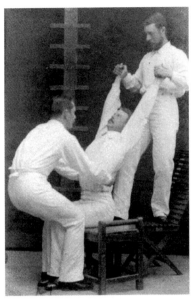

FIG. 1.3 Thoracic traction as performed by graduates of the Royal Central Institute of Gymnastics in the mid-1800s. (Reproduced with permission from Dr. Ottosson, http://www.chronomedica.se.)

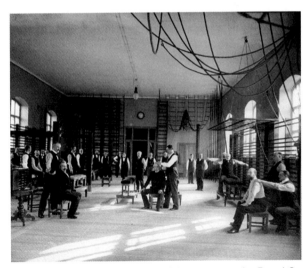

FIG. 1.4 Patients being treated by *sjukgymnast* at the Royal Central Institute of Gymnastics polyclinic in Stockholm, Sweden, 1896. (From Hansson N, Ottoson A. Nobel prize for physical therapy? Rise, fall, and revival of medico-mechanical institutes. *Phys Ther.* 201595(8):1184-1194.)

therapy), and esthetic gymnastics (philosophy). Ling systematized medical gymnastics into two divisions, massage and exercise, with massage defined as movements done on the body and exercise being movements done with a part of the body.[15,16] Ling may not have been the originator of medical gymnastics or massage, but he systematized these methods and attempted to add contemporary knowledge of anatomy and physiology to support medical gymnastics.[15,16]

Graduates of the RCIG earned the title "director of gymnastics" and in 1887 were licensed by Sweden's National Board of Health and Welfare, where physical therapists, until very recently, used the title *sjukgymnast* ("gymnast for the sick").[13,17,18] Throughout the 19th century, the RCIG provided its graduates with a scientific rationale, based on contemporary knowledge of anatomy and physiology, for the benefits of combining specific active, resistive, and passive movements and exercises, including variations of spinal manipulation, traction, and massage.[13] "Ling's doctrine of harmony" purported that the health of the body depended on the balance between three primary forms: mechanics (movement/exercise/manipulation), chemistry (food/medicine), and dynamics (psychiatry), and the Ling physical therapists were trained to restore this harmony through use of manual therapy. Ling, and the physical therapists who trained in his methods, wanted to revolutionize orthodox medicine, which they believed was too preoccupied with pharmacologic cures.[18] Ling believed that orthodox medicine should be oriented more toward mechanical modes of treating illness, such as his physical therapy movements and manipulations of the body.[18]

Graduates of RCIG immigrated to almost every major European city, Russia, and North America through the mid to late 1800s to establish centers of medical gymnastics and mechanical treatments.[13] Jonas Henrik Kellgren (1837–1916) graduated from the RCIG in 1865, eventually opened clinics in Sweden, Germany, France, and London, and is credited with development of many specific spinal and nerve manipulation techniques.[13] In addition, medical doctors from throughout Europe enrolled in the RCIG to add physical therapy methods to their treatment of human ailments and attained joint credentials as physician/physical therapist. Edgar F. Cyriax (1874–1955), the son-in-law of Kellgren and a graduate of RCIG before becoming a medical doctor, published more than 50 articles on Ling's and Kellgren's methods of physical therapy in international journals and advocated to include "mechano-therapeutics" in the curriculum and training of medical doctors in Britain.[13] In 1899, the Chartered Society of Physiotherapy was founded in England.[4] The first professional physical therapy association in the United States, which was the forerunner to the American Physical Therapy Association (APTA), was formed in 1921.[1]

Between 1921 and 1936, at least 21 articles and book reviews on manipulation were found in the physical therapy literature,[19] including the 1921 textbook, *Massage and Therapeutic Exercise,* by the founder and first president of the APTA, Mary McMillan. McMillan credits Ling and his followers with development and refinement of the methods used to form the physical therapy profession in the United States.[15,16] There is also evidence that the original six physical education schools in the United States, one of which was in Battle Creek, Michigan, where "reconstruction aides" were recruited and trained to treat the wounded soldiers during World War I, included Ling's principles in their curriculum.[18] In fact, prominent United States physical medicine physicians from the late 1800s, Harvey Kellogg and Douglas Graham, have connections to Ling and his physical therapy, with frequent references to him and his scientific principles in their publications.[20,21] Harvey Kellogg even had a "swedishroom" in his world-famous sanitarium in Battle

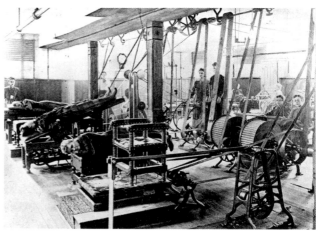

FIG. 1.5 "Swedishroom" at Dr. Havey Kellogg's world-famous sanitarium, Battle Creek, Michigan, where medico-mechanical machines developed by Jonas Zander were used to emulate Ling's principles of physical therapy movement and manipulation. (From Hansson N, Ottoson A. Nobel prize for physical therapy? Rise, fall, and revival of medico-mechanical institutes, *Phys Ther.* 2015;95(8):1184-1194.)

Creek where medico-mechanical machines developed by Swedish physician, Jonas Zander (1835–1920), were used to emulate Ling's principles of physical therapy movement and manipulation (Fig. 1.5). Interestingly, the textbook, *Swedish Movements on Medical Gymnastics*, written by the most authoritative author on Ling's physical therapy in the 19th century, the Swedish Professor T.J. Hartelius, was translated into English and published in Battle Creek, Michigan, with a foreword by Dr. Kellogg in 1896, which further shows Ling's physical therapy developing in the United States around the same time when chiropractic and osteopathy were in their infancy.[18,22]

In addition, McMillan devotes a 15-page chapter of her book to specific therapeutic exercise regimes developed by Ling, referred to as "A Day's Order," and states that the term *medical gymnastics* is synonymous with *therapeutic exercise*. In a subsequent editorial,[15] she wrote of the four branches of physiotherapy, which she identified as "manipulation of muscle and joints, therapeutic exercise, electrotherapy, and hydrotherapy."[16] Titles of articles during this period were quite explicit regarding manipulation, such as "The Art of Mobilizing Joints"[23] and "Manipulative Treatment of Lumbosacral Derangement."[24] The articles used phrases such as "adhesion . . . stretched or torn by this simple manipulation"[25] and "manipulation of the spine and sacroiliac joint."[26] This usage helps illustrate that manipulation has been part of physical therapy practice since the founding of the profession and through the 1930s.[19]

From 1940 to the mid-1970s, the word *manipulation* was not widely used in the American physical therapy literature.[4] This omission may have been caused in part by the American Medical Association's Committee on Quackery, which was formed in the 1960s and was active for the next 30 years in an attempt to discredit the chiropractic profession. The committee was forced to dissolve in 1990 because of Wilk's "restraint of trade" case, which was upheld in the US Supreme Court.[12] Because physical therapy remained within the mainstream medical model, the terms *mobilization* and *articulation* were used during this time frame to separate physical therapy from chiropractic. However, physical therapists continued to practice various forms of manipulation.

Through the early to mid-1900s, several prominent European Orthopaedic physicians influenced the practice of manipulation and the evolution of the physical therapist's role as a manipulative therapist. Between 1912 and 1935, James Mennell (1880–1957) provided advanced training in manipulation technique for physiotherapist at St. Thomas's Hospital in London.[27] In 1949, James Mennell published his textbook titled the *Science and Art of Joint Manipulation.* Mennell adapted knowledge of joint mechanics in the practice of manipulation and coined the phrase "accessory motion."[28] James H. Cyriax (1904–1985), son of Edgar Cyriax and grandson of Jonas Henrik Kellgren, published his classic *Textbook of Orthopaedic Medicine* in 1954. He made great contributions to Orthopaedic medicine with the development of detailed systematic examination procedures for extremity disorders, including refinement of isometric tissue tension signs, end feel assessment, and capsular patterns.[29] Cyriax attributed most back pain to disorders of the intervertebral disc and used aggressive general manipulation techniques that included strong manual traction forces to "reduce the disc."[29] Cyriax, who also taught and practiced Orthopaedic medicine at St. Thomas's Hospital until 1969 and was the successor of Mennell at St Thomas,[30] influenced many physiotherapists, including Stanley Paris and Freddy Kaltenborn, to carry on the skills and techniques required to effectively use manipulation.

Alan Stoddard[10] (1915–2002) was a medical and osteopathic physician in England who used skillful specific manipulation technique and also mentored many physical therapists, including Paris and Kaltenborn (Fig. 1.6). Stoddard authored two textbooks, *Manual of Osteopathic Technique* (1959) and *Manual of Osteopathic Practice* (1969), which became the cornerstone of osteopathic teaching in schools around the world.[31] Physical therapists, Kaltenborn[32] and Paris,[33] both believed that the Cyriax approach to extremity conditions was excellent, but they preferred Stoddard's specific manipulation techniques for the spine.

John Mennell (1916–1992), the son of James Mennell, first practiced Orthopaedic medicine in England. In the 1960s, he immigrated to the United States, where he held many educational programs for physical therapists through the 1970s and 1980s to promote manipulation within the physical therapy profession. He published several textbooks, including *Joint Pain, Foot Pain,* and *Back Pain,* and coined the phrase "joint play."[34] Mennell brought attention to sources of back pain other than the intervertebral disc.

In the 1960s, several physical therapists emerged as international leaders in the practice and instruction of manipulation. Physical therapist Freddy Kaltenborn (1923–2019), originally from Norway, developed what is now known as the Nordic

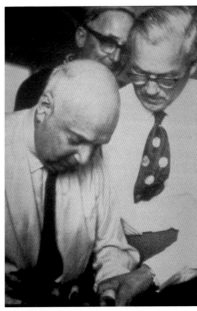

FIG. 1.6 Cyriax *(left)* and Stoddard *(right)* in Norway, 1965. (From Kaltenborn FM. *Manual Mobilization of the Joints: Volume II: the Spine.* Oslo, Norway: Norli; 2012).

approach. He published his first textbook on spinal manipulation in 1964 and was the first to relate manipulation to arthrokinematics.[33] His techniques were specific and perpetuated the importance of biomechanical principles, such as the concave/convex and arthrokinematic rules. Kaltenborn, in collaboration with physical therapist Olaf Evjenth, also developed extensive long-term training programs for physical therapists to specialize in manual therapy first in Norway and later throughout Europe, North America, and Asia.

Australian physical therapist, Geoffrey Maitland (1924–2010), published the first edition of his book *Vertebral Manipulation* in 1964.[35] Maitland was also influenced by the work of Cyriax and Stoddard but further refined the importance of a detailed history and comprehensive physical examination. He also developed the concept of treatment of "reproducible signs" and inhibition of joint pain with use of gentle oscillatory manipulation techniques. Maitland developed the I to IV grading system to further describe oscillatory manipulation techniques.[35] Maitland also established long-term manual therapy educational programs affiliated with universities in Australia, which subsequently facilitated the rapid growth of musculoskeletal physical therapy research.

Physical therapist, Stanley Paris, was originally from New Zealand. Early in his career, in 1961 and 1962, he was awarded a scholarship to study manipulation in Europe and the United States.[19] He had the opportunity to study with Cyriax, Stoddard, and Kaltenborn during this time and in 1965 published the textbook *Spinal Lesion.*[36] In the late 1960s, Paris immigrated to the United States, where he eventually completed his doctoral work in neuroanatomy of the lumbar spine and developed extensive educational programs for post-professional physical therapy education in manual physical therapy and manipulation that eventually resulted in the formation the University of St. Augustine for Health Sciences in St. Augustine, Florida. Paris also played key roles in formation of professional organizations in the United States, including the APTA Orthopaedic Section and the American Academy of Orthopaedic Manual Physical Therapists (AAOMPT), two professional organizations that have played roles in advocating for inclusion of manipulation within the scope of physical therapy practice and that have promoted education, practice, and research in manual physical therapy. Paris worked with physical therapists Maitland, Kaltenborn, and Gregory Grieve of the United Kingdom to form the International Federation of Orthopaedic Manipulative Physical Therapists (IFOMPT; Fig. 1.7).

The IFOMPT was founded in 1974 and represents organized groups of manual/manipulative physical therapists around the world that have established stringent postgraduation specialization educational programs in manual/manipulative physical therapy. The Federation sets educational and clinical standards and is a specialty subgroup of the World Confederation for Physical Therapy (WCPT). One organization of each WCPT country can be recognized by IFOMPT to represent that country if the organization meets IFOMPT criteria. The IFOMPT educational standards and international monitoring system has allowed physical therapists to be recognized as orthopaedic manual physical therapy (OMPT) specialists in countries beyond the country where they received their training.

The Academy of Orthopaedic Physical Therapy of the APTA represents all aspects of musculoskeletal physical therapy and is open to all members of the APTA, including physical therapist assistants. Before formation of the AAOMPT, no organization in the United States could meet the IFOMPT

criteria because no recognized educational system in manual therapy upheld standards of training and examination in manual therapy for physical therapists in the United States. However, by 1990, at least eight active manual therapy fellowship programs were operating independently within the United States.

In 1991, Freddy Kaltenborn invited representatives from these eight manual therapy fellowship programs to meet at Oakland University in Michigan to consider how the United States could develop educational standards in manual therapy and become a member organization of IFOMPT.[37] These eight physical therapists, Stanley Paris, Mike Rogers, Michael Moore, Kornelia Kulig, Bjorn Swensen, Dick Erhard, Joe Farrell, and Ola Grimsby, along with Trish King and Carol Jo Tichenor, became the founding members of the AAOMPT. The AAOMPT developed an educational standards document, bylaws, and a recognition process for manual therapy fellowship programs. In 1992, the AAOMPT was accepted as the member organization to represent the United States in IFOMPT.

Although prominent individuals, such as Paris, Kaltenborn, and Maitland, played a large role in development and advancement of manipulation and manual therapy within the physical therapy profession over the last half of the 20th century, the current practice and the future of the specialty area of OMPT are driven by evidence-based practice and the promotion of OMPT practice through professional associations, such as IFOMPT, AAOMPT, and the APTA.[37] A large and growing body of research evidence supports and guides the practice of manipulation within the scope of physical therapy practice and for other manual therapy practitioners.

There is evidence of overlap between the historical origins of the primary professions that practice manual therapy and manipulation to treat musculoskeletal conditions, and all developed, in part, as a viable alternative to the harmful and additive effects of drugs, such as opium, that the medical profession used to treat human ailments.[3] Since their inception, the professions have functioned independently and have at times politically challenged each other's growth, rights, and development.[3,27,32,37] Currently, there is recognition of another opioid crisis in the United States, Europe, and many parts of the developed world, and the manual therapy professions are beginning to work corporately to demonstrate the enhanced patient outcomes that can be obtained by seeing a nonpharmacologic manual therapy practitioner first, such as a physical therapist or chiropractor, in the episode of care for conditions such as low back pain.[38–40] This newfound cooperative relationship has the potential to yield stronger research evidence to support the Physical Therapy/Chiropractic First approach and to enhance the political status of both groups to influence healthcare policy in ways that will benefit patients and society.

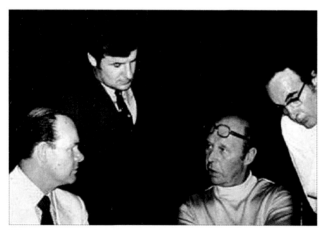

FIG. 1.7 Photograph was taken in 1967 at St. Thomas' Hospital, London to begin discussions for the formation of the International Federation of Orthopaedic Manipulative Physical Therapists (IFOMPT). Dr. Paris was Chair of the inaugural IFOMPT conference in 1974. The other three individuals were consultants to the process and served in that capacity for 7 years before this event. In 1978, IFOMPT became a subgroup of the World Confederation for Physical Therapy (WCPT). From left: Geoffrey Maitland, Stanley Paris, Freddy Kaltenborn, and Gregory Grieve. (From Paris SV. 37th Mary McMillan lecture: in the best interest of the patient. *Phys Ther.* 2006;86[11]: 1541-1553.)

ORTHOPAEDIC MANUAL PHYSICAL THERAPY TREATMENT PHILOSOPHY

IFOMPT defines OMPT as a specialized area of physiotherapy/physical therapy for the management of neuromusculoskeletal conditions, based on clinical reasoning, using highly specific treatment approaches including manual techniques and therapeutic exercises. OMPT also encompasses, and is driven by, the available scientific and clinical evidence and the biopsychosocial framework of each individual patient (see the IFOMPT Constitution 2012 at http://www.ifompt.com/site/ifompt/files/pdf//IFOMPT_Constitution.pdf).

IFOMPT considers the following terms as being interchangeable: *orthopaedic manual therapy, OMPT, orthopaedic manipulative therapy, musculoskeletal physical therapy*, and *orthopaedic manipulative physical therapy* (per IFOMPT Constitution 2020).

Paris[41] described a nine-point "Philosophy of Dysfunction" that summarizes the components of a traditional OMPT treatment philosophy (Box 1.1). Paris defines "dysfunction" as

---

BOX 1.1   Philosophy of Dysfunction as Described by Paris

I. That joint injury, including such conditions referred to as *osteoarthritis, instability*, and the aftereffects of sprains and strains, are dysfunctions rather than diseases.

II. That dysfunctions are manifest as either increases or decreases of motion from the expected normal or by the presence of aberrant movements. Thus dysfunctions are represented by abnormal movements.

III. That where the dysfunction is detected as limited motion (hypomobility), the treatment of choice is manipulation to joint structures, stretching to muscles and fascia and the promotion of activities that encourage a full range of movement.

IV. That when the dysfunction is manifest as increased movement (hypermobility), laxity, or instability, the treatment of the joint in question is not manipulation but stabilization by instruction of correct posture, stabilization exercises, and correction of any limitations of movement in neighboring joints that may be contributing to the hypermobility.

V. That the primary cause of degenerative joint disease is joint dysfunction. Therefore it may be concluded that its presence is caused by the failure or lack of accessibility to physical therapy.

VI. That the physical therapist's primary role is in the evaluation and treatment of dysfunction, whereas that of the physician is the diagnosis and treatment of disease. These are two separate but complementary roles in health care.

VII. That because dysfunction is the cause of pain, the primary goal of physical therapy should be to correct the dysfunction rather than the pain. When, however, the nature of the pain interferes with correcting the dysfunction, the pain will need to be addressed as part of the treatment program.

VIII. That the key to understanding dysfunction, and thus being able to evaluate and treat it, is understanding anatomy and biomechanics. It therefore behooves us in physical therapy to develop our knowledge and skills in these areas so that we may safely assume leadership in the nonoperative management of neuromusculoskeletal disorders.

IX. That it is the patients' responsibility to restore, maintain, and enhance their health. In this context, the role of the physical therapist is to serve as an educator, to be an example to the patient, and to reinforce a healthy and productive lifestyle.

Adapted from Paris SV. *Introduction to spinal evaluation and manipulation.* Atlanta: Institute Press; 1986.

---

increases or decreases of motion from the expected normal or as the presence of aberrant movements.[5] Therefore the primary focus of the OMPT's examination is the analysis of active and passive movement. If hypomobility is noted, joint mobilization and stretching techniques are used; if hypermobility is noted, stabilization exercises, motor control, and postural correction are emphasized. If aberrant movements are noted, a motor retraining exercise approach is appropriate. If localization of tissue reactivity and pain are noted, gentle oscillatory techniques, as described by Maitland, can be used to attempt to inhibit pain.[35] This is an "impairment-based approach," which is a foundation of physical therapy.

Manual physical therapy approaches place an emphasis on application of biomechanical principles in the examination and treatment of spinal disorders. Motion is analyzed with active and passive motion testing with visualization of the spinal mechanics; the motion is best described with standardized biomechanical terminology. Passive forces are applied, with passive accessory intervertebral motion testing and mobilization/manipulation techniques, along planes of movement parallel or perpendicular to the anatomic planes of the joint surfaces. Therefore knowledge of spinal anatomy and biomechanics is a prerequisite to learning a manual physical therapy approach for examination and treatment of the spine.

Orthopaedic manual physical therapists use a process of clinical reasoning that includes continual assessment of the patient, followed by application of a trail of manual therapy treatment or exercise, followed by further assessment of the patient's response to the treatment. This intimate relationship between examination, treatment, and reexamination provides useful clinical data for sound judgments regarding the patient's response to treatment and the need to modify, progress, or maintain the applied interventions.

Manual physical therapy is not a passive approach. The patient and therapist are both actively engaged in a therapeutic alliance to work toward pain modulation and restoration of active functional movements by the end of each treatment session. There are numerous studies that have illustrated that intrasession reduction of pain and restoration of motion translates into favorable intersession improvements in the same parameters and long-term positive clinical outcomes.[42–45]

Physical therapists have embraced the principles of evidence-based practice. When research evidence is available to guide clinical decisions, the physical therapist should follow the evidence-based practice guidelines. However, when research evidence is not clear, an impairment-based approach that includes a thorough evaluation and sound clinical reasoning should be used, with a focus on restoring function, reducing pain, and returning the patient to functional activities. In fact, a growing body of research evidence demonstrates the effectiveness of an impairment-based OMPT approach for the treatment of spine and extremity musculoskeletal conditions.[46–54] This textbook incorporates the best available evidence with an OMPT approach.

The evidence supports use of a classification system to guide the treatment of patients with spinal disorders.[55,56] An impairment-based classification system that is linked to the International Classification of Functioning, Disability, and Health (ICF) has been developed by the Orthopaedic Academy of the APTA for low back and neck pain conditions.[57,58] The ICF impairment-based terminology is incorporated within this textbook where appropriate. The impairment-based classification system recognizes that patients with spinal disorders are a heterogeneous group. However, subgroups of patients can be identified with common signs and symptoms that respond to interventions provided by physical therapists, including manipulation, specific directional exercises, neuromuscular control exercises, pain science education, and traction. A classification of common disorders is described in great detail for each anatomic region covered in this textbook.

For effective treatment of patients with spinal disorders, physical therapists complete a comprehensive physical examination that includes screening for red flags to ensure that physical therapy is appropriate to the patient's condition. The examination includes procedures with proven reliability and validity, and the results of the examination are correlated with patient questionnaire information and the patient's history to determine a diagnosis. The diagnosis places the patient in a classification and includes a problem list of noted impairments that affect the patient's condition. As treatment is implemented that specifically targets the impairments noted in the examination, the patient's condition is continually reassessed to determine the results of treatment and to determine whether modifications in diagnosis and treatment are necessary. The primary emphasis of the treatment is integration of manual therapy techniques and therapeutic exercise with principles of patient education to ultimately allow the patient to self-manage the condition.

Evidence-Based Practice

Evidence-based practice is defined as the integration of best research evidence with clinical expertise and patient values.[59] The research evidence considered in evidence-based practice is meant to be clinically relevant patient-centered research of the accuracy and precision of diagnostic tests, the power of prognostic markers, and the efficacy and safety of therapeutic, rehabilitative, and preventive regimens.[59] Clinical experience, the ability to use clinical skills and past experience, should also be incorporated into evidence-based practice to identify each patient's health state and diagnosis, risks and benefits of potential interventions, and the patient's values and expectations.[59] Patient values include the unique preferences, concerns, and expectations each patient brings to a clinical situation; these values must be integrated into clinical decisions if the therapist is to properly serve the patient.[59]

Evidence-based principles are incorporated throughout this textbook. When studies are identified to illustrate the accuracy and precision of diagnostic tests, this information is reported in the "notes" section of the examination technique description; when clinical outcome studies that use a specific intervention are identified, this information is included as well. The examination and treatment procedures included in this

textbook have been chosen based on the research evidence to support their use, on my clinical experience, and on safety considerations. The decision to use the examination and treatment techniques presented in this textbook should be made based on the clinician's knowledge of the evidence, competence in application of the intervention, and clinical experience combined with the patient's values and expectations. Although this textbook can establish a foundation for evidence-based practice for physical therapy management of spinal and temporomandibular disorders, new evidence continues to emerge regarding the best diagnostic and treatment procedures. Therefore the practitioner's responsibility is to stay abreast of new developments in research findings and to make appropriate changes in practice to reflect these new findings.

Many of the examination tests presented in this textbook have been tested for reliability and validity; this information is reported when available. Reliability is defined as the extent to which a measurement is consistent and free of error.[60] If an examination test is reliable, it is reproducible and dependable to provide consistent responses in a given condition.[60] Validity is the ability of a test to measure what it is intended to measure.[60] Both reliability and validity are essential considerations in determination of what tests and measures to use in the clinical examination of a patient.

Reliability is often reported as both interrater and intrarater reliability. Intrarater or intraexaminer reliability defines the stability or repeatability of data recorded by one individual across two or more trials.[60] Interrater reliability defines the amount of variability between two or more examiners who measure the same group of subjects.[60] For the statistical analysis of interval or ratio data, the intraclass correlation coefficient is the preferred statistical index because it reflects both correlation and agreement and determines the amount of variance between two or more repeated measures.[60,61] For ordinal, nominal, or categorical data, percent agreement can be determined and the kappa coefficient (k) statistic applied, which takes into account the effects of chance on the percent agreement.[61,62] Landis and Koch[63] have established a general guideline for interpretation of kappa scores (Table 1.1). Because the effect of chance is not affected by prevalence, the kappa coefficient can be deflated if the prevalence of a

TABLE 1.1	Kappa Coefficient Interpretation	
KAPPA STATISTIC	**STRENGTH OF AGREEMENT**
<0.00	Poor
0.00–0.20	Slight
0.21–0.40	Fair
0.41–0.60	Moderate
0.61–0.80	Substantial
0.81–1.00	Almost perfect

(From Landis JR, Koch GG. The measurement of observer agreement for categorical data. *Biometrics* 1977;33:159-174.)

TABLE 1.2	2 × 2 Contingency Table	
	DISEASE	**NO DISEASE**
Test positive	True positive A	False positive B
Test negative	False negative C	True negative D
	Sensitivity A/(A + C)	Specificity D/(B + D)

Table is used to compare results of reference standard with results of test under investigation; used to calculate sensitivity and specificity.
(Modified from Sackett DL, Straus SE, Richardson WS, et al. *Evidence-Based Medicine: How to Practice and Teach EBM,* ed 2. Edinburgh: Churchill Livingstone; 2000.)

particular outcome of the test or measure is either very high or very low.[59] "Acceptable reliability" must be determined by the clinician who uses the specific test or measure and should be based on which variable is tested, why a particular test is important, and on whom the test is to be used.[64]

Results of validity testing examination procedures are reported as sensitivity (Sens), specificity (Spec), positive likelihood ratio (+LR), and negative likelihood ratio (−LR). Sensitivity is the test's ability to obtain positive test results when the target condition is really present, or a true positive.[60] The 2 × 2 contingency table (Table 1.2) is used to calculate the sensitivity and specificity. "SnNout" is a useful acronym to remember that tests with high sensitivity have few false-negative results; therefore a negative result rules out the condition.[59] Specificity is the test's ability to obtain negative test results when the condition is really absent, or a true negative.[60] "SpPin" is a useful acronym to remember that tests with high specificity have few false–positive results; therefore a positive result rules in the condition.[59]

Likelihood ratios dictate the degree of the shift from the pretest probability that a patient has or does not have a condition to the posttest probability. A positive likelihood ratio is equal to Sensitivity/(1 − Specificity) and represents the amount of increase in odds favoring the condition if the test results are positive.[61] Positive likelihood ratios (+LR) of greater than 10 generate a large and often conclusive shift in probability; ratios of 5 to 10 generate moderate shifts in probability; and ratios of 2 to 5 generate small but sometimes important shifts in probability.[65] A likelihood ratio nomogram can be used to draw a line from the pretest probability through the likelihood ratio score and continue in a straight line to end at the posttest probability (Fig. 1.8).

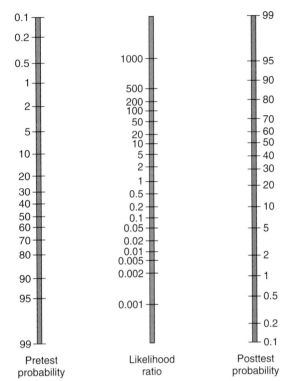

FIG. 1.8 Likelihood ratio monogram. (From Sackett DL, Straus SE, Richardson WS, et al. *Evidence-Based Medicine: How to Practice and Teach EBM,* ed 2. Edinburgh: Churchill Livingstone; 2000.)

A negative likelihood ratio (−LR) is equal to (1 − Sensitivity)/Specificity and represents the decrease in odds favoring the condition if the test results are negative.[61] Negative likelihood ratios of less than 0.1 generate large and often conclusive shifts in probability; ratios of 0.1 to 0.2 generate moderate shifts in probability; and ratios of 0.2 to 0.5 generate small but sometimes important shifts in probability (Table 1.3).[65]

The quality assessment of diagnostic accuracy studies (QUADAS) tool is an evidence-based tool.[66] It consists of a set of 14 items, phrased as questions, each of which should be scored as yes, no, or unclear (Table 1.4). The tool was developed for systematic reviews of research studies that assess the diagnostic accuracy of physical examination tests. The tool primarily assesses the studies bias, which limits the validity of the study results; and variability, which may affect the generalizability of study results; additional questions assess the quality of reporting.[66] The original intent of the QUADAS tool was

TABLE 1.3	Interpretation of Positive and Negative Likelihood Ratios	
POSITIVE LIKELIHOOD RATIO (+LR)	**EXPLANATION**	**NEGATIVE LIKELIHOOD RATIO (−LR)**
2–5	Alters posttest probability of a diagnosis by a small degree	0.2–0.5
5–10	Alters posttest probability of a diagnosis by a moderate degree	0.1–0.2
More than 10	Alters posttest probability of a diagnosis by a large degree	Less than 0.1

(Modified from Jaeschke R, Guyatt GH, Sackett DL. How to use an article about a diagnostic test. B. What are the results and will they help me in caring for my patients? *JAMA* 1994;271(9):703-707.)

TABLE 1.4	Quality Assessment of Diagnostic Accuracy Studies Tool			
ITEM		**YES**	**NO**	**UNCLEAR**
1	Was the spectrum of patients representative of the patients who will receive the test in practice?			
2	Were selection criteria clearly described?			
3	Is the reference standard likely to correctly classify the target condition?			
4	Is the time period between reference standard and index test short enough to be reasonably sure that the target condition did not change between the two tests?			
5	Did the whole sample or a random selection of the sample receive verification using a reference standard of diagnosis?			
6	Did patients receive the same reference standard regardless of the index test result?			
7	Was the reference standard independent of the index test (i.e., the index test did not form part of the reference standard)?			
8	Was the execution of the index test described in sufficient detail to permit replication of the test?			
9	Was the execution of the reference standard described in sufficient detail to permit its replication?			
10	Were the index test results interpreted without knowledge of the results of the reference standard?			
11	Were the reference standard results interpreted without knowledge of the results of the index test?			
12	Were the same clinical data available when test results were interpreted as would be available when the test is used in practice?			
13	Were uninterpretable/intermediate test results reported?			
14	Were withdrawals from the study explained?			

Adapted from Whiting P, Rutjes AWS, Reitsma JB, et al. The development of QUADAS: a tool for the quality assessment of studies of diagnostic accuracy included in systematic reviews. *BMC Med Res Methodol.* 2003;3:25.

to provide a qualitative assessment of the studies on diagnostic accuracy and not to provide a quality score.[66] However, many authors have interpreted use of the tool with QUADAS scores of 7 to 14 "yeses" to indicate a high-quality diagnostic accuracy study and a score of less than 7 as indicative of low quality.[67] Other authors have suggested that a score of 10 or more "yeses" is required to consider a study design as one of high quality.[68] Systematic reviews of diagnostic accuracy studies that use the QUADAS tool must incorporate the judgment of at least two independent reviewers, and disagreements between reviewers must be resolved by a third qualified individual or by discussion and consensus between the reviewers.[69] For this reason, only QUADAS scores that have been developed through a published systematic review are reported in this textbook.

Clinical prediction rules (CPRs) may be used to enhance the clinician's accuracy in predicting a diagnosis or in determining appropriate treatment strategies.[61] The rule is developed by applying an intervention to a group of patients and then identifying common characteristics in the group of patients who responded favorably to the intervention through calculation of positive and negative likelihood ratios. After the CPR is developed, it must be validated with an investigation of the accuracy of the CPR in a new group of patients with clinical tests or interventions performed by a different group of clinicians other than those who developed the rule.[60,70] Validation should also occur in multiple settings to enhance the rule's generalizability, and an impact study should be completed to determine what effect the rule has had on changing clinical behaviors and to assess whether economic benefits have resulted.[59,68]

The highest level of evidence to support interventions is based on the recommendations of systematic reviews and clinical practice guidelines, and clinicians should start their search to answer clinical management questions with identification of applicable systematic reviews.[59] A systematic review is a summary of the medical literature that uses explicit methods to systematically search, critically appraise, and synthesize the world literature on a specific issue.[59] The quality of systematic reviews is dependent on the quality of the randomized controlled trials (RCTs) that have been done to investigate the effectiveness of the interventions being studied. Sackett et al.[59] describe the essential questions to ask when reviewing the validity of RCTs:

1. Was the assignment of patients to treatment randomized? Was the randomization list concealed?
2. Was follow-up of patients sufficiently long and complete?
3. Were all patients analyzed in the groups to which they were randomized (even those who did not follow through on the prescribed treatment)?
4. Were patients and clinicians kept blind to treatment?
5. Were groups treated equally, apart from the experimental therapy?
6. Were the groups similar at the start of the trial?

If these questions are answered favorably, the results of the RCT can be used to assist with clinical decision making as long as the patient under consideration fits within the parameters of the patient population studied in the RCT. RCTs demonstrate the relative effectiveness and efficacy of one intervention compared with another or a control group that participated in the study. RCTs represent results at the population level. Within each comparison group, there are some individuals who improve and some who did not, but the RCT is unable to determine "why".[71] RCTs will also lack external validity for patient groups not included in the study, so review of the inclusion/exclusion criteria for a RCT is essential to determine if the results might hold true for an individual patient.[71] RCTs are also subject to unmeasured bias that commonly occurs after randomization, such as the Hawthorn effect, which is a change in behavior of the research subjects, administrators, and clinicians because they are participating in a study.[71] The care provided may not reflect what is typically done in clinical practice. RCTs provide useful information to help guide clinical practice but cannot replace sound clinical reasoning to determine the best approach for each individual patient.

Lower levels of evidence, such as case reports or case series, are useful for developing a hypothesis of the effect of a treatment approach, but a true cause and effect from the treatment used in the case reports and case series cannot be assumed without a control group. Often case series studies are used to support the need for an RCT and assist with development of the RCT methodology.

The literature is reviewed in each chapter related to the classification categories for subgrouping disorders commonly treated by physical therapists. One goal of this textbook is to promote an increase in the number of physical therapists, physicians, and other health professionals who follow the recommendations of high-quality clinical practice guidelines and systematic reviews for management of spinal disorders and to provide the necessary background and instructional information to assist in skill development to effectively implement the treatment recommendations related to manual therapy and exercise.

HOW TO USE THIS BOOK

The textbook has been organized by anatomic region as a useful and easy-to-use reference resource for students and clinicians. However, when this textbook is used as a resource to teach a course, students should be taught the principles and procedures of a detailed spinal examination and the clinical decision making required to appropriately classify and diagnose spinal disorders before learning the motor skills of spinal manipulation in that anatomic region. The advantage of teaching students the examination procedures before teaching manipulation techniques includes facilitation of safe application of the treatment procedures, and many of the passive intervertebral motion (PIVM) tests used in the spinal examination are converted to manipulation techniques. Therefore the process of learning the PIVM tests facilitates the motor skills required for proper performance of the manipulation techniques. The more proficient students become in the examination procedures, the easier the manipulation techniques are to learn.

The video clips can be used to assist the instructor in demonstration of the examination and manipulation techniques. Two or three cameras were used to film each technique, which provides unique angles of perspective and viewing that an individual viewing a demonstration in a large group of students cannot have. A live demonstration is still valuable, and the best use for the video clips may be for a second viewing or review of the technique during practice sessions. In addition, because all students have access to the video clips with the textbook, they can check the proper performance of the technique during practice sessions.

Definitions of Terms From the *Guide to Physical Therapist Practice*

Arthrokinematic: The accessory or joint play movements of a joint that cannot be performed voluntarily and that are defined by the structure and shape of the joint surfaces, without regard to the forces producing motion or resulting from motion. (APTA 2001) Accessory movement at joint surfaces. (APTA 2014)

Assessment: The measurement or quantification of a variable or the placement of a value on something. Assessment should not be confused with examination or evaluation.

Diagnosis: Diagnosis is both a process and a label. The diagnostic process includes integrating and evaluating the data that are obtained during the examination to describe the patient/client condition in terms that will guide the prognosis, the plan of care, and intervention strategies. Physical therapists

use diagnostic labels that identify the impact of a condition on function at the level of the system (especially the movement system) and at the level of the whole person.

Evaluation: A dynamic process in which the physical therapist makes clinical judgments based on data gathered during the examination.

Examination: A comprehensive screening and specific testing process leading to diagnostic classification or, as appropriate, to a referral to another practitioner. The examination has three components: the patient/client history, the systems review, and tests and measures.

Functional limitation: The restriction of the ability to perform, at the level of the whole person, a physical action, task, or activity in an efficient, typically expected, or competent manner.

Continued

Definitions of Terms From the *Guide to Physical Therapist Practice*—*Cont'd*

Impairment: Problems in the body functions and/or structures as a significant deviation or loss. (APTA 2014)

Intervention: The purposeful interaction of the physical therapist with the patient/client and, when appropriate, with other individuals involved in patient/client care, using various physical therapy procedures and techniques to produce changes in the condition.

Joint integrity: The soundness of the structure and function of the joint, which are classified in biomechanical terms as *arthrokinematic motion.* (APTA 2014)

Joint mobility: The capacity of the joint to be moved passively, for evaluating the structure and integrity of the joint surface and the characteristics of periarticular soft tissue. (APTA 2014)

Manual therapy techniques: Skilled hand movements and skilled passive movements of joints and soft tissue. (APTA 2014)

Mobilization/manipulation: A manual therapy technique comprising a continuum of skilled passive movements to the joints and/or related soft tissues that are applied at varying speeds and amplitudes, including a small-amplitude/high-velocity therapeutic movement. These interventions require immediate and continuous examination and evaluation throughout the intervention and, therefore are performed exclusively by the physical therapist. (APTA 2014)

Osteokinematics: Gross angular motions of the shafts of bones in sagittal, frontal, and transverse planes.

Passive accessory intervertebral motion (PAIVM) tests: A type of passive joint mobility assessment that uses passive joint play motions of the spine to induce spinal segment passive motion. The therapist judges the degree of passive mobility at the targeted spinal motion segment by sensing the amount of resistance to the passive joint play movement. Joint mobility, irritability, and end feel can be assessed with these procedures.

Passive intervertebral motion (PIVM) tests: A type of passive segmental joint mobility assessment of the spine that might include either passive accessory intervertebral motion tests or passive physiologic intervertebral motion tests. The therapist will make judgments of segmental passive motion, end feel, and pain provocation (i.e., irritability) assessment based on these procedures.

Passive physiologic intervertebral motion (PPIVM) tests: A type of passive joint mobility assessment that uses passive osteokinematic motions of the spine to induce spinal segment passive motion, which is palpated by the therapist to judge the degree of passive mobility at the targeted spinal motion segment

(Modified from American Physical Therapy Association. Guide to physical therapist practice, *Phys Ther.* 2001;81:9-746; American Physical Therapy Association. Guide to physical therapist practice, 2014 at guidetoptpractice.apta.org access January 12, 2019.)

Additional Definitions of Manual Therapy Terminology

Accessory motion: Those motions that are available in a joint that may accompany the classical movements or be passively produced isolated from the classical movement. Accessory movements are essential to normal full range of motion and painless function.

Component motion: Motions that take place in a joint complex or related joint to facilitate a particular active motion.

Close-packed position: Position of maximum congruency of a joint that is locked and statically efficient for load bearing but dynamically dangerous.

Joint dysfunction: A state of altered mechanics, either an increase or decrease from the expected normal, or the presence of an aberrant motion.

Joint play: Movements not under voluntary control that occur only in response to an outside force.

Kinematics: The study of the geometry of motion independent of the kinetic influences that may be responsible for the motion. In biomechanics, the two divisions of kinematics are osteokinematics and arthrokinematics.

Loose-packed position: Position of a joint where the capsule and ligaments are their most slack, which is unlocked, statically inefficient for load bearing, and dynamically safe.

(From Paris SV, Loubert PV. *Foundations of Clinical Orthopaedics.* St Augustine, FL: Institute Press;1990.)

REFERENCES

1. American Physical Therapy Association (APTA). *Referral for profit*. Available at http://www.apta.org/StateIssues/Manipulation/. Accessed December 17, 2014.

2. APTA CAPTE, editor. *Evaluative Criteria for the Accreditation of Education Programs for the Preparation of Physical Therapists*. Alexandria, VA: APTA; 2005.

3. MacDonald CW, Osmotherly PG, Parkes R, et al. The current manipulation debate: historical context to address a broken narrative, *J Man Manip Ther*. 2019;27(1):1-4.

4. Paris SV, Loubert PV. *Foundations of Clinical Orthopaedics*. St Augustine, FL: Institute Press; 1990.

5. Paris SV. A history of manipulative therapy. *J Man Manip Ther*. 2000;8(2):66-77.

6. Meeker WC, Haldeman S. Chiropractic: a profession at the crossroads of mainstream and alternative medicine. *Ann Intern Med*. 2002;136(3):216-227.

7. Hood W. On the so-called "bone-setting": its nature and results. *Lancet*. 1871;1:336-338.

8. Paget J. Clinical lecture on cases that bone-setters cure. *Br Med J*. 1867;1(314):1-4.

9. Hamonet C. Andrew Taylor still and the birth of osteopathy (Baldwin, Kansas, USA, 1855). *Joint Bone Spine*. 2003;70(1):80-84.

10. Stoddard A. *Manual of Osteopathic Practice*. London: Hutchinson; 1969.

11. Hart JF. Did DD Palmer visit at still in Kirksville? *Chiropr Hist*. 1997;17(2):49-55.

12. Peterson DH, Bergmann TF. *Chiropractic Technique: Principles and Procedures*, ed 2. St. Louis: Mosby; 2002.

13. Ottosson A. The manipulated history of manipulations of spines and joints? Rethinking orthopaedic medicine through the 19th century discourse of European mechanical medicine. *Med Studies*. 2011;3:83-116.

14. McMillan M. *Massage and Therapeutic Exercise*. Philadelphia: WB Saunders; 1921.

15. McMillan M. Change of name [editorial]. *PT Rev*. 1925;5(4):3-4.

16. McMillan M. *Massage and Therapeutic Exercise*, ed 2. Philadelphia: WB Saunders; 1925.

17. Kaltenborn KM. *Traction-Manipulation of the Extremities and Spine. Basic Thrust Techniques*, vol. 3. Oslo, Norway: Norli.

18. Hansson N, Ottoson A. Nobel prize for physical therapy? Rise, fall, and revival of medico-mechanical institutes. *Phys Ther*. 2015;95(8):1184-1194.

19. Paris SV. 37th Mary McMillan lecture: in the best interest of the patient. *Phys Ther*. 2006;86(11):1541-1553.

20. Kellogg JH. *The Art of Massage: Its Physiological and Therapeutic Applications*. Battle Creek, MI: Modern Medicine Publishing Co; 1885.

21. Graham D. *A Treatise on Massage, Theoretical and Practical: Its History, Mode of Application and Effects, Indications and Contra Indication*. New York: JH Vail & Co; 1890.

22. Hartelius TJ. *Swedish Movements or Medical Gymnastics*. Battle Creek, MI: Modern Medicine Publishing Co; 1896.

23. Herman RF. The art of mobilizing joints. *Phys Ther Rev*. 1936;16:94-95.

24. Thornhill MC. Manipulative treatment of lumbosacral derangement: report of a series of cases treated with technic described by Dr. B. S. Troedsson. *Phys Ther Rev*. 1938;18:65-67.

25. McKenzie RT. The place of manipulation and corrective gymnastics in treatment. *Phys Ther Rev*. 1929;9(6):240-242.

26. Swenson LL. Study of the intervertebral disc: with special reference to rupture of the nucleus pulposus and its relation to low back pain and to sciatica. *Phys Ther Rev*. 1941;21:179-184.

27. Pettman E. A history of manipulative therapy. *J Man Manip Ther*. 2007;15(3):165-174.

28. Mennell J. *The Science and Art of Joint Manipulation*. London: Churchill; 1949.

29. Cyriax J. *Textbook of Orthopaedic Medicine*, vol 1. London: Cassell; 1957.

30. Cyriax J. *Textbook of Orthopaedic Medicine*, vol 2. London: Baillierre Tindall; 1984.

31. Flint I, Hague S. Alan Stoddard. *BMJ*. 2002;325(7375):1305.

32. Huijbregts P. Orthopaedic manual physical therapy: history, development and future opportunities. Historical paper. *J Phys Ther*. 2010;1:11-24.

33. Kaltenborn FM. *The Spine Basic Evaluation and Mobilization Techniques*. Oslo, Norway: Olaf Norlis Bokhandel; 1964.

34. Mennell JM. *Joint Pain*. Boston: Little Brown; 1964.

35. Maitland GD. *Vertebral Manipulation*. London: Butterworth; 1964.

36. Paris SV. *Spinal Lesion*. Christchurch, New Zealand: Pegasus; 1965.

37. Olson KA. President's message: history is on our side. *Articulations*. 2005;11(2):1-3.

38. American Chiropractic Association (ACA). *Interprofessional Collaborative Spine Conference*. Pittsburgh, PA: American Chiropractic Association; 2019.

39. Magel J, Hansen P, Meier W, et al. Implementation of an alternative pathway for patients seeking care for low back pain: a prospective observational cohort study. *Phys Ther*. 2018;98(12):1000-1009.

40. Foster NE, Anema JR, Cherkin D, et al. Low back pain 2: prevention and treatment of low back pain: evidence, challenges, and promising directions. *Lancet*. 2018;391(10137):2368–2383.

41. Paris SV. *Introduction to Spinal Evaluation and Manipulation*. Atlanta: Institute Press; 1986.

42. Hahne AJ, Keating JL, Wilson SC. Do within-session changes in pain intensity and range or motion predict between-session changes in patients with low back pain? *Aust J Physiother*. 2004;50:17-23.

43. Tuttle N. Is it reasonable to use an individual patient's progress after treatment as a guide to ongoing clinical reasoning? *J Manip Physiol Ther*. 2009;32:396-403.

44. Wright AA, Abbott JH, Baxter D, et al. The ability of a sustained within-session finding of pain reduction during traction to dictate improved outcomes from a manual therapy approach on patients with osteoarthritis of the hip. *J Man Manip Ther*. 2010;18:166-172.

45. Cook C, Petersen S, Donaldson M, et al. Does early change predict long-term (6 months) improvements in subjects who receive manual therapy for low back pain? *Physiother Theory Pract*. 2017;33:716-724.

46. Bang MD, Deyle GD. Comparison of supervised exercise with and without manual physical therapy for patients with shoulder impingement syndrome. *J Orthop Sports Phys Ther*. 2000;30(3):126-137.

47. Bergman GJ, Winters J, Croesier KH, et al. Manipulative therapy in addition to usual medical care for patients with shoulder dysfunction and pain: a randomized, controlled trial. *Ann Intern Med*. 2004;141(6):432-439.

48. Cleland JA, Fritz JM, Kulig K, et al. Comparison of the effectiveness of three manual physical therapy techniques in a subgroup of patients with low back pain who satisfy a clinical prediction rule: a randomized clinical trial. *Spine*. 2009;34(25):2720-2729.

49. Deyle GD, Allison SC, Matekel RL, et al. Physical therapy treatment effectiveness for osteoarthritis of the knee: a randomized comparison of supervised clinical exercise and manual therapy procedures versus a home exercise program. *Phys Ther*. 2005;85(12):1310-1317.

50. Hoeksma HL, Dekker J, Ronday HK, et al. Comparison of manual therapy and exercise in osteoarthritis of the hip: a randomized clinical trial. *Arthritis Rheum*. 2004;51(5):722-729.

51. Hoving JL, Koes BW, de Vet HCW, et al. Manual therapy, physical therapy, or continued care by a general practitioner for patients with neck pain: a randomized controlled trial. *Ann Intern Med*. 2002;136:713-722.

52. Walker MJ, Boyles RE, Young BA, et al. The effectiveness of manual physical therapy and exercise for mechanical neck pain: a randomized clinical trial. *Spine*. 2008;33(22):2371-2378.

53. Whitman JM, Flynn TW, Childs JD, et al. A comparison between two physical therapy treatment programs for patients with lumbar spinal stenosis: a randomized clinical trial. *Spine*. 2006;31(22):2541-2549.

54. Vermeulen HM, Rozing PM, Obermann WR, et al. Comparison of high-grade and low-grade mobilization techniques in the management of adhesive capsulitis of the shoulder: randomized controlled trial. *Phys Ther*. 2006;86(3):355-368.

55. Brennan GP, Fritz JM, Hunter SJ, et al. Identifying subgroups of patients with acute/subacute "nonspecific" low back pain: results of a randomized clinical trial. *Spine*. 2006;31(6):623-631.

56. Fritz JM, Delitto A, Erhard RE. Comparison of a classification-based approach to physical therapy and therapy based on clinical practice guidelines for patients with acute low back pain: a randomized clinical trial. *Spine*. 2003;28:1363-1372.

57. Delitto A, George SZ, Van Dillen L, et al. Low back pain. *J Orthop Sports Phys Ther*. 2012;42(4):A1-A57.

58. Blanpied PR, Gross AR, Elliott JM, et al. Neck pain: revision 2017 Clinical Practice Guideline Linked to the International Classification of Functioning, Disability and Health from the Orthopaedic Section of the American Physical Therapy Association. *JOSPT*. 2017;47(7):A1-A83.

59. Sackett DL, Straus SE, Richardson WS, et al. *Evidence-Based Medicine: How to Practice and Teach EBM*, ed 2. Edinburgh: Churchill Livingstone; 2000.

60. Portney LG, Watkins MP. *Foundations of Clinical Research Applications to Practice*, ed 2. Upper Saddle River, NJ: Prentice Hall; 2000.

61. Cleland JA. *Orthopaedic Clinical Examination: an Evidence-Based Approach for Physical Therapists*. Carlstadt, NJ: Icon Learning Systems; 2005.

62. Cohen J. A coefficient of agreement for nominal scales. *Educ Psychol Meas*. 1960;20(1):37-46.

63. Landis JR, Koch GG. The measurement of observer agreement for categorical data. *Biometrics*. 1977;33:159-174.

64. Rothstein JM, Echternach JL. *Primer on Measurement: An Introductory Guide to Measurement Issues*. Alexandria, VA: American Physical Therapy Association; 1999.

65. Jaeschke R, Guyatt GH, Sackett DL. How to use an article about a diagnostic test. B. What are the results and will they help me in caring for my patients? *JAMA*. 1994;271:703-707.

66. Whiting P, Rutjes AWS, Reitsma JB, et al. The development of QUADAS: a tool for the quality assessment of studies of diagnostic accuracy included in systematic reviews. *BMC Med Res Methodol*. 2003;3:25.

67. De Graf I, Prak A, Bierma-Zeinstra S, et al. Diagnosis of lumbar spinal stenosis: a systematic review of the accuracy of diagnostic tests. *Spine*. 2006;31:1168-1176.

68. Cook C, Hegedus E. Diagnostic utility of clinical tests for spinal dysfunction. *Man Ther*. 2011;16:21-25.

69. Simoneau G. Editor-in-chief Personal communication. *J Orthop Sports Phys Ther*. 2014.

70. McGinn T, Guyatt GH, Wyer P, et al. Users' guides to the medical literature XXIIa: how to use articles about clinical decision rules. *JAMA*. 2000;284:79-84.

71. Cook CE, Thigpen CA. Five good reasons to be disappointed with randomized trials. *J Man Manip Ther*. 2019;27(2):63-65.

CHAPTER 2

Spinal Examination and Diagnosis in Orthopaedic Manual Physical Therapy

OVERVIEW

The purpose of this chapter is to provide a framework for completion of a comprehensive spinal examination, including systems medical screening, patient interview, disability assessment, and tests and measures. In addition, evaluation of the examination findings and principles involved in a diagnosis and plan of care are included. The tests and measures presented in this chapter are the basic examination procedures used in screening the spine, or they are techniques used across anatomic regions to complete a comprehensive spinal examination. Additional special tests and manual examination procedures, such as passive intervertebral motion tests, are presented in detail in subsequent chapters that focus on each anatomic region of the spine.

OBJECTIVES

1. Describe and implement the components of a comprehensive spinal examination.

2. Perform a medical screening as part of a spinal examination.

3. Describe common red flags and yellow flags that must be evaluated as part of a comprehensive spinal examination.

4. Explain the components of a patient interview, and provide interpretation of common responses to interview questions.

5. Use and interpret relevant questionnaires for pain, function, and disability.

6. Perform and interpret common tests and measures used in a spinal examination.

7. Explain the reliability and validity of common tests and measures used in a spinal examination.

8. Describe the clinical reasoning process used in the evaluation of clinical findings, diagnosis, and treatment planning for common spinal disorders, using the current best evidence with an impairment-based approach.

▶ *To view videos pertaining to this chapter, please visit the eBook.*

DIAGNOSIS IN PHYSICAL THERAPY PRACTICE

Physical therapy diagnostic classifications are based on clusters of patient signs and symptoms that guide treatment decisions. Because physical therapy interventions are designed for correction of physical impairments, such as hypomobility or poor neuromuscular control, the physical therapy diagnostic classifications are based on impairments that can be treated with physical therapy interventions. Other physical therapy diagnostic classifications may describe pain symptom location and behavior if these are the primary focus of the physical therapy

interventions. Patient management and education will be influenced by determination of the proportional contribution of the patient's musculoskeletal pain that can be attributed to nociceptive pain, peripheral neuropathic pain, or central sensitization (CS) pain.[1] Nociceptive pain refers to pain arising predominantly from somatic tissues in response to noxious chemical (inflammatory), thermal, or mechanical stimuli, as might occur in response to inflammation of traumatic, degenerative, or systemic origin or ischemia secondary to mechanical loading.[1] Peripheral neuropathic pain refers to pain arising from impairment of or a lesion within peripheral neural tissue (i.e., distal to and including the dorsal root ganglion), such as compressive neuropathies of spinal nerve roots, which may induce pathophysiologic changes that lead to neuronal hyperexcitability and/or acquired chemical or mechanical sensitivities.[1] CS pain refers to pain that arises or persists as a result of aberrant processing and/or hypersensitivity within the diffuse neural networks of the central nervous system (CNS) engaged in nociception, in the absence of or disproportionate to somatic tissue or peripheral nerve pathology.[2] Key pathophysiologic features include enhanced CNS synaptic efficacy, loss of spinal inhibitory interneurones, descending facilitation, and altered cortical processing.[3] Box 2.1 summarizes the key cluster of signs and symptoms based on an in-depth study of clinical expert physical therapists for the three main types of pain.

Medical diagnostic classifications focus on identification of disease and are determined by physicians. Although the physical therapist does not make a medical diagnosis, the physical therapist must determine whether the patient's condition is appropriate for physical therapy or whether the patient should be immediately referred for further medical diagnostic evaluation. The physical therapist may also identify signs of conditions that warrant further medical consultation but that may not be severe or progressive in nature so that physical therapy can still proceed while the patient seeks further medical evaluation. The patient will also commonly have medical conditions that have been diagnosed and are being appropriately managed. In this situation, physical therapy can proceed, but the condition should be monitored or taken into consideration as physical therapy treatment is implemented.

MEDICAL SCREENING

Medical screening is the evaluation of patient examination data to help determine whether further diagnostic tests and/or a patient's referral to a medical specialist is warranted.[7] Box 2.2 and Table 2.1 list common red flags for which patients should be screened before initiation of physical therapy. The screening process for *red flags*, which is a term used to describe signs or symptoms that are related to a serious underlying pathology and may indicate more diagnostic testing is necessary before the appropriate care can be delivered, has recently been questioned because of the poor diagnostic utility reported for most of the red flags published in low back pain (LBP) clinical prac-

---

BOX 2.1	Clinical Cluster of Signs and Symptoms to Diagnose the Three Primary Types of Pain

Nociceptive Pain[4] (Sensitivity 90.9%, Specificity 91.0%)
- Pain localized to the area of injury/dysfunction
- Clear, proportionate mechanical/anatomic nature to aggravating and easing factors
- Pain usually intermittent and sharp with movement/mechanical provocation
- May have a more constant dull ache or throb at rest
- The absence of:
  - pain associated with dysesthesias
  - night pain/disturbed sleep
  - pain described as burning, shooting, sharp or electric-shock-like
  - antalgic postures/movement patterns

Peripheral Neuropathic Pain[5] (Sensitivity 86.3%, Specificity 96.0%)
- Pain referred in a dermatomal or cutaneous distribution
- History of nerve injury, pathology, or mechanical compromise
- Pain/symptom provocation with mechanical/movement tests (e.g., active/passive, neurodynamic) that move/load/compress neural tissue

Central Sensitization Pain[6] (Sensitivity 91.8%, Specificity 97.7%)
- Disproportionate, nonmechanical, unpredictable pattern of pain provocation in response to multiple/nonspecific aggravating/easing factors
- Pain disproportionate to the nature and extent of injury or pathology
- Strong association with maladaptive psychosocial factors (e.g., negative emotions, poor self-efficacy, maladaptive beliefs, and pain behaviors)
- Diffuse/nonanatomic areas of pain/tenderness on palpation

BOX 2.2	Red Flags for the Cervical Spine

Cervical myelopathy
- Sensory disturbance of hand
- Muscle wasting of hand intrinsic muscles
- Unsteady gait
- Hoffmann reflex
- Inverted supinator sign
- Babinski sign
- Hyperreflexia
- Bowel and bladder disturbances
- Multisegmental weakness or sensory changes
- Age >45 years

Neoplastic conditions
- Age >50 years
- History of cancer
- Unexplained weight loss
- Constant pain; no relief with bed rest
- Night pain

Upper cervical ligamentous instability
- Occipital headache and numbness
- Severe limitation during neck active range of motion in all directions
- Signs of cervical myelopathy

Inflammatory or systemic disease
- Temperature >37° C
- Blood pressure >160/95 mm Hg
- Resting pulse >100 beats per minute
- Resting respiration >25 breaths per minute
- Fatigue

Vertebral artery insufficiency
- Drop attacks
- Dizziness
- Lightheadedness related to head movements
- Dysphagia
- Dysarthria
- Diplopia
- Cranial nerve signs

(Modified from Childs JD, Fritz JM, Piva SR, et al. Proposal of a classification system for patients with neck pain. *J Orthop Sports Phys Ther.* 2004;34(11):686-696.)

TABLE 2.1	Red Flags for Low Back Region
CONDITION	**RED FLAGS**
Back-related tumor	• Age >50 years • History of cancer (especially lung, breast, or prostate) • Unexplained weight loss • Failure of conservative therapy • Night pain
Back-related infection (spinal osteomyelitis)	• Pain • Fever • Neurologic dysfunction • Recent infection (e.g., urinary tract or skin) • Intravenous drug user/abuser • Concurrent immunosuppressive disorder • Poor living conditions • Recent spinal surgery
Cauda equine syndrome	• Urine retention or incontinence • Fecal incontinence • Saddle anesthesia • Global or progressive weakness in lower extremities • Sensory deficits in feet (i.e., L4, L5, and S1 areas) • Ankle dorsiflexion, toe extension, and ankle plantarflexion weakness • Leg pain—bilateral sciatica • Reduced anal tone
Spinal fracture	• History of trauma (including minor falls or heavy lifts for individuals who have osteoporosis or are elderly) • Prolonged use of steroids • Age >70 years

(From Boissonnault WG. *Primary Care for the Physical Therapist: Examination and Triage*. Philadelphia: Saunders; 2005. Updates from Finucane 2020.)

tice guidelines for screening spinal pathology.[8] The presence of one or two red flags alone should not be used as a reason to delay treatment or order advanced imaging, but instead should raise the therapist's suspicion of the potential for series pathology that should be factored into the clinical reasoning process to determine appropriate management of each individual patient. Presence of red flags also should heighten the clinician's attention to careful monitoring of changes of symptoms over time to shed further light on the patient's clinical presentation.[8] If the number of red flags increases over an episode of care and symptoms intensify, appropriate referral and diagnostic testing is more likely indicated than when a trial of a treatment proves successful in alleviation of symptoms.

There are comprehensive resources available that can assist in training clinicians to screen for pathologic conditions.[7,9,10] Conditions, such as gastrointestinal (GI) disease, psychosocial issues, or cardiovascular disease are cause for caution. If these conditions have not been diagnosed and treated by a physician, a referral is warranted. If these conditions are being medically managed, the physical therapist can proceed with evaluation and treatment while continuing to monitor these conditions.

Evidence-based screening strategies for serious conditions like cancer, fractures, cauda equina syndrome (CES), spinal infections, and abdominal pain that is nonmusculoskeletal in nature are completed by identification of a cluster of history and physical examination findings.[11] For example, LBP, advanced age, corticosteroid use, or pain caused by a traumatic incident may not be a concern when each finding is considered in isolation, but when these factors are clustered in an individual with back pain, they are highly predictive of a fracture.[11,12] Life-threatening conditions, such as fracture or malignant disease, are important conditions for identification; if suspected, these conditions warrant an immediate referral to the appropriate physician.

The results of a systematic review for assessment of the accuracy of clinical features and tests used to screen for malignant disease in patients with LBP found the prevalence rate of malignant disease ranged from 0.1% to 3.5%.[11] A history of cancer (positive likelihood ratio [+LR] = 23.7), an elevated erythrocyte sedimentation rate (ESR; +LR = 18.0), a reduced hematocrit level (+LR = 18.2), and overall clinician judgment (+LR = 12.1) increased the probability of identification of a malignant disease.[13] A combination of age of 50 years or more, history of cancer, unexplained weight loss, and no improvement after 1 month of conservative treatment showed a sensitivity of 100% for identification of malignant disease.[13] Therefore cancer as the cause of LBP can be ruled out with 100% sensitivity if the patient is younger than 50 years of age, does not exhibit unexplained weight loss, does not have a history of cancer, and is responding to conservative intervention.[14] Malignant disease is a rare cause of back pain, and the most useful features and tests to evaluate for it are a history of cancer, an elevated ESR, a reduced hematocrit level, and clinician judgment.[13]

The three most common primary cancers to metastasis to the spine are lung, breast, and prostate, and these three cancers make up 50% of metastatic spinal cord compression (MSCC).[15] MSCC occurs when there is pathologic vertebral body collapse or direct tumor growth causing compression of the spinal cord leading to irreversible neurologic damage.[16] In addition to severe pain and spinal instability, the condition can cause compression of the spinal cord leading to paraplegia, quadriplegia, and/or incontinence.[10] Approximately 25% of the individuals presenting with MSCC will present with MSCC as the first signs of cancer.[17] Early signs of epidural distention because of spinal malignancy include pain intensifying over time; worse on coughing, sneezing, straining (Valsalva maneuver); or on lying supine.[18] The UK National Institute for Health and Care Excellence (NICE) guideline recommends having a higher index of suspicion of spinal malignancy in those with a known cancer diagnosis or severe unremitting pain, especially if it is localized to the cervical or thoracic spine or the pain is aggravated by increased intraabdominal pressure.[19]

The natural history of metastatic disease with MSCC has an average survival of between 3 and 7 months with a probability of survival to 12 months of 36%.[20] Although breast, prostate, and lung cancers are the most common to metastasize to the spine, it is possible for other cancers, such as colorectal and lymphoma, to metastasize to the spine as well, and the

R	Referred pain that is multi-segmental or <u>band like</u>
E	<u>Escalating pain</u> which is poorly responsive to treatment (incl medication)
D	<u>Different</u> character or site to previous symptoms
F	Funny feelings, odd sensations or <u>heavy legs</u> (multi-segmental)
L	<u>Lying flat</u> increases back pain
A	<u>Agonising pain</u> causing anguish or despair
G	Gait disturbance, unsteadiness, especially on stairs (not just a limp)
S	Sleep <u>grossly</u> disturbed due to pain being worse at night

FIG. 2.1 Red flag mnemonic. Referred pain that is multisegmental or band like. Escalating pain that is poorly responsive to treatment (including medication). Different character or site to previous symptoms. Funny feelings, odd sensations, or heavy legs (multisegmental). Lying flat increases back pain. Agonizing pain causing anguish or despair. Gait disturbance, unsteadiness, especially on stairs (not just a limp). Sleep grossly disturbed because of pain being worse at night. (From Turnpenney J, Greenhalgh S, Richards L, et al. Developing an early alert system for metastatic spinal cord compression. *Prim Health Care Res Dev.* 2015;16(1):14-20.)

reoccurrence of these cancers may first show up with metastasis to the spine.[10] Magnetic resonance imaging (MRI) of the whole spine is the imaging method of choice for diagnosis of MSCC and has a sensitivity of 93% and specificity of 97%.[21] Early diagnosis is the key to improving outcomes and survival rates for patients with metastasis to the spine.[22] An 8-item red flag mnemonic (Fig. 2.1) has been developed to assist in early identification of MSCC and has been distributed in the United Kingdom as a credit card sized reminder to assist clinicians in early identification of MSCC.[22] The following three key statements about MSCC were also placed on the card along with reference to key sources of additional information (www.nice.org.uk; gmccn.nhs.uk):

- Past medical history of cancer (but note 25% patients do not have a diagnosed primary cancer).
- Early diagnosis is essential (as the prognosis is severely impaired once paralysis occurs).
- A combination of Red Flags increases suspicion (the more red flags, the higher the risk and greater urgency).[22] The red flags for patients at risk of or with MSCC are listed in Box 2.3.

Night pain is a red flag associated with metastatic bone disease, but it is also a common finding in benign back pain, which challenges its usefulness as a sign of serious pathology.[23] "Ominous" night pain symptoms are aggravated rather than relieved by lying down and is a concerning red flag if the patient describes the need to get up and walk to ease the pain during the night or that they are unable to sleep lying flat and routinely sleep upright in a chair.[24] Currently, there are no national guidelines on recognizing the signs and symptoms of metastatic bone disease for healthcare professions.[24] A "safety

BOX 2.3	Red Flags for Patients at Risk of or With Metastatic Spinal Cord Compression

- Limb weakness
- Difficulty walking
- Sensory loss
- Bladder or bowel dysfunction
- Neurological signs
- Progressive and unremitting lumbar spine pain
- Cervical or thoracic pain
- Pain increased with straining
- Night pain

(From Greenhalgh S, Selfe J. *Red Flags and Blue Lights, Managing Series Spinal Pathology,* ed 2. Elsevier; 2019.)

netting" process of closely observing patients at risk over time is an important consideration to effectively manage these potentially serious situations.[25] Using knowledge of a patient's risk of developing metastatic bone disease combined with ongoing assessment for red flags may help to raise a clinician's index of suspicion and result in timely investigation and management of the patient.[24]

Clinicians should also be on the lookout for early signs of CES because early identification can limit the extent of its long-term effects. CES occurs as a result of direct compression of the lumbosacral nerve roots distal to the conus medullaris.[10] The compression could be caused by a large central disc herniation at L4L5 or L5S1, or because of trauma, tumor, MSCC, spinal canal stenosis, epidural hematoma, abscess, or infection.[26] For diagnosis of CES, one or more of the following must be present:

1. Bladder and/or bowel dysfunction
2. Reduced sensation in the saddle area, and
3. Sexual dysfunction, with possible neurologic deficit in the lower limb (motor/sensory loss, reflex change)[27]

Bilateral lower extremity radicular pain is a symptom associated with CES, and when present, CES should be suspected and further inquiry should take place.[28] Urinary retention with overflow incontinence is a potential predictor of CES, with a sensitivity of 90% and a specificity of 95%.[29] In patients without urinary retention, the probability of CES is one in 10,000 for patients with LBP.[30] Clinical examination findings combined with MRI findings are required to make a diagnosis of CES. Fairbank (2014)[31] suggests that the following symptoms of CES should prompt immediate MRI:

- bilateral sciatica
- bilateral lower extremity paresthesia
- bilateral lower extremity motor deficit
- perineal pain
- perineal (saddle) paresthesia or anesthesia
- altered bladder/anal function
- bladder dysfunction

In a systematic review that pooled data from six studies ($n = 569$ participants) that compared the results of MRI with the presence of red flags associated with CES, including reduced anal tone, leg pain, back pain, saddle anesthesia, urinary retention, urinary incontinence and bowel incontinence,

Dionne et al.[32] reported pooled sensitivity for the signs and symptoms ranged from 0.19 to 0.43 and the pooled specificity ranged from 0.62 to 0.88. The authors concluded that red flags used to identify potential CES appear to be more specific than sensitive and when present should be considered justification for a prompt diagnostic workup.[32]

Greenhalgh and Selfe[10] have developed credit card–sized cue cards to assist clinicians and patients to avoid any embarrassment in asking the necessary CES–related questions and to make an early diagnosis of CES (Fig. 2.2). These cards have been translated into 28 languages and are available through the following website: https://eoemskservice.nhs.uk/.

In cases of spinal infection, there is often a prolonged period of time between onset and diagnosis, and people can remain relatively healthy until symptoms manifest in the later stages of the disease.[33] Spinal infection has a linear progression with back pain being the most common presenting symptom which can progress to neurologic symptoms.[34] If not treated in a timely manner, the condition can progress with serious complications, such as paralysis, instability of the spine, and even death.[34]

Spinal infections, such as tuberculosis (TB), discitis, and spinal abscesses are uncommon with an incidence of 0.2 to 2.4 cases per 100,000 annually in western societies.[35,36] The point prevalence of infection presenting as nonmechanical LBP is estimated at 0.01% in primary care[37] and 1.2% in a tertiary setting[38] with postprocedural discitis making up 30% of all cases of pyogenic spondylodiscitis.[39] The frequency of spinal infections presenting in a clinical setting depends on the demographics of the patient population. Because of the rarity of spinal infections in high–income countries, the diagnosis of spinal infections is often delayed because clinicians fail to recognize the relevant red flags and consider spinal infection as a potential differential diagnosis.[34]

The subjective history should consider determinants, which can be divided into comorbidities, environmental factors, and social factors that may affect the occurrence of spinal infection.[34] Yusuf[40] completed a metaanalysis that included 40 papers on spinal infection with a total of 2224 cases of spinal infection that were identified with spinal pain (72%), fever (55%), and neurologic dysfunction (33%) as the most common clinical features; diabetes (18%) and intravenous drug use (9%) were the most frequently occurring determinants.[40] Comorbidities that suppress a patient's immune system, such as diabetes, HIV, long-term steroid use, and smoking, put the person at risk of infection.[34] Social and environmental factors should be considered and include intravenous drug use, obesity, migrant born in a TB-endemic country, family history of TB, and poor living conditions.[34] Spinal surgery is a key risk factor for spinal infection, especially with the more complex multiple-level lumbar spine surgeries.[40] Discitis primarily affects the lumbar spine (58%) followed by the thoracic (30%) and cervical spine (11%).[41] TB lesions mainly affect the thoracic spine and often affect more than two levels.[41]

The literature describes a classic triad of clinical features for spinal infections, including back pain, fever, and neurologic dysfunction.[42] However, the reliance on people presenting

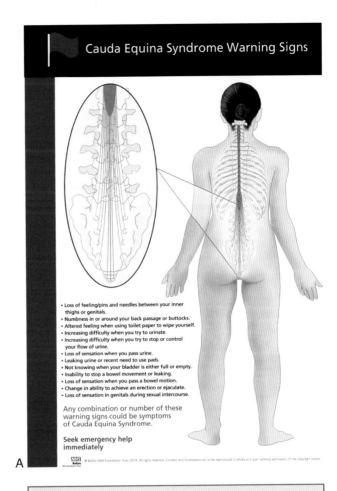

FIG. 2.2 Clinician's cauda equina syndrome (CES) cue card and patient's CES credit card. (From Greenhalgh S, Selfe J. *Red Flags and Blue Lights, Managing Series Spinal Pathology*, ed 2. Elsevier; 2019.)

with these features may result in missed cases or late diagnosis because not all people will present with all three features.[34] For example, only 50% to 55% of people report fever as a symptom[40,43] so a lack of fever cannot rule out spinal infection, and clinicians should not be reassured by the absence of fever.[34] Using both determinants and clinical features for spinal infection will assist clinicians in considering whether there is a need to request further investigations including blood tests and imaging (MRI) if spinal infection is suspected.[34]

A medical intake form is an essential component of a comprehensive initial patient examination. See Fig. 2.3 for an example of

To ensure you receive a complete and thorough evaluation, please provide us with the important background information on the following form. All information is considered confidential and will be released only to your physician unless prior written authorization is given. Thank you.

NAME: _____ OCCUPATION: _____

Have you seen any of the following for your current condition within the past year? (Check box)

☐ Physician (M.D., D.O.)   ☐ Psychiatrist/Psychologist   ☐ Attorney
☐ Dentist   ☐ Physical Therapist   ☐ Chiropractor

Have you EVER been diagnosed as having any of the following conditions?

☐ Cancer, If yes, describe what kind: _____

☐ Heart Problems	☐ Rheumatoid Arthritis	☐ Prostate Problems	☐ Restless Leg Syndrome*
☐ Pacemaker	☐ Other Arthritic Conditions	☐ Anxiety or Panic Attacks*	☐ Chronic Fatigue Syndrome*
☐ Circulation Problems	☐ Osteoporosis	☐ Depression	☐ Headaches*
☐ High Blood Pressure	☐ Kidney Disease	☐ Sexual Transmitted Diseases	☐ Irritable Bowel Syndrome*
☐ Lung Disease	☐ Thyroid Problems	☐ Fibromyalgia*	☐ Allergies
☐ Asthma	☐ Stroke	☐ Chemical Dependency	☐ Latex Allergy
☐ Diabetes	☐ Chemical Sensitivities*	☐ Whiplash*	☐ TMJ Disorder*
			☐ Other:_____

Please list any surgeries or other conditions for which you have been hospitalized within the last few years, including the approximate date of the surgery or hospitalization:

DATE   SURGERY/HOSPITALIZATION   DATE   SURGERY/HOSPITALIZATION

_____   _____   _____   _____

_____   _____   _____   _____

Please describe any injuries for which you have been treated (including fractures, dislocations, sprains) within the last few years and the approximate date of injury:

DATE   INJURY   DATE   INJURY

_____   _____   _____   _____

_____   _____   _____   _____

Have you recently noted:

☐ Weight loss/gain	☐ Nausea/vomiting	☐ Weakness	☐ Numbness/tingling
☐ Fatigue	☐ Dizziness	☐ Shortness of breath	☐ Headaches
☐ Fever/chills/sweats	☐ Pain at night	☐ Difficulty swallowing	☐ Change of appetite

Please provide your current height: _____ inches   weight: _____ lbs.

Have you fallen within the past 12 months?   Yes   No

During the past month, have you often been bothered by feeling down, depressed, or hopeless?   Yes   No
During the past month, have you often been bothered by little interest or pleasure in doing things?   Yes   No
Have you had any recent changes in your bowel or bladder function?   Yes   No

How many packs of cigarettes do you smoke a day?   _____

If one drink equals one beer or glass of wine, how much alcohol do you drink in a week?   _____

How are you able to sleep at night?   ☐ Fine   ☐ Moderate difficulty*   ☐ Only with medications*

OVER

FIG. 2.3 Medical intake form.

On the scales below, please circle the number which best represents your pain levels:

At Worst: No Pain 0   1   2   3   4   5   6   7   8   9   10 Worst Pain Imaginable

Current: No Pain 0   1   2   3   4   5   6   7   8   9   10 Worst Pain Imaginable

At Best: No Pain 0   1   2   3   4   5   6   7   8   9   10 Worst Pain Imaginable

Aggravating Factors: Identify up to 3 important activities that you are unable to do or are having difficulty with as a result of your problem. List them below:

1. _____

2. _____

3. _____

Exercise/Physical Activity Level

Completely Sedentary   High Level Training Program

      0   1   2   3   4   5   6   7   8   9   10

Would you like education/advice on how to safely improve your exercise/activity level? _____ Yes _____ No

Body Chart: Please mark your present symptoms on the Body Chart.

Please list any PRESCRIPTION medication (including dosages) you are currently taking (INCLUDING injections, and/or skin patches):

MEDICATION   DOSAGE   MEDICATION   DOSAGE
_____   _____   _____   _____

_____   _____   _____   _____

Which of the following OVER-THE-COUNTER medications have you taken in the last week? (Check the box.)

    ☐ Aspirin   ☐ Laxatives   ☐ Vitamins/mineral supplements
    ☐ Tylenol   ☐ Antacids   ☐ Advil/Motrin/Ibuprofen
    ☐ Decongestants   ☐ Antihistamines   ☐ Other

Have you been seen by a home health agency within the last 60 days? _____ yes _____ no

How did you hear about Northern Rehab?
    ☐ Physician   ☐ Family/Friend _____   ☐ Previous Patient   ☐ Social Media _____
    ☐ Newspaper   ☐ Saw us at an Event _____   ☐ Internet Search   ☐ Drive-by

Therapist Use
Form reviewed with patient? YES ☐   NO ☐

_____   _____
Date   Therapist signature

FIG. 2.3, cont'd Medical intake form.

a medical intake form. Symptoms of medical conditions, such as increased muscle tone and pain, may mimic symptoms of musculoskeletal dysfunctions. In addition, identification of risk factors for certain medical conditions affects the precautions to and progression of physical therapy interventions. For instance, a patient with cardiovascular disease risk factors, such as hypertension, needs close monitoring as therapeutic exercise programs are

initiated and progressed. However, if the patient's hypertension is managed with beta blocker therapy, which lowers heart rate and dampens or eliminates the pulse response to exercise, the pulse rate is not an effective means for monitoring the patient's response to exercise.[44] Instead, perception of the patient's level of exertion needs to be used to monitor patients who exercise while undergoing beta blocker therapy. Likewise, a diagnosis of osteoporosis is a precaution to excessive strain through the skeletal system with strong stretching or manipulation procedures. However, skilled gentle manual therapy and soft tissue techniques used with precautions to protect the skeletal system and gradual progressive loading of the skeletal system with a monitored exercise program benefit patients with osteoporosis.

A complete list of medications that the patient is taking is also an important component of the medical screening. This information can provide insights into the medical conditions for which the patient is undergoing treatment, and the therapist may find that the combination of prescription and over-the-counter medications is causing an overdosage situation that could result in medical complications. A common example is the use of antiinflammatory drugs. Boissonnault and Meek[45] found that 79% of 2433 patients who were treated in a sample of outpatient physical therapy clinics reported use of antiinflammatory drugs during the week before the survey. Nearly 13% of these patients had two or more risk factors for development of GI disease, and 22% reported combined use of aspirin and another antiinflammatory drug.[45] The risk factors for development of GI complications from nonsteroidal antiinflammatory drugs include advanced age (>61 years), history of peptic ulcer disease, use of other drugs known to damage or exacerbate damage to the GI tract, consumption of or high doses of multiple antiinflammatory drugs or aspirin, and serious systemic illness, such as rheumatoid arthritis.[46]

The physical therapist should review the medical intake form with the patient for follow-up questions regarding medical conditions and medications to obtain greater detail concerning the nature of each condition. This review can also provide insight into the level of understanding the patient has of the medical conditions and medications. The physical therapist can assist the physician in identification of patient needs regarding further education on the medical management of the patient's conditions; the physical therapist also can make referrals for further consultation regarding identified risk factors for medical complications that may inhibit the rehabilitation process.

Psychosocial issues or yellow flags, as listed in Box 2.4, are indications that the rehabilitation approach should be modified.[47] Fear-avoidance beliefs associated with chronic LBP have been shown to be effectively treated with an active exercise program monitored by a physical therapist combined with a behavior modification program that provides positive reinforcement for functional goal attainment.[48] A gradual introduction of activities that the patient fears in a monitored therapeutic environment has yielded favorable results in patients with chronic LBP.[48]

Patients with chronic whiplash-associated disorder (WAD) with moderate to severe ongoing symptoms have been shown to have higher levels of unresolved posttraumatic stress and high levels of persistent fear of movement and reinjury.[49] Heightened anxiety levels in patients after a whiplash injury have been associated with a greater likelihood of long-term pain and a poorer prognosis.[49] When these factors are identified in a patient with acute WAD, an early psychologic consultation is indicated.[49]

Heightened anxiety and fear-avoidance beliefs should not prevent a physical therapist from providing interventions to address the physical impairments identified with these patients, but should

---

BOX 2.4 Clinical Yellow Flags That Indicate Heightened Fear-Avoidance Beliefs

Attitudes and Beliefs
- Belief that pain is harmful or disabling, which results in guarding and fear of movement
- Belief that all pain must be abolished before return to activity
- Expectation of increased pain with activity or work; lack of ability to predict capabilities
- Catastrophizing; expecting the worst
- Belief that pain is uncontrollable
- Passive attitude toward rehabilitation

Behaviors
- Use of extended rest
- Reduced activity with significant withdrawal from daily activities
- Avoidance of normal activity and progressive substitution of lifestyle away from productive activity
- Reports of extremely high pain intensity
- Excessive reliance on aids (braces, crutches, and so on)
- Sleep quality reduced after onset of pain
- High intake of alcohol or other substances with an increase since onset of back pain
- Smoking

(Data from Childs JD, Fritz JM, Piva SR, et al. Proposal of a classification system for patients with neck pain. *J Orthop Sports Phys Ther.* 2004;34(11):686-696; Kendall NAS, Linton SJ, Main CJ. *Guide to Assessing Psychosocial Yellow Flags in Acute Low Back Pain: Risk Factors for Long-Term Disability and Work Loss.* Wellington, New Zealand: Accident Rehabilitation and Compensation Insurance Corporation of New Zealand and the National Health Committee; 2002.)

---

elevate the clinician's awareness that an active exercise approach combined with psychologically informed pain management strategies (see Ch. 4) should be incorporated into the treatment plan.

Depression can also affect the health status and the rehabilitation potential of patients. Clinicians have demonstrated a poor ability to identify depressive symptoms in patients being treated for LBP.[50] To enhance clinicians' ability to properly identify the signs of depression, the medical intake form should include the following two questions to screen for depression:
- During the past month, have you often been bothered by feeling down, depressed, or hopeless? Yes No
- During the past month, have you often been bothered by little interest or pleasure in doing things? Yes No

If the patient answers "yes" to these two questions, the follow-up "help" question should be asked:
- Is this something with which you would like help? Yes, Yes but not today, No

Arrol et al.[51] reported a sensitivity of 79% and a specificity of 94% for detection of major depression with the two screening questions with the "help" question, for a positive predictive value of 41% and a negative predictive value of 98.8%.[51] If the patient answers "yes" to all three questions, the patient should be referred for further assessment and treatment of the depression as an adjunct to the physical therapy treatment. Use of these questions are an effective, valid means of screening for depressive symptoms, has correlated well with a more comprehensive screening tool for depression (Depression Anxiety Stress Scale-21), and should be incorporated into the initial physical therapist examination.[50]

Major clinical depression has a lifetime prevalence rate of 10% to 25% for women and 5% to 12% for men.[52] Up to 15% of people with major clinical depression commit suicide.[48] In addition, depression is common in patients with chronic back and neck pain, and a multidisciplinary approach that includes counseling, medical management, and exercise is needed to successfully treat these conditions. Wideman et al.[53] tracked depressive symptoms in a group of patients with work-related musculoskeletal injuries and depressive symptoms who received 7 weeks of physical therapy and found that depressive symptoms resolved in 40% of the patients. The patients whose depressive symptoms did not resolve during physical therapy were more likely to have had elevated levels of depressive symptoms, pain catastrophizing at pretreatment, and lack of improvement in pain and depressive symptoms at midtreatment.[53]

Disability and Psychosocial Impact Questionnaires

Disability, function, and pain indexes have been shown to be more accurate measures of response to treatment for spinal disorders than impairment measures.[54] Disability index and screening questionnaires, such as the STarT Back, Fear-Avoidance Beliefs Questionnaire (FABQ), the Central Sensitization Inventory (CSI), the Modified Oswestry Disability Index (mODI), and the Neck Disability Index (NDI), assist in quantification of a patient's perception of disability, the psychosocial impact of the disability, and the prognosis for recovery. The Patient-Specific Functional Scale (PSFS) and the Numeric Pain Rating Scale (NPRS) can also assist in quantification of a patient's level of perceived functional limitations and pain perception. These instruments can be used to track outcomes and determine the level of success of a treatment approach for both clinical practice and research situations.

Hill et al.[55] have developed and validated a screening tool referred to as the STarT Back Screening Tool (Fig. 2.4) that has been advocated as an excellent screening tool in primary care situations to triage patients into three subgroups; low, medium, and high risk, for potential development of chronic LBP. The tool includes nine items: bothersomeness, referred leg pain, comorbid pain, catastrophizing, disability (2 items), fear, anxiety, and depression. Overall tool scores are produced by summing positive items (items 1–9). The psychosocial subscale score is a sum of bothersomeness, fear, catastrophizing, anxiety, and depression items (items 5–9). The tool demonstrated good reliability and validity and was acceptable to patients and clinicians.[55] Tool overall scores of 0 to 3 are classified as low risk, and those scoring 4 or 5 on a psychosocial subscale are classified as high risk. The remainder are classified as medium risk (overall tool score >3 but <4 on the psychosocial subscale).[55]

The research group that developed this tool advocates targeted treatment inventions based on the results of the STarT Back Screening tool. The low-, medium-, and high-risk groups should all receive education and advice on back care emphasizing positive messages about activity, pain relief, and work.[56] The medium- and high-risk groups should also receive evidence-based physical therapy to address the impairments identified from a clinical examination.[56] The high-risk group should also receive treated for biopsychosocial risk factors by adopting cognitive behavioral principles to address unhelpful beliefs and behaviors.[56] This approach has been tested with a randomized controlled trial with 851 patients with LBP with the intervention group ($n = 568$) receiving the stratified care based on risk level and the control group ($n = 283$) receiving usual patterns of care. At 12 months, stratified care was associated with a mean increase in generic health benefit and cost savings compared with the control group lending support for the use of this tool in management of patients with LBP.[57]

Waddell et al.[58] have stated that fear of pain and what we do about it may be more disabling than the pain itself. Individuals react to pain on a continuum from confrontation to avoidance. Confrontation is an adaptive response in which an individual views pain as a nuisance and has a strong motivation to return to normal levels of activity.[59] An avoidance response may lead to a reduction in physical and social activities, excessive fear avoidance behaviors, prolonged disability, and adverse physical and psychologic consequences.[59]

The FABQ was developed and tested by Waddell and colleagues[58] as a way to quantify a patient's fear of physical activity, work, and risk of reinjury and their beliefs about the need to change behavior to avoid pain (Fig. 2.5). The questionnaire consists of 16 statements that the patient rates on a scale from 0 (completely disagree) to 6 (completely agree). The FABQ work (FABQW) subscale is calculated by adding items 6, 7, 9, 11, 12, and 15. The FABQ physical activity subscale is calculated by adding items 2, 3, 4, and 5. Test-retest reliability when used with patients with chronic LBP and sciatica had a kappa score of 0.74; all results reached a 0.001 level of significance.[59] The Pearson product-moment correlation coefficients for the two scales were 0.95 and 0.88.[59] The FABQ was found to correlate with levels of psychologic distress, and the FABQW subscale was strongly related to work loss from LBP over a 1-year period, even with a control for pain intensity and location.[59]

Fear of movement and activity is suspected to be a primary factor in the transition from acute LBP to chronic long-term disability associated with LBP. Fritz[59] found that fear-avoidance beliefs were present in patients with acute LBP and were a significant predictor of disability and work status at a 4-week follow-up. In other words, Fritz[59] found that patients with higher levels of fear of work (FABQW >34; sensitivity = 55%; specificity = 84%; +LR = 3.33; negative likelihood ratio [−LR] = 0.54) at the initial evaluation were less likely to return to full work status after 4 weeks of treatment for the LBP condition. Higher scores on the FABQ are an indication to use an active exercise–based approach in which the feared activities are gradually introduced to the patient in a controlled environment to assist the patient in overcoming fears.[60] Low scores for the work subscale (FABQW <19) have been associated with an improved likelihood to succeed with lumbopelvic spinal manipulation.[61] In a cohort of patients without work-related LBP, the FABQW subscale was a better predictor of 6-month outcomes, compared with the FABQ physical activity subscale, with the FABQW subscale scores of greater than 20 demonstrating an increased risk of reporting no improvement with 6-month Oswestry Disability Index (ODI) scores.[62] Therefore the FABQ should be completed at the

The Keele STarT Back Screening Tool

Patient name: _____   Date: _____

Thinking about the **last 2 weeks** tick your response to the following questions:

	Disagree 0	Agree 1
1. My back pain has **spread down my leg(s)** at some time in the last 2 weeks	☐	☐
2. I have had pain in the **shoulder** or **neck** at some time in the last 2 weeks	☐	☐
3. I have only **walked short distances** because of my back pain	☐	☐
4. In the last 2 weeks, I have **dressed more slowly** than usual because of back pain	☐	☐
5. It's not really safe for a person with a condition like mine to be physically active	☐	☐
6. **Worrying thoughts** have been going through my mind a lot of the time	☐	☐
7. I feel that **my back pain is terrible** and **it's never going to get any better**	☐	☐
8. In general I have **not enjoyed** all the things I used to enjoy	☐	☐

9. Overall, how **bothersome** has your back pain been in the **last 2 weeks**?

Not at all	Slightly	Moderately	Very much	Extremely
☐	☐	☐	☐	☐
0	0	0	1	1

Total score (all 9): _____   **Sub Score (Q5-9):**_____

© Keele University 01/08/07
Funded by Arthritis Research UK

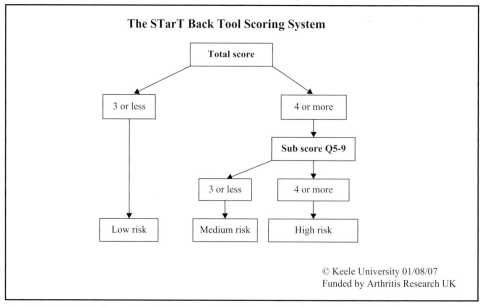

FIG. 2.4 STarT Back Screening Tool. (From Hill JC, Dunn KM, Lewis M, et al. A primary care back pain screening tool: identifying patient subgroups for initial treatment. *Arthritis Rheum.* 2008;59(5):632–641.)

Name: _____   Date: _____

Here are some of the statements that other patients have made to us about their pain. For each statement, please circle a number from 0 to 6 to describe how much physical activities (such as, bending, lifting, walking, or driving) affect or would affect your back pain.

	Completely disagree		Unsure			Completely agree
1. My pain was caused by physical activity.	0	1	2	3	4	5	6
2. Physical activity makes my pain worse.	0	1	2	3	4	5	6
3. Physical activity might harm my back.	0	1	2	3	4	5	6
4. I should not do physical activities that (might) make my pain worse.	0	1	2	3	4	5	6
5. I cannot do physical activities that (might) make my pain worse.	0	1	2	3	4	5	6

The following statements are about how your normal work affects or would affect your back pain.

6. My pain was caused by my work or by an accident at work.	0	1	2	3	4	5	6
7. My work aggravated my pain.	0	1	2	3	4	5	6
8. I have a claim for compensation for my pain.	0	1	2	3	4	5	6
9. My work is too heavy for me.	0	1	2	3	4	5	6
10. My work makes or would make my pain worse.	0	1	2	3	4	5	6
11. My work might harm my back.	0	1	2	3	4	5	6
12. I should not do my normal work with my present pain.	0	1	2	3	4	5	6
13. I cannot do my normal work with my present pain.	0	1	2	3	4	5	6
14. I cannot do my normal work until my pain is treated.	0	1	2	3	4	5	6
15. I do not think that I will be back to my normal work within 3 months.	0	1	2	3	4	5	6
16. I do not think that I will ever be able to go back to my normal work.	0	1	2	3	4	5	6

FIG. 2.5 The Fear-Avoidance Beliefs Questionnaire (FABQ).

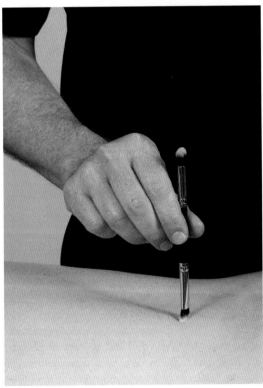

FIG. 2.6 Test for allodynia. Allodynia can be tested by gently touching the patient with a soft make up brush.

intake of all patients with LBP-related conditions to assist in guiding treatment decisions. The FABQ has also been validated and can be used for patients with musculoskeletal conditions of the neck, upper extremity, and lower extremity with slight modifications for the appropriate anatomic location.[63,64]

CS is a neurophysiologic phenomenon in which CNS neurons become hyperexcitable, resulting in hypersensitivity to both noxious and nonnoxious stimuli with abnormal and intense enhancement of pain.[65] The term central sensitivity syndrome (CSS) describes a group of medically indistinct (or nonspecific), interrelated disorders, such as fibromyalgia, chronic fatigue syndrome, temporomandibular joint (TMJ) disorder, tension headache/migraine, restless leg syndrome, and irritable bowel syndrome for which CS may be a common etiology[65] (www.pridedallas.com/questionnaires).

CS is associated with allodynia (pain response from a normally nonpainful stimulation, such as touch with a soft brush (Fig. 2.6), hyperalgesia (excessive sensitivity to a normally painful stimulus), expansion of the receptive field (pain extending beyond the area of peripheral nerve supply), and often prolonged pain after a painful stimulus has been removed (usually throbbing, burning, tingling, or numbness)[65,66] (www.pridedallas.com/questionnaires). Patients with LBP who were classified as having predominantly CS pain have been found to have more severe pain, poorer physical and mental health status, and greater levels of pain-related disability, depression and anxiety compared with patients classified as having nociceptive or peripheral neuropathic pain.[1]

Experimental studies have used a variety of stimuli to test for CS, including thermal stimuli: thresholds for cold pain, heat pain, cold detection, and heat detection; tactile stimuli: pressure pain thresholds (PPTs) (Box 2.5); vibratory or vibrotactile stimuli: detection thresholds for vibration or combination of tactile and vibratory stimuli, for example, electric toothbrush; electrical stimuli: reaction to electrical pulses with electrodes; ischemic stimuli: ischemic compression of the arm with a cuff; and reaction on specific pain mediators, for example, reaction on injection with hypertonic saline.[66] Other than PPT, these stimuli have not been standardized or validated for widespread clinical utilization. See Box 2.5 for illustration of the PPT procedure and Tables 2.2 and 2.3 for normal values.

Common sites for testing PPT include: (1) the suprascapular region, (2) the anterior tibialis muscle belly, and (3) the C4 articular pillar. Pain detection and tolerance thresholds are measured with a digital pressure algometer (Wagner Instruments FDX-25 algometer, USA) using a probe with 1 cm^2 surface to the targeted muscle. The pressure is increased from 0 at a rate of 30 to 50 kPa/s to a maximum pressure of 1000 kPa. Pain detection threshold is defined as the point at which the pressure sensation turns to pain and is intolerable ($\geq$8/10). If the patient does not stop the test before reaching 1000 kPa, this value is considered the threshold.

The reliability for testing PPTs has been reported by Jorgensen et al.[67] as good to excellent for all variables with intraclass correlation coefficient (ICC) values of 0.86 for anterior tibialis, 0.89 for C3C4, and 0.83 for infraspinatus muscle sites. Another study that tested 60 health subjects and 40 subjects with neck pain reported intrarater reliability was almost perfect (ICC = 0.94–0.97), interrater reliability was substantial (ICC = 0.79–0.90), and test-retest reliability was substantial (ICC = 0.76–0.79).[68] The mean value for PPT at the upper trapezius muscle for healthy subjects ($n = 60$) was 251.8 kPa (2.57 kgf), with a standard deviation of 102.3 kPa and a 95% confidence interval (CI) of 225.5 to 278.0 kPa.[68] Jorgensen[67] also found significant correlations between PPT and neck pain disability measures, the authors concluded that this test has satisfactory psychometric properties to be recommended for clinical use.[67]

CSS have been described as having higher levels in blood and urine cytokines and neurotrophines causing low-grade inflammation of glia cells.[66] In patients with fibromyalgia, reports of higher serum levels of tumor necrosis factor-α and proinflammatory interleukins (IL-1, IL-6, IL-8) and a reduction of antiinflammatory ILs (IL-4, IL-10) have been observed.[66] In chronic musculoskeletal pain and overactive bladder, serum or urine levels of neurotrophins such as nerve growth factor and brain-derived neurotrophic factor have been found increased.[66] Functional MRI have also shown changes in brain morphology (global and regional gray matter volumes) and changes in density and signaling in patients with CSSs.[66] Because physical therapists do not typically have access to laboratory or imaging studies, use of a validated questionnaire to screen for CS will be more clinically useful.

The CSI is a screening questionnaire instrument for clinicians to help identify patients with a CSS (Fig. 2.4). Part A has 25 items scored from 0 to 4. Total scores range from 0 to 100.

BOX 2.5   Pressure Pain Threshold

a. Pressure pain threshold (PPT) at the upper trapezius and supraspinatus muscle in sitting

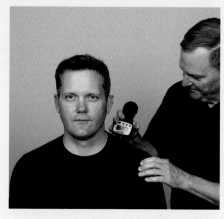

b. PPT at the anterior tibialis muscle belly in supine

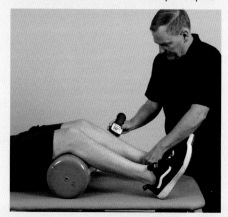

c. PPT at the right C4 articular pillar in prone

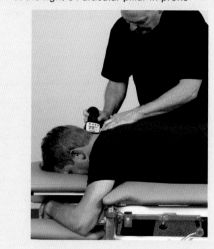

Part B (which is not scored) asks if one has previously been diagnosed with one or more specific disorders, including seven separate CSSs and three CSS-related disorders (www.pridedallas.com/questionnaire). The CSI has now been translated, and psychometrically validated, in a number of different languages that can be found at www.pridedallas.com/questionnaires. If a patient indicates on the medical screening form (Fig. 2.3) that they have been

CENTRAL SENSITIZATION INVENTORY: PART A

Name: _____ Date: _____

Please circle the best response to the right of each statement.

1. I feel tired and unrefreshed when I wake from sleeping.
   Never   Rarely   Sometimes   Often   Always

2. My muscles feel stiff and achy.
   Never   Rarely   Sometimes   Often   Always

3. I have anxiety attacks.
   Never   Rarely   Sometimes   Often   Always

4. I grind or clench my teeth.
   Never   Rarely   Sometimes   Often   Always

5. I have problems with diarrhea and/or constipation.
   Never   Rarely   Sometimes   Often   Always

6. I need help in performing my daily activities.
   Never   Rarely   Sometimes   Often   Always

7. I am sensitive to bright lights.
   Never   Rarely   Sometimes   Often   Always

8. I get tired very easily when I am physically active.
   Never   Rarely   Sometimes   Often   Always

9. I feel pain all over my body.
   Never   Rarely   Sometimes   Often   Always

10. I have headaches.
    Never   Rarely   Sometimes   Often   Always

11. I feel discomfort in my bladder and/or burning when I urinate.
    Never   Rarely   Sometimes   Often   Always

12. I do not sleep well.
    Never   Rarely   Sometimes   Often   Always

13. I have difficulty concentrating.
    Never   Rarely   Sometimes   Often   Always

14. I have skin problems such as dryness, itchiness, or rashes.
    Never   Rarely   Sometimes   Often   Always

15. Stress makes my physical symptoms get worse.
    Never   Rarely   Sometimes   Often   Always

16. I feel sad or depressed.
    Never   Rarely   Sometimes   Often   Always

17. I have low energy.
    Never   Rarely   Sometimes   Often   Always

18. I have muscle tension in my neck and shoulders.
    Never   Rarely   Sometimes   Often   Always

19. I have pain in my jaw.
    Never   Rarely   Sometimes   Often   Always

20. Certain smells, such as perfumes, make me feel dizzy and nauseated.
    Never   Rarely   Sometimes   Often   Always

21. I have to urinate frequently.
    Never   Rarely   Sometimes   Often   Always

22. My legs feel uncomfortable and restless when I am trying to go to sleep at night.
    Never   Rarely   Sometimes   Often   Always

23. I have difficulty remembering things.
    Never   Rarely   Sometimes   Often   Always

24. I suffered trauma as a child.
    Never   Rarely   Sometimes   Often   Always

25. I have pain in my pelvic area.
    Never   Rarely   Sometimes   Often   Always

Total=_____

FIG. 2.7 Central Sensitization Inventory

BOX 2.6	Jenkins Sleep Questionnaire

HOW OFTEN IN THE PAST MONTH DID YOU:	(0) NOT AT ALL	(1) 1–3 DAYS	(2) 4–7 DAYS	(3) 8–14 DAYS	(4) 15–21 DAYS	(5) 22–31 DAYS
1. Have trouble falling asleep?						
2. Wake up several times per night?						
3. Have trouble staying asleep? (including waking up too early)						
4. Wake up after your usual amount of sleep feeling tired and worn out?						

TABLE 2.2	Pressure Pain Threshold Mean Values for Subjects With and Without Neck Pain		
PRESSURE PAIN THRESHOLD (PPT)	MEAN PPT FOR HEALTHY CONTROL SUBJECTS ($n = 60$)	MEAN PPT FOR SUBJECTS WITH NECK PAIN ($n = 40$)	MINIMUM DETECTABLE CHANGE FOR SUBJECTS WITH NECK PAIN
Upper trapezius	251.8 kPa (2.57 kgf)	238.9 kPa (2.44 kgf)	121.9 kPa (1.19 kgf)
Anterior tibialis	334.1 kPa (3.41 kgf)	401.7 kPa (4.10 kgf)	132.0 kPa (1.29 kgf)

(Modified from Walton DM, Macdermid JC, Nielson W, et al. Reliability, standard error, and minimal detectable change of clinical pressure pain threshold testing in people with and without acute neck pain. *J Orthop Sports Phys Ther.* 2011;41(9):644-650.)

TABLE 2.3	Pressure Pain Thresholds Reference Values for Hyposensitivity and Hypersensitivity						
PRESSURE PAIN THRESHOLDS (kPa)	AGE	FEMALE MEAN (SD)	REFERENCE VALUES FOR HYPERSENSITIVITY (p^5, p^{10}, p^{25})	REFERENCE VALUES FOR HYPOSENSITIVITY (p^{75}, p^{90}, p^{95})	MALE MEAN	REFERENCE VALUES FOR HYPERSENSITIVITY (p^5, p^{10}, p^{25})	REFERENCE VALUES FOR HYPOSENSITIVITY (p^{75}, p^{90}, p^{95})
Detection suprascapular	20-49	212(74)	(118, 123, 153)	(258, 309, 360)	313(94)	(150, 168, 243)	(395, 428, 451)
	50-80	314(80)	(199, 210, 250)	(379, 417, 451)	355(105)	(223, 246, 279)	(415, 474, 544)
Tolerance Suprascapular	20-49	684(107)	(556, 573, 607)	(752, 857, 917)	777(102)	(606, 632, 700)	(869, 891, 927)
	50-80	832(83)	(688, 713, 785)	(885, 930, 974)	851(78)	(736, 763, 798)	(904, 966, 1000)

p^5, 5th percentile (0.05 quantile); p^{10}, 10th percentile (0.10 quantile); p^{25}, 25th percentile (0.25 quantile); p^{75}, 75th percentile (0.75 quantile); p^{90}, 90th percentile (0.90 quantile); p^{95}, 95th percentile (0.95 quantile). Data is based on testing 300 pain-free volunteers. Hypersensitivity values below the 25th percentile may be indicative of central sensitization. Hyposensitivity values above the 75th percentile may categorize patients as pain hyposensitive.
(From Neziri AY, Scaramozzino P, Andersen OK, et al. Reference values of mechanical and thermal pain tests in a pain-free population. *Eur J Pain* 2010;15(4):376-383.)

previously diagnosed with one of the conditions commonly associated with CSS, which are marked with an asterisks (*) on the medical screening form, the CSI should be administered.

The CSI has high reliability and validity (test-retest reliability = .82; Cronbach's alpha = .88).[65] In a follow-up study, 121 patients who were referred to a multidisciplinary pain center found that a large percentage of patients ($n = 89$, 74%) met clinical criteria for one or more CSSs, and CSI scores were positively correlated with the number of diagnosed CSSs.[69] A CSI score of 40 out of 100 best distinguished between the CSS patient group and a nonpatient comparison sample ($n = 129$) (area under the curve = .86, sensitivity = 81%, specificity = 75%).[69] The following severity ranges have been recommended: Subclinical = 0 to 29; Mild = 30 to 39; Moderate = 40 to 49; Severe = 50 to 59; and Extreme = 60 to 100.[69] Higher total CSI scores have been reported to be associated with higher pain intensity and wider pain distribution. Associations have also been reported between CSI scores and biologic markers of CS, including brain gamma amino butyric acid levels and brain-derived neurotrophic factor.[70]

Cuesta-Vargas et al.[70] pooled CSI data from studies conducted in seven countries with 2093 subjects and determined that the internal consistency was excellent for the CSI total score (Cronbach alpha = 0.92). Another systematic review of 14 CSI studies determined to have good to excellent quality of evidence concluded that the CSI generates reliable and valid data to quantify the severity of CS related symptoms.[71]

If a patient indicates that they get less than the recommended 7 to 8 hours of sleep per night, have moderate or severe difficulty with sleep, or can only sleep with medication, a sleep questionnaire, such as the Jenkins Sleep Questionnaire, should be administered to further quantify the nature and degree of sleep impairment (Box 2.6).[72] The Jenkins Sleep Questionnaire includes four questions on quality of sleep that are rated 0 to 5 based on the number of days out of the past 30 the individual has experienced sleep difficulty, and it has been determined to be a reliable and valid method (internal reliability 0.79) of quantifying sleep impairments.[72] A score of 12 or more out of a possible 20 is considered significant for diagnosis of sleep impairment because this indicates difficulty with at least three aspects of sleep for 15 or more days of the month.[72,73] Selection of 15 or more nights in 1 month as the cut-off point for diagnosing a sleep disturbance on any one of the four items has also been used to diagnose sleep disorders in sleep studies. This is based on criteria from the Diagnostic and Statistical Manual of Mental Disorder, Fourth Edition (DSM-IV-TR),[52] which stipulates to diagnose a sleep disorder that difficulty maintaining/initiating sleep or nonrestorative sleep should be present for three or more nights per week for at least 1 month.[74–77] Chronic insomnia has been defined as difficulty falling asleep, maintaining sleep, or waking up too early at least three nights/week for the past 3 months.[78]

Sleep disturbances are very common in individuals with depression and anxiety.[79,80] About 75% of people with depression experience symptoms of insomnia, and insomnia in nondepressed patients is a risk factor for later development of depression.[79] A large survey study from a community sample across the adult age span showed that those with insomnia had greater depression and anxiety levels than people not having insomnia and were 9.82 and 17.35 times as likely to have clinically significant depression and anxiety.[80]

Difficulty falling asleep has been correlated with signs of anxiety, and difficulty staying asleep has been correlated with depression.[72,80] Awaking tired and fatigued is a sign of poor sleep quality. Symptoms of insomnia among older adults are also associated with decrease in health-related quality of life.[81] Sleep contributes to modulation of pain and addressing sleep disturbances may impact pain perception severity.[82,83] Sleep impairments are common with patients with chronic pain, fibromyalgia, and/or CS, and sleep hygiene education should be addressed in the comprehensive care of these patients (see Box 4.18).[84] Anxiety and depression can be screened with the Four-Item Patient Health Questionnaire for Anxiety and Depression as described in Chapter 7 (see Table 7.4), and this questionnaire should be administered with the Jenkins Sleep Questionnaire in patients with chronic pain, CS, or difficulty sleeping.

The mODI (Fig. 2.8) is a region-specific disability scale for patients with LBP. The modified scale substitutes the Employment/Homemaking category for the Sex Life category in the original scale.[85,86] The mODI has been used in numerous LBP studies. The questionnaire consists of 10 items that address different aspects of function and disability, each scored from 0 to 5, with higher values representing greater disability. The total score is obtained with a sum of the responses, which are then expressed as a percentage (range, 0%–100%). For example, 25/50 = 50%. If all items are answered, the point total can be doubled to obtain the percentage score (i.e., 25 × 2 = 50%).

The purpose of the mODI is assessment of change of perceived disability over time, and the reliability over a 4-week period has been reported as quite good (ICC = 0.90; 95% CI = 0.78–0.96).[59] Validity and responsiveness are good for construct and content.[59,87] The minimal clinically important

difference (MCID) is 6 percentage points (sensitivity = 0.91; specificity = 0.83) and is defined as the amount of change that best distinguishes between patients who have improved conditions and those whose conditions remain stable.[59] The minimal detectable change (MDC) for the mODI has been reported as 10.5 percentage points, which would be the amount of change that should be seen in an individual patient to be 90% confident that real change has occurred.[88] The mODI is easy to administer and easy to score. The mODI was developed primarily for patients with acute LBP, and the properties may differ for patients with chronic LBP.

The NDI (Fig. 2.9) is a condition-specific questionnaire that has been shown to be reliable and valid with patients with neck pain.[89] This scale has been used in numerous neck pain studies and is structured and scored similarly to the mODI. The questionnaire consists of 10 items that address different aspects of function and disability, each scored from 0 to 5, with higher values representing greater disability. The total score is obtained with a sum of the responses, which are then expressed as a percentage (range, 0%–100%). For example, 25/50 = 50%. If all items are answered, the point total can be doubled to obtain the percentage score (i.e., 25 × 2 = 50%).

The NDI has also been tested for reliability and responsiveness for patients with cervical radiculopathy.[64] Cleland et al.[64] reported test-retest reliability as moderate, with an ICC of 0.68 and a 95% CI of 0.30 to 0.90. The MDC for the NDI is 10.2 percentage points, and the MCID for the NDI was 7.0 percentage points. Sterling et al.[49] used data from whiplash clinical studies to define patients who had recovered as having NDI scores of less than 8%, those with mild disability as having scores of 10% to 28%, and those with moderate to severe disability as having scores of greater than 30%. A systematic review of the NDI suggested use of an MDC of 10% and concluded that the NDI has acceptable reliability for use with patients with neck pain and cervical radiculopathy.[90]

Cleland et al.[91] found that a PSFS exhibited superior reliability, construct validity, and responsiveness in a cohort of patients with cervical radiculopathy compared with the NDI. The PSFS has also been found to be the most responsive measurement of disability in patients with chronic whiplash compared with four other disability measures.[92]

The PSFS is a patient-specific outcome measure for investigation of functional status with the patient asked to nominate activities (up to three) that are difficult to perform because of their condition and then to rate the level of limitation for each activity on a 0- to 10-point scale with 0 representing unable to perform and 10 representing able to perform at same level as before (Fig. 2.3). The ratings are averaged for the three activities. The PSFS has been shown to be valid and responsive to change for patients with several different clinical conditions, including neck pain, cervical radiculopathy, knee pain, upper extremity musculoskeletal problems, and LBP.[93–97] For patients with cervical radiculopathy, the test-retest reliability was high for the PSFS with an ICC of 0.82 and a 95% CI of 0.54 to 0.93.[64] The MDC for the PSFS was 2.1, and the MCID was 2 on a 0 to 10 scale.[64] The PSFS can be used for patients with

Section 1: To be completed by patient

Name: _____ Age: _____ Date: _____

Occupation: _____ Number of days of back pain: _____ (this episode)

Section 2: To be completed by patient

This questionnaire has been designed to give your therapist information as to how your back pain has affected your ability to manage in everyday life. Please answer every question by placing a mark on the line that best describes your condition today. We realize you may feel that two of the statements may describe your condition, but **please mark only the line that most closely describes your current condition.**

Pain intensity
_____ The pain is mild and comes and goes.
_____ The pain is mild and does not vary much.
_____ The pain is moderate and comes and goes.
_____ The pain is moderate and does not vary much.
_____ The pain is severe and comes and goes.
_____ The pain is severe and does not vary much.

Personal care (washing, dressing, etc.)
_____ I do not have to change the way I wash and dress myself to avoid pain.
_____ I do not normally change the way I wash or dress myself even though doing these tasks causes some pain.
_____ Washing and dressing increase my pain, but I can do these tasks without changing how I do them.
_____ Washing and dressing increase my pain, and I find it necessary to change the way I do these tasks.
_____ Because of my pain I am partially unable to wash and dress without help.
_____ Because of my pain I am completely unable to wash or dress without help.

Lifting
_____ I can lift heavy weights without increased pain.
_____ I can lift heavy weights but doing so causes increased pain.
_____ Pain prevents me from lifting heavy weights off of the floor, but I can manage if they are conveniently positioned (e.g., on a table, etc.).
_____ Pain prevents me from lifting heavy weights off of the floor, but I can manage light to medium weights if they are conveniently positioned.
_____ I can lift only very light weights.
_____ I cannot lift or carry anything at all.

Walking
_____ I have no pain when walking.
_____ I have pain when walking, but I can still walk my required normal distances.
_____ Pain prevents me from walking long distances.
_____ Pain prevents me from walking intermediate distances.
_____ Pain prevents me from walking even short distances.
_____ Pain prevents me from walking at all.

Sitting
_____ Sitting does not cause me any pain.
_____ I can sit as long as I like provided that I have my choice of seating surfaces.
_____ Pain prevents me from sitting for more than 1 hour.
_____ Pain prevents me from sitting for more than a half hour.
_____ Pain prevents me from sitting for more than 10 minutes.
_____ Pain prevents me from sitting at all.

Standing
_____ I can stand as long as I want without increased pain.
_____ I can stand as long as I want, but my pain increases with time.
_____ Pain prevents me from standing for more than 1 hour.
_____ Pain prevents me from standing for more than a half hour.
_____ Pain prevents me from standing for more than 10 minutes.
_____ I avoid standing because it increases my pain right away.

Sleeping
_____ I get no pain when I am in bed.
_____ I get pain in bed, but it does not prevent me from sleeping well.
_____ Because of my pain, my sleep is only 3/4 of my normal amount.
_____ Because of my pain, my sleep is only 1/2 of my normal amount.
_____ Because of my pain, my sleep is only 1/4 of my normal amount.
_____ Pain prevents me from sleeping at all.

Social life
_____ My social life is normal and does not increase my pain.
_____ My social life is normal, but it increases my level of pain.
_____ Pain prevents me from participating in more energetic activities (e.g., sports, dancing, etc.).
_____ Pain prevents me from going out very often.
_____ Pain has restricted my social life to my home.
_____ I have hardly any social life because of my pain.

Traveling
_____ I get no increased pain when traveling.
_____ I get some pain while traveling, but none of my usual forms of travel make the pain any worse.
_____ I get increased pain while traveling, but the pain does not cause me to seek alternative forms of travel.
_____ I get increased pain while traveling, and the pain causes me to seek alternative forms of travel.
_____ My pain restricts all forms of travel except that which is done while I am lying down.
_____ My pain restricts all forms of travel.

Employment/homemaking
_____ My normal job/homemaking activities do not cause pain.
_____ My normal job/homemaking activities increase my pain, but I can still perform all that is required of me.
_____ I can perform most of my job/homemaking duties, but pain prevents me from performing more physically stressful activities (e.g., lifting, vacuuming).
_____ Pain prevents me from doing anything but light duties.
_____ Pain prevents me from doing even light duties.
_____ Pain prevents me from performing any job or homemaking chores.

Section 3: To be completed by physical therapist/provider

Score: _____ or _____ % (SEM 11, MDC 16) Initial FU ___ weeks   discharge

Number of treatment sessions: _____ Gender: _____Male _____Female

Diagnosis _____

Adapted from Hudson-Cook N, Tomes-Nicholson K, Breen A: A revised Oswestry disability questionnaire. In Roland M, Jenner J, editors: *Back pain: new approaches to rehabilitation and education,* New York, 1989, Manchester University Press. [Prepared May 1999]

FIG. 2.8 The Modified Oswestry Disability Index (mODI).

Name: _____

Date: _____

This questionnaire has been designed to give your therapist information as to how your neck pain has affected you in your everyday life activities. Please answer each section, marking only ONE box that best describes your status today.

Section 1 — Pain Intensity
☐ I have no pain at the moment.
☐ The pain is very mild at the moment.
☐ The pain is moderate at the moment.
☐ The pain is fairly severe at the moment.
☐ The pain is very severe at the moment.
☐ The pain is the worst imaginable at the moment.

Section 2 — Personal Care (washing, dressing, etc.)
☐ I can look after myself normally without causing extra pain.
☐ I can look after myself normally but doing so causes me extra pain.
☐ It is painful to look after myself, and I am slow and careful.
☐ I need help every day in most aspects of self-care.
☐ I do not get dressed, wash with difficulty, and stay in bed.

Section 3 — Lifting
☐ I can lift heavy weights without extra pain.
☐ I can lift heavy weights but doing so gives extra pain.
☐ Pain prevents me from lifting heavy weights off the floor, but I can manage light to medium weights if they are conveniently positioned.
☐ I can lift only very light weights.
☐ I cannot lift or carry anything at all.

Section 4 — Reading
☐ I can read as much as I want, with no pain in my neck.
☐ I can read as much as I want, with slight pain in my neck.
☐ I can read as much as I want, with moderate pain in my neck.
☐ I cannot read as much as I want because of moderate pain in my neck.
☐ I can hardly read at all because of severe pain in my neck.
☐ I cannot read at all.

Section 5 — Headache
☐ I have no headache at all.
☐ I have slight headaches, which come infrequently.
☐ I have moderate headaches, which come infrequently.
☐ I have moderate headaches, which come frequently.
☐ I have severe headaches, which come frequently.
☐ I have headaches almost all the time.

Section 6 — Concentration
☐ I can concentrate fully when I want, with no difficulty.
☐ I can concentrate fully when I want, with slight difficulty.
☐ I have a fair degree of difficulty in concentrating when I want to.
☐ I have a lot of difficulty in concentrating when I want to.
☐ I have a great deal of difficulty in concentrating when I want to.
☐ I cannot concentrate at all.

Section 7 — Work
☐ I can do as much as I want.
☐ I can only do my usual work but no more.
☐ I can do most of my usual work but no more.
☐ I cannot do my usual work.
☐ I can hardly do any work at all.
☐ I cannot do any work at all.

Section 8 — Driving
☐ I can drive my car without any neck pain.
☐ I can drive my car as long as I want, with slight pain in my neck.
☐ I can drive my car as long as I want, with moderate pain in my neck.
☐ I cannot drive my car as long as I want because of moderate pain in my neck.
☐ I can hardly drive at all because of severe pain in my neck.
☐ I cannot drive my car at all.

Section 9 — Sleeping
☐ I have no trouble sleeping.
☐ My sleep is slightly disturbed (less than 1 hour sleep loss).
☐ My sleep is mildly disturbed (1-2 hours sleep loss).
☐ My sleep is moderately disturbed (2-3 hours sleep loss).
☐ My sleep is greatly disturbed (3-5 hours sleep loss).
☐ My sleep is completely disturbed (5-7 hours sleep loss).

Section 10 — Recreation
☐ I am able to engage in all my recreational activities, with no neck pain at all.
☐ I am able to engage in all my recreational activities, with some pain in my neck.
☐ I am able to engage in most but not all of my usual recreational activities because of pain in my neck.
☐ I am able to engage in a few of my usual recreational activities because of pain in my neck.
☐ I can hardly do any recreational activities because of pain in my neck.
☐ I cannot do any recreational activities at all.

FIG. 2.9 The Neck Disability Index (NDI).

many different conditions, whereas the mODI is intended to be used with patients with lumbar conditions and the NDI is designed for patients with cervical spine and cervical radiculopathy conditions.

A pain drawing on a body chart is a helpful clinical assessment tool. The patient is advised to complete a body chart as part of a medical screening form (Fig. 2.3), and the therapist should also complete one as part of the initial interview. Patients may draw symptoms in anatomic areas on the body diagram that were not included in the initial medical diagnosis; these symptoms need to be further explored by the therapist to determine whether the symptoms are from a visceral or somatic structure and to determine whether the multiple pain complaints are linked to the same underlying condition or are separate. In addition, patients may express extreme emotional reactions with their pain symptoms by drawing in pain markings across the entire body or by circling the entire body. In these cases, other questionnaires, such as the FABQ, should be completed by the patient to further quantify the psychosocial components of the patient's symptoms, and a multidisciplinary approach that includes both active exercise physical therapy and psychologic counseling may be necessary for patient rehabilitation.

The 11-point NPRS is a measure of pain in which patients rate pain ranging from 0 (no pain) to 10 (worst imaginable pain); this scale has been shown to have concurrent and predictive validity as a measure of pain intensity (Fig. 2.3).[98–100] In clinical situations, it is informative to have the patient consider a 48-hour time frame and rate their pain on three NPR scales based on consideration of the worst, best, and current level of pain. Responsiveness refers to the ability of a measure to detect change accurately when it has occurred.[101] The NPRS shows adequate responsiveness for use in both a clinical and a research setting. A two-point change on the NPRS represents a clinically meaningful change in a patient's perceived level of pain that exceeds the bounds of measurement error.[101]

Patient Interview and History

The purpose of the initial patient interview is to develop a rapport with the patient, establish a chronology of events, screen for red flags, establish whether physical therapy is appropriate for the patient, develop hypotheses regarding the cause of the patient's symptoms, and begin to narrow down the appropriate impairment classification or diagnosis for the patient. Expert physical therapist clinicians spend a greater amount of time on the interview portion of the examination than novice clinicians. In fact, experts tend to split their time equally between the subjective examination and the physical examination, which is in contrast to novices who tend to spend more than twice as much time on the physical examination as they spend on the patient interview and history.[102] The experts tend to generate the majority of their hypotheses during the subjective examination and tend to have a clearer idea of the patient's problems before starting the physical examination compared with novices.[102] These are skills that can best be developed

through clinical mentoring in clinical internship, residency, and fellowship experiences.

In the beginning of the interview, open-ended questions should be asked, such as the following:
- "When did you first notice this problem?"
- "Where did the pain start?"
- "Explain how this problem started."

Next, the location and character of the symptoms should be determined. The therapist should use a body chart to mark interpretation of the pain location, to indicate the focal point of the pain, and to mark where the pain tends to spread. Notes can be made on the body chart regarding the nature of the symptoms, such as sharp pain, burning, numbness, or tingling.

Next, the symptom behavior is determined. The therapist should ask questions such as, "What makes your pain worse?" and "What makes your pain better?" The symptoms associated with common musculoskeletal conditions typically are intensified with certain positions or activities and are relieved with other positions and activities. If the patient is unable to identify positions or activities that affect the intensity and nature of the symptoms, either a strong psychosocial component exists with the pain symptoms or an underlying visceral condition may be causing the symptoms. On occasion, however, the patient is simply a poor historian. These questions also assist with medical screening. For instance, if the patient has throbbing midthoracic pain that intensifies in frequency and intensity with exertion (such as shoveling snow or climbing stairs), a cardiovascular condition (such as an aortic aneurysm) may be suspected and should be further evaluated by a physician.

In response to these open-ended questions, more specific follow-up questions should be asked to further outline the symptom behavior as possible diagnostic hypotheses are considered. For instance, with lumbar spinal stenosis, lower extremity symptoms are commonly provoked with standing and walking and relieved with sitting. In contrast, lumbar radicular symptoms caused by a lumbar herniated disc are commonly provoked with standing and sitting. Specific follow-up questioning to make this distinction can assist in development of the diagnosis.

Another important question is, "How does your pain vary through the course of the day and night?" Most musculoskeletal conditions can be relieved with rest and the use of recumbent positions. If the pain wakes the patient at night, the therapist should inquire whether the patient can quickly return to sleep by changing positions or whether the pain is unremitting regardless of position. The latter answer is a red flag and warrants further medical investigation in most circumstances, because malignant diseases can cause intense unremitting night pain. Generally speaking, most musculoskeletal-related pain should improve with rest. However, the patient may feel stiff in the morning, and with activity, a reduction in stiffness is commonly reported. Severe multiple-joint morning stiffness is common with rheumatoid arthritis. If the back pain intensifies before mealtime and is relieved after eating, a gastric ulcer may be suspected; or if shoulder girdle or thoracic pain is intensified after a heavy meal, a gallbladder problem may be evident.

Determination of functional limitations and establishment of functional goals can assist with documentation and with measurement of progress. Development of a gauge of the level of normal functional activity and how these activities are limited by the current condition can assist in development of the treatment plan, especially regarding duration of treatment. For instance, if the patient wants to return to heavy work or vigorous exercise and currently is very inactive because of a spinal condition, the duration of treatment might be longer than that of a patient who has lesser physical goals.

Inquiries about past treatments for the current condition may assist in development of a treatment plan as well. For instance, if a patient with LBP has received extensive chiropractic "adjustments" for back pain symptoms with minimal benefit, a stabilization exercise program may be indicated, especially if signs and symptoms of instability (i.e., movement coordination impairments) are noted.

A neurologic screen can also start with the initial interview, with asking the patient about tingling, numbness, or loss of skin sensation. If peripheral symptoms are present, a full neurologic examination is warranted, including deep tendon reflexes, sensation, and myotomal strength testing (Boxes 2.11, 2.12, and 2.13). In addition, saddle paresthesia or numbness is an indication of a central spinal lesion caused by neurologic involvement of the S4 nerve. Presence of this symptom is a red flag and warrants further diagnostic testing, such as MRI for assessment of the integrity of the cauda equina. Follow-up questions regarding bladder function are also indicated with the presence of saddle paresthesia or numbness. Isolation of the specific nerve root that is affected cannot be reliably determined by the location of a patient's reports of peripheral pain or paresthesia. Even in patients with proven nerve root compression caused by a prolapsed intervertebral disc in the lumbar spine, more than 50% of the patient's peripheral symptoms will fall outside the corresponding dermatome in more than 85% of the patients.[103] The dermatomes map out areas of sensation that correspond with spinal level nerve roots. Dermatomes are not intended for interpretation of pain patterns. The function of the nerve roots is best determined by interpretation of a cluster of neurologic screening findings, including sensation, deep tendon reflexes, and myotomal strength testing. Diagnostic testing, such as electromyogram (EMG) and MRI, can further clarify spinal nerve root involvement and function.

Inquiry about history of similar conditions can provide insight into the underlying diagnosis. For instance, instability and discogenic conditions tend to recur with intermittent flare-ups reported over many years. Simple muscle and joint sprains and strains are more likely to be a result of a first-time episode of acute back pain.

Medical history can be explored by asking the patient an open-ended question such as, "Other than this problem, how is your overall health?" In addition, the medical intake form should be reviewed with the patient, and follow-up questions should be asked for each condition and medication listed to gain further insight into the patient's health status and to screen each system.

Therapists should also inquire what are the patient's expectations for physical therapy, because patient satisfaction and outcomes are increasingly being linked to the level in which the physical therapist meets the patient's expectations.[104,105] Lastly, the patient should be asked to establish functional therapy goals and asked one last open-ended question, such as, "Is there anything else you would like to tell me before I begin the examination?" These questions give the patient another opportunity to provide pertinent medical history that may have been previously missed.

TESTS AND MEASURES
Postural Inspection

Visual inspection of the patient from anterior, posterior, oblique, and lateral views can assist the therapist in determination of postural deviations that may contribute to spinal impairments (Box 2.7). The anterior and posterior views can provide clues of asymmetries in leg length or pelvic height or scoliosis (Fig. 2.10A,B,C). The lateral view shows alterations in anterior to posterior curves and head, shoulder, and pelvic positions (Fig. 2.10D). Kendall's plumb line assessment of posture can be used as a reference standard against which to describe deviations from ideal posture.[106] The oblique views are also important for further analysis of spinal contour (Fig. 2.10E,F). Areas of excessive muscle tone and guarding may also be noted as signs of underlying instability or tissue irritation. Visual assessment should precede structural examination and palpation.

Structural Examination

Structural examination is an extension of the visual inspection but involves palpation of bony landmarks for assessment of alteration in symmetry or positioning of the bony structures of the spine and pelvis. Structural examination findings have greater significance in the diagnostic process if the findings can be correlated with other positive examination findings, such as limitations in active and passive motion and positive pain provocation testing.

BOX 2.7 | Postural Inspection

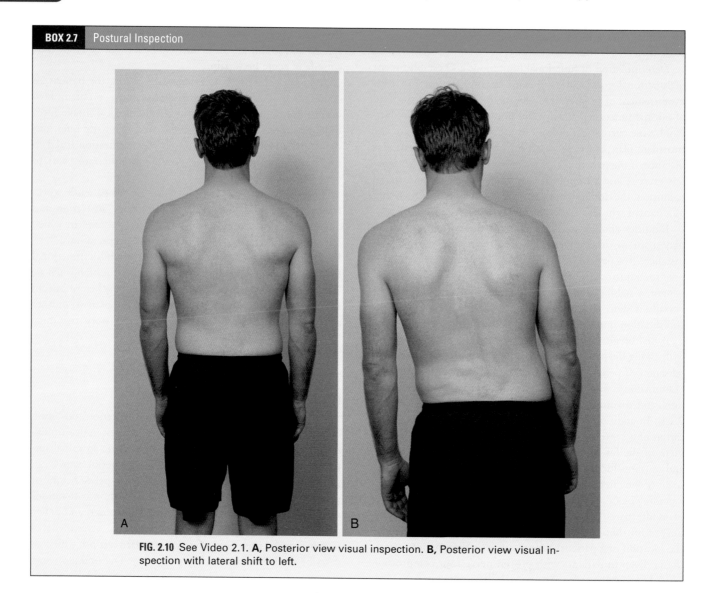

FIG. 2.10 See Video 2.1. **A,** Posterior view visual inspection. **B,** Posterior view visual inspection with lateral shift to left.

BOX 2.7 Postural Inspection—cont'd

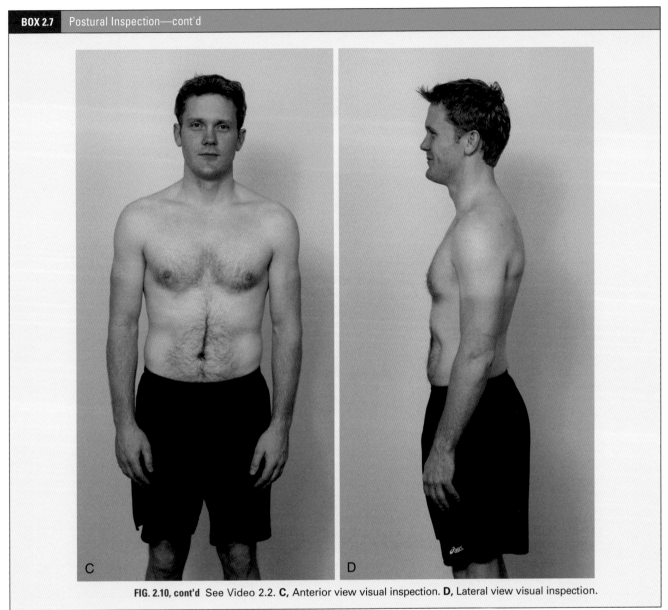

FIG. 2.10, cont'd See Video 2.2. **C,** Anterior view visual inspection. **D,** Lateral view visual inspection.

Continued

BOX 2.7   Postural Inspection—cont'd

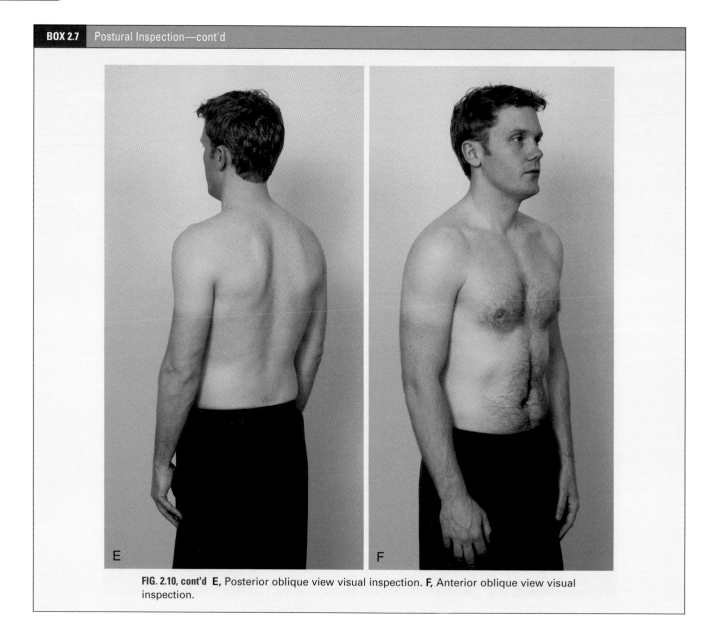

FIG. 2.10, cont'd E, Posterior oblique view visual inspection. **F,** Anterior oblique view visual inspection.

BOX 2.7   Postural Inspection—cont'd

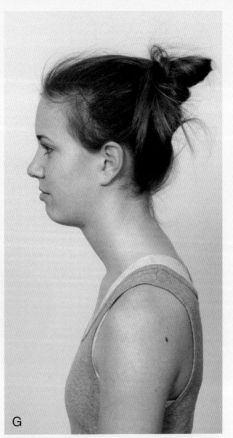

G

FIG. 2.10, cont'd See Video 2.3. **G,** Lateral view postural assessment: forward head posture. Visualize plum line standard that ideally runs vertically through the lobe of the ear and middle lateral portion of acromion process of the shoulder. This subject has a moderate level of forward head posture positioning.

▶ Palpation of Level of Mastoid Processes

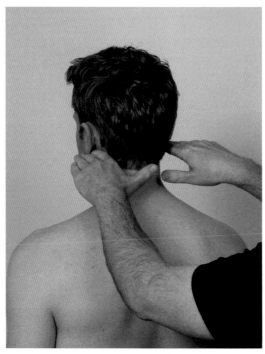

FIG. 2.11 See Video 2.4. Level of mastoid processes.

PATIENT POSITION	The patient stands facing away from the therapist.
THERAPIST POSITION	The therapist stands directly behind the patient with eyes level with the patient's occiput.
PROCEDURE	With palms kept parallel to floor and fingers firmly together, the therapist uses the index fingers to palpate the mastoid processes.
NOTES	The therapist should observe for symmetry in the position of the mastoid processes to assess for a sidebent position of the head that could indicate the presence of a possible craniovertebral dysfunction.

▶ Palpation of Level of Shoulder Girdles and Scapulae

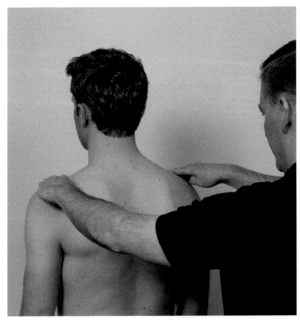

FIG. 2.12 See Video 2.5. Level of shoulder girdles.

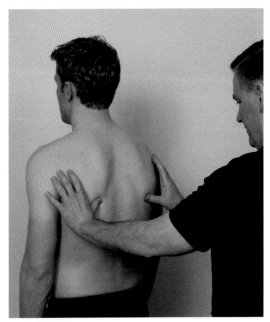

FIG. 2.13 See Video 2.6. Level of scapulae.

PATIENT POSITION	The patient stands facing away from the therapist.
THERAPIST POSITION	The therapist stands directly behind the patient with eyes level with the patient's shoulders.
PROCEDURE	With palms kept parallel to floor and fingers firmly together, the therapist uses the pads of digits 2 to 5 to palpate the superior aspect of the shoulder girdle. Next, the thumbs are used to palpate the inferior angle of each scapula.
NOTES	The therapist should observe for asymmetry in the position of the shoulder girdles and scapulae that may be a sign of underlying thoracic spine scoliosis or muscle imbalances of the shoulder girdle, such as shortened upper trapezius or levator scapulae muscles and weak lower trapezius or serratus anterior muscles.

▶ Palpation of Iliac Crest Height in Standing

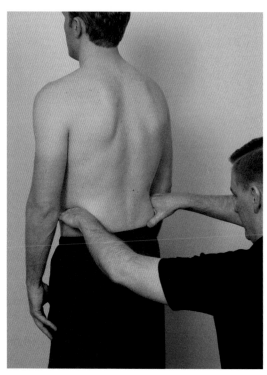

FIG. 2.14 See Video 2.7. Palpation of iliac crest height in standing.

PATIENT POSITION	The patient stands facing away from the therapist.
THERAPIST POSITION	The therapist kneels directly behind the patient with eyes level with the patient's iliac crest.
PROCEDURE	With palms kept parallel to the floor and fingers firmly together, the therapist uses the index fingers to palpate the superior aspect of iliac crests. The therapist should observe for symmetry in heights of iliac crests.
NOTES	Asymmetry may be an indication of either a leg length difference, a sacroiliac displacement, a structural hip malformation (coxa vara, coxa valga), a hip injury (such as a slipped capital epiphysis), or a structural malformation of an innominate bone. Flynn et al.[61] reported interexaminer reliability with a kappa value of 0.23.

▶ Palpation of Posterior Superior Iliac Spines in Standing

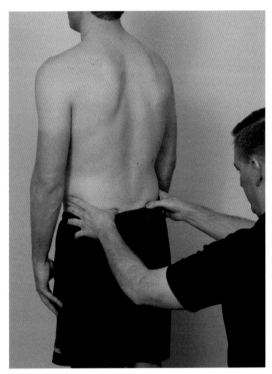

FIG. 2.15 See Video 2.8. Palpation of posterior superior iliac spines in standing.

PATIENT POSITION	The patient stands facing away from the therapist.
THERAPIST POSITION	The therapist kneels directly behind the patient with eyes level with the patient's posterior superior iliac spines (PSIS).
PROCEDURE	The therapist first finds the sacral dimples and moves slightly lateral and inferior to locate the PSIS on each side with each thumb. The thumbs are used to palpate the inferior aspect of the PSIS (palpate "up and under" PSIS). The therapist should observe for symmetry in heights of the PSIS.
NOTES	Asymmetry may be an indication of either a leg length difference, a sacroiliac displacement, a structural hip malformation (coxa vara, coxa valga) or a hip injury (such as a slipped capital epiphysis), or a structural malformation of an innominate bone. Flynn et al.[61] reported an interexaminer reliability of 0.13 in standing and of 0.23 in sitting in tests on 71 patients with LBP referred to physical therapy.

▶ Palpation of Greater Trochanter Height

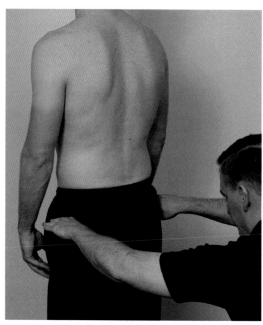

FIG. 2.16 See Video 2.9. Palpation of greater trochanter height.

PATIENT POSITION	The patient stands facing away from the therapist.
THERAPIST POSITION	The therapist kneels directly behind the patient with eyes level with the patient's greater trochanters.
PROCEDURE	With palms kept parallel to the floor, the therapist uses the radial aspect of the index fingers to palpate the inferior edge of the greater trochanters (palpate "up and under" the greater trochanters). The therapist may need to ask the patient to sway side to side to help with accurate location of the greater trochanters. The therapist should observe for symmetry in heights of the greater trochanters.
NOTES	Asymmetry may be an indication of a leg length discrepancy or a structural deviation in the shape of the greater trochanters. A leg length discrepancy of half an inch or greater has been positively correlated with a greater incidence rate of LBP and should be addressed as part of the treatment program.[107] Palpation of the height of the fibular head and assessment of height of the medial arch of each foot can assist with determination of the portion of the lower extremity where the asymmetry originates.

▶ Palpation of Iliac Crest Height in Sitting

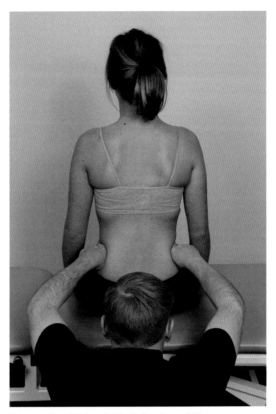

FIG. 2.17 See Video 2.10. Palpation of iliac crest height in sitting.

PATIENT POSITION	The patient sits with legs over the edge of the table and facing away from the therapist.
THERAPIST POSITION	The therapist kneels directly behind the patient with eyes level with the iliac crests.
PROCEDURE	With palms kept parallel to the floor and fingers firmly together, the therapist uses the index fingers to palpate the superior aspect of the iliac crests. The therapist should observe for symmetry in height of the iliac crests.
NOTES	Palpation of the pelvic structures with the patient sitting on a firm level surface can assist with differentiation of the cause of asymmetries noted in the standing structural examination. For example, if the iliac crest height is level in sitting but asymmetry is noted in standing, the cause is likely a lower extremity asymmetry rather than a pelvic dysfunction. However, if the same amount of pelvic height asymmetry is noted both in sitting and in standing, the cause is likely pelvic asymmetry rather than lower extremity structural asymmetry.

▶ Palpation of Posterior Superior Iliac Spines in Sitting

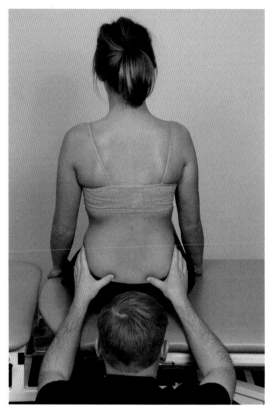

FIG. 2.18 See Video 2.11. Palpation of posterior sacroiliac spines in sitting.

PATIENT POSITION	The patient sits with legs over the edge of the table and facing away from the therapist.
THERAPIST POSITION	The therapist kneels directly behind the patient with eyes level with the PSIS.
PROCEDURE	The therapist first finds the sacral dimples and moves slightly lateral and inferior to locate the PSIS on each side with each thumb. The therapist uses the thumbs to palpate the inferior aspect of the PSIS (palpate "up and under" the PSIS). The therapist should observe for symmetry in heights of the PSIS.
NOTES	Palpation of the pelvic structures with the patient sitting on a firm level surface can assist with differentiation of the cause of symmetries noted in the standing structural examination. For example, if the PSIS height is level in sitting but asymmetry is noted in standing, the cause is likely lower extremity asymmetries rather than a pelvic dysfunction. However, if the same degree of PSIS asymmetry is noted both in sitting and in standing, the cause is likely pelvic asymmetry rather than lower extremity structural asymmetry or leg length difference.
	Documentation of structural examination findings can be quickly noted with marking the observed findings on a body chart diagram (Fig. 2.19). When writing about or describing the findings, consistency with description of the asymmetry by the side that is lower is best. For example: "The structural examination reveals a lowered iliac crest, PSIS, and greater trochanter palpated in the standing position."

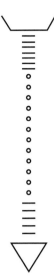

FIG. 2.19 Structural examination documentation: a spine diagram can be used to mark structural examination findings. Slash marks can be used to mark relative positions of bony landmarks, and spinal curvatures can be drawn in.

Active Range of Motion Examination

The purpose of the active range of motion (AROM) examination is to document the amount of motion impairment present at the time of the examination, to identify pain provocation with motion, and to develop a hypothesis on the cause of the pain and limited motion. Signs of spinal instability, such as aberrant motion patterns, may also be noted with AROM examination. Identification of regions of spinal stiffness with the AROM examination can assist in locating and isolating hypomobile spinal segments that respond favorably to spinal manipulation. The AROM findings are correlated with other examination findings to determine the appropriate spinal disorder classification to guide management of the patient's condition.

▶ Cervical Forward-Bending Active Range of Motion

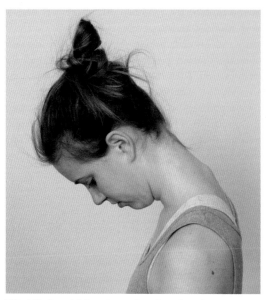

FIG. 2.20 See Video 2.12. Cervical forward-bending active range of motion (AROM).

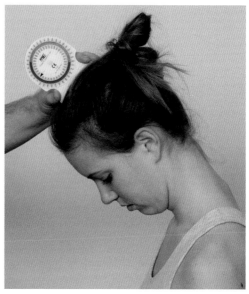

FIG. 2.21 See Video 2.13. Cervical forward-bending measured with inclinometer.

PATIENT POSITION	The patient stands (or sits) with good posture and arms relaxed at the sides.
THERAPIST POSITION	The therapist stands to the side and slightly behind the patient to clearly observe cervical motion.
PROCEDURE	The patient is instructed to slowly nod the head and bend the cervical spine forward. The motion should start in the upper cervical spine and continue down to approximately the level of T3. A straightening or reversal of the cervical lordosis should occur on forward bending. The chin should also be near the sternum. Motion can be measured with an inclinometer placed in a midsagittal position on the top of the head.
NOTES	Whether or not the motion reproduces the patient's symptoms should be noted. If a segmental restriction is caused by a unilateral facet restriction, forward bending may deviate to the ipsilateral side of the restriction. Piva et al.[108] used a gravity inclinometer to measure cervical forward bending on 30 subjects and found a mean of 60 degrees forward bending, with an ICC of 0.78 (0.59:0.89), a standard error of the mean (SEM) of 5.8 degrees, a MDC of 16 degrees, and a kappa value for symptom reproduction of 0.87 (0.81:0.94).

▶ Cervical Backward-Bending Active Range of Motion

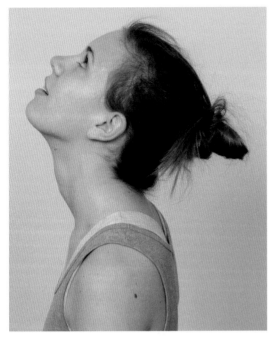

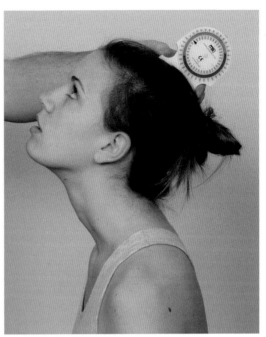

FIG. 2.22 See Video 2.14. Cervical backward-bending active range of motion (AROM).

FIG. 2.23 See Video 2.15. Cervical backward-bending measured with inclinometer.

PATIENT POSITION	The patient stands (or sits) with good posture and arms relaxed at the sides.
THERAPIST POSITION	The therapist stands to the side and slightly behind the patient to clearly observe the cervical motion.
PROCEDURE	Patient is instructed to slowly look up and bend the cervical spine backward as far as he or she can move comfortably. Motion can be measured with an inclinometer placed in a midsagittal position on the top of the head.
NOTES	Whether or not the motion reproduces the patient's symptoms is noted. If a segmental restriction caused by a facet restriction is present, backward bending may deviate to the contralateral side of the restriction. Patients are guarded in case they become dizzy during the backward-bending motion. Reproduction of neck pain may be from facet joint compression/irritation, and a reproduction of referred symptoms into the arm could be from nerve root irritation or from a referral pattern from structures of the cervical spine. Piva et al.[108] used a gravity inclinometer to test reliability on 30 subjects and found a mean of 48 degrees of backward bending, an ICC of 0.86 (0.73:0.93), an SEM of 5.6 degrees, an MDC of 16 degrees, and a kappa value for symptom reproduction of 0.65 (0.54:0.76).

Cervical Sidebending (Lateral Flexion) Active Range of Motion Right and Left

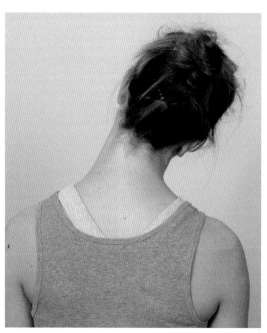

FIG. 2.24 See Video 2.16. Cervical side bending (lateral flexion) active range of motion (AROM) right and left.

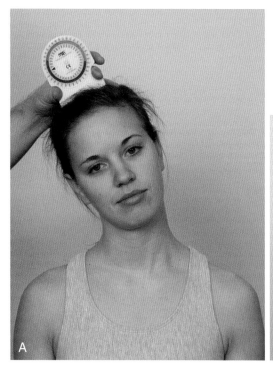

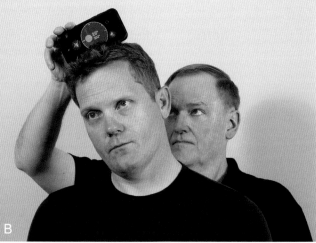

FIG. 2.25 See Video 2.17. **A,** Cervical spine lateral flexion measured with inclinometer. **B,** Cervical spine lateral flexion measured with a mobile phone goniometer application.

Cervical Sidebending (Lateral Flexion) Active Range of Motion Right and Left—cont'd

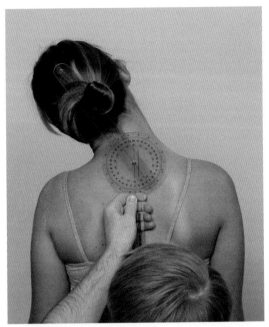

FIG. 2.26 See Video 2.18. Cervical spine lateral flexion measured with goniometer.

PATIENT POSITION	The patient stands (or sits) with good posture and arms relaxed at the sides.
THERAPIST POSITION	The therapist stands directly behind the patient.
PROCEDURE	The patient is instructed to side bend (lateral flexion) the cervical spine by slowly dropping the head and neck toward the right shoulder. Motion can be measured with a goniometer (C7 as fulcrum point) or an inclinometer (placed in the frontal plane on top of the head).
NOTES	The therapist should observe for a smooth curve throughout the cervical spine. Any fulcruming throughout the spinal segments should be noted. The amount of motion available in each direction is compared and noted if the motion reproduces the patient's symptoms. Piva et al.[108] used a gravity inclinometer to measure cervical side bending on 30 subjects and found a mean AROM of 39 degrees left lateral flexion and of 41 degrees right lateral flexion, with an ICC of 0.85 left and 0.87 right, an SEM of 4.2 left and 3.7 right, an MDC of 12 left and 10 right, and a kappa value for pain reproduction of 0.28 left and 0.75 right.

Cervical Sidebending (Lateral Flexion) Active Range of Motion Right and Left With Shoulder Girdle Supported

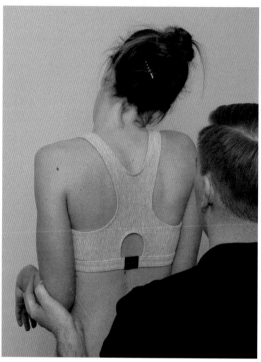

FIG. 2.27 See Video 2.19. Cervical side bending (lateral flexion) active range of motion (AROM) right and left with shoulder girdle supported.

PATIENT POSITION	The patient stands with good posture and arms relaxed at the sides.
THERAPIST POSITION	The therapist stands directly behind the patient.
PROCEDURE	The patient's arms are supported at the elbows (with elbows flexed to approximately 90 degrees to the side) to passively elevate the patient's shoulders to place the cervical spine soft tissues on slack. The patient is instructed to side bend the cervical spine by slowly dropping the head and neck toward the right shoulder.
NOTES	The therapist should observe for a smooth curve throughout the cervical spine. Any fulcruming throughout the spinal segments is noted. The therapist observes side bending to the left and the right with the arms supported. The amount of motion available in each direction is compared. The findings of this examination procedure are compared with the findings of the side-bending AROM test with unsupported arms at the side. If the patient is able to achieve significantly greater range of motion with the arms supported, the limitation is most likely the result of soft tissue (i.e., myofascial) tightness. However, if the patient has the same limitation in the amount of range of motion, the limitation is most likely from facet joint restriction.

▶ Cervical Rotation Active Range of Motion

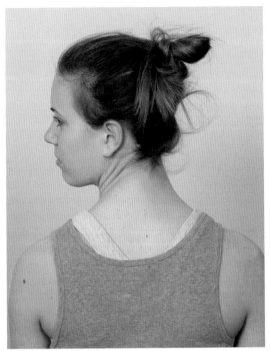

FIG. 2.28 See Video 2.20. Cervical rotation active range of motion (AROM) right and left.

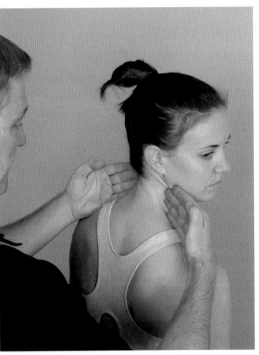

FIG. 2.30 See Video 2.21. Therapist hand positioning used to enhance visual estimate of cervical rotation active range of motion (AROM).

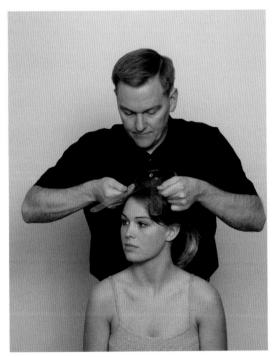

FIG. 2.29 Cervical spine rotation active range of motion (AROM) measured with goniometer.

Cervical Rotation Active Range of Motion—cont'd

PATIENT POSITION	The patient stands (or sits) with good posture and arms relaxed at the sides.
THERAPIST POSITION	The therapist stands directly behind the patient.
PROCEDURE	The patient is instructed to rotate the cervical spine by slowly turning the head and neck to look over the right shoulder. The procedure is repeated with rotation to the left. Motion can be measured with a goniometer with the moving arm lined up with the nose, the stationary arm facing straight ahead, and the fulcrum at the center crown of the cranium.
NOTES	The chin should near the plane of the shoulder with the end range of rotation. The amount of motion available in both directions is compared and noted if the motion reproduces the patient's symptoms and the location/nature of the symptoms. The visual estimate of cervical rotation can be enhanced by placement of the ulnar border of both hands along the superior aspect of the upper trapezius (Fig. 2.28). Full range of cervical rotation includes having the patient's mandible touching the therapist's proximal phalanx of the index finger. Eighty percent of full range of motion involves the mandible touching the middle phalanx, and 70% of full cervical rotation involves the patient's mandible just touching the distal phalanx. Youdas et al.[109] reported an ICC for measurements of cervical spine AROM of 60 patients with a universal goniometer that ranged from 0.78 to 0.95 for intratester reliability. When the motion was measured with a cervical range of motion (CROM) inclinometer or universal goniometer, intertester reliability ranged from 0.54 to 0.92. For visual estimates of cervical AROM, ICC values for intertester reliability ranged from 0.42 for flexion/extension to 0.82 for rotation.

▶ Upper Thoracic Rotation Active Range of Motion

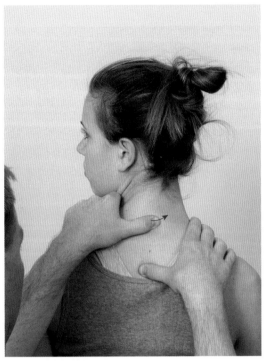

FIG. 2.31 See Video 2.22. Cervical spine rotation active range of motion (AROM) with palpation of upper thoracic rotation.

PATIENT POSITION	The patient stands (or sits) with good posture and arms relaxed at the sides.
THERAPIST POSITION	The therapist stands directly behind the patient.
PROCEDURE	With testing of upper thoracic rotation, the therapist uses one thumb to palpate the apex of the patient's C7 spinous process. The other thumb is used to palpate the apex of the patient's T4 spinous process. The patient is instructed to rotate the upper thoracic spine by slowly turning the head and neck to look over the right shoulder. The therapist should observe for the C7 spinous process to move to the opposite side of the rotation with a slight upswing at the end of the movement. The procedure is repeated with the thumb moved from C7 to T1 and then to T2.
NOTES	Whether or not the motion reproduces symptoms is noted, as are the location and nature of the symptoms. The thumb position is maintained to assess rotation in the opposite direction. The amount of motion available in each direction at each spinal segment is compared.

Active Range of Motion Cervical Spine Rotation in Supine Measured With Inclinometer

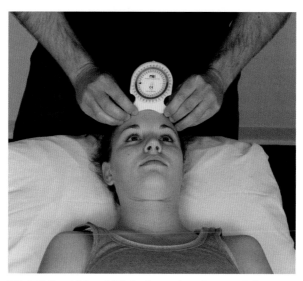

FIG. 2.32 See Video 2.23. Inclinometer placement for measurement of supine cervical spine rotation.

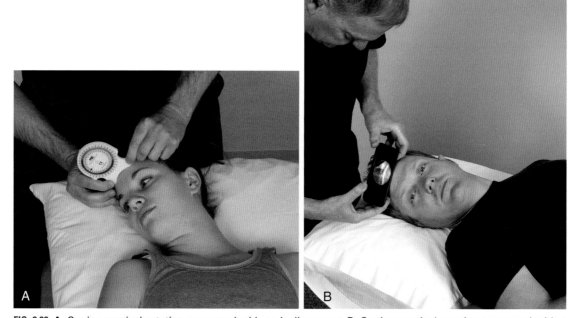

FIG. 2.33 **A**, Supine cervical rotation measured with an inclinometer. **B**, Supine cervical rotation measured with a mobile phone goniometer application.

Active Range of Motion Cervical Spine Rotation in Supine Measured With Inclinometer—cont'd

PATIENT POSITION	The patient is supine with the head resting on a small- to medium-sized pillow to support the head and neck in a neutral position with the face parallel with the plane of the treatment table.
THERAPIST POSITION	The therapist stands at the head of the table.
PROCEDURE	The patient is instructed to rotate the cervical spine by slowly turning the head and neck to look over the right shoulder. A gravity inclinometer can be positioned on the forehead and used to measure the motion.
NOTES	The amount of motion available in both directions is compared. Whether or not the motion reproduces the patient's symptoms is noted, as are the location and nature of the symptoms produced. If neck pain is reported on the ipsilateral side of the most restricted rotation direction, cervical downglide restrictions are suspected on the symptomatic side. If neck pain is reported on the contralateral side of motion restriction, cervical upglide restrictions are suspected on the symptomatic side. Passive intervertebral motion (PIVM) testing must be completed to isolate the passive segmental mobility. Supine rotation testing is a quick way to assess premanipulation and postmanipulation range of motion. Piva et al.[108] used a gravity inclinometer to test cervical spine rotation AROM in supine and reported an ICC of 0.86 (0.74:0.93) for right rotation and of 0.91 (0.82:0.96) for left rotation, an SEM of 4.8 degrees (right) and 4.1 degrees (left), an MDC of 13 degrees (right) and 11 degrees (left), and a kappa value of 0.76 (right) and 0.74 (left) for symptom reproduction.

▶ Thoracolumbar Forward-Bending Active Range of Motion

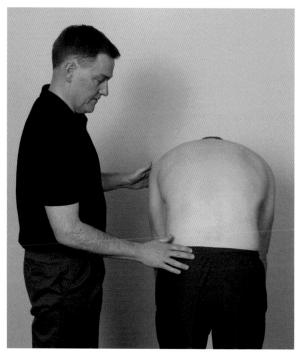

FIG. 2.34 See Video 2.24. Lumbar and thoracic forward-bending visual inspection.

PATIENT POSITION	The patient stands with good posture and arms relaxed at the sides.
THERAPIST POSITION	The therapist stands behind or just lateral to the patient with a clear view of the thoracic and lumbar spine.
PROCEDURE	The patient is instructed to forward bend the thoracic and lumbar spine by slowly forward bending the head and neck, then the shoulders, followed by the thoracic and lumbar spine. The patient is guarded during the examination to prevent loss of balance and falling forward. The therapist should observe for a smooth forward curve in the thoracic spine and a straightening or reversal of the lordosis in the lumbar spine.
NOTES	Whether or not the motion reproduces the patient's symptoms is noted. The therapist should observe and palpate for any shaking, juddering, or trick (i.e., aberrant) movements during the motion because these may indicate instability (i.e., movement coordination impairments) in the lumbar spine. Also, the presence of lateral deviation with forward bending is noted because this may be a sign of a facet joint restriction. The motion may be repeated up to 10 times to determine whether symptoms centralize or peripheralize with the active motion. Once symptoms centralize or peripheralize, the repeated movements are discontinued for that test direction.

▶ Lumbar Forward-Bending Measurement

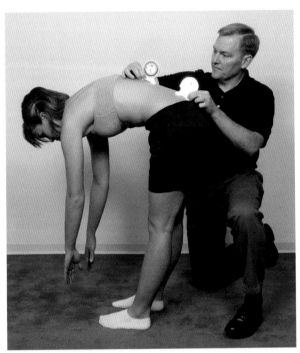

FIG. 2.35 See Video 2.25. Lumbar forward-bending measurement—double inclinometer method.

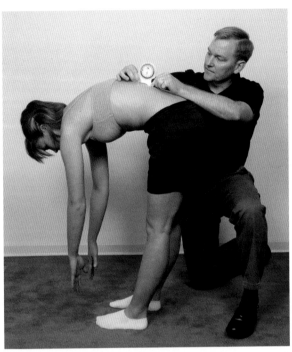

FIG. 2.36 See Video 2.26. Lumbar forward-bending measurement—single inclinometer method.

PATIENT POSITION	The patient stands with feet shoulder width apart, good posture, and arms relaxed at the sides. For the double inclinometer method, inclinometers are placed at midline of the spine in line with the PSIS and 15 cm above the baseline mark. The starting position angles of both inclinometers are zeroed. For the single inclinometer method, place the inclinometer at the T12 spinous process.
THERAPIST POSITION	The therapist stands just lateral to the patient with a clear view of the thoracic and lumbar spine and inclinometers.
PROCEDURE	The patient is instructed to forward bend the thoracic and lumbar spine by slowly forward bending the head and neck, then the shoulders, followed by the thoracic and lumbar spine. The angle of both inclinometers at the end position is noted, and the degree of forward bending is calculated by subtracting the angle of the lower inclinometer (represents hip motion) from the upper inclinometer (represents total motion). For the single inclinometer method, simply document the degree of forward bending from the start position.
NOTES	Nitchke et al.[110] found ICC levels for intertester reliability to be 0.35 and for intratester reliability to be 0.52. Maher and Adams[111] found a strong correlation between the inclinometer method of measuring lumbar forward-bending and backward-bending motion and radiographic assessment. A single inclinometer method has also shown good reliability when performed with placing a single inclinometer at the T12 vertebra.[112]

Thoracolumbar Backward-Bending Active Range of Motion

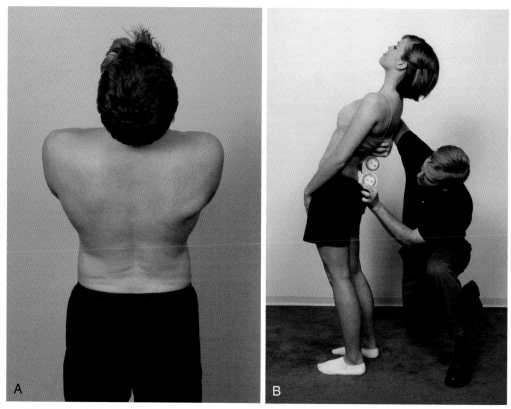

FIG. 2.37 See Video 2.27. **A,** Thoracolumbar backward bending active range of motion (AROM). **B,** Thoracolumbar backward bending active range of motion—double inclinometer method.

PATIENT POSITION	The patient stands with good posture and arms folded across the chest.
THERAPIST POSITION	The therapist stands behind or just lateral to the patient with a clear view of the thoracic and lumbar spine.
PROCEDURE	The patient is instructed to backward bend the thoracic and lumbar spine by slowly leaning backward as far as comfortable. The therapist should be sure to guard the patient during the examination to prevent loss of balance and falling backward.
NOTES	The therapist should observe for symmetry in the motion and an increase in lumbar lordosis. Whether the motion reproduces the patient's symptoms is noted. The motion may be repeated up to 10 times to determine whether the symptoms centralize or peripheralize. Once a change in symptoms is noted (i.e., centralization or peripheralization), the repeated movements are discontinued for that test direction. Lumbar backward bending can be measured with either a single or double inclinometer method similar to that described for lumbar forward bending.

▶ Thoracolumbar Lateral Flexion Active Range of Motion

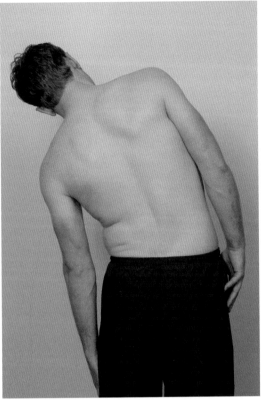

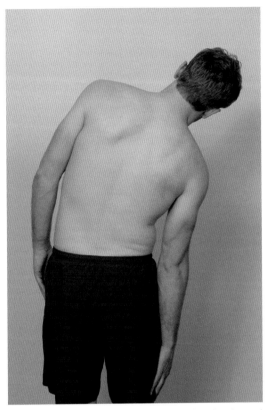

FIG. 2.38 See Video 2.28. Left thoracolumbar lateral flexion (side bending).

FIG. 2.39 See Video 2.28. Right thoracolumbar lateral flexion (side bending).

PATIENT POSITION	The patient stands with good posture and arms relaxed at the sides.
THERAPIST POSITION	The therapist stands directly behind the patient.
PROCEDURE	The patient is instructed to side bend the thoracic and lumbar spine by slowly side bending the head and neck, then the shoulders, followed by the thoracic and lumbar spine to the right. The therapist should observe for a smooth curve throughout the thoracic and lumbar spine. Any fulcruming throughout the spinal segments is noted, as is whether the motion reproduces the patient's symptoms. The procedure is repeated with side bending to the left. The amount of motion available in each direction is compared.
NOTES	A flat area may be an indication of muscle or joint tightness, and a fulcrum point in the range of motion may indicate greater mobility at that spinal level compared with the segments above and below the fulcrum point.

▶ Thoracolumbar Rotation Active Range of Motion

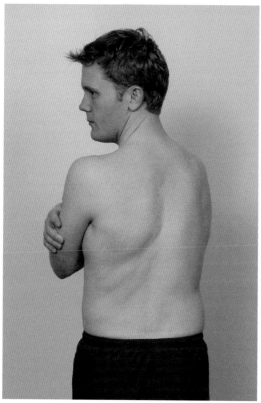

FIG. 2.40 See Video 2.29. Left thoracolumbar rotation.

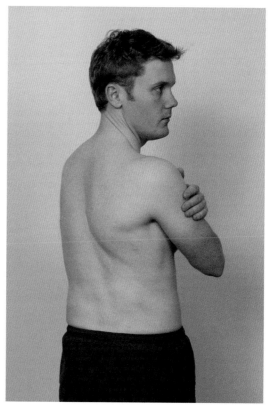

FIG. 2.41 See Video 2.29. Right thoracolumbar rotation.

PATIENT POSITION	The patient stands with good posture and arms folded across the chest.
THERAPIST POSITION	The therapist stands directly behind the patient, gently stabilizing the patient's pelvis.
PROCEDURE	The patient is instructed to rotate the thoracic and lumbar spine by slowly turning the head and neck to look over the right shoulder and by continuing to rotate the shoulders to include the thoracic and lumbar spine. The therapist should observe for side bending of the thoracic and lumbar spine to the left (the opposite direction of the rotation). Whether the motion reproduces the patient's symptoms is noted. The procedure is repeated with rotating to the right. The amount of motion available in each direction is compared.
NOTES	The therapist can provide overpressure through the pelvis to determine the reactivity of the stretched tissues with this motion. Thoracolumbar rotation AROM can also be tested in the seated position to reduce the influence of hip and pelvic motion.

⏵ Hook-Lying Lower Trunk Rotation

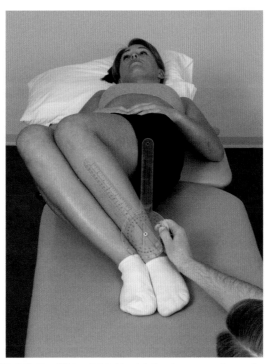

FIG. 2.42 See Video 2.30. Hook-lying lower trunk rotation.

PATIENT POSITION	The patient is supine in a hook-lying position with knees flexed to 90 degrees and feet flat on the table.
THERAPIST POSITION	The therapist kneels at the foot end of the table.
GONIOMETER ALIGNMENT	The stationary arm is perpendicular to the table or parallel to a plumb line or straight edge on the wall at the head of the treatment table. The axis point is 3 inches superior to the talus of the superior lower extremity with the bottom edge of the 14-inch plastic goniometer resting on the talus. The moving arm is parallel to the shaft of the tibia, pointing to the tibial tuberosity.
PROCEDURE	The angle of the top leg to the stationary arm represents the degree of lower trunk rotation. The patient can be asked to perform the motion with three repetitions in each direction as a warm-up before the measurement is taken. As the patient moves the legs to her right, left rotation of the lumbar spine is produced.
NOTES	Olson and Goerhing[113] tested the reliability of this goniometric measurement and found Pearson correlation coefficients for intrarater reliability that ranged from 0.59 to 0.82 for right rotation ($P < .001$) and 0.76 to 0.82 for left rotation ($P < .001$) and interrater reliability that ranged from 0.62 to 0.83 with right rotation ($P < .001$) and 0.75 to 0.77 for left rotation ($P < .001$). Asymmetry in lower trunk rotation is an impairment that can be treated with lumbar rotation manipulation techniques directed in the direction of the limitation. This method can be used as a pre- and postmanipulation AROM assessment.

Documentation

When measured with a goniometer or inclinometer, AROM can be documented by writing the motion and the corresponding degree measurement. AROM visual estimates are documented with stating the percentage of the expected range of motion that is observed. A chart with lines for each motion can also be used as a shorthand method of documentation, with the end of the stem representing 100% of expected motion (Fig. 2.43).

PALPATION

Palpation is the process of examining the body by means of touch and is a fundamental physical therapist skill that provides information about bony landmark location, tissue temperature, texture, resilience, and motion.[114] Palpation can be divided into palpation for tissue condition, palpation for bony landmark position, and palpation for passive intervertebral motion.

Palpation for Passive Intervertebral Motion

Physical therapists generally examine PIVM as part of the examination of patients with spinal disorders. PIVM testing involves the process of passively inducing spinal segmental motion while simultaneously attempting to palpate and judge the amount and quality of motion. PIVM tests can also be used as

pain provocation tests. Some authors separate PIVM tests into two subcategories: passive physiologic intervertebral motion (PPIVM) testing and passive accessory intervertebral motion (PAIVM) testing.[115] The PPIVM tests involve induction and palpation of motion in the cardinal planes of movement, such as forward bending, side bending, and rotation. PAIVM tests involve induction and judgment of joint play movements that require an outside force to produce the motion, such as a posterior to anterior gliding motion of the spinal segment. In addition to being used as a passive motion assessment, PAIVM tests are more likely to be used for assessment of end feel and pain provocation. PPIVM tests are primarily used for assessment of segmental passive movements and at times end feel but less commonly for pain provocation.

The results of PIVM test mobility judgments can be graded and documented simply as hypomobile, normal, or hypermobile for each motion direction and each spinal segment tested. Another common mobility scale first published by Gonnella et al.[116] incorporates a 7-point (0–6) grading scale, with 0 mobility denoting a fused spinal segment and 6 mobility used to describe an unstable spinal segment. A 3/6 on the mobility scale is used to denote a normal degree of mobility judgment for the individual tested. See Table 2.4 for further description of each category on the mobility scale.

The results of pain provocation assessments from PIVM tests are commonly described as the level of tissue or joint reactivity.[117] Table 2.5 outlines three levels of joint reactivity that are based on when the sequence of pain provocation is produced in relation to range of mobility assessment. For instance, a high level of reactivity is described as when pain provocation is reported before resistance to passive motion is

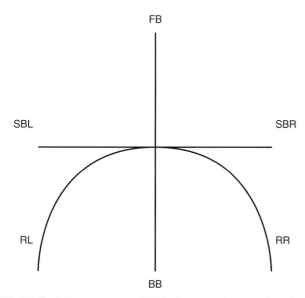

FIG. 2.43 Each line represents 100% of expected range of motion. A *slash mark* at the corresponding length of the line can be made at the observed visual estimate of percent of expected motion in each direction tested. *Three slash marks* can be used when myofascial limitations are suspected of causing limitation in motion. *X* is used at point of limitation when pain provocation is reported with motion. Additional written notes of pain location with each motion can also be made. Deviations in motion direction or muscle shakiness can also be drawn on motion diagram. *BB,* Backward bending; *FB,* forward bending; *RL,* rotation left; *RR,* rotation right; *SBL,* side bending left; *SBR,* side bending right.

TABLE 2.4	Passive Intervertebral Motion Grading System	
GRADE	**DESCRIPTION**	**TREATMENT**
0	Ankylosis or no detectable movement	No treatment
1	Considerable limitation in movement	Mobilization/manipulation
2	Slight limitation in movement	Mobilization/manipulation
3	Normal	No treatment
4	Slight increase in motion	No treatment or stabilization exercises
5	Considerable increase in motion	Stabilization exercises and treatment of neighboring hypomobility
6	Unstable	Stabilization exercises and treatment of neighboring hypomobility; external support; fusion

(Modified from Gonnella C, Paris SV, Kutner M. Reliability in evaluating passive intervertebral motion. *Phys Ther.* 1982;62(4):436-444.)

TABLE 2.5	Reactivity
LEVEL OF REACTIVITY	**DESCRIPTIONS**
High reactivity	Pain is reported before detection of resistance to passive motion
Moderate reactivity	Pain is reported synchronous to detection of resistance to passive motion
Low reactivity	Pain is reported after detection of resistance to passive motion (pain only with overpressure to passive motion)

Level of reactivity is used to describe relationship of pain provocation as it relates to sense of tissue resistance during passive motion, accessory motion, or passive intervertebral motion (PIVM) testing.
(Modified from Paris SV. *Introduction to Spinal Evaluation and Manipulation.* Atlanta: Institute Press; 1986.)

detected. A moderate level of reactivity is described as when pain provocation is reported synchronous to detection of resistance to passive motion. A low level of reactivity is described as when pain provocation is reported after resistance to passive motion is detected. In other words, pain is reported only with overpressure to passive motion.

In addition, PIVM tests can be used to make judgments on end feel, which is the quality of resistance that the clinician feels when passively taking a joint to the clinical limits of range. The type of end feel depends on the anatomic structure of the joint tested. The end feel can be judged as normal or abnormal for that joint. The spinal segments typically are restrained by capsular and ligamentous tissues. Therefore the end feel with performance of PAIVM tests for the spine tends to be a firm capsular or tissue stretch end feel. Box 2.8 outlines and describes normal and abnormal end

BOX 2.8	End Feel Classifications

Normal End Feel
- Soft tissue approximation: soft tissue presses against soft tissue at the end of mobility
- Tissue stretch: firm end feel that gives with overpressure at end of expected mobility
- Bone to bone: hard end feel at the end of mobility as a result of normal anatomic structure

Abnormal End Feel
- Muscle guarding: muscle holding or tension limiting the passive mobility
- Hard capsular: a firm tissue stretch felt before expected passive mobility
- Bone to bone: hard end feel felt before expected passive mobility
- Empty: minimal resistance felt but motion stopped because of severe pain
- Springy block: a springy rebound to passive mobility from internal joint derangement

(Data from Paris SV, Loubert PV. *FCO Foundations of Clinical Orthopaedics.* Atlanta: Institute Press; 1990; McGee DJ. *Orthopaedic Physical Assessment,* ed 4. Philadelphia: Saunders;2002; and Cyriax J. *Textbook of Orthopaedic Medicine: Diagnosis of Soft Tissue Lesions,* vol 1, ed 8. London: Balliere Tindall; 1982.)

feels. Olson et al.[118] found that the reliability of end feel testing was higher than the reliability for mobility judgments with testing of PIVM for craniovertebral side bending. Patla and Paris[119] showed fair to good interrater reliability for testing end feel of the elbow joint, with a kappa value of 0.40 for testing end feel of elbow flexion and a kappa value of 0.73 for testing end feel of elbow extension. Most reliability studies on PIVM testing have focused on judgments of mobility or pain provocation or both.

Manual physical therapists use the results of PIVM tests to guide which interventions will be used. Therapists who use the examination of PIVM as part of the comprehensive examination of spinal conditions are able to formulate intervention plans that achieve positive patient outcomes.[120–128] In addition, clinical prediction rules that predict patient success from lumbar manipulation and lumbar stabilization exercise programs to treat LBP include the results of posterior to anterior PAIVM tests in the set of criteria that comprise the rules,[60,61] which validates the clinical utility of the PAIVM testing in clinical decision making to enhance treatment outcomes for patients with LBP. However, when PIVM testing has been studied in isolation, both interrater and intrarater reliability results have been poor.[116,118,129–131]

In clinical situations, therapists rarely use passive joint mobility examinations in isolation. Rather, they combine the results of passive mobility examinations with other examination procedures, such as patient history, observation, palpation for position and condition, AROM, and various other selected special tests. With use of the results of a cluster of examination procedures that have adequate reliability, rather than those of only a single examination procedure, the therapist can determine the patient's specific impairments and generate an intervention plan. Professional standards are not met with an intervention plan based on the results of only one examination procedure. However, most studies that have looked at rater reliability have studied specific examination procedures in isolation.[116,118,129–131]

Gonnella et al.[116] assessed passive intervertebral forward bending of levels T12 to S1 and found reasonably good intrarater reliability but poor interrater reliability. They suggested that reliability might be increased by better clarifying the patient position and determining whether the therapists were assessing range of motion or end feel during the examination.[116]

In the chiropractic literature, Nansel et al.[130] concluded that motion-based palpation showed poor reliability ($z < .05$; kappa coefficient, 0.013) and found that it may not be an internally valid predictor of vertebral joint dysfunction in otherwise healthy asymptomatic individuals.[131] Strender et al.[131] looked at seven different examination procedures of the cervical spine, some of which were PIVM tests, and showed poor interrater reliability (kappa coefficients for mobility testing were C0–C1 = 0.091; C1–C2 = 0.15; C2–C3 = 0.057).

Maher and Adams[111] studied the reliability of pain and stiffness assessments with a posteroanterior PAIVM test of the lumbar spine and found poor reliability in determining stiffness (ICC values of 0.03–0.37) but good reliability in pain reproduction. Binkley et al.[129] studied lumbar postero-anterior PAIVM testing and showed poor reliability (ICC = 0.25) and suggested that caution should be used with the results of this assessment in the absence of other data. Hicks et al.[132] studied interrater reliability in identification of lumbar segmental instability. Again, the segmental mobility interrater reliability was poor (–0.02 to 0.26), and the interrater reliability for pain provocation was more acceptable (0.25–0.55).

Abbott et al.[133] reported on the validity of the use of lumbar forward and backward bending PIVM testing and lumbar posterior to anterior PAIVM testing to detect lumbar spinal instability (LSI) and used lumbar flexion/extension radiographs as the reference standard on 138 patients with LBP. Flexion PIVM tests were highly specific for the diagnosis of translation LSI but showed very poor sensitivity. Likelihood ratio statistics for flexion PPIVM tests were not statistically significant. Extension PIVM tests performed better than flexion PIVM tests, with slightly higher sensitivity resulting in a +LR of 7.1 for radiographic evidence of translation LSI. This research demonstrates that PIVM test procedures have moderate validity for detecting passive segmental motion instability.[133]

Olson et al.[118] assessed interrater reliability of craniovertebral side bending in five different positions of 10 healthy subjects and found poor interrater (kappa values of –0.03 to 0.18) and intrarater (kappa values of –0.02 to 0.14) reliability in all positions. Interrater reliability of C1 to C2 rotation, C2 to C3 lateral flexion, C7 to T1 flexion/extension, and first rib spring test was assessed by Smedmark et al.[134] These results were somewhat better, showing fair to moderate reliability (kappa scores ranged from 0.28–0.43).[134] Patients were used in this study, and efforts were made to standardize the testing protocol.[134]

Jull et al.[135] were able to show excellent symptom reproduction with palpation and isolation of upper cervical facet joints, and validation of the palpation findings was confirmed (100% agreement) with pain relief produced with anesthetic nerve blocks to the targeted symptomatic joints.

In clinical situations, therapists rarely use passive joint mobility examinations in isolation. Rather, they combine the results of the assessment with the results of other examination procedures. Cibulka and Koldehoff[136] showed excellent interrater reliability in assessment of the sacroiliac joint (kappa value of 0.88) with use of a cluster of four examination procedures, with the requirement that three of the four have positive results to consider the patient to have a sacroiliac dysfunction. However, Potter and Rothstein[137] showed poor reliability when studying each of those same four examination procedures in isolation.

The design of Cibulka and Koldehoff's[136] study more closely emulates how therapists actually assess patients in the clinic. Likewise, Arab et al.[138] reported substantial to excellent intraexaminer and interexaminer reliability of clusters of motion palpation and provocation tests to diagnose sacroiliac joint impairments with kappa scores ranging from 0.44 to 1.00 and 0.52 to 0.92. This supports that clusters of motion palpation combined with provocation tests have adequate reliability for use in clinical assessment of the sacroiliac joint.

Jarett et al.[139] assessed the reliability of use of a cluster of four examination procedures to diagnose craniovertebral dysfunctions if three of four procedures had positive results. The four criteria included resting head position measured with a CROM inclinometer device, a pattern of AROM restriction characteristic of craniovertebral dysfunction, asymmetric position of the C1 transverse process with palpation, and limitation of motion or abnormal end feel assessment with passive craniovertebral side-bending test. For the composite test results, the kappa coefficient for the symptomatic group was 0.524 with an 87% agreement between the two therapists. For the individual tests, the kappa scores ranged from –0.047 (palpation of the transverse process of C1) to 0.516 (resting CROM position) with percent agreements ranging from 77% to 90%. Overall, this study showed higher kappa values with use of a cluster of examination findings (categorized as fair to moderate) to determine an impairment compared with the kappa values of the individual examination findings (categorized as poor to moderate).[139]

In general, the interrater reliability of PIVM testing is poor; and at times, the intrarater reliability has reached a more acceptable moderate level. Use of palpation and PIVM testing for symptom reproduction has shown acceptable and, at times, very good levels of reliability. There is also preliminary evidence that PIVM testing is a valid method to assist in diagnosis of lumbar spine instability and can be used to assist in screening for cervical facet joint pain. In addition, inclusion of PIVM testing in a cluster of findings to arrive at a diagnosis has shown more acceptable levels of reliability; and inclusion of posteroanterior PAIVM test findings in the clinical prediction rules for lumbar manipulation and stabilization helps to further validate the clinical usefulness of these procedures.[60,61]

The clinical implications of this body of research on reliability of PIVM testing are that PIVM tests that focus on mobility assessment should not be used in isolation to determine an impairment diagnosis or to guide treatment decisions. Instead, these examination procedures must be used as part of a cluster of findings to arrive at a diagnosis; the other examination procedures should include symptom reproduction, AROM testing, results of disability and fear avoidance questionnaires, and symptom location and behavior. In addition, the motor learning processes used by student therapists to master PIVM testing can enhance the ease of learning manipulation procedures. Student physical therapists are suggested to develop competence on the manual examination skills, such as PIVM testing before being taught spinal manipulation.[140]

Detailed illustrations and descriptions of PIVM tests are included in Chapters 4, 5, and 6 for each region of the spine. When available, the reliability and validity of each test are included with the description of the technique. Box 2.9 outlines general performance recommendations for clinicians to consider when performing PIVM testing. Palpation for tissue condition and position procedures are included in this chapter

BOX 2.9	Passive Intervertebral Motion Technique Considerations

- Patient positioning
  - Relaxed and well supported
  - Spinal neutral position
- Position of therapist
  - Good body mechanics with table at appropriate height
  - As close to patient as possible
  - Firm and professional contact
- Performance of technique
  - Slow, rhythmic, relaxing movements
  - Relax palpating hand
  - Palpate for, do not create or block, movements
  - Consider starting away from restricted and painful segments

(Modified from Paris SV, Loubert PV. *FCO Foundations of Clinical Orthopaedics.* Atlanta: Institute Press; 1990.)

because these procedures are often included as part of the general spinal examination.

Palpation for Tissue Condition

The layers of connective tissue should be carefully palpated and assessed as part of the comprehensive spinal examination. First, the therapist should start with inspection and palpation of the skin. The therapist needs to look for any skin lesions, scars, or areas of discoloration and ask the patient follow-up questions on the history of any significant findings. The skin is palpated for extensibility, temperature, and moisture. Increased temperature is an indication of an inflammatory process. Poor skin extensibility may be an indication of a connective tissue disorder or of a chronically stiff back. Subcutaneous tissues should also be assessed for tissue mobility.

Careful palpation of skeletal muscles can yield valuable information. The muscle palpation should begin with the more superficial muscles and gradually proceed to include the deeper muscles in the anatomic areas of interest. Of particular interest is identification of taut bands within the muscle tissue commonly associated with trigger points. Trigger points are "hyperirritable spots in a taut band of a skeletal muscle that is painful on compression, stretch, overload, or contraction of the tissue that usually responds to palpation with a referred pain that is perceived to be distant to the spot."[141] Trigger points are located within taut bands, which are bands of contractured muscle fibers that feel like tense strings within the belly of the muscle and can be palpated with the pads of the fingers.[142]

Trigger points can be further classified as active or latent. Direct palpation of an active trigger point reproduces the local or referred pain that is familiar to the patient for which the latter is seeking treatment.[142] In latent trigger points, the palpation produces local or referred pain that is not familiar to the patient.[142] The latent trigger points do not actively produce symptoms while not being palpated. For instance, a patient with low back and leg pain may have active trigger points in the gluteus medius muscle of the symptomatic extremity but

may also have latent trigger points in the gluteus medius muscle on the asymptomatic extremity. Both active and latent trigger points can provoke motor dysfunctions (such as muscle weakness, inhibition, increased motor irritability, muscle imbalances, and altered motor recruitment) in either the affected muscle or in functionally related muscles.[141–143]

Chemical muscle holding involves muscles with multiple trigger points and taut bands that cause myofascial pain that is associated with tissue ischemia and hypoxia (Box 2.10). This causes an increased release of the neurotransmitter acetylcholine (ACh) at the motor endplate and leads to a decrease of the local pH. A low pH downregulates acetylcholinesterase at the neuromuscular junction and can trigger the release of neurotransmitters (such as substance P, interleukins, adenosine triphosphate, and prostaglandins) that result in activation of

BOX 2.10	Dysfunctional Muscle Holding States

Muscle Spasm
- Pathologic involuntary (electrogenic) muscle contraction
- Observe twitching of the muscle

Involuntary Muscle Holding
- Increased muscle tone caused by an underlying dysfunction (e.g., instability)
- Disappears when adequately supported
- Hypertonic but otherwise normal to touch

Chemical Muscle Holding
- Increased tone remains in multiple positions
- Increased muscle tone to touch that is nonelastic, thickened, dense tissue (taut bands and trigger points)
- Limited range of motion and extensibility
- May be caused by sustained involuntary muscle holding
- Retention of metabolites and tissue fluids cause further nociception

Taut Band
- Tense strings within the muscle belly
- A contracture within muscle fibers independent of electromyogenic activity that does not involve the entire muscle

Trigger Point
- Hyperirritable spot in a taut band of a skeletal muscle that is painful on compression, stretch, overload, or contraction of the tissue that usually responds with a referred pain that is perceived to be distant to the spot

Voluntary Muscle Holding
- Increased muscle tone from pain or fear of pain
- Voluntary movements are restrained

Adaptive Shortening
- Normal tone
- Limited range of motion from shortened muscle
- Loss of sarcomeres
- Can be caused by postural adaptation or sustained muscle holding states

(Modified from Paris SV, Loubert PV. *FCO Foundations of Clinical Orthopaedics.* Atlanta: Institute Press; 1990; Dommerholt J, Fernandez-de-las-Penas C. *Trigger Point Dry Needling: an Evidenced and Clinical-Based Approach.* Edinburgh: Churchill Livingstone/Elsevier; 2013; and Simons DG, Travell JG, Simons LS. *Myofascial Pain and Dysfunction: the Trigger Point Manual,* vol 1. Philadelphia: Lippincott Williams and Wilkins; 1999.)

peripheral nociceptive receptors.[142] A lowered pH activates the transient receptor potential vanilloid receptors and acid-sensing ion channels via hydrogen ions and protons.[142] These channels are nociceptive, so they initiate pain, hyperalgesia, and CS.[142] This tends to sensitize the CNS to nociceptive input and leads to patient perception of local and referred pain originating from the muscle trigger points.

The clinical characteristics of referred pain from muscle include the following: muscle referred pain is described as deep, diffuse, burning, tightening, or pressing pain; the location of the referred pain from muscle can be quite similar to the location of referred pain from joint impairments; the referred pain from muscle can spread cranial/caudal or ventral/dorsal; the intensity of the muscle referred pain and the size of the referred pain area tend to be positively correlated to the degree of irritability or sensitization of the CNS; other referred symptoms from muscle trigger points can include burning, tingling, numbness, coldness, stiffness, fatigue, weakness, or muscle motor fatigue; inactivation of active trigger points should relieve the referred pain.[142,144]

Trigger point diagnosis is associated with the following: (1) presence of a palpable taut band in a skeletal muscle when accessible to palpation; (2) presence of a hyperirritable spot in the taut band; (3) palpable local twitch response on snapping palpation (or dry needling) the trigger point; and (4) presence of referred pain elicited by stimulation or palpation of the hyperirritable spot.[141] The minimum acceptable criteria for trigger point diagnosis are the presence of a hyperirritable spot within a palpable taut band of the skeletal muscle combined with the patient's recognition of the referred pain elicited by the trigger point.[141] When experienced clinicians apply these criteria, good interexaminer reliability has been reported with kappa scores from 0.84 to 0.88.[145]

Treatment of underlying joint and muscle impairments may alleviate muscle holding states and trigger points. In more chronic situations, direct treatment of the myofascial tissue and trigger points needs to be included in the treatment program, such as soft tissue mobilization and massage techniques. Trigger point dry needling can also provide an effective intervention for trigger points, and comprehensive resources on this clinical intervention commonly performed by physical therapists are available.[142,144] Dry needling can be an effective treatment adjunct to the manual physical therapy approach provided in this textbook (Fig. 2.44).

Fig. 2.45 provides a grid for documentation of PIVM findings and also provides a body diagram and key for shorthand notation of palpation findings.

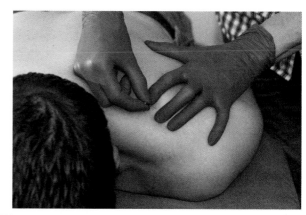

FIG. 2.44 Dry needling of the supraspinatus muscle in prone. (Reprinted with permission from Dommerholt J, Fernandez-de-las-Penas C. *Trigger Point Dry Needling: an Evidenced and Clinical-Based Approach.* Edinburgh: Churchill Livingstone Elsevier; 2013.)

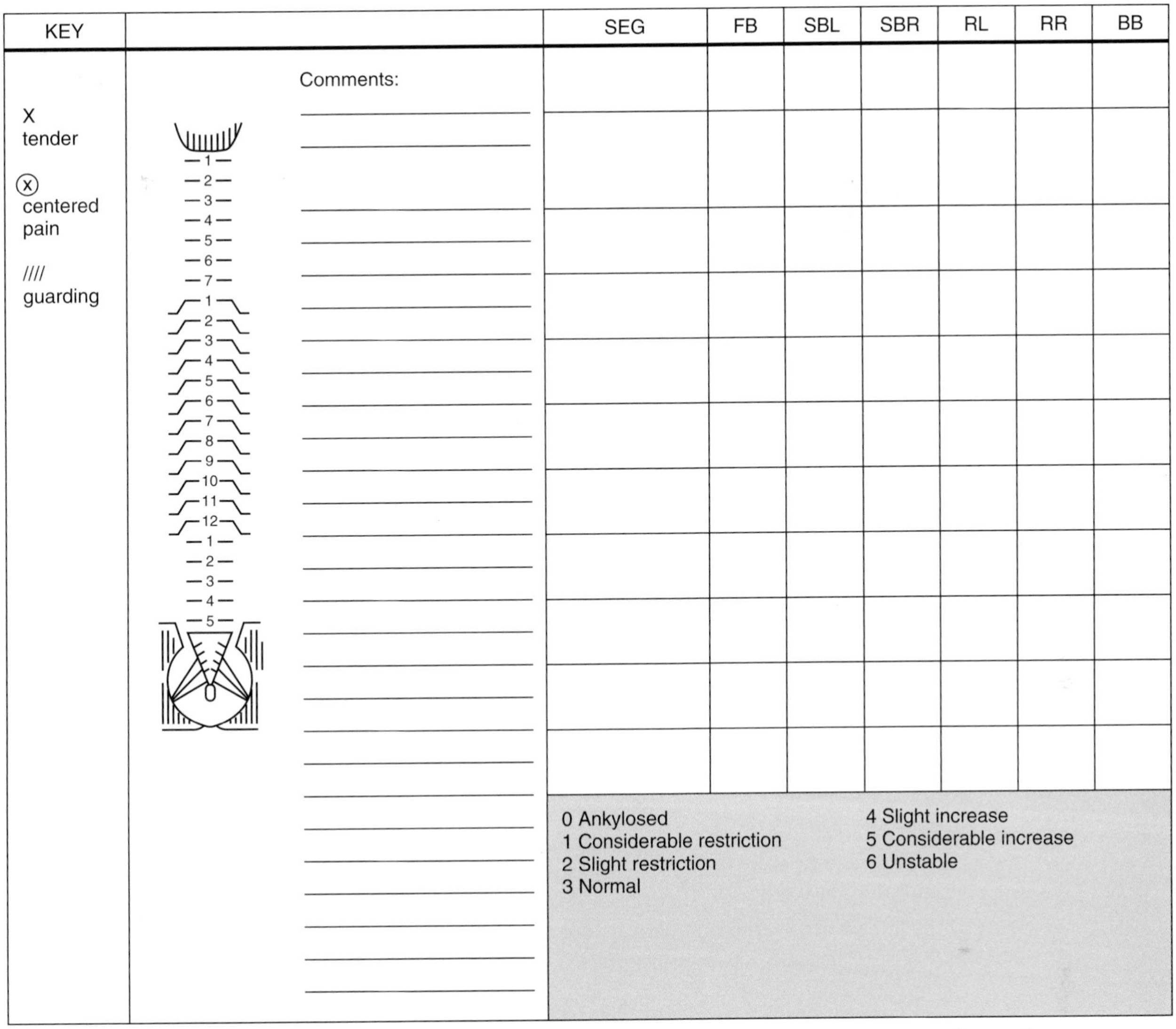

KEY			SEG	FB	SBL	SBR	RL	RR	BB
X tender		Comments:							
Ⓧ centered pain									
//// guarding									

0 Ankylosed   4 Slight increase
1 Considerable restriction   5 Considerable increase
2 Slight restriction   6 Unstable
3 Normal

FIG. 2.45 The body chart can be used to document palpation findings, and the grid can be used to document passive intervertebral motion (PIVM) test findings. *BB,* Backward bending; *FB,* forward bending; *RL,* rotation left; *RR,* rotation right; *SBL,* side bending left; *SBR,* side bending right; *SEG,* spinal segment.

▶ Skin Palpation for Temperature and Moisture

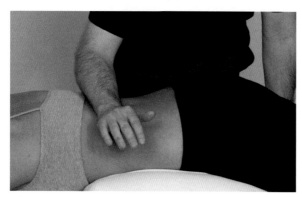

FIG. 2.46 See Video 2.31. Skin temperature and moisture assessment with forearm.

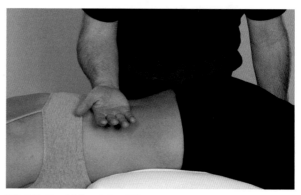

FIG. 2.47 See Video 2.31. Skin temperature and moisture assessment with dorsum of the hand.

PATIENT POSITION	The patient is prone with a pillow under the chest/trunk.
THERAPIST POSITION	The therapist stands next to the patient.
PROCEDURE	Starting in the cervical region, the therapist uses the dorsum of the hand or the volar aspect of the forearm to palpate the entire length of the spine for temperature and moisture. Both the right and left sides of the back are palpated.
NOTES	The temperature of the back should be warm in the cervical region, slightly warmer in the thoracic region, and slightly cooler in the lumbar region. The therapist should observe for deviations from this pattern and for differences between right and left sides. Increases in temperature and moisture could be a sign of inflammation, and decreases in temperature and moisture could be a sign of a chronic disorder.

▶ Subcutaneous Tissue Assessment: Skin Rolling

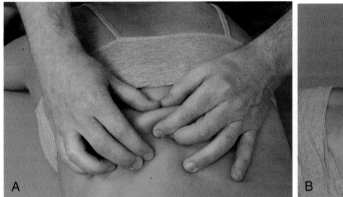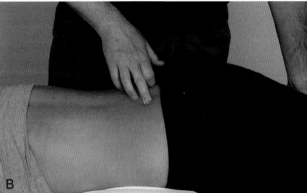

FIG. 2.48 See Video 2.32. **A,** Skin rolling. **B,** See Video 2.33. Skin mobility assessment: cross motions

PATIENT POSITION	The patient is prone with a pillow under the chest/trunk.
THERAPIST POSITION	The therapist stands next to the patient.
PROCEDURE	The therapist uses the thumb and index finger to gently pinch and lift the skin just lateral to the spine. The skin between the thumb and index finger is gently "rolled" to assess for mobility. The entire length of the spine is assessed, with comparison of right and left sides.
NOTES	The skin and subcutaneous tissue should be soft and easy to move. The therapist should note any tenderness, abnormal amounts of fat, fluid, edema, or nodules. The skin and subcutaneous tissues are typically more mobile around the lumbosacral junction, the cervical/thoracic junction, and the scapula. Skin extensibility can also be tested with the pads of the index and long fingers to move the skin in small X shapes along the lateral aspect of the spine.

Thoracic and Lumbar Muscle Palpation: Tone/Guarding Assessment

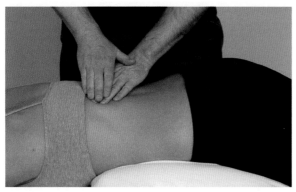

FIG. 2.49 See Video 2.34. Palpation of specific spinal muscles of various depth.

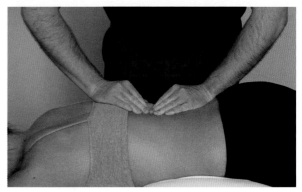

FIG. 2.50 See Video 2.35. "Muscle splay."

PATIENT POSITION	The patient is prone with a pillow under the chest/trunk.
THERAPIST POSITION	The therapist stands next to the patient.
PROCEDURE	First, the therapist uses the pads of the index and long fingers to palpate the layers of muscle tissue with assessment for signs of muscle holding, tenderness, or edema. Next, the index/long fingers and thumbs are used to make a triangle and gently grasp the musculature just lateral to the spine. The therapist assesses how the musculature moves by alternately "pushing" with the thumbs and "pulling" with the fingers. This technique is called "muscle splay."
NOTES	The muscles should be soft and easy to move. The therapist should note any areas of tenderness or muscle guarding. The right and left sides are compared. See Box 2.10 for an outline of dysfunctional muscle holding states that can be identified with palpation of muscle tissue condition, and when found, may be an indication to assess the anatomic region for additional impairments.

Anterior Neck Muscle Palpation

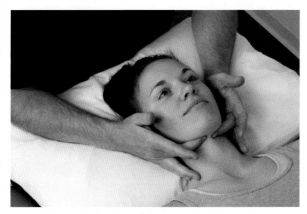

FIG. 2.51 Palpation of the suprahyoid muscles.

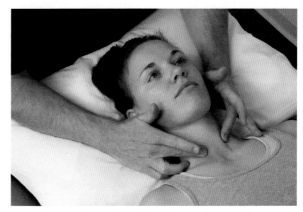

FIG. 2.52 Palpation of the infrahyoid muscles.

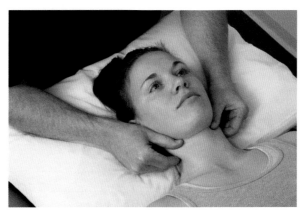

FIG. 2.53 Palpation of the sternocleidomastoid muscles.

PATIENT POSITION	The patient is supine with a small pillow supporting the patient's head and neck in a neutral position.
THERAPIST POSITION	The therapist sits or stands at the head of the table.
PROCEDURE	The therapist first palpates the thyroid cartilage and the hyoid bone. Next, the therapist palpates the suprahyoid and infrahyoid muscles to identify areas of tenderness, guarding, or loss of tissue extensibility. The sternocleidomastoid muscle can also be palpated for tenderness, guarding, or loss of extensibility by gently grasping the muscle distal to the mastoid process and gliding the tissue anterior to posterior.
NOTES	In patients with cervical or TMJ dysfunction, these muscles may develop loss of tissue extensibility, tenderness, or muscle guarding and require soft tissue mobilization techniques to address these impairments.

Posterior Neck Muscle Palpation

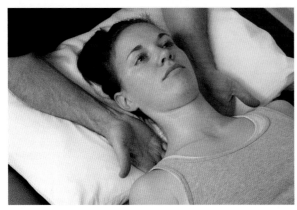

FIG. 2.54 Palpation of the posterior upper thoracic muscles.

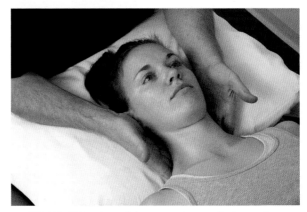

FIG. 2.55 Palpation of the posterior cervical muscles.

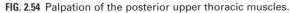

PATIENT POSITION	The patient is supine with a small pillow supporting the patient's head and neck in a neutral position.
THERAPIST POSITION	The therapist sits or stands at the head of the table.
PROCEDURE	The therapist first palpates the spine of the scapula and using the pads of the fingers and moves superiorly to palpation the upper thoracic muscles. The fingers are gradually moved medially and superiorly to palpate the posterior cervical muscles at each spinal level up to the occiput.
NOTES	In patients with cervical impairments, these muscles may develop loss of tissue extensibility, tenderness, or muscle guarding and require soft tissue mobilization techniques to address these impairments.

▶ Palpation of Supraspinous and Interspinous Ligaments

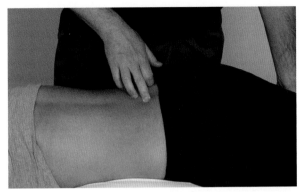

FIG. 2.56 See Video 2.36. Palpation of supraspinous and interspinous ligaments.

PATIENT POSITION	The patient is prone with a pillow under the chest/trunk.
THERAPIST POSITION	The therapist stands next to the patient.
PROCEDURE	To palpate the supraspinous ligament, the therapist uses the pad of the long finger and palpates the interspinous space. The ligament should be springy and nontender. To palpate the interspinous ligament, the therapist uses the pad of the long finger and palpates just deep and lateral to the supraspinous ligament. Both right and left sides of the ligament are palpated. The ligament should be springy and nontender. The interspinous ligaments are short and strong and connect the adjoining spinous processes throughout the thoracic and lumbar spine.
NOTES	Ligaments should normally feel smooth and taut with a springy suppleness. If tenderness is reported, especially if combined with a feeling of swelling, the ligament is likely inflamed. If the ligament feels thickened, hard, and tight, hypomobility likely will be present at that spinal segment. Strender et al.[147] reported a kappa value of 0.55 for intertester reliability for reproduction of tenderness between spinous processes of the lumbar vertebra in examination of patients with LBP.

Palpation for Position

For diagnosis of a positional fault of a vertebra, mobility deficits must be noted with PIVM testing with an attempt to move the spinal segment out of the suspected faulty vertebral position. Mobility deficits must be found at the spinal segment to warrant manipulation to correct a positional fault. In theory, a positional fault of a spinal segment may occur when a vertebra is unable to return to its neutral or rest position. Paris[117] describes three suspected theoretic causes:

1. A vertebra may get caught on a rough surface of the joint.
2. An impacted meniscus may lock the facet joints.
3. The facet joints may stiffen in a position after an injury.

Although the three theories are physiologically possible, very little to no evidence is available to prove that positional faults exist, can be reliably detected, or can be corrected with manipulation techniques. This may be due to the lack of a device that can detect and measure positional faults in a reliable and valid manner combined with the fact that a great deal of normal anatomic variability may be misinterpreted as a positional fault. In an evidence informed clinical reasoning framework, significantly greater emphasis must be placed on findings of mobility deficits and pain provocation than suspected positional findings. Care must be taken to restrict explanations of suspected positional faults to patients to avoid perpetuating fear and anxiety in patients with back pain.

▶ Pinch Test: Thoracic and Lumbar Spines

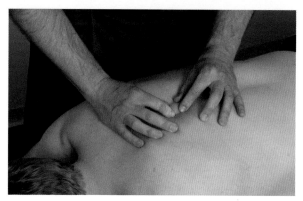

FIG. 2.57 See Video 2.37. Pinch test assessment of relative positions of spinous processes.

PATIENT POSITION	The patient is prone with a pillow under the chest/trunk.
THERAPIST POSITION	The therapist stands next to the patient.
PROCEDURE	The therapist uses the pad of the long finger to palpate each interspinous space in the lumbar and thoracic spine. Palpation should begin in the lumbar spine and continue cranially. Any forward-bent or backward-bent positional faults are noted. Also, any swelling or tenderness is noted. The therapist uses the thumb and index finger to pinch adjacent spinous processes in the lumbar and thoracic spine. Any rotational positional faults are noted, as well as swelling or tenderness.
NOTES	Because anatomic variations in spinous process length and angulation are common, deviations of relative positioning of the spinous processes of the thoracic and lumbar spine must be interpreted with caution.

▶ Palpation of Articular Pillars and Facet Joints of the Cervical Spine

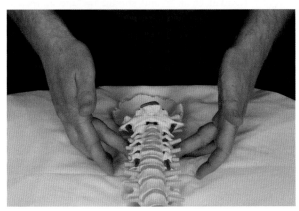

FIG. 2.58 See Video 2.38. Finger placement for palpation of articular pillars and facet joints of cervical spine.

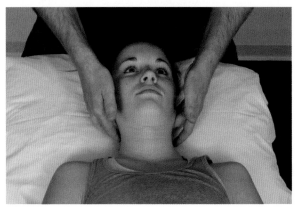

FIG. 2.59 See Video 2.38. Palpation of articular pillars and facet joints of the cervical spine.

PATIENT POSITION	The patient is supine with the head on a pillow.
THERAPIST POSITION	The therapist stands at the head of the patient.
PROCEDURE	The therapist uses the pads of the long fingers to palpate the spine of the scapula and adjacent soft tissues, noting any tenderness or muscle guarding. For palpation of the articular pillars and facet joints of the cervical spine, the spinous process of C2 is located with the pad of one long finger. With the pads of both long fingers, the therapist slides laterally around the neck until the middle fingers are directly inferior to the mastoid processes. From this position, the pads of the middle fingers are used to palpate the articular pillars and facet joints. The facet joints feel like small peaks and lie deep beneath the muscle tissue. The articular pillars feel like small valleys between each facet joint. Each facet joint and articular pillar is palpated from C2–C3 to C6–C7.
NOTES	Any swelling or tenderness is noted, and right and left sides are compared. The therapist notes any signs of tenderness, swelling, muscle holding, or tissue thickening. The patient's head should remain on the pillow throughout the procedure. Patient relaxation is the key to palpation of the facet joints and articular pillars. This technique allows for palpation of tissue condition and vertebral position of the cervical spine. Deviations in vertebral position are suspected with comparison of the relative position of the left and right articular pillar of each vertebra as the head and neck rest in the neutral position.

Neurologic Examination

The neurologic examination can be divided into tests for sensation, strength, and deep tendon reflexes and an upper motor neuron screening. If positive findings are noted, further diagnostic testing, such as a nerve conduction study or MRI, may be indicated to confirm the findings. See Boxes 2.11, 2.12, and 2.13 for illustrations of neurologic examination procedures. Sensation testing should include assessment of light touch and sharp/dull perception and should include testing of each dermatomal area (Figs. 2.60E–G and 2.61A–C). See

Figs. 2.63 and 2.64 for illustrations of the common dermatomes. Strength tests can be graded on a 0 to 5 scale as described by Kendall et al.[106] and should include at least one muscle (i.e., myotome) that corresponds to the anatomic nerve roots in the region of the spine assessed. For instance, in the examination of the cervical spine, myotomal strength should be assessed for the cervical nerve roots; for lumbar spine examination, the lumbar nerve root myotomes should be evaluated. See Tables 2.6 and 2.7 for details on nerve root levels and corresponding muscles for each level.

| BOX 2.11 | Upper Quarter Neurologic Examination |

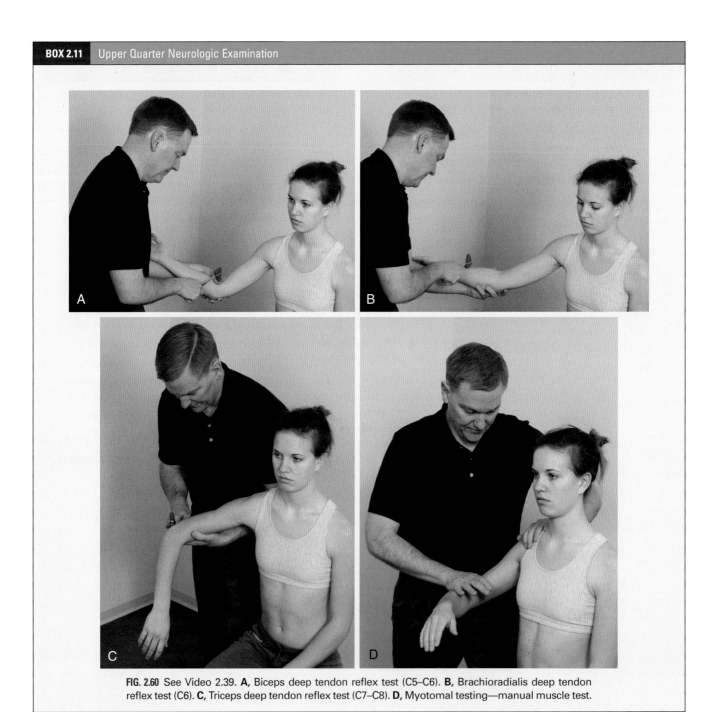

FIG. 2.60 See Video 2.39. **A,** Biceps deep tendon reflex test (C5–C6). **B,** Brachioradialis deep tendon reflex test (C6). **C,** Triceps deep tendon reflex test (C7–C8). **D,** Myotomal testing—manual muscle test.

BOX 2.11   Upper Quarter Neurologic Examination—cont'd

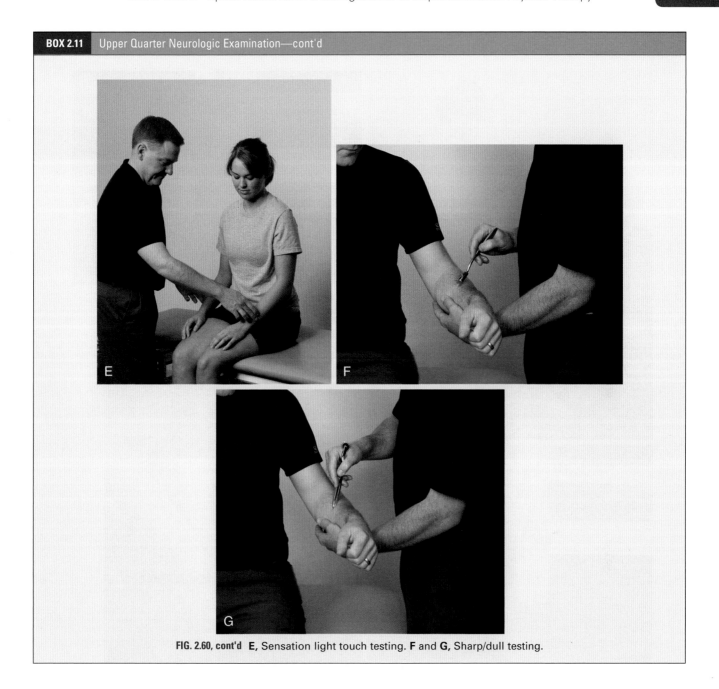

FIG. 2.60, cont'd E, Sensation light touch testing. **F** and **G,** Sharp/dull testing.

BOX 2.12 Lower Quarter Neurologic Examination

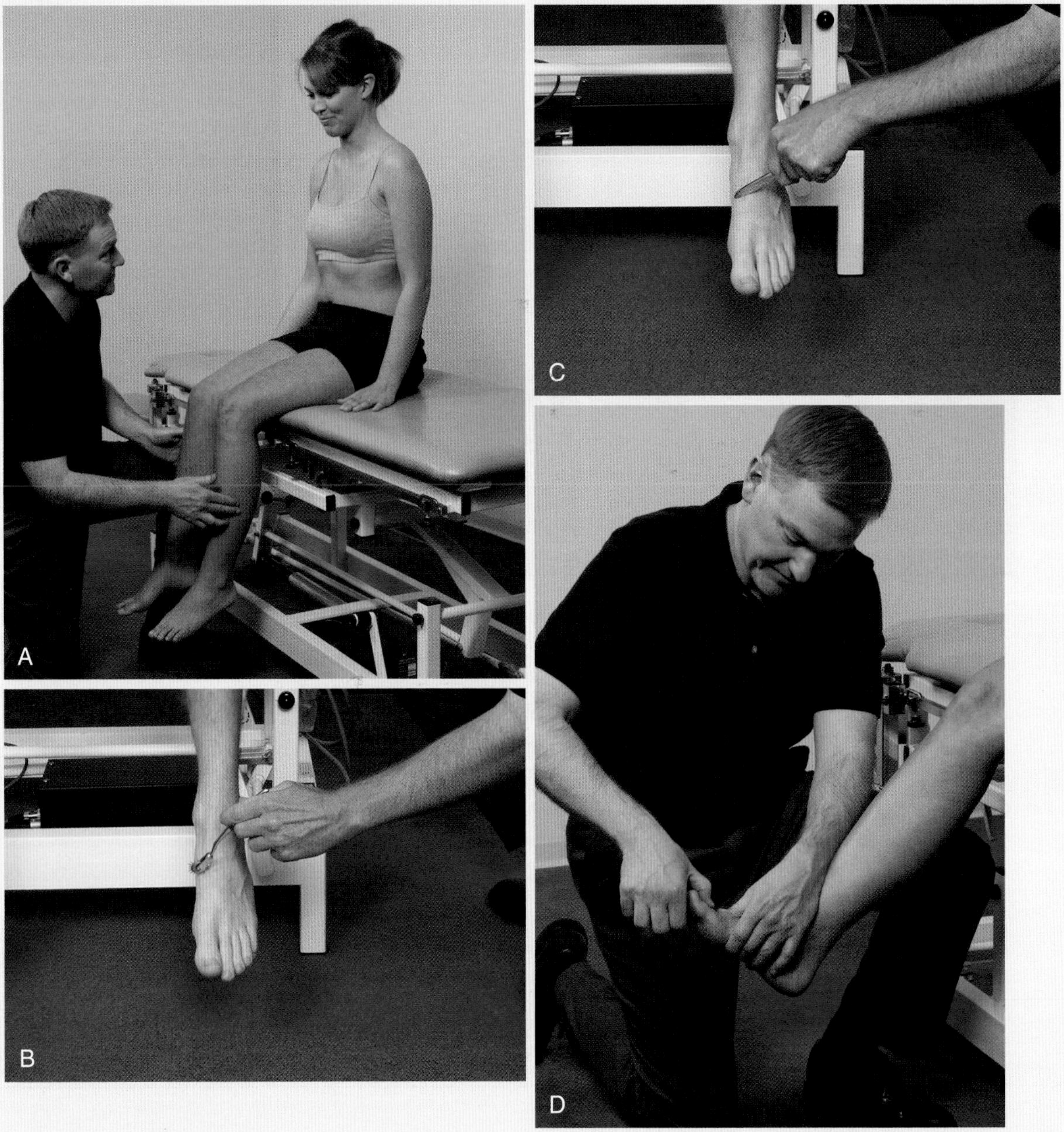

FIG. 2.61 A, Sensation light touch testing. **B** and **C,** Sharp/dull testing. **D,** Myotomal strength testing.

BOX 2.12 Lower Quarter Neurologic Examination—cont'd

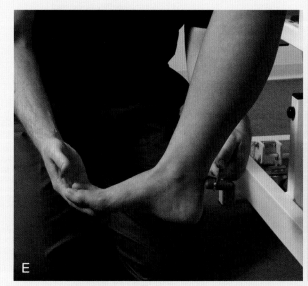

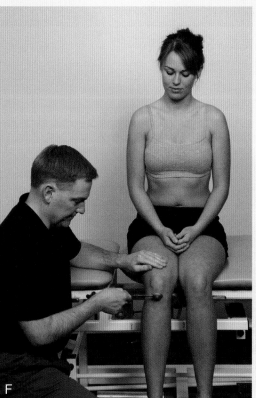

FIG. 2.61, cont'd **E,** See Video 2.40. Achilles deep tendon reflex (S1). See Video 2.40. **F,** Patella deep tendon reflex (L4).

BOX 2.13 Upper Motor Neuron Screen for Cervical Myelopathy

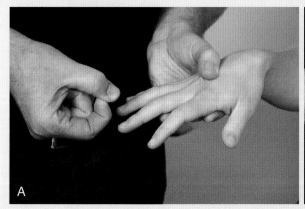

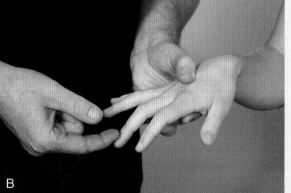

FIG. 2.62 See Video 2.41. **A,** Hoffman reflex start position. **B,** Hoffman reflex procedure: With the patient standing or sitting, the therapist stabilizes the proximal interphalangeal joint of the middle finger and applies a stimulus to the patient's finger by "flicking" the fingernail with his finger into distal interphalangeal flexion as the middle phalanx is stabilized. A positive test is reflexive adduction, flexion of the thumb, or flexion of the other fingers.

Continued

BOX 2.13 Upper Motor Neuron Screen for Cervical Myelopathy—cont'd

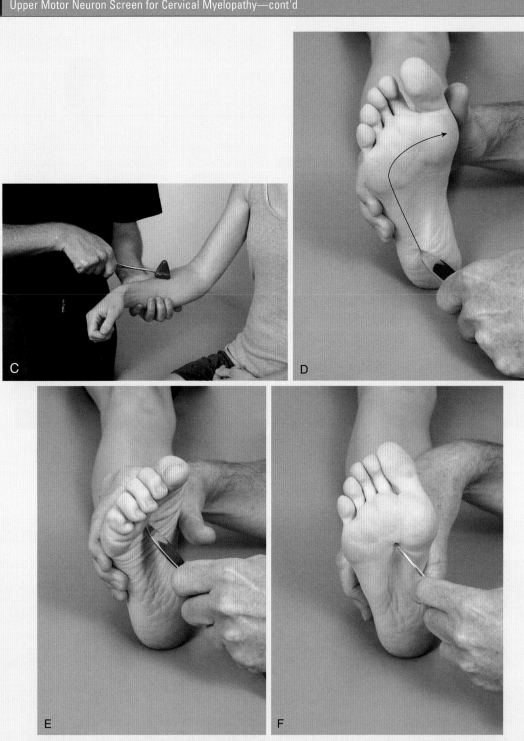

FIG. 2.62, cont'd See Video 2.42. **C,** Inverted supinator sign procedure: With the patient in a seated position, the therapist supports the patient's slightly pronated forearm on his forearm. The therapist applies a quick strike with a reflex hammer at the distal one-third of the radius near the attachment of the brachioradialis tendon. The test is performed in the same manner as a brachioradialis tendon reflex test. A positive test is reflexive finger flexion or reflexive elbow extension rather than the normal elbow flexion that occurs with deep tendon reflex test of the brachioradialis. See Video 2.43. **D,** Start position of Babinski sign. **E,** Negative Babinski sign. **F,** Positive Babinski sign. Babinski sign procedure: with the patient in a supine position, the therapist supports the patient's foot in neutral and applies stimulation to the lateral plantar surface of the foot from the heel to metatarsals and across the metatarsal heads with the blunt end of a reflex hammer. A positive test is reflexive great toe extension and fanning of the second through fifth toes rather than the negative response of flexion of the toes.

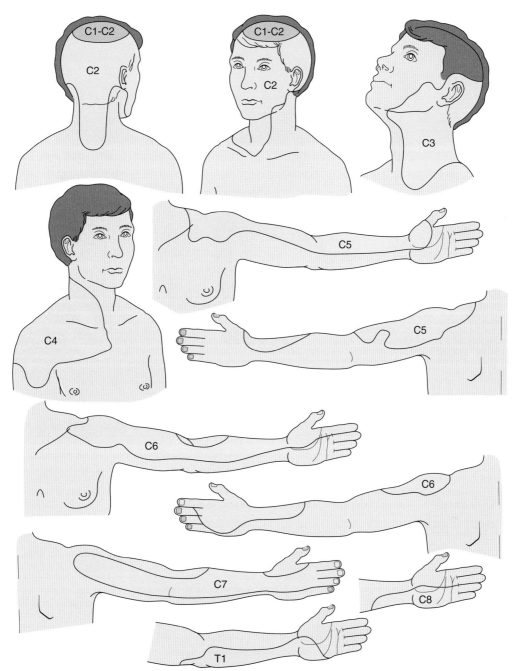

FIG. 2.63 Cervical dermatomes.

Deep tendon reflexes are graded 0 to 4, with a grade 2 considered normal, a grade 4 hypertonic, and a grade 0 absent, and they should be tested if neurologic involvement is suspected. Boxes 2.11 and 2.12 illustrate proper deep tendon reflex testing technique and provide the corresponding nerve root level for each deep tendon reflex (Figs. 2.60A–C and 2.61E,F). Vroomen et al.[148] reported reliability for testing Achilles and patella deep tendon reflexes on patients with lumbar radiculopathy as kappa values of 0.53 and 0.42.

Lauder et al.[149] used needle electrodiagnostic procedures as the gold standard for diagnosis of nerve root involvement as the cause of radiculopathy that included a motor nerve conduction study, a sensory nerve conduction study, and a standard 10-muscle EMG and compared the diagnosis with the results of the history and examination findings. The presence of numbness has a high sensitivity for cervical radiculopathy (79%), and subjects with weakness or a reduced reflex were two to five times more likely to have abnormal results on electrodiagnosis.[149] Reduced reflexes combined with weakness are associated with subjects having a ninefold increase in the likelihood of cervical radiculopathy, and subjects with a reduced biceps reflex were 10 times more likely to have a cervical radiculopathy with needle EMG.[149] For deep

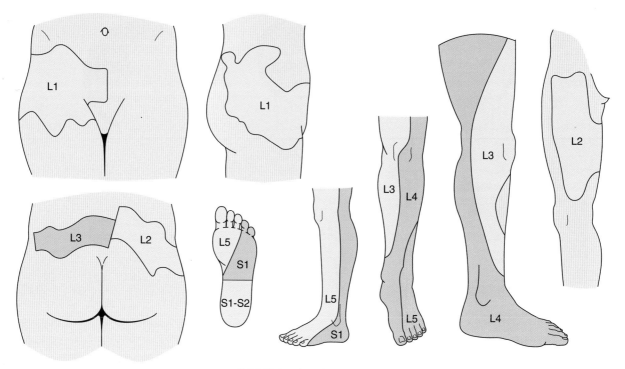

FIG. 2.64 Lumbar dermatomes.

TABLE 2.6	Myotomes of Upper Limb	
NERVE ROOT	**TEST ACTION**	**MUSCLES[a]**
C1–C2	Neck flexion	Rectus lateralis, rectus capitis anterior, longus capitis, longus colli, longus cervicis, and sternocleido-mastoid
C3	Neck side flexion	Longus capitis, longus cervicis, trapezius, and scalenus medius
C4	Shoulder elevation	Diaphragm, trapezius, levator scapulae, scalenus anterior, and scalenus medius
C5	Shoulder abduction	Rhomboid major and minor, deltoid, supraspinatus, infraspinatus, teres minor, biceps, and scalenus anterior and medius
C6	Elbow flexion and wrist extension	Serratus anterior; latissimus dorsi; subscapularis; teres major; pectoralis major (clavicular head); biceps; coracobrachialis; brachialis; brachioradialis; supinator; extensor carpi radialis longus; and scalenus antiori, medius, and posterior
C7	Elbow extension and wrist extension	Serratus anterior, latissimus dorsi, pectoralis major (sternal head), pectoralis minor, triceps, pronator teres, flexor carpi radialis, flexor digitorum superficialis, extensor carpi radialis longus, extensor carpi radialis brevis, extensor digitorum, extensor digiti minimi, and scalenus medius and posterior
C8	Thumb extension and ulnar deviation	Pectoralis major (sternal head), pectoralis minor, triceps, flexor digitorum superficialis, flexor digitorum profundus, flexor pollicis longus, pronator quadrates, flexor carpi ulnaris, abductor pollicis longus, extensor pollicis brevis, extensor indicis, abductor pollicis brevis, flexor pollicis brevis, opponens pollicis, and scalenus medius and posterior
T1	Hand intrinsic	Flexor digitorum profundus, intrinsic muscles of hand (except extensor pollicis brevis), flexor pollicis brevis, and opponens pollicis

[a]Muscles listed may be supplied by additional nerve roots; only primary nerve root sources are listed.
(From Magee DJ. *Orthopaedic Physical Assessment,* ed 5. Philadelphia: Saunders; 2007.)

tendon reflex testing, the biceps muscle sensitivity was 0.10, the specificity was 0.99, the +LR was 10.0, and the −LR was 0.91; the triceps deep tendon reflex muscle sensitivity was 0.10, the specificity was 0.95, the +LR was 2.0, and the −LR was 0.95; and the brachioradialis deep tendon reflex muscle sensitivity was 0.08, the specificity was 0.99, the +LR was 8.0, and the −LR was 0.93.[149] Neurodynamic tension tests are also considered part of the standard neurologic examination, and detailed descriptions are included in the lumbopelvic and cervical spine chapters (see Chapters 4 and 6).

TABLE 2.7	Myotomes of Lower Limb	
NERVE ROOT	**TEST ACTION**	**MUSCLES**
L1–L2	Hip flexion	Psoas, iliacus, sartorius, gracilis, pectineus, adductor longus, and adductor brevis
L3	Knee extension	Quadriceps; adductor longus, magnus, and brevis
L4	Ankle dorsiflexion	Tibialis anterior, quadriceps, tensor fasciae latae, adductor magnus, obturator externus, and tibialis posterior
L5	Toe extension	Extensor hallucis longus, extensor digitorum longus, gluteus medius and minimus, obturator internus, semimembranosus, semitendinosus, peroneus tertius, and popliteus
S1	Ankle plantar flexion Ankle eversion Hip extension Knee flexion	Gastrocnemius, soleus, gluteus maximus, obturator internus, piriformis, biceps femoris, semitendinosus, popliteus, peroneus longus and brevis, and extensor digitorum brevis
S2	Knee flexion	Biceps femoris, piriformis, soleus, gastrocnemius, flexor digitorum longus, flexor hallucis, and intrinsic foot muscles
S3	Toe plantar flexion	Intrinsic foot muscles (except abductor hallucis), flexor hallucis brevis, flexor digitorum brevis, and extensor digitorum brevis

(From Magee DJ. *Orthopaedic Physical Assessment,* ed 5. Philadelphia: Saunders; 2007.)

Cervical spine myelopathy results in upper motor neuron lesions of the spinal cord and is caused by space-occupying lesions of the central cervical vertebral canal, most commonly as a result of severe degenerative changes of the cervical spine that compress the spinal cord. Cook et al.[150] analyzed the data from 249 patients with cervical spine dysfunctions to determine which clinical tests and measures, when clustered together, were most diagnostic for cervical spine myelopathy compared with MRI findings of cervical spine myelopathy. Using multivariate regression analyses and calculations for sensitivity, specificity, and positive and negative likelihood ratios, a cluster of five clinical signs were identified: (1) gait deviation (wide-based gait, ataxia, or spastic gait); (2) presence of Hoffmann reflex (Fig. 2.62A,B); (3) inverted supinator sign (Fig. 2.62C); (4) positive Babinski test (Fig. 2.62D,E,F); and (5) age greater than 45 years[150] (Box 2.13). Any one positive of the five tests yielded a sensitivity of 0.94 (0.89–0.97) and a −LR of 0.18 (0.12–0.42).[150] This suggests that therapists who identify only one or fewer of the five positive test findings can be confident that the patient does not have cervical spine myelopathy. Three of five positive findings from the cluster were able to rule in cervical spine myelopathy (sensitivity = 0.19, specificity = 0.99, +LR = 30.9, and −LR = 0.81) with a posttest probability of 94%.[150]

EVALUATION OF EXAMINATION FINDINGS AND THE DIAGNOSIS

Clinical decision making in orthopaedic manual physical therapy should use an evidence-based approach. Research evidence supports the effectiveness of treating spinal disorders by subgrouping patients based on identification of key physical impairments, patient characteristics, and symptoms.[151] The treatment is based on the subgroup classification that the patient fits into at the time of the examination, and the subgrouping may change through the course of the treatment duration based on reexamination findings. With clinical situations in which the research evidence is not clear, use of an impairment-based approach is the foundation of physical therapy treatment of musculoskeletal disorders.

An impairment-based approach can guide clinical decision making when specific physical impairments (such as mobility deficits, joint hypermobility, and muscle weakness or tightness) are identified through the clinical examination, and appropriate interventions are administered based on the examination findings. For instance, identification of joint stiffness or hypomobility is an indication for spinal manipulation, and joint hypermobility and weakness are indications for spinal stabilization exercises. The presence of muscle or myofascial tightness is an indication for soft tissue mobilization techniques and stretching. In this way, a problem list can be generated, and a specific intervention for each impairment can be included in the plan of care. The overall management of the patient's condition is based on identification of clusters of signs and symptoms characteristic of a diagnosis or classification.

Fritz et al.[152] showed a correlation between patients who were judged as having lumbar hypomobility with PAIVM testing to respond favorably to spinal manipulation. In other words, patients with lumbar stiffness are more likely to respond favorably to spinal manipulation. In addition, a strong correlation for a positive response to a spinal stabilization exercise program was correlated with hypermobility noted with posteroanterior PAIVM testing of the lumbar spine. This correlation offers further support for an impairment-based approach and validates the use of posteroanterior PAIVM testing as an important component of a physical therapist examination scheme to determine the most effective intervention for spinal disorders.[152]

Typically, medical practitioners have based a diagnosis either on the patient's symptoms, such as neck pain or LBP, or on results of imaging studies, such as degenerative disc disease or osteoarthritis of the neck. Both of these types of diagnoses are inadequate to guide clinical decision making in physical therapy. The location of symptoms is only one finding that must be correlated with the behavior of the symptoms with activity and other important clinical findings, such as movement restrictions, joint restrictions, muscle length impairments, and muscle recruitment patterns. The location of the symptoms alone cannot be the sole guide for determination of the most effective intervention.

In one report, patients were given a symptom-based diagnosis at 64% of all visits to family physicians and emergency departments.[153] A symptom-based diagnosis was given at 91% of all emergency department visits for neck pain.[153] When a physician cannot identify a serious pathologic condition, the physician makes a diagnosis of sprain, strain, neck pain, or back pain 90% of the time, which is a symptom-based diagnosis that does nothing to guide the proper intervention.[153] These findings suggest that classification systems are needed to guide interventions for neck and back pain.

Likewise, the findings on imaging studies, such as MRI and radiographs, are commonly provided as the primary diagnosis. Although degenerative changes found on imaging studies of the spine could be contributing factors to the patient's set of signs and symptoms, they are unlikely to be the only factor. The presence or absence of degenerative changes in the spine cannot be the sole finding to guide physical therapy interventions. A wide range of spinal pathologic conditions have been shown on MRI results of asymptomatic persons, including degenerative changes, disc protrusions, disc herniations, free fragments, and annular tears.[98,154–157]

Most physical therapy interventions do not likely change the degenerative findings seen on imaging studies, but often improvements in mobility, pain, and function can be attained with physical therapy. The imaging findings often are the same at the end of the duration of the physical therapy treatment even when significant clinical improvements are noted. Therefore the imaging findings cannot be used to guide nonsurgical treatment in most cases.

Most evidence-based guidelines for treatment of spine conditions suggest use of imaging only when a patient has a red flag, has a recent history of significant trauma, or has not responded to at least 4 weeks of conservative management.[158] In these circumstances, imaging is indicated and typically starts with plain radiographs. If the patient has neurologic signs, an MRI may be indicated.

Completion of a comprehensive physical examination to determine whether the symptom behavior and physical impairments follow a typical musculoskeletal pattern can greatly assist in the medical screening and diagnostic process. In the evaluation, the physical therapist must state the clinical impression that best classifies or diagnoses the patient's condition.

Next, a problem list should be included that outlines the most significant impairments that contribute to the perpetuation of the patient's primary symptoms. The impairment-based classification system affords a great deal of guidance in clinical decision making in patients with spinal and TMJ disorders and is described in detail in Chapters 4 to 7.

PLAN OF CARE AND PROGNOSIS

Interventions must be identified in the plan of care to address the impairments and to best manage the patient's diagnosed condition. These clinical decisions should be based first on research evidence to support the interventions within the therapist's scope of practice and based on the therapist's clinical knowledge and experience regarding how to best address the impairments and manage the patient's condition. For each anatomic area addressed in Chapters 4 to 7, the clinical research is presented to assist in the clinical decision making for each classification.

The decision regarding frequency and duration of treatment is also based on clinical experience and research evidence. Typically, 4 to 6 weeks is needed to make significant progress in reducing the intensity of pain and severity of disability associated with many spinal conditions. An additional 4 to 6 weeks may be needed to fully restore strength and function. The duration of treatment and the prognosis are influenced by the general health and the psychosocial status of the patient as much as by the diagnosis. For instance, a patient who smokes, is diabetic, or has cardiovascular risk factors tends to recover at a slower rate. Psychosocial factors (such as elevated fear-avoidance beliefs, anxiety, and depression) can affect the rehabilitation process and delay return to work.[159] Job satisfaction before injury can affect the likelihood of recovery from a spine injury and return to work.[160] In addition, patient compliance with the therapist's recommendations and the patient's level of motivation to return to the prior level of function can affect the rate of recovery. All these factors must be considered as a prediction of duration of treatment and prognosis are made at the time of the initial examination.

In explanations of the findings of the examination and treatment plan to the patient with back or neck pain, efforts should be made to offer reassurance of a favorable prognosis and to assure the patient that most back injuries are not serious. The impact of reassurance and patient education provided by a healthcare worker has been shown to effect positive outcomes in treatment of back pain.[161] Spending time with the patient to answer questions, to reassure that conservative treatment can help improve the condition and to explain the plan of care can assist in development of a therapeutic alliance with the patient and in creating a favorable treatment outcome. Likewise, continuity of care by the same therapist working consistently with the same patient throughout the episode of care has been shown to result in improved treatment outcomes, to lower subsequent healthcare costs, and to lower the incidence of surgical procedures in patients with LBP.[162]

REFERENCES

1. Smart KM, Blake C, Staines A, et al. Self-reported pain severity, quality of life, disability, anxiety and depression in patients classified with 'nociceptive', peripheral neuropathic' and 'central sensitisation' pain. The discriminant validity of mechanisms-based classifications of low back (+leg) pain. *Man Ther.* 2012; 17:119-125.

2. Costigan M, Scholz J, Woolf CJ. Neuropathic pain: a maladaptive response of the nervous system to damage. *Annu Rev Neurosci.* 2009;32:1-32.

3. Latremoliere A, Woolf CJ. Central sensitization: a generator of pain hypersensitivity by central neural plasticity. *J Pain.* 2009; 10:895-926.

4. Smart KM, Blake C, Staines A, et al. Mechanisms-based classifications of musculoskeletal pain: part 3 of 3: symptoms and signs of nociceptive pain in patients with low back (leg) pain. *Man Ther.* 2012;17:352-357.

5. Smart KM, Blake C, Staines A, et al. Mechanisms-based classifications of musculoskeletal pain: part 2 of 3: symptoms and signs of peripheral neuropathic pain in patients with low back (leg) pain. *Man Ther.* 2012;17:345-351.

6. Smart KM, Blake C, Staines A, et al. Mechanisms-based classifications of musculoskeletal pain: part 1 of 3: symptoms and signs of central sensitisation in patients with low back (leg) pain. *Man Ther.* 2012b;17:336-344.

7. Boissonnault WG, Goodman C. Physical therapists as diagnosticians: drawing the line on diagnosing pathology. *J Orthop Sports Phys Ther.* 2006;36(6):351-353.

8. Cook CE, George SZ, Reiman MP. Red flag screening for low back pain: nothing to see here, move along: a narrative review. *Br J Sports Med.* 2018;52(8):493-496.

9. Boissonnault WG. *Primary Care for the Physical Therapist: Examination and Triage*, ed 2. Philadelphia: Saunders; 2010.

10. Greenhalgh S, Selfe J. *Red Flags and Blue Lights, Managing Series Spinal Pathology*, ed 2. London: Elsevier; 2019.

11. Ross MD, Boissonnault WG. Red flags: to screen or not to screen? *J Orthop Sports Phys Ther.* 2010;40(11):682-684.

12. Henschke N, Maher CG, Refshauge KM, et al. Prevalence of and screening for serious spinal pathology in patients presenting to primary care settings with acute low back pain. *Arthritis Rheum.* 2009;60:3072-3080.

13. Henschke N, Maher CG, Refshauge KM. Screening for malignancy in low back pain patients: a systematic review. *Eur Spine J.* 2007;16(10):1673-1679.

14. Deyo RA, Diehl AK. Cancer as a cause of back pain: frequency, clinical presentation, and diagnostic strategies. *J Gen Intern Med.* 1988;3(3):230-238.

15. Coleman R, Holen I. *Bone Metastases*, ed 5. Philadelphia, PA: Elsevier; 2014: Chapter 51.

16. Levack P, GrahamJ, Collie D, et al. *A prospective audit of the diagnosis, management, and outcome of malignant cord compression (CRAG 97/08).* Edinburgh: CRAG: West of Scotland NHS; 2001.

17. NICE. *Metastatic spinal cord compression in adults: risk assessment, diagnosis and management clinical guideline (CG75).* 2008.

18. Al-Qurainy R, Collis E. Metastatic spinal cord compression: diagnosis and management. *BMJ.* 2016;353(i2539):1-7.

19. National Institute for Health and Care Excellence (NICE). National Collaborating Centre for Cancer. National Institute for Health and Care Excellence clinical guideline 75. Metastatic spinal cord compression: Diagnosis and management of adults at risk of or with metastatic spinal cord compression. 2008. www.nice.org.uk/guidance/cg75.

20. Sutcliffe P, Connock M, Shyangdan D, et al. A systematic review of evidence on malignant spinal metastases: natural history and technologies for identifying patients at high risk of vertebral fracture and spinal cord compression. *Health Technol Assess.* 2013;17(42):1-274.

21. Loblaw DA, Perry J, Chambers A, et al. Systematic review of the diagnosis and management of malignant extradural spinal cord compression: the Cancer Care Ontario Practice Guidelines Initiative's Neuro-Oncology Disease Site Group. *J Clin Oncol.* 2005;23:2028-2037.

22. Turnpenney J, Greenhalgh S, Richards L, et al. Developing an early alert system for metastatic spinal cord compression. *Prim Health Care Res Dev.* 2015;16(1):14-20.

23. Harding I, Davies E, Buchannon E, et al. The symptom of night pain in a back pain triage clinic. *Spine.* 2005;30:1985-1988.

24. Finucane L, Greenhalgh S, Selfe J. What are the red flags to aid the early detection of metastatic bone disease as a cause of back pain? *Physiother Pract Res.* 2017;38(2):73-77.

25. Coleman R. Clinical features of metastatic bone disease and risk of skeletal morbidity. *Clin Cancer Res.* 2006;12:6243s-6249s.

26. Douraiswami B, Muthuswamy K, Naidu D, et al. Indeterminate cauda equine syndrome: a case report. *J Clin Ortho Trauma.* 2016;1(7):50-54.

27. Fraser S, Roberts L, Murphy E. Cauda equina syndrome: a literature review of its definition and clinical presentation. *Arch Phys Med Rehabil.* 2009;11:1964-1968.

28. Todd N, Dickson D. Standards of care in cauda equina syndrome. *Br J Neurosurg.* 2016;30(5):518-522.

29. Abrahm JL. Assessment and treatment of patients with malignant spinal cord compression. *J Support Oncol.* 2004;2:377-388, 391, discussion 391-393, 398, 401.

30. Deyo RA, Rainville J, Kent DL. What can the history and physical examination tell us about low back pain? *JAMA.* 1992;268(6):760-765.

31. Fairbank J. Cauda equina syndrome – risk management. *J Trauma and Orthop.* 2014;2(3):49-50.

32. Dionne N, Adefolarin A, Kunzelman D, et al. What is the diagnostic accuracy of red flags related to cauda equine syndrome (CES), when compared to magnetic resonance imaging (MRI)? A systematic review. *Musculoskelet Sci Pract.* 2019; 42:125-133.

33. Wainwright A. Infections of the spine. In: Bartley R, ed. *Management of low back pain in primary care.* Oxford: Butterworth-Heinemann; 2001.

34. Finucane L, Mercer C, Greenhalgh S, et al. International framework for red flags for potential serious spinal pathology. *JOSPT.* 2020;50(7):350-372.

35. Lam KS, Webb JK. Discitis. *Hosp Med.* 2004;65(5):280-286.

36. Hopkinson N, Stevenson J, Benjamin S. A case ascertainment study of septic discitis: clinical, microbiological and radiological features. *QJM.* 2001;94(9):465-470.

37. Jarvik JG, Deyo RA. Diagnostic evaluation of low back pain with emphasis on imaging. *Ann Intern Med.* 2002;137(7): 586-597.

38. Premkumar A, Godfrey W, Gottschalk MB, et al. Red flags for low back pain are not always really red: a prospective evaluation of the clinical utility of commonly used screening questions for low back pain. *J Bone Joint Surg Am.* 2018;100(5):368-374.

39. Duarte RM, Vaccaro AR. Spinal infection: state of the art and management algorithm. *Eur Spine J.* 2013;22(12):2787-2799.

40. Yusuf M, Finucane L, Selfe J. Red flags for the early detection of Spinal Infection in back pain patients a Scoping Review. *BMC Musculoskelet Disord.* 2019;20:606.

41. Gouliouris T, Aliyu SH, Brown NM. Spondylodiscitis: up- date on diagnosis and management. *J Antimicrob Chemother.* 2010; 65(Suppl 3):iii11-iii24.

42. Davis DP, Wold RM, Patel RJ, et al. The clinical presentation and impact of diagnostic delays on emergency department patients with spinal epidural abscess. *J Emerg Med.* 2004;26(3):285-291.

43. Lener S, Hartmann S, Barbagallo GMV, et al. Management of spinal infection: a review of the literature. *Acta Neurochir (Wien).* 2018;160:487-496.

44. Boissonnault WG, Koopmeiners MB. Medical history profile: orthopaedic physical therapy outpatients. *J Orthop Sports Phys Ther.* 1994;20(1):2-10.

45. Boissonnault WG, Meek PD. Risk factors for anti-inflammatory-drug or aspirin-induced gastrointestinal complications in individuals receiving outpatient physical therapy services. *J Orthop Sports Phys Ther.* 2002;32(10):510-517.

46. Wolfe MM, Lichtenstein DR, Singh G. Gastrointestinal toxicity of nonsteroidal antiinflammatory drugs. *N Engl J Med.* 1999; 340(24):1888-1899.

47. Childs JD, Fritz JM, Piva SR, et al. Proposal of a classification system for patients with neck pain. *J Orthop Sports Phys Ther.* 2004;34(11):686-700.

48. George SZ, Fritz JM, Bialosky JE, et al. The effect of a fear-avoidance-based physical therapy intervention for patients with acute low back pain: results of a randomized clinical trial. *Spine.* 2003;28(23):2551-2560.

49. Sterling M, Jull G, Kenardy J. Physical and psychological factors maintain long-term predictive capacity post-whiplash injury. *Pain.* 2006;122(1-2):102-108.

50. Haggman S, Maher CG, Refshauge KM. Screening for symptoms of depression by physical therapists managing low back pain. *Phys Ther.* 2004;84(12):1157-1166.

51. Arrol B, Goodyear-Smith F, Kerse N, et al. Effect of the addition of a "help" question to two screening questions on specificity for diagnosis of depression in general practice: diagnostic validity study. *BMJ.* 2005;331:884.

52. American Psychiatric Association (APA). *Diagnostic and Statistical Manual of Mental Disorders,* ed 4. Washington, DC: APA; 2000.

53. Wideman TH, Scott W, Martel MO, Sullivan MJL. Recovery from depressive symptoms over the course of physical therapy: a prospective cohort study of individuals with work-related orthopaedic injuries and symptoms of depression. *J Orthop Sports Phys Ther.* 2012;42(11):957-967.

54. Pengal LHM, Refshauge KM, Maher CG. Responsiveness of pain, disability, and physical impairment outcomes in patients with low back pain. *Spine.* 2004;29(8):879-883.

55. Hill JC, Dunn KM, Lewis M, et al. A primary care back pain screening tool: identifying patient subgroups for initial treatment. *Arthritis Rheum.* 2008;59(5):632-641.

56. Hay EM, Dunn KM, Hill JC, et al. A randomized clinical trial of subgrouping and targeted treatment for low back pain compared with best current care. The STarT Back Trail study protocal. *BMC Musculoskelet Disord.* 2008;9(58):1-9.

57. Hill JC, Whitehurst DG, Lewis M, et al. Comparison of stratified primary care management for low back pain with current best practice (STarT Back): a randomized controlled trial. *Lancet.* 2011;378:1560-1571.

58. Waddell G, Newton M, Henderson I, et al. A Fear-Avoidance Beliefs Questionnaire (FABQ) and the role of fear-avoidance beliefs in chronic low back pain and disability. *Pain.* 1993; 52(2):157-168.

59. Fritz JM. A comparison of a modified Oswestry low back pain disability questionnaire and the Quebec Back Pain Disability Scale. *Phys Ther.* 2001;81(2):776-788.

60. Hicks GE, Fritz JM, Delitto A, et al. Preliminary development of a clinical prediction rule for determining which patients with low back pain will respond to a stabilization exercise program. *Arch Phys Med Rehabil.* 2005;86(9):1753-1762.

61. Flynn T, Fritz J, Whitman J, et al. A clinical prediction rule for classifying patients with low back pain who demonstrate short-term improvement with spinal manipulation. *Spine.* 2002;27(24): 2835-2843.

62. George SZ, Fritz JM, Childs JD. Investigation of elevated fear-avoidance beliefs for patients with low back pain: a secondary analysis involving patients enrolled in physical therapy clinical trials. *J Orthop Sports Phys Ther.* 2008;38(2):50-58.

63. George SZ, Stryker SE. Fear-avoidance beliefs and clinical outcomes for patients seeking outpatient physical therapy for musculoskeletal pain conditions. *J Orthop Sports Phys Ther.* 2011; 41(4):249-259.

64. Cleland JA, Fritz JM, Whitman JM, et al. The reliability and construct validity of the Neck Disability Index and the patient specific functional scale in patients with cervical radiculopathy. *Spine.* 2006;31(5):598-602.

65. Mayer TG, Neblett R, Cohen H, et al. The development and psychometric validation of the central sensitization inventory. *Pain Pract.* 2012;12:276-285.

66. Den Boer C, Dries L, Terluin B, et al. Central Sensitization in chronic pain and medically unexplained symptom research: a systematic review of definitions, operationalizations and measurement instruments. *J Psychom Res.* 2019;117:32-40.

67. Jorgensen R, Ris I, Falla D, et al. Reliability, construct and discriminate validity of clinical testing in subjects with and without chronic neck pain. *BMC Musculoskelet Disord.* 2014;15:408.

68. Walton DM, Macdermid JC, Nielson W, et al. Reliability, standard error, and minimal detectable change of clinical pressure pain threshold testing in people with and without acute neck pain. *J Orthop Sports Phys Ther.* 2011;41(9):644-650.

69. Neblett R, Cohen H, Choi Y, et al. The central sensitization inventory (CSI): establishing clinically significant values for identifying central sensitivity syndromes in an outpatient chronic pain sample. *J Pain.* 2013;14(5):438-445.

70. Cuesta-Vargas AI, Neblett R, Chiarotto A, et al. Dimensionality and reliability of the central sensitization inventory in a pooled multicountry sample. *J Pain.* 2018;19(3):317-329.

71. Scerbo T, Colasurdo J, Dunn S, et al. Measurement properties of the central sensitization inventory: a systematic review. *Pain Pract.* 2018;18(4):544-554.

72. Jenkins CD, Stanton BA, Niemcryk SJ, et al. A scale for the estimation of sleep problems in clinical research. *J Clin Epidemiol.* 1988;41(4):313-321.

73. Ornat L, Martinez-Dearth R, Chedraui P, et al. Assessment of subjective sleep disturbance and related factors during female mid-life with the Jenkins Sleep Scale. *Marturitas.* 2014;77: 344-350.

74. Jerlock M, Gaston-Johansson F, Kjellgren KI, et al. Coping strategies, stress, physical activity and sleep in patients with unexplained chest pain. *BMC Nurs.* 2006;5:7.

75. Lallukka T, Rahkonen O, Lahelma E. Workplace bullying and subsequent sleep problems—the Helsinki Health Study. *Scand J Work Environ Health.* 2011;37:204-212.

76. Lallukka T, Haaramo P, Lahelma E, et al. Sleep problems and disability retirement: a register-based follow-up study. *Am J Epidemiol.* 2011;173:871-881.

77. Lallukka T, Dregan A, Armstrong D. Comparison of a sleep item from the general health questionnaire-12 with the Jenkins Sleep Questionnaire as measures of sleep disturbance. *J Epidemiol.* 2011;21(6):474-480.

78. American Academy of Sleep Medicine. *International Classification of Sleep Disorders, Revised: Diagnostic and Coding Manual.* Chicago, IL: American Academy of Sleep Medicine; 2001.

79. Nutt D, Wilson S, Paterson L. Sleep disorders as core symptoms of depression. *Dialogues Clin Neurosci.* 2008;10:329-336.

80. Taylor DJ, Lichstein KL, Durrence HH, et al. Epidemiology of insomnia, depression, and anxiety. *Sleep.* 2005;28:1457-1464.

81. Shubert CR, Cruickshanks KJ, Dalton DS, et al. Prevalence of sleep problems and quality of life in an older population. *Sleep.* 2001;25:889-893.

82. Smith MT, Haythornthwaite JA. How do sleep disturbance and chronic pain inter-relate: insights from the longitudinal and cognitive-behavioral clinical trials literature. *Sleep Med Rev.* 2004;8:119-132.

83. Smith MT, Quartana PJ, Okonkwo RM, et al. Mechanisms by which sleep disturbance contributes to osteoarthritis pain: a conceptual model. *Current Pain Headache Rep.* 2009;13:447-454.

84. Siengsukon CF, Al-dughmi M, Stevens S. Sleep health promotion: practical information for physical therapists. *Phys Ther.* 2017;97:826-836.

85. Fairbank JC, Couper J, Davies JB, et al. The Oswestry low back pain disability questionnaire. *Physiotherapy.* 1980;66(8):271-273.

86. Hudson-Cook N, Tomes-Nicholson K, Breen A. A revised Oswestry disability questionnaire. In: Roland MO, Jenner JR, editors. *Back Pain: New Approaches to Rehabilitation and Education.* New York: Manchester University Press; 1989.

87. Beurskens AJ, de Vet HC, Koke AJ. Responsiveness of functional status in low back pain: a comparison of different instruments. *Pain.* 1996;65(1):71-76.

88. Davidson M, Keating JL. A comparison of five low back disability questionnaires: reliability and responsiveness. *Phys Ther.* 2002;82(1):8-24.

89. Vernon H, Mior S. The Neck Disability Index: a study of reliability and validity. *J Manipulative Physiol Ther.* 1991;14(7):409-415.

90. MacDermid JC, Walton DM, Avery S, et al. Measurement properties of the neck disability index: a systematic review. *J Orthop Sports Phys Ther.* 2009;39(5):400-417.

91. Cleland JA, Childs JD, Fritz JM, et al. Development of a clinical prediction rule for guiding treatment of a subgroup of patients with neck pain: use of thoracic spine manipulation, exercise, and patient education. *Phys Ther.* 2007;87(1):9-23.

92. Stewart M, Maher MG, Refshauge KM. Responsiveness of pain and disability measures for chronic whiplash. *Spine.* 2007;32(5):580-585.

93. Chatman A, Hyams S, Neel J, et al. The patient-specific functional scale: measurement properties in patients with knee dysfunction. *Phys Ther.* 1997;77:820-829.

94. Stratford P, Gill C, Westaway M, et al. Assessing disability and change in individual patients: a report of a patient-specific measure. *Physiother Can.* 1995;47:258-263.

95. Westaway M, Stratford P, Binkley J. The patient-specific functional scale: validation of its use in persons with neck dysfunction. *J Orthop Sports Phys Ther.* 1998;27(5):331-338.

96. Hefford C, Abbott JH, Arnold R, et al. The patient-specific functional scale: validity, reliability, and responsiveness in patients with upper extremity musculoskeletal problems. *J Orthop Sports Phys Ther.* 2012;42(2):56-65.

97. Horn KK, Jennings S, Richardson G, et al. The patient-specific functional scale: psychometrics, clinimetrics, and application as a clinical outcome measure. *J Orthop Sports Phys Ther.* 2012;42(1):30-42.

98. Jensen MC, Brant-Zanwadzki MN, Obuchowski N, et al. Magnetic resonance imaging of the lumbar spine in people without back pain. *N Engl J Med.* 1994;331(2):69-73.

99. Jensen MP, Turner JA, Romano JM. What is the maximum number of levels needed in pain intensity measurement? *Pain.* 1994;58(3):387-392.

100. Jensen MPT, Turner JA, Romano JM, et al. Comparative reliability and validity of chronic pain intensity measures. *Pain.* 1999;83(2):157-162.

101. Childs JD, Piva SR, Fritz JM. Responsiveness of the numeric pain rating scale in patients with low back pain. *Spine.* 2005;30(11):1331-1334.

102. Doody C, McAteer M. Clinical reasoning of expert and novice physiotherapists in an outpatient orthopaedic setting. *Physiotherapy.* 2002;88:258-268.

103. Taylor CS, Coxon AJ, Watson PC. Do L5 and S1 nerve root compressions produce radicular pain in a dermatomal pattern? *Spine.* 2013;38:995-998.

104. Bishop MD, Mintken P, Bialosky JE, et al. Patient expectations of benefit from interventions for neck pain and resulting influence on outcomes. *J Orthop Sports Phys Ther.* 2013;43(7):457-465.

105. Puentedura EJ, Cleland JA, Landers MR, et al. Development of a clinical prediction rule to identify patients with neck pain likely to benefit from thrust joint manipulation to the cervical spine. *J Orthop Sports Phys Ther.* 2012;42(7):577-592.

106. Kendall FP, McCreary EK, Provance PG. *Muscles Testing and Function with Posture and Pain*, ed 4. Baltimore: Williams and Wilkins; 1993.

107. Giles L, Taylor J. Low back pain associated with leg length inequality. *Spine.* 1981;6(5):510-521.

108. Piva SR, Erhard RE, Childs JD, et al. Inter-rater reliability of passive intervertebral and active movements of the cervical spine. *Man Ther.* 2006;11(4):321-330.

109. Youdas JW, Carey JR, Garrett TR. Reliability of measurements of cervical spine range of motion: comparison of three methods. *Phys Ther.* 1991;71(2):98-106.

110. Nitchke J, Nattrass C, Disler P, et al. Reliability of the American Medical Association guides' model for measuring spinal range of motion. *Spine.* 1999;24(3):262-268.

111. Maher C, Adams R. Reliability of pain and stiffness assessments in clinical manual lumbar spine examination. *Phys Ther.* 1984;74(9):809-811.

112. Cleland JA. *Orthopaedic Clinical Examination: an Evidence-Based Approach for Physical Therapists.* Carlstadt, NJ: Icon Learning Systems; 2005.

113. Olson KA, Goehring M. Intra and inter-rater reliability of a goniometric lower trunk rotation measurement. *J Back Musculoskelet Rehabil.* 2009;22:157-164.

114. Downey BJ, Taylor NF, Niere KR. Manipulative physiotherapists can reliably palpate nominated lumbar spinal levels. *Man Ther*. 1999;4(3):151-156.

115. Maitland G. *Vertebral Manipulation*, ed 5. London: Butterworth; 1986.

116. Gonnella C, Paris SV, Kutner M. Reliability in evaluating passive intervertebral motion. *Phys Ther*. 1982;62(4):436-444.

117. Paris SV. *Introduction to Spinal Evaluation and Manipulation*. Atlanta: Institute Press; 1986.

118. Olson K, Paris S, Spohr C, et al. Radiographic assessment and reliability study of the craniovertebral sidebending test. *J Man Manipulative Ther*. 1998;6(2):87-96.

119. Patla C, Paris SV. Reliability of interpretation of the Paris classification of normal end feel for elbow flexion and extension. *J Man Manipulative Ther*. 1993;1(2):60-66.

120. Bigos S, Bowyer O, Braen G, et al. Acute low back problems in adults. In: *Clinical practice guideline no. 14, Agency for Health Care Policy and Research (AHCPR) Publication No. 95–0642*. Rockville, MD: US Department of Health and Human Services; 1994.

121. Blomberg S, Hallin G, Grann K, et al. Manual therapy with steroid injections: a new approach to treatment of low back pain. *Spine*. 1994;19(5):569-577.

122. DiFabio R. Manipulation of the cervical spine: risks and benefits. *Phys Ther*. 1999;79(1):50-65.

123. Koes B, Bouter L, VanMameren H, et al. The effectiveness of manual therapy, physiotherapy, and treatment by the general practitioner for nonspecific back and neck complaints. *Spine*. 1992;17(1):28-35.

124. Meade T, Dyer S, Browne W, et al. Low back pain of mechanical origin: randomised comparison of chiropractic and hospital outpatient treatment. *BMJ*. 1990;300:1431-1437.

125. Nilsson N, Christensen H, Hartvigsen J. The effect of spinal manipulation in the treatment of cervicogenic headache. *J Manipulative Physiol Ther*. 1997;20(5):326-330.

126. Nwuga V. Relative therapeutic efficacy of vertebral manipulation and conventional treatment in back pain management. *Am J Phys Med*. 1982;61(6):273-278.

127. Schoensee S, Jensen G, Nicholson G, et al. The effect of mobilization on cervical headaches. *J Orthop Sports Phys Ther*. 1995;21(4):184-196.

128. Twomey L, Taylor L. Spine update: exercise and spinal manipulation in the treatment of low back pain. *Spine*. 1995;20(5):615-619.

129. Binkley J, Stratford PW, Gill C. Interrater reliability of lumbar accessory motion mobility testing. *Phys Ther*. 1995;75(9):786-792.

130. Nansel D, Peneff A, Jansen R, et al. Interexaminer concordance in detecting joint-play asymmetries in the cervical spines of otherwise asymptomatic subjects. *J Manipulative Physiol Ther*. 1989;12(6):428-433.

131. Strender L, Lundin M, Nell K. Interexaminer reliability in physical examination of the neck. *J Manipulative Physiol Ther*. 1997;20(8):516-520.

132. Hicks GE, Fritz JM, Delitto A, et al. Interrater reliability of clinical examination measures for identification of lumbar segmental instability. *Arch Phys Med Rehabil*. 2003;84:1858-1864.

133. Abbott JH, McCane B, Herbison P, et al. Lumbar segmental instability: a criterion-related validity study of manual therapy assessment. *BMC Musculoskelet Disord*. 2005;6(56):1-10.

134. Smedmark V, Wallin M, Arvidsson I. Inter-examiner reliability in assessing passive intervertebral motion of the cervical spine. *Man Ther*. 2000;5(2):97-101.

135. Jull G, Bogduk N, Marsland A. The accuracy of manual diagnosis of for cervical zygapophyseal joint pain syndromes. *Med J Aust*. 1988;148(5):233-236.

136. Cibulka M, Koldehoff R. Clinical usefulness of a cluster of sacroiliac joint tests in patients with and without low back pain. *J Orthop Sports Phys Ther*. 1999;29(2):83-92.

137. Potter N, Rothstein J. Intertester reliability for selected clinical tests of the sacroiliac joint. *Phys Ther*. 1985;65(11):1671-1675.

138. Arab AM, Abdollahi I, Joghataei MT. Inter- and intra-examiner reliability of single and composites of selected motion palpation and pain provocation tests for sacroiliac joint. *Man Ther*. 2009;14:213-221.

139. Jarett LL, Olson KA, Bohannon RW. *Reliability in Examining Craniovertebral Sidebending* (Master's thesis). St Augustine, FL: University of St Augustine; 2005.

140. Manipulation Education Committee. *Manipulation Education Manual for Physical Therapist Professional Degree Programs*. Alexandria, VA: APTA; 2004.

141. Simons DG, Travell JG, Simons LS. *Myofascial Pain and Dysfunction: the Trigger Point Manual*, vol. 1. Philadelphia: Lippincott Williams and Wilkins; 1999.

142. Dommerholt J, Fernandez-de-las-Penas C. *Trigger Point Dry Needling: an Evidenced and Clinical-Based Approach*. Edinburgh: Churchill Livingstone/Elsevier; 2013.

143. Lucas KR, Rich PA, Polus BI. Muscle activation patterns in the scapular positioning muscles during loaded scapular plane elevation: the effects of latent myofascial trigger points. *Clin Biomech*. 2010;25(8):765-770.

144. Fernandez-de-las-Penas C, Ge HY, Arendt-Neilsen L. Referred pain from muscle/myofascial trigger points. In: Fernandez-de-las-Penas C, Cleland J, Heijbregts P, editors. *Neck and Arm Pain Syndromes: Evidence-Informed Screening, Diagnosis, and Conservative Management*. London: Churchill Livingstone/Elsevier; 2011:404–418.

145. Gerwin RD, Shannon S, Hong CZ, et al. Interrater reliability in myofascial trigger point examination. *Pain*. 1997;69(1-2):65-73.

146. Neziri AY, Scaramozzino P, Andersen OK, et al. Reference values of mechanical and thermal pain tests in a pain-free population. *Eur J Pain*. 2010;15(4):376-383.

147. Strender L, Sjoblom A, Ludwig R, et al. Interexaminer reliability in physical examination of patients with low back pain. *Spine*. 1997;22(7):814-820.

148. Vroomen PC, de Krom MC, Knottnerus JA. Consistency of history taking and physical examination in patients with suspected lumbar nerve root involvement. *Spine*. 2000;25(1):91-97.

149. Lauder TD, Dillingham TR, Andary M, et al. Predicting electrodiagnostic outcome in patients with upper limb symptoms: are the history and physical examination helpful? *Arch Phys Med Rehabil*. 2000;81(4):436-441.

150. Cook C, Brown C, Isaacs R, et al. Clustered clinical findings for diagnosis of cervical spine myelopathy. *J Man Manipulative Ther*. 2010;18(4):175-180.

151. Brennan GP, Fritz JM, Hunter SJ, et al. Identifying subgroups of patients with acute/subacute "nonspecific" low back pain: results of a randomized clinical trial. *Spine*. 2006;31(6):623-631.

152. Fritz J, Whitman JM, Childs JD. Lumbar spine segmental mobility assessment: an examination of validity for determining intervention strategies in patients with low back pain. *Arch Phys Med Rehabil.* 2005;86(9):1745-1752.

153. Riddle DL, Schappert SM. Volume and characteristics of inpatient and ambulatory medical care for neck pain in the United States: data from three national surveys. *Spine.* 2007;32(1): 132-140.

154. Gore DR. Roentgenographic findings in cervical spine in asymptomatic persons: a ten-year follow-up. *Spine.* 2001;26(22): 2463-2466.

155. Petren-Mallmin M, Linder J. MRI cervical spine findings in asymptomatic fighter pilots. *Aviat Space Environ Med.* 1999; 70(12):1183-1188.

156. Siivola SM, Levoska S, Tervonen O, et al. MIR changes of cervical spine in asymptomatic and symptomatic young adults. *Eur Spine J.* 2002;11(4):358-363.

157. Stadnik TW, Lee RR, Coen HL, et al. Annular tears and disk herniation: prevalence and contrast enhancement on MR images in the absence of low back pain or sciatica. *Radiology.* 1998; 206:49-55.

158. Koes BW, van Tulder MW, Oselo R, et al. Clinical guidelines for the management of low back pain in primary care: an international comparison. *Spine.* 2001;26(22):2504-2514.

159. Fritz JM, Delitto A, Erhard RE. Comparison of classification-based physical therapy with therapy based on clinical practice guidelines for patients with acute low back pain: a randomized clinical trial. *Spine.* 2003;28(13):1363-1371.

160. Hoogendoorn WE, van Poppel MN, Bongers PM, et al. Systematic review of psychosocial factors at work and private life as risk factors for back pain. *Spine.* 2000;25(16):2114-2125.

161. Waddell G. *The Back Pain Revolution.* Edinburgh: Churchill Livingstone; 2004.

162. Magel J, Jaewhan K, Thackeray A, et al. Associations between physical therapy continuity of care and health care utilization and costs in patients with low back pain: a retrospective Cohort Study. *Phys Ther.* 2018;98(12):990-999.

CHAPTER 3

Manipulation Theory, Practice, Clinical Reasoning, and Education

OVERVIEW

The purpose of this chapter is to present principles related to the practice of mobilization/manipulation. Theories are described that attempt to explain the effects of mobilization/manipulation. A brief overview of the evidence that supports the use of mobilization/manipulation is presented, but further detail on the evidence is provided in the anatomic regional chapters. In addition, potential adverse effects and contraindications to manipulation are discussed, and concepts of learning and teaching manipulation are also presented. An introduction to psychologically informed language and pain neuroscience education are also included to assist in the clinical reasoning and management of patients with musculoskeletal conditions.

OBJECTIVES

- Describe the theories that explain the effects of manipulation.
- Present an overview of the evidence for the effectiveness of manipulation.
- Explain the clinical reasoning framework used by manual and musculoskeletal physical therapists.
- Explain the likelihood of adverse effects and contraindications and precautions to manipulation.
- Describe the guiding principles of hand/body placement and handling skills for the performance of manipulation technique.
- Describe the components of effective motor learning principles that facilitate learning performance of manipulation.
- Use psychologically informed language and pain neuroscience education to effectively manage pain-related musculoskeletal conditions.

INTRODUCTION OF MANIPULATION

The *Guide to Physical Therapist Practice*[1] considers manipulation as an interchangeable term with mobilization and defines mobilization/manipulation as a manual therapy technique comprising "a continuum of skilled passive movements to joints and/or related soft tissues that are applied at varying speeds and amplitudes, including a small-amplitude/high-velocity therapeutic movement."[1] The American Physical Therapy Association (APTA) Manipulation Education Committee further refined the definition of high-velocity thrust manipulation as "high-velocity, low-amplitude therapeutic movements within or at end range of motion (ROM)."[2] These definitions are used throughout this textbook.

The International Federation of Orthopaedic Manipulative Physical Therapists (IFOMPT) defines manipulation as "a passive, high velocity, low amplitude thrust applied to a joint complex within its anatomical limit with the intent to restore optimal motion, function, and/or to reduce pain."[3] IFOMPT further defines mobilization as "a manual therapy technique comprising a continuum of skilled passive movements that are applied at varying speeds and amplitudes to joints, muscles or nerves with the intent to restore optimal motion, function, and/or to reduce pain.[3] The National Center for Complementary and Integrative Health uses the term *spinal manipulative therapy* (SMT) and states that SMT is another term for spinal manipulation that is practiced by healthcare professionals, such as chiropractors, osteopathic physicians, and physical therapists, and practitioners perform spinal manipulation by using their hands or a device to apply a controlled force to a joint of the spine (National Institutes of Health). Therefore

SMT is a term used in interprofessional context by practitioners and researchers related to the practice and study of spinal manipulation.

Some manual physical therapy clinicians and researchers prefer to use the term *manipulation* for the high-velocity, low-amplitude thrust techniques and the term *mobilization* for the nonthrust techniques.[4] Both the IFOMPT and the APTA definitions imply that there is overlap between the definitions of mobilization and manipulation. Therefore the terms *thrust* and *nonthrust* will precede manipulation and mobilization when this level of clarity is required for the description of a specific manual therapy technique. Mintken et al.[5] have proposed that six categories of information should be included in a thorough description of a manipulation technique: (1) rate of force application, (2) location in range of available movement, (3) direction of force, (4) target of force, (5) relative structural movement, and (6) patient position.[5]

An infinite variety of manipulation procedures is possible throughout the spine. Slight variations in hand placement and patient positioning combined with variations in velocity, rhythm, and depth of force application can be made to meet the therapeutic goals of the manual therapy procedure. The techniques included in this text have been chosen based on application of biomechanical principles, their ability to be modified to meet specific patient needs, the evidence to support the use of the techniques, and the clinical usefulness and safety of the techniques. Maitland[6] has provided a framework for description of various grades of mobilization/manipulation based on the depth within the ROM that the force is applied and the rate of oscillation application. Table 3.1 provides further description of the grades of mobilization/manipulation. Fig. 3.1 has useful diagrams to assist in understanding the application of various depths of force with each grade of

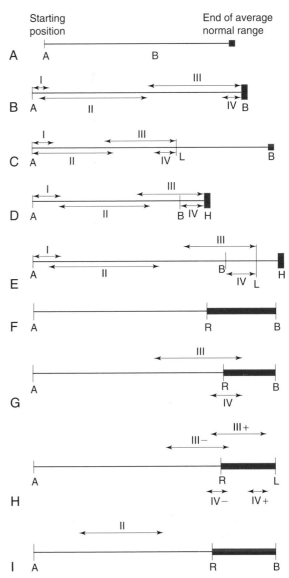

FIG. 3.1 A, Depiction of range of movement. **B,** Grades in normal range with hard end feel. **C,** Grades in hypermobile joint. **D,** Grades in relation to hypermobile asymptomatic range. **E,** Grades in hypermobile range with slight limitation and hard end feel. **F,** Depiction of soft end feel. **G,** Grades III and IV under soft end feel. **H,** Depiction of techniques taken into resistance in grades III and IV under soft end feel. **I,** Grade II movements are always resistance-free movements. *A,* Starting position; *B,* range of movement beyond normal average range; *H,* end of hypermobile range; *L,* pathologic limit of range (hard end feel); *N,* normal hypermobile range; *R,* beginning of resistance. (Modified from Maitland G, Hengeveld E, Banks K, et al. *Maitland's Vertebral Manipulation,* ed 7. Edinburgh: Elsevier; 2005.)

TABLE 3.1	Types of Mobilization/Manipulation Techniques
TYPE	**DESCRIPTION**
Grade I oscillation	Small-amplitude movement performed near starting position of range
Grade II oscillation	Large-amplitude movement performed within range but not reaching limit of range; can occupy any part of range that is free of stiffness or muscle guarding
Grade III oscillation	Large-amplitude movement performed up to limit of range and moving into stiffness or muscle guarding
Grade IV oscillation	Small-amplitude movement performed at limit of range, stretching into stiffness or muscle guarding
High-velocity thrust	High-velocity, low-amplitude therapeutic movements within or at end range of motion
Isometric	Patient's muscles are used to mobilize a joint by performing an isometric contraction against operator's resistance

manipulation. Grades I and II are within the range that is free of resistance, and grades III and IV are passive movements that move up to the point of resistance. Grades III+ and IV+ are passive movements that stretch into the resistance of a joint with a mobility deficit.

Paris[7] has described a progressive oscillation manipulation force application that provides a useful way to sequentially and gradually increase the force deeper into the range of allowable passive mobility. Once the end of the available range is reached, further end-range oscillations (i.e., grade III+ or IV+), sustained stretch, or short-amplitude, high-velocity thrust may be applied. The treatment effect of reducing pain and restoring mobility can be attained with end-range oscillatory techniques, progressive oscillation, or a small-amplitude, high-velocity thrust. Grade I and II mobilization techniques tend to be used for pain inhibition because of the neurophysiologic effects of manipulation. The advantage of the thrust manipulation is that the patient is less able to actively guard against a thrust and the mechanical and neurophysiologic effects of the manipulation can be maximized.

Isometric manipulation, or muscle energy technique (MET), is a form of manipulative treatment in which the patient actively uses muscles on request from the therapist as the therapist holds the patient's joint in a precisely controlled position, in a specific direction, and against a specific counterforce.[8] The technique is carried out with gradually increasing tension and the technique application is similar to a hold relax stretch technique as described by Knott and Voss,[9] but increased emphasis on positioning focuses the forces at a targeted joint. The joint is positioned at the point of a barrier to further movement. This position is held as the patient is asked to actively move out of the position but is held in the position by the therapist. After the isometric contraction, the joint is moved actively or passively further into the desired ROM. Isometric manipulations use the local muscles attached at the motion segment to theoretically stretch the joint and reflexively inhibit the local muscle tone at the spinal segment to allow easier application of an end-range manipulation. The effectiveness of these techniques may also be linked to muscle facilitation at the spinal motion segment.

Mobilizations with movement (MWM) are manual therapy techniques developed and popularized by physiotherapist Brian Mulligan in which a sustained passive accessory joint mobilization is combined with an active or functional movement.[10] Mulligan[11] refers to the MWM of the spine as "*SNAGs,*" which stands for sustained natural apophyseal glides. SNAGs are MWM performed in a weight-bearing position in which the direction of the mobilization forces is applied along the plane of the targeted facet joint.[11] The SNAGs are typically repeated for up to three sets of 10 repetitions, as long as the range of pain-free motion continues to improve throughout the treatment session.[10] SNAGs are a useful adjunct to other mobilization/manipulation and therapeutic exercise procedures.

EVIDENCE FOR MANIPULATION

The highest level of evidence to support interventions is based on the recommendations of clinical practice guidelines, systematic reviews, and metaanalysis.[12] Numerous clinical practice guidelines have recommended manipulation for the treatment of spinal disorders.[13–15] The strongest support in the literature for thrust manipulation is for the treatment of acute low back pain (LBP). Numerous clinical practice guidelines recommend

the inclusion of manipulation within the first 4 to 6 weeks of acute LBP without radiculopathy.[13–15] The first such guideline to recommend manipulation for acute LBP was the U.S. Agency for Health Care Policy and Research,[13] which provided the highest ranking of evidence for manipulation for any intervention included in the review. Since that time, multiple clinical practice guidelines have arrived at the same conclusion.[13–15] In a systematic review of national guidelines for the treatment of LBP, the vast majority, but not all, of the guidelines recommend spinal manipulation for acute and chronic LBP.[16] A recent metaanalysis of randomized controlled trials (RCTs) on benefits of SMT for chronic LBP concluded that SMT results in a modest beneficial effect.[17] Likewise, a systematic review and metaanalysis of the effects of SMT for acute LBP concluded that SMT was associated with modest improvements in pain and function.[18] The Low Back Pain Clinical Practice Guideline from the Orthopaedic Academy of the APTA provided a strong endorsement for using thrust manipulative procedures to reduce pain and disability in patients with mobility deficits and acute low back and back-related buttock or thigh pain and further recommend that thrust manipulation and nonthrust mobilization procedures can be used to improve spine and hip mobility and reduce pain and disability in patients with subacute and chronic low back and back-related lower extremity pain.[19]

In regard to treatment of neck pain, the clinical practice guidelines tend to support a multimodular approach that combines nonthrust mobilization or thrust manipulation with specific therapeutic exercise programs.[20] A 2010 Cochrane systematic review attempted to delineate whether thrust manipulation or nonthrust mobilization used alone has a therapeutic effect on adults experiencing neck pain.[21] The authors concluded that moderate-quality evidence showed cervical thrust manipulation and nonthrust mobilization produced similar effects on pain, function, and patient satisfaction at intermediate follow-up.[21] Recent systematic reviews and clinical practice guidelines conclude that multimodal care including education, exercise, and manual therapy can benefit patients with neck pain and whiplash associated disorders.[22,23] Greater evidence is found in the literature to support the use of mobilization/manipulation and therapeutic exercise than most other interventions provided by physical therapists. The evidence for mobilization/manipulation is reviewed in greater detail in Chapters 4 to 7, which address each region of the spine and the temporomandibular joint (TMJ).

EFFECTS OF MANIPULATION

During the past 200 years, many theories have been developed and perpetuated that attempt to explain the effects of manipulation. From the bonesetter explanation that the cracking sound associated with a manipulation is a "bone being put back into place" to the modern exploration of the hypoalgesic effects of manipulation, practitioners have attempted to establish theories to explain the mechanism for the beneficial effects of skilled passive movements to joints and surrounding soft tissues. Some theories, such as the chiropractic subluxation theory, have been widely criticized as lacking biologic feasibility;[24] other theories, such as the central nervous system mechanism for pain modulation, continue to gain supportive evidence.[25] This model suggests that a mechanical force from mobilization/manipulation initiates a cascade of neurophysiologic responses from the peripheral and central nervous system that are then responsible for favorable clinical outcomes.[26]

From a physical therapist's perspective, the two primary indications for spinal mobilization/manipulation are pain caused by musculoskeletal tissue nociception and mobility deficits. Therefore the two primary effects of spinal mobilization/manipulation are improvement in mobility and reduction of pain. Paris[27] has outlined the effects of mobilization/manipulation into three main categories: mechanical, neurophysiologic, and psychologic. This outline establishes a useful framework for exploration of the evidence to support the theoretic effects of mobilization/manipulation (Box 3.1). It should also be noted that there is overlap between these three categories, and it is impossible to totally separate the effects of mobilization/manipulation without consideration of the clinical effects on each individual patient.

Mechanical Effects

The mechanical effects of mobilization/manipulation include the restoration of tissue extensibility and ROM of hypomobile joints. The evidence to support the mechanical effects of mobilization/manipulation can be divided into studies that

---

| BOX 3.1 | Theoretical Effects of Spinal Joint Mobilization/Manipulation |

Mechanical Effects
- Restoration of mobility and range of motion
- Elongation of connective tissues under a load (stress/strain curve)
- Disrupting the cross linkages between the collagen fibersStretching of capsular adhesions
- Release entrapment of a joint menisci
- Correction of a position fault

Neurophysiologic Effects
- Reduction of pain perception; local and regional pain inhibition (hypoalgesia)
  - Type I and type II mechanoreceptor activation
  - Activation of the periaqueductal gray area of the midbrain
  - Trigger descending pain inhibitory pathways of the central nervous system
  - Sympathetic nervous system analgesic response
  - Peripheral/spinal cord mechanism at dorsal horn
- Influence on muscle activation (neuromuscular responses)
  - Activation of type III mechanoreceptors
  - Inhibition of global/superficial muscle tone
  - Facilitation of local/deep muscle activation
  - Facilitation of regional/extremity muscle activation

Psychologic Effects
- Placebo effects
- Influence of therapist instructions/interactions
- Influence of patient expectations

---

show that mobilization/manipulation can increase ROM and animal studies that examine how joints and connective tissues respond to immobilization, injury/repair, and mobilization/manipulation.

Restoration of Mobility and Range of Motion

Many studies have shown improved ROM after spinal mobilization/manipulation; the following are a sampling of these studies. Nansel et al.,[28] who reported on a study of 24 asymptomatic subjects with asymmetric neck side-bending motion, showed a significant increase in cervical ROM after thrust joint manipulation to the lower cervical spine compared with subjects who received placebo manipulation. In another study of 16 subjects with chronic neck pain, subjects showed an improvement in cervical ROM after a thrust joint manipulation to restricted C5–C6 and C6–C7 segments.[29] In a randomized trial of 100 subjects with neck pain, one group received thrust manipulation and the other nonthrust techniques to the cervical spine; both groups had similar improvements in ROM.[30] The effect of a single thoracic spine thrust manipulation was studied in 78 asymptomatic subjects who were randomly assigned to receive thrust manipulation to a restricted segment, mobility testing only, or no intervention. Thoracic thrust manipulation was associated with an increase in ROM, but no improvements were noted in the two other groups.[31]

Campbell and Snodgrass[32] used a biomechanical devise to measure segmental thoracic stiffness before and after application of a thoracic spine thrust manipulation technique performed on 24 asymptomatic adults. Reduction of spinal stiffness was noted at the targeted spinal level in the majority of the subjects, but not at the adjacent spinal levels.[32] Sims-Williams et al.[33] reported on 94 subjects who were randomly assigned to receive a lumbar thrust manipulation or a placebo. Improvements in ROM were noted after the treatment, but no differences in ROM were noted compared with the placebo group at a 1-year follow-up examination. Shum et al.[34] demonstrated reduction of pain and lumbar stiffness in 19 subjects with LBP immediately following posteroanterior (PA) grade III mobilization at the L4 level for three 60-second cycles. The lumbar stiffness improved to a degree similar to asymptomatic subjects immediately following the mobilization and was measured with a biomechanical analysis based on the force plate measurement of force application and the resultant degree of angular deformation of the spine.[34] Powers et al.[35] demonstrated reduced pain with standing lumbar extension and increased lumbar extension ROM (17.8%) with a prone press up, as measured with a magnetic resonance imaging (MRI) analysis, immediately following PA grade III mobilizations targeting symptomatic lumbar spine segments in 15 people with nonspecific LBP.

Tuttle et al.[36] developed a measurement devise for the cervical spine that reliably measures manual force application and spinal displacement during movement produced by a force applied manually by a therapist.[37] In a study using this devise, Tuttle et al.[37] demonstrated that in patients with neck pain PA mobilization techniques to the cervical spine can positively change cervical active ROM (AROM) and PA stiffness when the technique is applied to a previously identified symptomatic spinal segment, and these positive effects on AROM and stiffness did not occur if the nonthrust mobilization was applied to other random spinal segments. Likewise, Snodgrass et al.[38] found a greater reduction in spinal stiffness and pain following a larger force magnitude (90 N) PA force cervical nonthrust mobilization than both a lighter force mobilization (30 N) or placebo treatment with patients with neck pain 4 days after treatment. These studies support the concept that changes in spinal stiffness with improvement in spinal ROM can occur when mobilization techniques are specifically applied to stiffened, symptomatic spinal segments.

Use of isometric manipulation, also known as MET, has been advocated for treatment of joint hypomobility conditions. Schenk, MacDiarmid, and Rousselle[39] showed improvements in lumbar backward-bending ROM in a group of 13 asymptomatic subjects after lumbar isometric manipulation techniques performed 2 times per week for 4 weeks compared with a control group. The same researchers[40] showed improvement in cervical ROM in a group of asymptomatic subjects who received isometric manipulation to the cervical spine 2 times per week for 4 weeks compared with a control group. Lenehan et al.[41] demonstrated significant increase on ROM of asymptomatic volunteers ($n = 30$) with restricted trunk ROM immediately following one application of a seated thoracic spine MET to correct a rotation restriction. The improvement in ROM was not seen in the control group ($n = 18$).[41] Collectively, these findings indicate that isometric manipulation, thrust manipulation, and nonthrust mobilization techniques can be used to improve spinal mobility and reduce stiffness.

Joint and Connective Tissue Response to Immobilization, Injury/Repair, and Mobilization/ Manipulation

In theory, the mechanical effects of mobilization/manipulation occur when techniques are used that apply adequate force to apply tensile loads to the connective tissues that comprise and surround the joint capsule and to stretch capsular adhesions that may have formed in response to the injury and repair process.

Connective tissues are made up of a framework of collagen and elastin fibers, and the proportion of collagen and elastin fibers varies from tissue to tissue depending on tissue function.[42] If the tissue's primary function is to transmit loads (such as tendons) or to restrain joint displacement (such as a ligament or joint capsule), the tissue framework is almost exclusively collagen; but if a great degree of elasticity is needed (such as, in the ligamentum flavum), a greater percentage of the tissue is made up of elastin.[42] These connective tissue structures respond to a tensile load with various degrees of viscoelastic properties depending on the structural framework.

Woo et al.[43] have described the effects of prolonged immobilization (9 weeks) as creation of a loss of extracellular molecules and water in the ground substance that leads to an increase in the number of collagen cross-links, which creates inhibition of free-gliding collagen fibers and resultant loss of ROM. Forced passive motion restores ROM of the immobilized joint of an animal model with the greatest amount of force necessary with the first cycle of passive ROM.[43] Woo et al.[43] explain that the first cycle of passive motion disrupts the cross-linkages between the collagen fibers, which allows the fibers to glide more freely with subsequent passive motion cycles.

Viscoelastic properties are illustrated with a stress/strain or load/elongation (Fig. 3.2) curve that illustrates the effect on tissue elongation or strain that is created with a gradually increasing load or stress. The first phase of the stress/strain curve is the toe region; this initial elongation in the tissue occurs with the application of a low load and is created by the straightening of the collagen crimp or waviness of the fibers. Once the fibers are straightened and oriented in the direction of the stress, an increase in load is needed to create a proportional lengthening of the tissue. This second linear phase represents the elastic component of the tissue; if the load is released during this phase, the tissue returns to its original length. Therefore if a stretch is applied to a tissue with just enough force to elongate the tissue into the elastic phase, the tissue returns to its original length once the stretch is released without producing a long-term increase in tissue length.

If the intensity of the load is gradually increased over time, microfailure of the collagen begins to occur; and when the load is removed, a proportional increase in tissue resting length remains.[42] This third phase of the stress/strain curve is referred to as the plastic phase. The plastic phase must be reached with stretching/mobilizing to create a long-lasting increase in length of connective tissue. The viscoelastic property of hysteresis occurs when the tissue is stressed into the plastic phase. Hysteresis is characterized by a greater amount

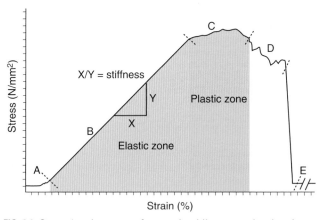

FIG. 3.2 Stress/strain curve of an excised ligament that has been stretched to a point of mechanical failure (disruption). The ligament is considered an elastic tissue. *Zone A* shows the nonlinear region. *Zone B* (elastic zone) shows the linear relationship between stress and strain, demonstrating the stiffness of the tissue. *Zone C* indicates the mechanical property of plasticity. *Zones D* and *E* demonstrate the points of progressive mechanical failure of the tissue. (Modified from Neumann DA. *Kinesiology of the Musculoskeletal System: Foundations for Physical Rehabilitation*, ed 2. St Louis: Mosby; 2010.)

of energy being absorbed by the tissue during the loading than is dissipated during the unloading.[44] This energy is likely absorbed by the connective tissues in the form of heat. Warren, Lehmann, and Koblanski[45,46] have shown that heat can be used to decrease the amount of force needed to elongate collagen tissue. The heat production associated with hysteresis can be used to assist in tissue elongation.

With further increase in the strain over time, a progressive failure of collagen bundles occurs. Eventually, the tissue continues to elongate without needing an increased load,[44] which is referred to as the creep phase. If the load is sustained past the creep phase, tensile mechanical failure or rupture of the tissue occurs.[44] Therefore when a stretch/mobilization is applied to a tissue for the purpose of creating permanent elongation of that tissue, the load must be of sufficient intensity and duration to reach the plastic phase on the stress/strain curve; but the failure point must be avoided if excessive tissue damage or rupture is to be prevented.

The stress/strain curve varies between tissues depending on the proportion of collagen and elastin in the tissue. A more elastic tissue tends to elongate to a greater extent before microfailure occurs, but complete failure occurs abruptly with a shorter plastic phase.[47] If a tissue is stretched only within the elastic phase and the plastic phase is never reached, permanent elongation of the tissue does not occur. With repetition of the stretching in the elastic range of the tissue, the connective tissue progressively becomes stronger and more resistant to microfailure. This phenomenon was shown by Tipton et al.[48] who found that dogs that received regular exercise needed a greater degree of force to create failure and rupture of the experimental group's muscle tendon units compared with a control group. However, Tipton et al.[48] also found that dogs that had been immobilized for 6 weeks had a significantly weaker transitional zone in bone-tendon-bone and bone-ligament-bone preparations. The results of this study need to be considered in the stretching of connective tissues. Based on this animal research, caution must be taken to avoid rupture of previously immobilized tissues.

Precautions must be taken in attempts to mobilize traumatized connective tissues depending on the stage of inflammation and repair. This is particularly important to consider in postsurgical situations. The stages of repair of dense connective tissue include acute inflammation, fibroplastic, and remodeling phases. Acute inflammation lasts 2 to 14 days and is characterized by pain, redness, heat, swelling, and loss of function. A vascular/chemical response occurs with vasodilation, exudate formation, and clotting and a cellular response with phagocytosis to clean the wound. Cummings, Crutchfield, and Barnes[49] recommend resting damaged tissues for the first 24 to 48 hours after trauma to allow the repair process to begin and to avoid excessive inflammation and bleeding. As the repair process continues, the wound is invaded by fibroblasts, which lay down collagen fibers in a random arrangement.[49] The new collagen fibers are held together by weak hydrogen bonds during the first 8 to 10 days, and the collagen can be easily stretched and molded during the first 8 to 10 days.[49]

The fibroblastic phase begins at day 4 and lasts up to 21 days. As the wound matures, the hydrogen bonds are replaced by covalent bonding that strengthens the scar.[49] Reepithelialization and fibroplasia with neovascularization occur during this phase with random strands of fibrin being laid down.[30] Myofibroblasts also enter the wound site as early as 3 to 5 days after trauma and bond to collagen fibers to create shrinkage of the wound.[49,50]

The final phase of healing is the remodeling phase and includes consolidation (day 21 to day 60), with a change from cellular to more fibrous tissue, and finally maturation (day 60 to day 360), in which collagen fibers are slowly aligned and strengthened and the weak hydrogen bonds transition to stronger covalent bonds. Loading and stressing the connective tissue during the maturation phase affects the shape, strength, and pliability of the tissue. The collagen bundles organize along lines of stress, and the fibroblasts also orient to stress. Stress to the connective tissue stimulates glycosaminoglycan and proteoglycan production.[51] However, too much stress pulls apart newly formed collagen bundles and causes acute inflammation.

Based on this knowledge of the healing process of injured dense connective tissues, Box 3.2 outlines general clinical recommendations to facilitate healing of the connective tissues. Excessive scar tissue formation and myofibroblastic activity are created by excessive inflammation at the area surrounding the wound site; therefore overstressing a healing wound site with an excessive amount of stretching or exercise could potentially create excessive inflammation and adhesion formation of the adjacent connective tissues.[49] Adhesions could cause a progressive loss of motion for as long as 6 months to 1 year as the scar tissue matures.[49] Mechanical principles, such as an understanding of the stress/strain curve, can be applied clinically to stretch joint capsular adhesions.

Facet Joint Meniscoid Entrapment and Positional Faults

Other theories to explain the mechanical effects of mobilization/manipulation that have less supporting evidence include correction of a facet joint meniscoid entrapment and positional faults. Acute facet joint locking is a condition with a sudden loss of joint mobility that is often caused by a nontraumatic event. The joints that tend to lock have meniscoids. The

---

BOX 3.2	General Clinical Recommendations to Facilitate Healing of Dense Connective Tissues After Severe Injury or Surgery

- Ensure relative rest for the first 24 to 48 hours
- Low-load, high-repetition exercise can stimulate healing
- Use only very gentle range of motion for the first 10 to 14 days (grade I and II mobilizations)
- Often, 4 to 8 weeks is needed before loading injured tissue to end range
- Continue to exercise and stretch for 1 year

mechanism of the locking seems to involve either entrapment of a meniscoid in a groove formed in the articular cartilage or a piece of meniscus that may break loose and form a loose body, with the loose body creating the entrapment.[52,53] Intracapsular meniscoid structures are present in spinal facet joints. Facet menisci are believed to be capable of becoming entrapped, or impinged, between the two facet surfaces, causing the joint surfaces to lock, which is associated with pain with movements that downglide and load the facet joint. Manipulation techniques that gap the joint or isometric manipulation techniques that theoretically pull the facet joint capsule laterally are believed to dislodge the impingement, and patients show immediate improvement in joint motion and reduction of pain with movement.[52,53] No studies have specifically addressed the effect of spinal mobilization/manipulation on meniscoid impingement.[54] However, anatomic plausibility of the meniscoid impingement or entrapment theory has been refuted by anatomists after a review of the literature on the topic.[55,56]

Although traditional chiropractic philosophy is based on detection and correction of spinal subluxations and realignment of these spinal subluxations, no valid research has shown that subluxations/positional faults correlate with pain or are a cause of hypomobility in the spine.[54] Spinal facet subluxations of less than 4.5 mm are not detectable with radiography. When comparing radiographic results at pre- and postmanipulation time points, clinicians were not capable of detecting a change in vertebral position after a chiropractic spinal thrust joint manipulation. In a study by Tullberg et al.,[57] joint manipulation did not cause a detectable change in the relative position of the ilium on the sacrum when measured with roentgen stereo-photogrammetric analysis.

Therefore, although the positional fault and meniscoid theories are somewhat plausible, the ability to detect these impairments in clinical practice is not feasible and no reliable valid measurement tool is sensitive enough to detect and measure the presence of these impairments in clinical practice. Thus these conditions are considered theoretic. In a clinical commentary on the effects of manual therapy, Bialosky et al.[58] criticize theories related to the identification and correction of a specific biomechanical dysfunction with manual therapy techniques calling these theories "unsubstantiated and counterproductive."

Neurophysiologic Effects of Manipulation

Spinal AROM is influenced by not only connective tissue and myofascial mobility but also by pain perception, fear of pain,[59] and neuromotor control. The neurophysiologic effects of mobilization/manipulation have been associated with a reduction in pain intensity (hypoalgesia) and influence on muscle tone and motor control.[26] Mobilization/manipulation has been reported to exert both local[60,61] and distal[62,63] neurophysiologic effects based on the anatomic region of application. The neurophysiologic effects of mobilization/manipulation likely provide the most feasible explanation for the beneficial effects of manipulation.[58] In a systematic review on the mechanisms

of action of spinal mobilizations, the authors conclude that the evidence suggests that mobilizations cause a neurophysiologic effect that results in sympathoexcitation, decreased neural mechanosensitivity, mechanical hypoalgesia (both locally and distally to the targeted mobilization site), and normalized muscle activity, endurance and pain-free strength.[64] Before providing a sampling of the research on the neurophysiologic effects of manipulation on the sympathetic nervous system and motor system, an explanation of the involved neuroanatomy and physiology is necessary.

The tissues of the spine, including the skin, fascia, muscle, tendon, joints, ligaments, and intervertebral disc (outer annulus), are well innervated and provide afferent input to the central nervous system.[65] Extensive numbers of type I and II mechanoreceptors and free nerve endings (type IV receptors) have been noted in the cervical facet joints[66] and in the muscle spindles of the cervical spine.[67,68] Similar receptors are found in the thoracic and lumbar spine, but in fewer numbers and with a more inconsistent distribution than in the cervical spine.[69] The type I mechanoreceptors provide afferent input to the central nervous system regarding static joint position and increase their rate of firing in response to movement. The type II mechanoreceptors remain inactive as long as joints are immobile. When joints are moved actively or passively, they emit brief bursts of impulses.[70] Therefore with joint movement caused by spinal mobilization/manipulation, these receptors fire and provide afferent input to the central nervous system.

The afferent nerves from the receptors terminate in the spinal cord, synapsing in the dorsal horn to signal both proprioceptive and nociceptive information.[71] As spinal mobilization/manipulation produces movement of the vertebral column and its associated structures, multiple receptors are influenced to generate afferent input to ascend up the spinal cord. In the cervical spine, additional complex interactions occur with other systems, such as vestibular and optic systems, that may also activate in response to manipulation techniques.[72] As a result, a neuroanatomic basis is seen through which a multifaceted neurophysiologic response may occur with manipulation.

Antinociception is suppression of nociception in response to stimulation that normally would be painful.[73] The phenomenon of antinociception can be summarized by a five-level model (Fig. 3.3):

- Level I occurs in the periphery by desensitizing nociceptive C fibers with interventions, such as topical menthol.[73]
- Level II occurs in the dorsal horn via inhibitory neurons releasing encephalin and dynorphin which is referred to as the counterirritant effect (Fig. 3.4). Examples include superficial heat, massage, mobilization, and TENS that stimulate activity in collateral branches of nonnociceptive afferents to decrease or prevent transmission at the dorsal horn of nociceptive information to the second-order neuron in the spinal cord.[73]
- Level III is the fast-acting neuronal descending system involving the periaqueductal gray (PAG), the rostral ventromedial medulla, and the locus coeruleus. Activity in this area is naturally occurring and can be triggered with

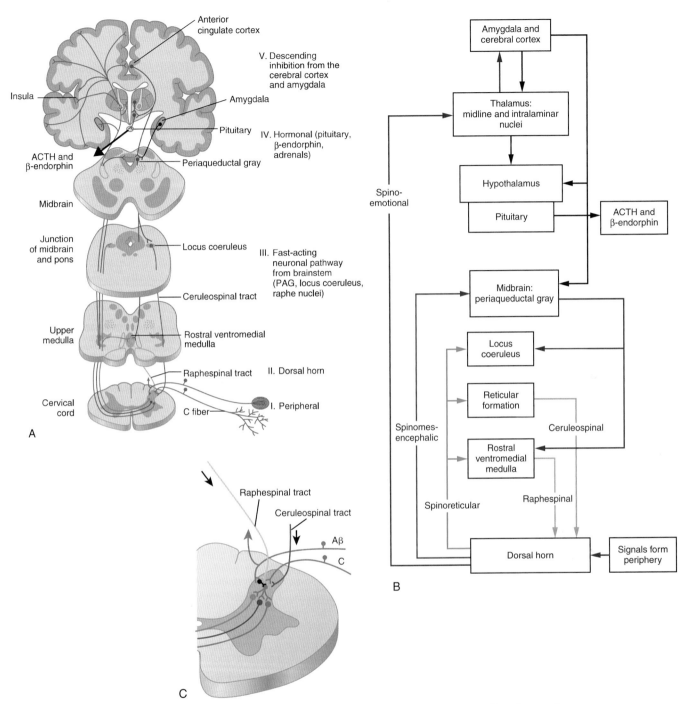

FIG. 3.3 Antinociceptive systems. **A,** On the left side, tracts that convey ascending slow nociceptive information are shown: spinoemotional *(blue),* spinomesencephalic *(red),* and spinoreticular *(green)* tracts. Structures indicated in the coronal section are not in the same plane (anterior cingulate and amygdala are anterior to the section of thalamus illustrated). On the right, the five levels of the nervous system involved in pain inhibition are shown. The emotion areas of the cortex include the anterior cingulate, insular, prefrontal, and ventrolateral orbitofrontal cortex. All tracts are bilateral. Signals in the spinoreticular tract facilitate the locus coeruleus neurons. **B,** Flowchart illustrating the same pathways as in **A.** The flow of slow nociceptive information upward is shown on the left, and the descending antinociceptive pathways are shown on the right. **C,** A segment of the spinal cord. The raphespinal tract synapses with an interneuron *(black)* that inhibits the transmission of nociceptive information in the dorsal horn of the spinal cord. The ceruleospinal tract directly inhibits the primary nociceptive afferent. *ACTH,* Adrenocorticotropic hormone. (From Lundy-Ekman L. *Neuroscience Fundamentals for Rehabilitation,* ed 5. Elsevier, 2018.)

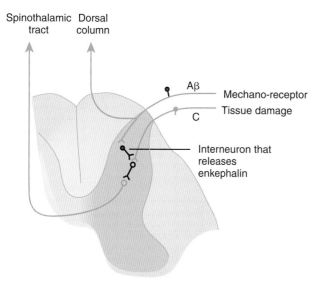

Spinothalamic tract   Dorsal column

Aβ — Mechano-receptor

C — Tissue damage

Interneuron that releases enkephalin

FIG. 3.4 Counterirritant mechanism. Circuits in the dorsal horn that may produce inhibition of nociceptive signals. Collaterals of mechanoreceptive afferents stimulate interneurons that release enkephalins. Enkephalin binding inhibits the transmission of nociceptive messages by primary afferents and interneurons in the nociceptive pathway. (From Lundy-Ekman L. *Neuroscience Fundamentals for Rehabilitation*, ed 5. Elsevier, 2018.)

mobilization/manipulation techniques or stimulated with narcotics binding to opioid receptors.[73]

- Level IV is the hormonal system involving the periventricular gray in the hypothalamus, the pituitary gland that releases B-endorphin, and the adrenal medulla. Stress-induced antinociception actives the raphespinal tracts plus releases hormonal endorphins from the pituitary gland and the adrenal medulla. The hormonal endorphins bind to opiate receptors in the pain matrix and spinal cord.[73]

- Level V is the amygdala and cortical level. The amygdala mediates emotional aspects of pain, and at the cortical level, expectations, excitement, distraction, and placebo all play a role in adjusting the transmission of nociceptive signals.[73]

Bialosky[26] has established a model for the neurophysiologic mechanisms of manual therapy that corresponds in various proportions to the five levels of antinociception. The supraspinal cord mechanisms involve activation of pain modulatory circuitry triggered within the brain in response to the intervention or the psychologic expectations and experiences associated with the intervention. The spinal cord level mechanism is linked with synaptic connections at the spinal cord level (i.e., dorsal horn) in response to the peripheral nerve response to the manipulation[26] (Fig. 3.5). The model of the mechanisms of manual therapy has been updated to include three zones by the same research group[58] (Fig. 3.6). The first zone encompasses the interaction between the provider and the patient, including their beliefs and expectations, as well as the stimulus at the targeted tissue. Zone two encompasses the nervous system response of the patient receiving a manual therapy intervention similar to the original model, and zone three includes the clinical outcomes of the manual therapy interventions, such as inhibition of pain and emotional distress.[58]

Analgesic Response to Mobilization/Manipulation

Both animal and human studies have shown that a key locus of control for mediation of endogenous analgesia is the PAG area of the midbrain.[74–76] The PAG area plays an important integrative role for behavioral responses to pain, stress, and other stimuli by coordinating responses of a number of systems, including the nociceptive system, autonomic nervous system, and motor system.[77–79] Animal studies have shown that when key regions of the PAG area are stimulated, a sympathetic nervous system (fight or flight) response is evoked combined with a nonopioid form of analgesia[72] (see Fig. 3.3). Type I and II mechanoreceptors from joints and muscles project primary afferent neurons to the dorsal horn which synapse with second-order neurons that ascend to the PAG area.[80] A series of studies is presented to show a postmanipulation sympathetic response (skin conductance) combined with analgesia (pressure pain threshold) in symptomatic and asymptomatic subjects, which provides preliminary evidence that the analgesic response to spinal manipulation is likely the result of the stimulation of mechanoreceptors that provide afferent impulses to the central nervous system to trigger descending pain inhibitory (i.e., antinociceptive) pathways originating from the PAG area of the midbrain.[81]

Several different sensory modalities have been used to assess pain sensitivity (e.g., thermal, electrical, and mechanical) associated with the application of manual therapy procedures, but mechanical pressure pain threshold testing offers several distinct advantages. For example, elevated pressure pain threshold has been found to be a valid measure of hypoalgesia, and administering pressure pain threshold testing in the clinical setting is feasible for clinicians (see Box 2.5) Skin conductance is monitored as a measure of sympathetic nervous system response to manipulation; when this response is increased because of increased moisture on the skin, it is a measure of the sympathetic nervous system excitatory response of manipulation. Thermal pain thresholds have also been used to study hypoalgesic and hyperalgesic responses to manipulation in normal subjects[61,63] and clinical populations.[60,82,83]

Sterling, Jull, and Wright[84] studied 30 subjects with cervical pain of insidious onset. These subjects received an anterior glide grade III mobilization to the C5 facet on the painful side, a placebo condition that consisted of manual contacts, or a control condition that consisted of no physical contact between subject and clinician. After the mobilization technique, subjects had a significant increase in pressure pain thresholds and a decrease in visual analog scores compared with the other two conditions. La Touche et al.[85] provided supine upper cervical (C0–C3) anterior to posterior nonthrust mobilization over three treatment sessions compared with placebo mobilizations for 32 patients with neck and craniofacial pain and reported that pressure pain thresholds in the craniofacial and cervical regions significantly increased and pain intensity significantly decreased in the treatment group compared with

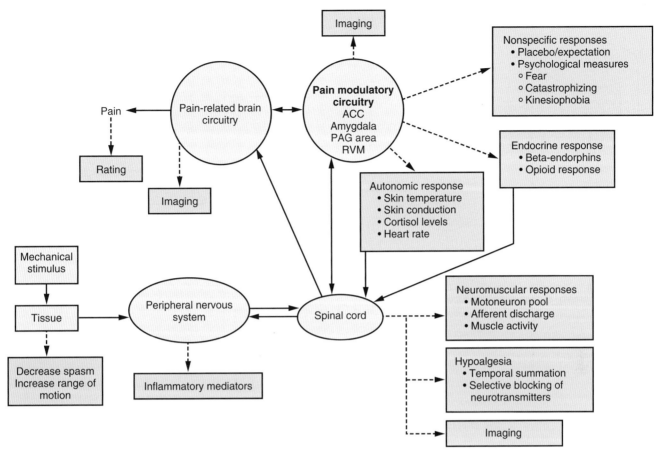

FIG. 3.5 Comprehensive model of the mechanisms of manual therapy. The model suggests a transient, mechanical stimulus to the tissue produces a chain of neurophysiologic effects. *Solid arrows* denote a direct mediating effect. *Broken arrows* denote an associative relationship, which may include an association between a construct and its measure. *Blue boxes* indicate the measurement of a construct. *ACC,* Anterior cingulate cortex; *PAG,* periaqueductal gray; *RVM,* rostral ventromedial medulla. (Modified from Bialosky JE, Bishop MD, Price DD, et al. The mechanisms of manual therapy in the treatment of musculoskeletal pain: a comprehensive model. *Man Ther.* 2009;14(5):531-538.)

placebo. The upper cervical nonthrust mobilization also produced a sympathoexcitatory response demonstrated by a significant increase in skin conductance, breathing rate, and heart rate ($P < .001$) after application of the technique compared with placebo.[85]

Peterson, Vicenzino, and Wright[86] evaluated the effect of grade III PA mobilization to the C5–C6 spinal segment and showed an increase of skin conductance of 60% from baseline during the treatment intervention versus a 20% increase for the placebo group, with a significant difference between groups. This study showed that PA mobilization produces an initial immediate sympathoexcitatory effect that starts within 15 seconds after initiation of treatment.[86]

Vicenzino et al.[87] tested the interaction between changes in mechanical pain threshold and skin conductance during the cervical lateral gliding procedure and found a significant correlation between the time taken to achieve the maximum increase in peripheral skin conductance and the increase in

mechanical pain thresholds. Those subjects who had the most rapid sympathoexcitatory response also showed the greatest increase in pain threshold (relative hypoalgesia),[87] which may explain why some individuals respond more dramatically to manipulation than others. The authors hypothesize that those individuals with more direct neural connections from the peripheral to the PAG area have the more rapid sympathoexcitatory response and the greater hypoalgesia effect with manipulation.[87]

McGuiness, Vicenzino, and Wright[88] showed a highly significant increase in both respiratory rate and blood pressure after a grade III PA mobilization applied to the C5–C6 motion segment; the placebo group showed a slight decrease in these measures. Vicenzino et al.[89] measured factors related to the sympathetic nervous system function, including heart rate and blood pressure, during application of a C5–C6 lateral glide nonthrust mobilization on 24 asymptomatic subjects and found a significant increase in heart rate and blood pressure of

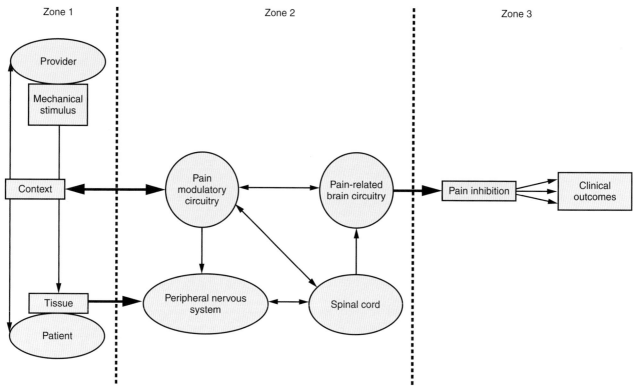

FIG. 3.6 Updated comprehensive model of the mechanisms of manual therapy. The model suggests that a transient, mechanical stimulus to the tissue produces a chain of neurophysiological effects. Zone 1 represents the mechanical stimulus from the provider to the tissue, as well as the interaction between the patient and provider. Zone 2 represents potential nervous system responses to the mechanical stimulus, as well as the patient-provider interaction. Zone 3 represents the potential outcomes. (From Bialosky JE, Beneciuk JM, Bishop MD, et al. Unraveling the mechanisms of manual therapy: modeling an approach. *J Orthop Sports Phys Ther.* 2018;48(1):8-18.)

14% compared with 1% to 2% in the placebo and control conditions. The respiratory rate increased 36%. These studies add support for a sympathoexcitatory response to mobilization/manipulation procedures.

The effect of cervical lateral glide nonthrust mobilization has also been evaluated in patients with lateral epicondylitis.[90] Measures of mechanical pain threshold, pain-free grip pressure, range of shoulder abduction in upper limb neurodynamic (ULND) test 2b, and visual analog scale (VAS) measures of pain and function were obtained before and after treatment and placebo and control interventions. Treatment resulted in significant improvements in most measures obtained, which indicates that lateral glide cervical nonthrust mobilization procedures produced a relative hypoalgesic effect of the lateral elbow region a few minutes after the treatment. The mean increase in mechanical pain threshold was approximately 26%, the mean increase in pain-free grip pressure was 29%, and the mean increase in shoulder abduction with ULND test 2b was 44%.[90] Marks et al.[91] demonstrated similar enhanced treatment outcomes following cervical nonthrust mobilization techniques with improvement in the ULND test 1, pain, and cervical ROM in an RCT comparing use of cervical nonthrust mobilization techniques to ULND mobilization for 20 patients with neck and upper extremity symptoms.

In a retrospective analysis of 112 patients who underwent treatment for lateral epicondylalgia, Cleland, Whitman, and Fritz[92] found that patients who received mobilization/manipulation to the cervical spine combined with local treatment for the lateral epicondylalgia were seen for significantly fewer visits with positive outcomes compared with the patients who only received local therapy for the lateral epicondylalgia. A grade III PA rotatory mobilization technique applied to the T4 vertebra at a frequency of 0.5 Hz produced a side-specific sympathoexcitatory increase in skin conductance in the hand, which was significantly greater than the response after a placebo mobilization technique, and the opposite hand demonstrated a similar sympathoexcitatory effect but to a slightly lesser extent.[93]

A significant change in skin conductance was also demonstrated after a unilaterally applied PA nonthrust mobilization to the left L4–L5 zygapophyseal joint that was specific to the side treated for the treatment group during the intervention period compared with placebo and control conditions in 45 normal participants.[94] This study demonstrated side-specific peripheral sympathetic nervous system changes in the lower limbs with the lumbar nonthrust mobilization technique.[94]

Temporal summation is a clinical measure of central sensitization in which "a high frequency of action potentials in the presynaptic neuron elicits postsynaptic potentials that overlap and

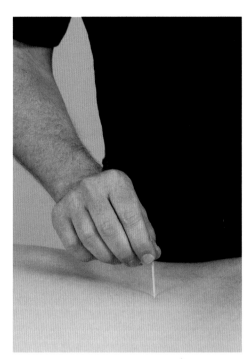

FIG. 3.7 Temporal summation. One method of testing temporal summation is to repeatedly prick the skin with a tooth pick 20 times for 1 minute. A normal response is for the patient to report an equal of amount of mild discomfort with each prick. Hypersensitivity with temporal sensation occurs when the patient reports intensification of pain with the repeated skin prick and may be a sign of central sensitization.

summate with each other."[60] Temporal summation occurs when an individual reports an increase perception of pain from repetitive painful stimuli (e.g., thermal pain, electrical stimulation, or gentle prick with a toothpick) that are applied at the same intensity at a low frequency (e.g., <3 seconds), and individuals with central sensitization report increased intensity of pain with the repeated noxious stimuli (Fig. 3.7). Temporal summation has been used as a proxy measure of central sensitization for studies investigating the mechanisms of spinal manipulation in both healthy subjects and those experiencing chronic pain.[60] For example, Bialosky et al.[58] measured thermal pain sensitivity in 36 patients with LBP immediately after a lumbopelvic thrust manipulation and found inhibition of temporal summation in participants who received the manipulation. This was not observed in patients after exercise on a stationary bicycle or after back extensor exercises. Because activation of the dorsal horn of the spinal cord has been directly observed with temporal summation in animal studies, inhibition of temporal summation suggests modulation of dorsal horn excitability because it was observed primarily in the lumbar innervated area of the lower extremity.[60] Randoll et al.[95] induced temporal summation pain at the thorax in normal subjects with repeated electrical stimulation and found reduction in temporal summation following thrust manipulation of the T4 spinal level. This adds further support for short-term spinal cord level analgesic effects of thoracic thrust manipulation and suggests that thoracic spinal thrust manipulation may offer some benefit for patients with central sensitization.

Willet et al.[96] studied three different frequency rates of application of lumbar PA nonthrust mobilizations on the degree of pressure pain threshold at the lumbar spine and at multiple sites throughout the body and found significant widespread hypoalgesic effect, regardless of the rates of mobilization in asymptomatic subjects. Sparks et al.[97] used functional MRI (fMRI) of the brain and found a significant reduction in participants' perception of pain, as well as a reduction in cerebral blood flow to areas associated with the pain matrix after a thoracic spine thrust manipulation.

These studies support the concept that mobilization/manipulation procedures can produce a hypoalgesic effect both in healthy participants and in patients. In a systematic review of the literature, Wirth et al.[98] concluded that there was evidence for an association between thrust manipulation and immediate, short-term changes in the autonomic nervous system reflected in heart rate variability and skin conductance, but the effects seem to depend on the spinal level that is targeted with the thrust manipulation with the most pronounced effects occurring with upper thoracic and cervical thrust manipulation techniques. The autonomic nervous system effects also are more pronounced in patients with pain rather than normal subjects.[98] Because the response to mobilization/manipulation is coupled with a sympathoexcitatory response and the hypoalgesic effect is both local and regional, convincing support exists that the mechanism for the neurophysiologic effects of manipulation lies in the stimulation of descending pain inhibitory systems of the central nervous system projecting from the midbrain to the spinal cord (central pathway). There is also preliminary evidence that spinal manipulation causes a regional hypoalgesic mechanism by inhibition of a temporal summation effect in the dorsal horn of the spinal cord (peripheral pathway). Therefore there is evidence that spinal manipulation has an immediate effect on pain modulation via both central and peripheral pathways. Further research is warranted to determine how the immediate hypoalgesic effects of manipulation relate to long-term clinical improvements and to attempt to link how the change in pain sensitivity caused by mobilization/manipulation relates to meaningful clinical outcomes.[62]

Analgesic Effect Caused by Biochemical Changes
A systematic review concluded that there is a moderate level of evidence in normal subjects that spinal manipulation can increase biochemical biomarkers, including substance-p, neurotensin, oxytocin, and interleukin levels and may influence cortisol levels postintervention.[99] These biomarkers are involved in pain perception, pain modulation, and play an important role in inflammation, tissue healing, and immune response.[99] However, this research is preliminary and has not been replicated in symptomatic subjects or correlated with positive clinical outcomes. At this point, no clinical implications can be drawn from the preliminary biomarker research.

Another proposed explanation of the analgesic effect of joint mobilization/manipulation is stimulation of release of endogenous opioid peptides that bind to receptor sites in the nervous system and produce analgesia. One such opiate is beta-endorphin. Vernon et al.[100] measured the plasma levels of beta-endorphin at 5-minute intervals after thrust manipulation of the cervical spine of asymptomatic participants. The findings showed an increase in the plasma levels of beta-endorphin in the experimental group 5 minutes after the thrust compared with a control group that received a similar but less aggressive mobilization technique.[100] At 15 minutes after thrust manipulation, the beta-endorphin level was back to a baseline level.[100] However, other investigators have performed similar studies and have been unable to measure differences in beta-endorphin levels after a spinal manipulation compared with control and sham treatment groups in both symptomatic and asymptomatic groups.[101,102]

For further investigation of the premise that endogenous opioids are involved in analgesia after spinal manipulation, Zusman, Edwards, and Donaghy[103] compared the effects of a spinal manipulation on VAS pain scores for participants who were given naloxone or a saline solution control. Naloxone is an opioid antagonist and reverses the effect of endogenous opioids. Equal improvements in VAS pain scores were seen for both groups, which suggests that endogenous opioids are not the physiologic mechanism of postmanipulation analgesia.[103] Similar results were noted by Vicenzino et al.[104] in a similar study design that used naloxone with the experimental group and found that after lateral glide cervical mobilization techniques, the hypoalgesia response was the same between the experimental, sham, and control groups.

Animal studies with rats and injections of various medications to either block or enhance the effects of neurotransmitters found that the hypoalgesic effects of manipulation likely involve the descending pain inhibitory mechanisms that use serotonin and noradrenaline rather than opioid or gamma-aminobutyric acid receptors.[105] These studies taken together suggest very little evidence to support the involvement of the opioid system in manipulation-induced analgesia.

Influence on Muscle Activation

Speculation exists that the isometric manipulation causes the Golgi tendon organ to fire, which inhibits the antagonistic movement pattern to allow a greater degree of movement into the agonist movement pattern.[44,106] The effect of isometric manipulation techniques is also explained by Sherrington's principle of reciprocal innervation, which states that with an isometric contraction of the agonistic muscles, the antagonistic muscles are inhibited to allow greater freedom of movement into the agonist movement pattern.[107] In addition to these possible explanations of the effects of an isometric manipulation, speculation exists that an isometric contraction of the local muscles attached to the targeted spinal facet joint (e.g., multifidus muscle) applies a stretch to the joint capsule[4] or corrects slight positional faults by either pulling directly on the joint capsule or moving the adjacent bone.[108] Further research is needed to fully understand the mechanical and neurophysiologic effects of isometric manipulation techniques.

Several studies have investigated the effect of manipulation (usually thrust) on the motor system to determine whether spinal manipulation can inhibit muscle tone, increase muscle tone, or enhance muscle performance. The findings have been variable. Theoretically, muscle tone inhibition occurs with a strong end-range stretch of a joint from firing type III joint mechanoreceptors, which create a reflexive inhibition of the local muscle tone of the muscles overlying the joint. Pecos-Martin[109] demonstrated a reduction in electromyography (EMG) activity during active prone trunk extension and an increase in pressure pain threshold of the thoracic erector spinae muscles immediately following 3 minutes of a grade III central mobilization of the most symptomatic thoracic spinal level in people ($n = 17$) with thoracic pain. The reduction in EMG activity was not noted in the placebo group ($n = 17$) who received sham (less than a grade I) mobilizations of the T7 vertebrae.

The effect of thrust manipulation of the thoracic and lumbar spine was studied on 34 patients with joint hypomobility with and without musculoskeletal pain. Participants were randomly assigned to either receive the thrust manipulation or no intervention. Participants who received the thrust manipulation had on average a 20% reduction in paraspinal muscle activity as measured with EMG activity compared with control participants.[110] Similar results have been reported in reduction of hamstring muscle activity in patients with unilateral LBP, with comparison before and after a lumbar thrust manipulation.[111]

Dishman, Cunningham, and Burke[112] used electrodiagnostic testing to compare the effects of spinal manipulation at the cervical and lumbar spines on the tibial nerve H-reflex to investigate the relationship between potential cortical and segmentally controlled responses to spinal manipulation. A clinician performed a unilateral manipulation at either L5–S1, C5–C6, or both levels. They showed a small but significant decrease in the size of the H-reflex after the lumbar manipulation, but this effect only lasted 60 seconds after the manipulation and no effect was noted from the cervical manipulation.[112] The authors suggest a segmental rather than a global effect produced by spinal manipulation on the motor neuron pool.[112] Speculation also exists that spinal manipulation can increase muscle activation and force output. In one study performed on 16 patients with chronic neck pain, biceps muscle strength improved after a thrust joint manipulation to restricted C5–C6 and C6–C7 spinal segments.[29] A similar study demonstrated increased bilateral biceps muscle-resting EMG activity after a C5–C6 thrust manipulation in 54 asymptomatic participants.[113] An increase in lower trapezius strength occurred after a thoracic spine nonthrust mobilization in a study of 40 asymptomatic participants.[114] These participants were randomly assigned to receive either grade IV or grade I anterior glide mobilizations to T6–T12. Participants who received grade IV mobilization had a significant increase in lower trapezius muscle strength compared with those who received grade I mobilizations.[114] Cleland et al.[115] were able to show a significant increase in strength output

(14%) of the lower trapezius muscle immediately after a thoracic spine thrust manipulation compared with a control group. Suter et al.[116] studied 18 patients with knee pain and sacroiliac joint dysfunctions. After a manipulation that targeted the sacroiliac joint, a significant increase in knee extension torque occurred on the symptomatic side.

Keller et al.[117] was able to demonstrate a significant increase in maximum voluntary contraction and surface EMG activity of the erector spinae muscles with prone trunk extension immediately after a lumbar manipulation technique compared with a control and placebo manipulation group in 40 patients with LBP.[117] Rehabilitative ultrasound imaging has also been used to demonstrate enhanced activation of the lumbar multifidus muscle during a prone upper extremity lifting task immediately after and 24 hours after a lumbar thrust manipulation technique in a male patient with chronic LBP.[118] Bicalho et al.[119] assessed the surface EMG activity in 40 patients with nonspecific chronic LBP who were randomly assigned to two groups, manipulation ($n = 20$) and control ($n = 20$). The manipulation group received a side-lying lumbar rotation thrust manipulation at the L4–L5 level. The control group remained in the side-lying position without receiving a manipulation. EMG surface signals from the right and left paraspinal muscles (L5–S1 level) were acquired during trunk flexion/extension cycles before and after the thrust manipulation, and the manipulation group had a more normalized muscle activation pattern with trunk flexion/extension after the thrust manipulation.[119]

Sterling, Jull, and Wright[84] used nonthrust mobilization of the cervical spine in patients with neck pain to assess the effects on motor responses, sympathetic nervous system function, and analgesia. The effect of PA cervical technique on the craniocervical flexion test (see Box 6.1) was assessed. Decreased activation of the superficial muscles of the cervical spine was reported with the craniocervical flexion test and was interpreted as facilitation of the deep neck flexor muscles.[84] These results provides preliminary evidence that spinal manipulation can alter motor responses and facilitate muscle function that was previously inhibited because of pain or impairment.

The effect of spinal mobilization/manipulation on the motor system is inconclusive. Some studies support both facilitation and inhibition of the motor system after mobilization/manipulation. The response may vary depending on the technique, the location and nature of the pain, and the muscles that are tested.[72] In general, spinal mobilization/manipulation tends to facilitate the deep, local spinal muscles that assist in coordination of spinal neuromuscular control and tends to inhibit the more global, superficial spinal muscles that tend to tense and guard with spinal impairments. The neurophysiologic effects of spinal mobilization/manipulation tend to occur locally at the targeted spinal region and distally at the corresponding extremity with shared innervation of the targeted spinal segments. A growing body of knowledge exists regarding the effects on the sympathetic nervous system in response to spinal mobilization/manipulation and the hypoalgesic effects that accompany the sympathetic responses. However,

absolutely no scientific validation supports the long-held tenet of the chiropractic profession that spinal manipulation alters autonomic nervous system outflow to the organs and viscera or that this can rectify dysfunction of the end organs.[72,120]

Psychologic Effects

Few studies have specifically addressed and measured the psychologic effects of manipulation. In a systematic review, 129 RCTs of spinal manipulation were identified, but only 12 adequately reported psychologic outcomes.[121] The psychologic outcome measures might include assessment of fear, anxiety, catastrophizing, and kinesophobia. Based on six of these studies, it was concluded that there is evidence that spinal manipulation improved psychologic outcomes compared with verbal interventions.[121]

One aspect of the psychosocial context of patients that physical therapists must consider is the patient's expectations of the treatment. Bishop et al.[122] were able to demonstrate through a secondary analysis of a clinical trial for treatment of neck pain with thrust manipulation and exercise that patients' expectations for success of physical therapy interventions have a strong influence on outcomes. More than 80% of the 140 patients in the study expected moderate pain relief of symptoms, prevention of disability, the ability to do more activity, and to sleep better.[122] The manual therapy interventions of massage (87%) and manipulation (75%) had the highest proportion of patients who expected significant improvement.[122] At 1 month, the patients who were unsure of experiencing complete relief of pain had lower odds of reporting successful outcome than the patients expecting complete relief.[122] Believing that manipulation would help and not receiving manipulation lowered the odds of success compared with believing manipulation would help and receiving manipulation.[122] The authors conclude that having expectations of benefit has a strong influence on clinical outcomes for patients with neck pain.[122] A clinical prediction rule (CPR) development study for patients who respond favorably to cervical thrust manipulation found that one of the key factors in the CPR was a positive expectation that manipulation will help.[123]

In addition, the expectation effect can be affected by the manner in which the intervention is delivered and the words used to describe the expected outcome from the intervention. In fact, a negative effect can be produced in some patients by suggesting that the intervention tends to have a negative effect on pain. This is referred to as "nocebo."[124] Bialosky et al.[125] studied the effects of positive, negative, or neutral expectation instructional sets on 60 healthy participants regarding the effects of a lumbopelvic thrust manipulation technique on pain perception associated with thermal pain threshold testing at the low back and leg. Subjects who were given a negative expectation instructional set (i.e., the subjects were told before the manipulation that the procedure "is an ineffective form of manipulation used to treat LBP and we expect it to temporarily worsen your perception of heat pain") demonstrated significant hyperalgesia (increased pain) in their low back, but no change in pain perception was noted in the neutral or positive expectation instructional sets. Hypoalgesia in the leg was noted with all three treatment groups, which replicates prior findings of hypoalgesia in the lower extremity after lumbar spine thrust manipulation, and this occurred regardless of expectation.[125] This study provides preliminary evidence that expectations of manipulation can be influenced by the physical therapist and that these expectations can influence pain perception at the body area to which the expectation is directed.[125]

New theories on placebo mechanisms have shown that placebo represents the psychosocial aspect of every treatment, and the study of placebo is essentially the study of psychosocial context that surrounds the patient.[126] Therefore understanding placebo is essential for researchers and all medical practitioners, particularly those dealing with patients with pain, depression, and motor disorders.[126]

Many controlled studies on the effects of mobilization/manipulation have used a sham or placebo treatment that might include manual touch or positioning for a manipulation without actually imparting a manipulative force. In these studies, slight improvements can often be measured in pain and disability levels for the participants in the sham treatment groups. The effect of touch and reassurance from a medical professional can have powerful effects on easing the patient's fear and anxiety, which can translate into reduced pain and disability. The placebo effect size can be measured for a particular intervention if the participants are divided into three groups: treatment group, placebo treatment group, and control group.[125] The difference between the control and the placebo groups will provide data on the placebo effect.[125] The placebo effect is variable in both the number of responders and the magnitude of the effect. The percentage of placebo responders has been estimated to be as high as 35%, but lesser response ranges have been reported.[124]

George and Robinson's[124] summary of the literature on the placebo effect of physical therapy interventions highlighted that the placebo effect triggers a neurophysiologic mechanism recorded with fMRI of the brain demonstrating activity in the cortical areas directly associated with pain inhibition. Studies have also confirmed involvement of the endogenous opioid system by demonstrating that the placebo response is naloxone (opioid receptor antagonist) reversible, which means that the reduction of pain from a placebo response can be reversed with the opioid receptor antagonist.[124] These studies provide preliminary data to support that the psychologic factors of manual therapy interventions may trigger supraspinal cord pain modulatory mechanisms similar to the neurophysiologic effects of spinal manipulation.

In summary, the psychologic effects of manipulation are dependent on the psychosocial context of the patient, including the patient's values and expectations of the treatment. In general, if patients have a positive attitude and expectation of an intervention and they receive that intervention, the positive effects of the treatment tend to be the greatest. The therapist's bias and expectations, as well as the words used by the therapist can impact the outcome. The therapist/patient interaction can influence the patient's expectations of the treatment and therefore can affect the magnitude of the placebo and psychologic effects of the intervention. The extent that joint manipulation has on psychologic outcomes requires further investigation.

Psychologically Informed Language and Pain Neuroscience Education

Therapists must develop an awareness of the impact that the language used in interactions with patients in pain has on the patients' psychologic and emotional state. In a survey of 130 participants with chronic and recurrent LBP, Setchell et al.[127] reported that the vast majority of the patients described the cause of their pain as resulting from the body being like a "broken machine" with permanent damage, and in general, they used very negative words to describe their condition. Nearly 90% of the participants reported learning these beliefs from health professionals.[127] Clinicians tend to be unaware of the harm their words can cause. By focusing solely on pathoanatomic factors as the cause of the pain, clinicians can actually worsen psychologic factors by increasing the magnitude of the perceived threat of the condition.[128]

Early advanced imaging (such as MRI) of patients with LBP seems to be a factor in increased healthcare expense downstream in the patient's care, including increased incidence of emergency department visits, opioid prescriptions, and surgery.[129] Once the patient becomes focused on the results of the image and the words used to describe the findings on the image, the magnitude of perceived threat is intensified and symptoms worsen. For instance, a term like "degenerative disc disease" may sound catastrophic to the patient conjuring feelings of hopelessness and despair. A better approach may be to describe the imaging findings of degeneration as "normal age changes" analogous to having a dermatologist inform a patient that they have developed "wrinkles on their skin." This description puts the finding in proper perspective because a high percentage of nonsymptomatic individuals in the patient's age range will demonstrate similar findings.[130]

Another area to be very cautious with use of language is in describing theoretic, biomechanical findings with patients. For instance, using a spine model to demonstrate how the therapist thinks that the patient has a "displaced sacroiliac joint" or a "malaligned spine" can potentially increase the magnitude of the perceived threat from the condition and result in fear of movement and intensification of pain perception. The patient will become extra cautious of movement and activity to avoid "redisplacing" their pelvis or putting their "spine out of place" from moving the wrong way. It is best to keep the explanation as simple and straight forward as possible with a positive outlook of how the therapist and patient can work together to restore mobility and reduce pain as they proceed through the rehabilitation program. Therefore the therapist should simply describe the region of stiffness and tissue sensitivity and explain that manual therapy techniques will be used to "improve mobility and send signals to brain to dampen the pain." Explain to the patient that they will, "feel better and move better" following a particular manipulation technique or exercise to enhance the therapeutic outcome[131] through positively influencing the patient's expectations.

There is positive evidence of the benefits of education, movement, and exercise on the management of spinal conditions.[132] Instead of describing the effects of manual therapy as "fixing a structure," patients should be educated on the current scientific understanding of the neurophysiologic mechanisms of action of manual therapy techniques in terms that are understandable to the patient.[60,121] The therapist should explain that manual therapy techniques will be used to help modulate the patient's pain and restore their mobility which should enable the patient to move and function more comfortably, and the patient can use a home exercise program for similar effects.[133] Explain to the patient that "movement and exercise will not only loosen and strengthen your back but also send good signals to your brain that can dampen your pain" and "the best thing we can do for your back is to get it moving and keep it moving." Repeating simple phrases throughout the treatment sessions, such as "motion is lotion" can help to reinforce the positive therapeutic effects of both the manual therapy and the exercise program, and repeating statements, such as "the spine is a strong structure" can also help to minimize fear and anxiety.[134]

Therapists must be aware of the impact of the language they use with patients in all professional situations. Heightened emphasis on pain coping strategies and pain neuroscience education should be included in the plan of care when patients express high levels of fear and anxiety about their pain and/or score at or above a moderate level on the Central Sensitization Inventory (Fig. 2.7) or a high level on the STarT Back questionnaire (Fig. 2.4) as described in Chapter 2.[135–137]

Pain neuroscience education is a cognitive-based educational intervention performed by physical therapists that aims to desensitize the central nervous system and consequently reduce pain and disability by providing a broader biopsychosocial understanding to conceptualize the meaning of the pain experience.[138,139] Pain neuroscience education instructs patients in the role of neurophysiologic (e.g., central and peripheral nervous system sensitization), psychologic, social, and environmental factors to better understand the pain experience.[139] For chronic musculoskeletal pain disorders, there is evidence from multiple systematic reviews that an educational strategy addressing neurophysiology and neurobiology of pain can have a positive effect on pain, disability, catastrophizing, physical performance, and minimizing healthcare utilization.[138,140,141] The objectives include to decrease the threat value of pain, increase the patients' knowledge about pain neuroscience, and to reconceptualize pain into a broader biopsychosocial perspective.[139] To achieve this, the patient needs to understand that all pain is produced, constructed, and modulated by the brain and that once a normal inflammatory and healing response has occurred, their pain symptoms are created by hypersensitivity of the nervous system rather than ongoing tissue damage.[139] Through metaanalysis, Watson et al.[141] reported that the treatment effect of pain neuroscience education for kinesiophobia was clinically significant in the short

term and for pain catastrophizing in the medium term. The pain neuroscience education should be an interactive educational process with the patient. For instance, allowing a patient to tell his own pain story has been identified as a key component to enhance the outcomes of pain neuroscience education[141] and motivational interviewing methods have been proposed as an effective means to enhance pain reconceptualization.[139]

Patients with musculoskeletal-related nociceptive pain should receive elements of the following pain neuroscience education: nociceptors are specialized sensory neurons that can be stimulated in three ways: mechanically, thermally, and chemically (Fig. 3.8). Nociceptors pass information via the peripheral nervous system (i.e., primary afferent nerves) regarding the intensity, duration, and location of peripheral noxious stimulation.[142] The primary afferent sends a message to the dorsal horn of the spinal cord which interacts with the interneuron, followed by a second-order neuron that sends the message to the brain (Fig. 3.3). The nerve axon will respond and adapt (via opening ion channels) to stimuli applied to the nerve, such as temperature, stress, movement, pressure, immune changes, or blood flow.[73,142] If enough ion channels open because of one type of stimulus, the signals reach the brain and are interpreted as pain. Nociception is interpreted by the brain as pain based on the brain's interpretation of the relative threat associated with the information transmitted and the intensity and magnitude of the impulses.[142] Inflammation exposes the peripheral nerves to inflammatory mediators called

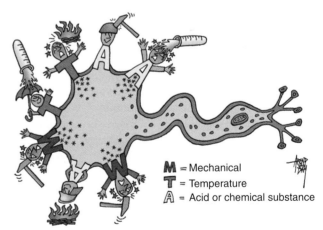

FIG. 3.8 Illustration used to explain basic principles of acute nociception. This illustration presents a neuron, with on the left its "sensors" which are capable of sensing temperature changes (indicated by the letter "T"), chemical substances ("A") and mechanical pressure ("M"). Activation of such a sensor opens the corresponding ion channel in the cell membrane of the neuron. This enables an influx of sodium ions into the neuron ('positive charges enter the cell'), possibly resulting in an action potential ("the danger message"). It is important for the patient to realize that the presence of an action potential does not necessarily imply that pain is or will be experienced. (From Nijs J, van Wilgen CP, Van Oosterwijck J, et al. How to explain central sensitization to patients with unexplained chronic musculoskeletal pain: practice guidelines. *Man Ther.* 2011;16:413-418.)

cytokines that create peripheral nerve sensitization that is manifest as hypersensitivity of the injured/inflamed and surrounding tissues.[143] This is part of the body's normal protective mechanism. There are descending fibers from the brain that supply endogenous chemicals that allow for a modulation (i.e., dampening or downregulation) of nociception and the pain experience.[142] Other brain activity, such as thoughts, memories, emotions, stress, and anxiety can influence the interpretation of these signals, the up- or down-modulation of pain, and the brain's pain output.

With patients with signs of central sensitization, pain neuroscience education should include additional elements, such as the following: a common phenomenon in treating individuals with musculoskeletal related pain is for the pain to continue or even intensify beyond the natural healing timeline. A likely explanation for this phenomenon is associated with changes of the primary and second-order afferent nerve fibers and where they intersect at the dorsal horn of the spinal cord.[142] Ion channels of the nerve fibers are continuously changing so that one type can drop out and another can take its place depending on input provided to the body and the brain that may positively or negatively affect the neuroplasticity, which is the ability of neurons to change their function, chemical profile (quantities and types of neurotransmitters produced), and/or structure.[73,142] At the primary afferent nerve fibers, an abnormal concentration of ion channels located in the axon can develop an ability to generate its own impulses and can fire in response to adrenaline (fear, anxiety, stress, or anger), movement or mechanical pressure, or temperature changes in the environment.[142,144] The ion channel changes of the nerve axon are one explanation for persistent hyperalgesia that can occur with peripheral sensitization (i.e., nociceptive chronic pain)[142,144] (Fig. 3.9). Neuropathic pain occurs when injury of a peripheral nerve results in ephaptic transmission (abnormal cross-talk between neurons) and ectopic foci (added action potentials where myelin is damaged), making the nerve hypersensitive to mechanical and chemical stimuli.[73] With persistent input from the periphery to the dorsal horn because of peripheral sensitivity or neuropathic pain, changes occur in the second-order neurons (glial cell modification), the dorsal horn (enhanced receptors and neurotransmitters), and brain pathways (i.e., neuroplasticity) leading to heightened central sensitization and a reduced ability to modulate nociceptive impulses.[145] In response to these persistent danger signals that the brain interprets as a threat, receptors at the dorsal horn can be added and replaced with new ones that stay open longer to further intensify the sensitivity (i.e., upregulation) leading to a lower threshold for activation and central sensitization.[145] These changes can lead to a reduced pain threshold, an increase in the magnitude and duration of responses to noxious input (pain spreading), and can permit normally innocuous inputs to generate pain sensations (i.e., allodynia)[145,146] (Fig. 3.10).

Patients should be informed that understanding the way that the brain processes pain can help to begin to reduce the sensitivity of the nervous system. Exercise and manual therapy techniques, as well as localization training, will send positive signals to the brain that can trigger a pain modulation (i.e., downregulation) response and dampen nervous system sensitivity and reduce pain perception. Specific areas of the brain (primary sensory cortex) provide interpretation of somatosensory stimulation, such as light touch creating a cortical body map that can be illustrated by the homunculus (Fig. 3.11). When the body part is not moved normally or regularly because of pain or fear of pain, the cortical body map can be altered as part of the neuroplastic changes occurring with central sensitization with consequences, such as inhibited two-point discrimination, difficulty with left-right discrimination, and reduced ability to localize light touch.[142] Localization training could include showing a patient with chronic LBP a body diagram with a nine-box grid on the low back (Fig. 3.12) and asking them to identify which box is being touched on their back.[147] Louw et al.[147] demonstrated immediate improvement in pain and lumbar forward bending following a 5-minute localization train session in a series of 16 patients with chronic LBP. Normally, individuals should be accurate 80% of the time, and if they are not, localization training can help improve neuroplasticity and brain mapping.[142]

Positive effects of pain neuroscience education on pain perception, disability, and catastrophizing can allow patients to apply this new view of their pain state by reappraising their ability to move.[138] With the therapist's reassurance of the decreased threat of additional tissue injury and a realization that pain may be caused by neural sensitivity rather than tissue injury, patients may be able to actively move further and allow therapists to passively move them further.[138] Patients tend to learn pain neuroscience education most effectively via metaphors, examples, and images.[140] More comprehensive resources are available elsewhere for therapists to expand their knowledge on pain neuroscience education.[73,142,148,149]

Pain neuroscience education aims to describe how the nervous system, through peripheral nerve sensitization, central sensitization, synaptic activity, and brain processing, interprets information from the tissues, and that neural activation, as either upregulation or downregulation, has the ability to modulate the pain experience.[138] Patients are thus educated that the nervous system's processing of their injury, in conjunction with various psychosocial factors, determines their pain experience and that pain is not always a true representation of the status of the tissues.[138] Pain neuroscience education aims at reconceptualizing pain, by explaining that all pain is in the brain and that, rather than local tissue damage, hypersensitivity of the central nervous system may be the cause of the pain problem and enables patients to understand their pain.[150] By reconceptualizing pain as the brain's interpretation of the threat of the injury, rather than an accurate measure of the degree of injury in their tissues, patients may be more inclined to move, exercise, and push into some discomfort.[138]

Pain should be conceptualized as a highly complex, subjective human experience that is felt in tissues but interpreted by the mind as a response to a perceived threat.[151] In this context, because the degree of pain intensity is influenced by the

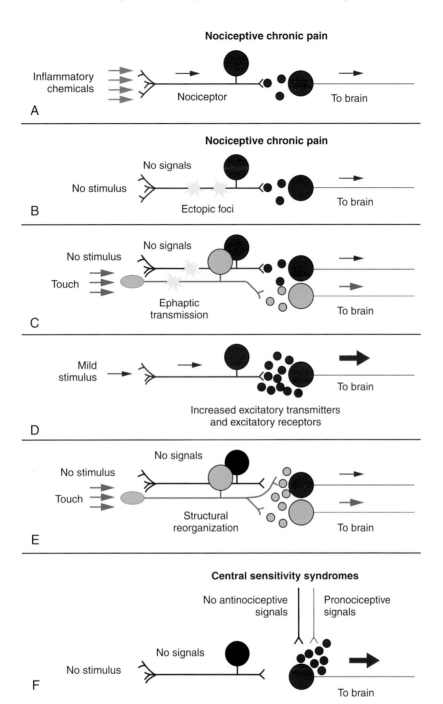

FIG. 3.9 Mechanisms of nociceptive and neuropathic pain and central sensitivity syndromes. *Red* indicates activity in the nociceptive pathway. *Black* indicates that the neuron or part of a neuron is inactive. *Green* indicates activity in the light touch pathway. **A,** Normal physiologic function of the pain system: inflammatory chemicals at the site of injury have sensitized peripheral nociceptors, and signals indicating tissue damage travel to the brain. **B** to **E** illustrate neuropathic mechanisms: **B,** Ectopic foci. **C,** Ephaptic transmission from an Aβ tactile neuron to nociceptive fibers. **D,** Central sensitization, created by increased excitatory transmitter availability and an increased number of excitatory receptors. **E,** Structural reorganization, in this case, the retraction of C-fiber proximal endings from nociceptive tract neurons and growth of Aβ tactile endings to synapse with nociceptive tract neurons. **F,** Central sensitivity syndromes cause changes in pain matrix top-down regulation, with silence of antinociceptive signals and excessive pronociceptive signals. (From Lundy-Ekman L. *Neuroscience Fundamentals for Rehabilitation*, ed 5. Elsevier; 2018.)

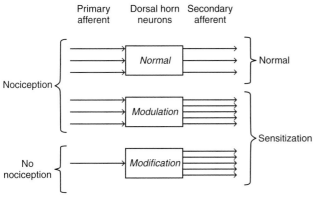

FIG. 3.10 Illustration used to explain the difference between acute nociception and central sensitization in chronic pain. This illustration explains one of the essential features of central sensitization in chronic pain. The situation on top represents the normal situation, with primary afferents transporting three danger messages to the dorsal horn neurons, as is the case when you cut your finger. Next, the dorsal horn neurons activate the secondary afferents that transport the same three danger messages to the brain for processing. However, in many cases dorsal horn neurons modulate the incoming danger messages, as illustrated in the middle and below. The situation in the middle represents 'real' nociception, with three danger messages entering the spinal cord neurons, and five being sent to the brain. This implies that the incoming messages are amplified in the spinal cord before entering the brain. The situation illustrates central sensitization in patients with chronic pain. Even in absence of nociception, messages from the periphery (e.g., touching the skin above the painful region or moving the affected limb) are amplified in a powerful way such that the dorsal horn neurons send several danger messages to the brain. (From Nijs J, van Wilgen CP, Van Oosterwijck J, et al. How to explain central sensitization to patients with unexplained chronic musculoskeletal pain: practice guidelines, *Man Ther.* 2011;16:413-418.)

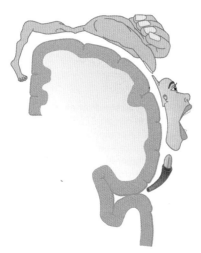

FIG. 3.11 Primary sensory cortex. Areas of the right postcentral gyrus responding to somatosensory stimulation from the left body/face are indicated by the homunculus. (From Lundy-Ekman L. *Neuroscience Fundamentals for Rehabilitation*, ed 5. Elsevier; 2018.)

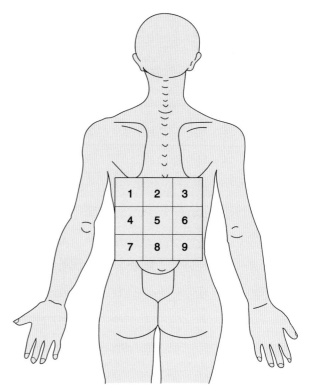

FIG. 3.12 Localization treatment grid. (From Louw A, Farrell K, Wettach L, et al. Immediate effects of sensory discrimination for chronic low back pain: a case series. *N Z J Physiother.* 2015; 43(2):58-63.)

magnitude of the perceived threat, it may help the patient cope with their condition more effectively if the therapist can provide an example of the severe pain intensity reported by a violin player getting stuck with a pin in their finger compared with a truck driver. The violin player's occupation is threatened by a finger injury where the truck driver's is not to the same extent. This can be further related to the patient's particular situation by asking patients how they may feel threatened by their current pain situation.

Another example that can be made to further educate patients on the interaction of threat, attention, and pain, is to tell a story about a person who steps on a nail. Normally, when a person steps on a nail, nociception impulses travel to the brain, the brain interprets the nail in the foot as a threat to their wellbeing and they experience pain. If the person stepped on the nail in the middle of a road and looked up to see a bus about to hit them, they would forget about the nail pain and jump out of the way of the bus. The bus becomes the larger threat and overrides the pain from the nail in the foot. Reassuring patients with chronic pain conditions that their body is structurally strong and movement and activity are not going to cause further threat to their wellbeing but will ultimately help dampen the pain and make them stronger so they can return to normal activities, can help to lessen the threat associated with their injury and pain.

Moseley[152] advocates that therapists must educate patients that pain provides the tissues a protective buffer. The protective buffer offered by pain can change with a huge range of variables including inflammation, cognitive and social cues.[152] The pain system over time can learn to become more protective and overly sensitized, and the best way to retrain this protective pain system is by learning about pain, adopting active management strategies, gradually loading the painful tissue through movement and activity, and using psychologically informed therapies.[152] Likewise, pain can be explained to patients as the nervous system's alarm system. Because of a variety of social and psychologic factors, such as stress, anxiety, or depression, the nervous system can become sensitized so that the alarm system goes off in response to activities that normally would not be interpreted as painful. You can ask the patient if they had a fire alarm that was going off in their house with no sign of a fire, at what point should they stop looking for a fire, but instead, give attention to the problem with the alarm (i.e., sensitized nervous system). Therefore treatments that downregulate the nervous system (such as exercise and manual therapy) are needed to lower the threshold for triggering the pain alarm system. The best treatment for this is to understand that this is occurring (i.e., pain neuroscience education) and to work toward desensitizing the nervous system through movement, exercise, gentle manual therapy techniques, and gradual progression of activity.

A dialog with the patient to confirm that the patient understands that pain, behavior, thoughts, and emotions influence and maintain each other is vital before beginning an exercise program designed to progressively guide the patient to overcome their fears of movement induced pain.[127] As patients are guided through exercises that specifically target isolated muscle contractions or specific directions of movement, reassurance must be provided to the patient that the perceived pain is not related to the muscle or movement itself, but rather a product of the brain and an enhanced central nociceptive processing. Ultimately, the enhanced central nociceptive processing can be dampened through reconceptualizing the pain and guided prescribed exercise.

It is best to change the underlying metaphor with patients to "life is a journey" rather than attempting to "fix a broken machine," and the emphasis of physical therapy should become helping the patient manage their condition and move on with their life so that the chronic pain can be managed in the background of their life without dominating the foreground and distracting them from their life goals and valued activities.[128] Ultimately, once red flags have been screened, the therapist's job is to alleviate the patient's fears, which will reduce the perceived threat and minimize the pain perception. This can be accomplished through pain neuroscience education, manual therapy, exercise, and reassurance throughout the rehabilitation process.

THE AUDIBLE JOINT "POP"

The physiology of an audible joint pop or crack phenomenon associated with a joint manipulation has been investigated in three principal studies: Roston and Haines,[153] Unsworth, Dowson, and Wright,[154] and Kawchuk et al.[155] with application of increasing tension at the metacarpal-phalangeal joint of the third finger and monitoring of the amount of joint separation with intermittent radiographs, Roston and Haines[153] were able to show that the amount of joint separation increases very gradually in a linear fashion as the tension on the joint is increased. However, when a critical amount of tension is reached to produce a joint "pop," a sudden increase in the amount of joint separation is noted. Roston and Haines[153] interpreted the space noted after the cracking as a "partial vacuum occupied by water vapor and blood gases under reduced pressure." A joint that has been "cracked" is not capable of being recracked for approximately 20 minutes,[153,154] which is referred to as the refractory period; the belief is that gas must be reabsorbed before the joint can be cracked again.[153]

Unsworth, Dowson, and Wright[154] performed a similar study and described the formation of vapor-filled bubbles in the joint as a result of cavitation, which is the process of fluid converted to gas from a critical reduction in pressure. In the case of the joint, the synovial fluid is vaporized once negative 2.5 atmospheric pressure is reached as a result of tension placed on the joint.[154] Unsworth, Dowson, and Wright[154] further explain the cracking phenomenon as the result of not just the formation of a gas bubbles in the joint cavity from negative pressure but the explosion of these gas bubbles to cause the noise. The gas bubbles seem to collapse instantly once formed as the bubbles come into contact with the remaining synovial fluid, which is of a higher pressure. Unsworth, Dowson, and Wright[154] also identified a sudden jump in joint separation just after the crack and noted that the reloading and noncracking joints have a more gradual separation but separate to the same distance.

The joint surfaces must be close to give the correct preloading conditions for cavitation to occur, and Unsworth, Dowson, and Wright[154] found that the joint separation takes 15 minutes to return to its precracking value. They calculated that reabsorption of the gas, which is believed to be primarily carbon dioxide, may take 30 minutes.[154] These factors may help to explain the refractory period. Unsworth, Dowson, and Wright[154] noted that the joints that did not crack in the study had a resting joint separation 25% greater than the cracking joints. The joints that did not crack separated when under tension in a similar fashion as the cracking joints in their refractory period, and the common denominator seems to be the amount of joint separation before application of the load.

Kawchuk et al.[155] used real-time cine MRI at a rate of 3.2 frames per second to visualize the audible joint sound of 10 metacarpophalangeal joints caused by application of long axis traction by inserting the finger into a flexible tube tightened around the length of a cable. As the traction force increased, real-time cine MRI demonstrated gradual increase in joint space until a rapid joint cavity separation occurs concurrently with sound production, after which the resulting cavity remained visible.[155] The space remained as long as the traction force was maintained, but returned to normal with release of the force.[155] These results offer direct experimental evidence that joint cracking is associated with joint cavity creation rather than collapse of a preexisting bubble.[155] These observations are consistent with tribonucleation, a process where opposing surfaces resist separation until a critical point where they then separate rapidly creating a sustained gas cavity.[155]

Flynn et al.[156] compared the immediate effects of a lumbopelvic manipulation for patients who were noted as having an audible joint sound (i.e.,"pop") with the manipulation and for those who did not. In comparison of the response between the two groups, Flynn et al.[156] reported no difference in outcomes (disability, pain, lumbar flexion AROM) between the group of patients who had an audible pop with the manipulation and the group of those who did not. In a secondary analysis of 40 participants who underwent thermal pain sensitivity testing of their leg and low back, Bialosky et al.[157] found the same degree of hypoalgesia at the low back and the lower extremity immediately after a lumbopelvic thrust manipulation independent of perception of an audible pop. However, the inhibition of lower extremity temporal summation was greater in individuals in whom an audible pop was perceived.[157]

Silevis and Cleland[158] found that the immediate effects of a T3–T4 thrust manipulation on pain reduction and activity of the autonomic nervous system were the same whether or not the thrust manipulation resulted in one audible pop, multiple audible pops, or no audible pop for 50 patients with chronic neck pain who received the intervention. Likewise, a study that demonstrated increased bilateral biceps muscle resting EMG activity after a C5–C6 thrust manipulation in 54 asymptomatic participants found that this occurred whether or not an audible pop occurred with the manipulation.[113]

Based on these studies,[113,156–158] the beneficial effects of manipulation do not appear to be dependent on the production of a joint sound. Therefore creation of a joint sound should not be the primary goal of a manipulation technique. There may be some placebo-related treatment effect with achieving a joint sound, especially if this is a component of a patient's expectations for a positive treatment experience, but further study is needed to better understand the psychologic impact of the joint sounds. Outcome measures other than production of joint sounds appear to be more important, including reduction in pain, reduction in perceived disability, and improvement in mobility and function.

CLINICAL REASONING IN USE OF SPINAL MANIPULATION

Clinical reasoning in musculoskeletal and manual physical therapy requires development of a model in which a detailed patient history is obtained through use of intake forms, medical screening forms, and a patient interview. The initial patient interview is an important component to establishing a therapeutic alliance with the patient, and with utilization of active listening skills, the therapist can begin to develop a rapport with the patient that can translate to positive clinical outcomes. The therapist will interpret the data from the intake forms and interview to develop multiple diagnostic hypotheses

and to screen for risk factors and red and yellow flags. Consideration for medical, neurologic, and vascular screening is developed and implemented based on the presenting data. Expert physical therapists will use both hypothetico-deductive reasoning and pattern recognition in the clinical reasoning process to arrive at an initial working diagnosis.[159] The physical examination should be planned based on the information obtained in the history and interview to support or refute the hypotheses.

The physical examination should include tests and measures with sound reliability and validity, and the therapist will consider patterns and clusters of positive and negative findings to test the hypotheses. These data are further evaluated to arrive at an impairment-based classification/diagnosis and to develop a plan of treatment management in collaboration with the patient.

The therapist must continue to evaluate and reevaluate the patient throughout each treatment session to progress or modify the treatment accordingly with the intention of achieving the most optimal clinical outcomes. Manual physical therapists have the ability to further test hypotheses based on patient response to manual therapy procedures.[159] Between-session changes in pain intensity and ROM are more likely to occur in patients who demonstrate within session changes in the same parameters.[160,161] Therefore evaluation and reevaluation of key subjective and objective findings throughout each treatment session should be used to guide clinical decisions on which treatments are most effective and will result in the most positive outcomes. Manual therapy is not a passive intervention. When applied properly, manual therapy interventions actively engage the patient in the therapeutic alliance to determine effective response to the treatment. Commonly, the manual therapy interventions will be coupled with therapeutic exercises that can be used to reinforce and further assess the effects of the manual therapy.

An Impairment-Based Biomechanical Approach to Clinical Decision Making

Biomechanical approach is a term for an impairment-based approach of management of spinal disorders in which clinical decisions are based on the results of clinical tests and measures that analyze active and passive motion. The clinical decisions on the depth, location, and direction of manipulation procedures are based on knowledge of spinal mechanics for interpretation of these clinical findings. Pain provocation and tissue reactivity are assessed in a similar manner, and this clinical information is factored into the decision of manipulation technique selection. For instance, if a joint is both hypomobile and highly reactive, techniques are selected with adequate depth and force to stretch the joint, but less vigorous techniques (grades I and II) may precede the stretch manipulation procedure to first attempt to inhibit pain, especially if the patient reflexively holds against the manipulation forces. A thrust technique can often be successful in this situation because the speed of the technique can precede the muscle guarding reaction, and if successful, pain reduction and muscle inhibition result at the targeted spinal segment. If a spinal segment is found to be hypermobile, it is treated with motor control exercises, and perhaps grade III or IV manipulation techniques may be used at hypomobile regions above or below the hypermobile spinal segment.

Cleland and Childs[162] have challenged the validity of use of a biomechanical model as a basis for clinical reasoning manual physical therapy. Historically, a biomechanical model has been the basis for most manual physical therapy clinical approaches, and the foundations of these approaches are what clinicians have used to show positive outcomes from manual therapy interventions applied in clinical trials.[163–165] Therefore one could argue that the biomechanical model works well clinically, but the rationale for the effectiveness is now being challenged.

One argument against the use of a biomechanical model relates to evidence with use of dynamic MRI that accessory PA manipulation forces directed to the spine are less localized than originally thought. Kulig, Landel, and Powers[166] assessed spinal dynamics with PA mobilization (grade IV force) techniques of the lumbar spine and showed that sagittal plane motion occurs at all the lumbar spinal levels with this technique.

The results of the study from Kulig, Landel, and Powers[166] revealed a consistent pattern of lumbar spine motion during PA mobilization procedures. The amount of motion was greatest at the targeted spinal segment where the PA force was applied, and the PA force produced motion directed toward extension. In addition, two patterns of motion were observed at the nontargeted segments. With force applied at L5, L4, or L3, all lumbar segments generally moved toward extension (Figs. 3.13 and 3.14). With force applied at L2 or L1, the three most cranial lumbar segments (L1–L2, L2–L3, and L3–L4) moved toward extension, and the two most caudal segments (L4–L5 and L5–S1) moved toward flexion (see Figs. 3.13 and 3.14). The magnitude of extension motion was greatest at the targeted segment.[166]

Although the dynamic MRI study illustrates that more than one spinal segment moves with PA force application, the pattern of induced passive motion to the lumbar spine was unique with each targeted segmental application. As an assessment tool, unique information is obtained with assessment of PA mobility at each spinal level and clinical decisions can still be based on this information. Further, if a particular spinal level is painful with PA force application, oscillatory techniques can be applied to adjacent spinal levels to induce some motion at the painful segment. Likewise, if mechanical effects are desired, the greatest extension movement can be applied by mobilizing at the targeted hypomobile segment. If passive motion is contraindicated at a spinal level (such as after a recent lumbar fusion), PA mobilization techniques should not be used at the adjacent spinal segments. Therefore the manual physical therapist can use this knowledge to enhance the biomechanical approach but, at the same time, must understand that the ability to segment specific with manual therapy assessment and treatment procedures is limited.

The forces applied to specific vertebrae create a motion at more spinal levels than just the targeted segment. At the same time, the pattern and magnitude of motion are unique to localization of force application. Clinically useful information can be attained by applying forces at each vertebra to assess mobility and reactivity. These results must be interpreted as spinal region specific versus spinal segment specific. However, for documentation purposes and for the purpose of finding the location to reapply the technique in the future, documentation of the segment where the force was applied is still acceptable. In the end, correlation of findings is needed to determine the best intervention. Clinicians should never rely on the results of one assessment to make a clinical decision. In the case of PA passive accessory intervertebral motion (PAIVM) tests, this examination finding should be correlated with symptom behavior, AROM, tissue palpation, muscle strength/length testing, and other passive intervertebral motion (PIVM) tests.

Tuttle et al.[167] demonstrated that that PA mobilization techniques to the cervical spine for patients with neck pain positively changed cervical AROM and spinal stiffness only when the technique was applied to a previously identified symptomatic spinal segment, but these positive effects of AROM and stiffness did not occur if the mobilization was applied to other random spinal segments. In a follow-up review paper, Tuttle[167] used computer-based modeling combined with biomechanical measurement studies of spinal stiffness to highlight that differences in PA stiffness are most apparent and detectable at levels of force between 10 N to 20 N, which are below the forces commonly used in teaching manual therapy techniques.[167] Therefore more gentle PA forces will tend to be more effective at detecting PA mobility deficits. These studies further highlight the importance of development of skilled, specific gentle handling skills to maximize the therapeutic benefits of manual therapy techniques.

A second argument against the use of a biomechanical model is the evidence that random selection of manipulation techniques may be just as effective as techniques selected based on a clinical assessment that incorporates a biomechanical model.[162] McCarthy et al.[168] completed a RCT in 60 patients

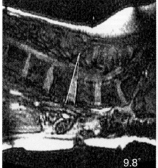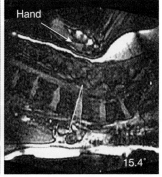

FIG. 3.13 The intervertebral angle was measured as the angle formed by lines defining the end plates of adjacent vertebrae. Segmental lumbar motion was defined as the difference in the intervertebral angle between the resting position *(left)* and intervertebral angle from the end range image *(right)*. The *arrow* identifies the hand of the examiner.

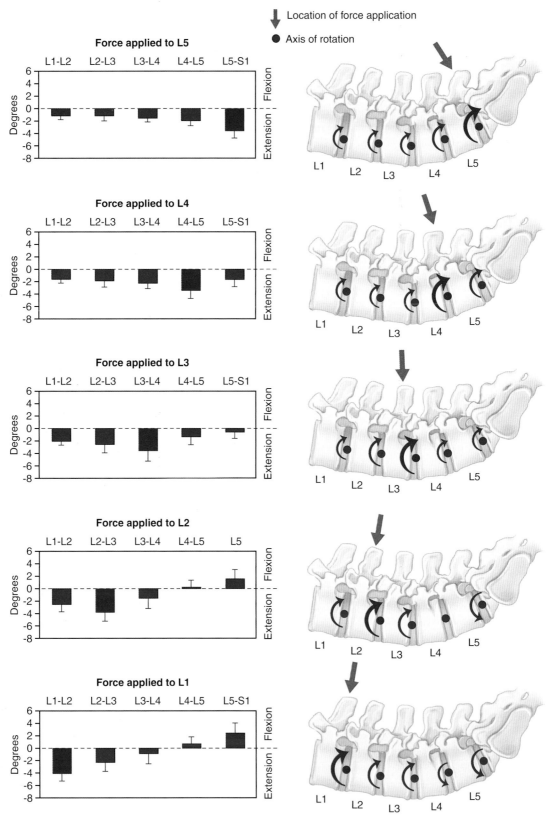

FIG. 3.14 *Left column,* Mean segmental motion at each lumbar segment during a posterior-to-anterior spine mobilization technique applied to the spinous process of a single vertebra. *Error bars* represent 1 standard deviation. *Right column,* Motion represented graphically. *Arrows* indicate the vertebra at which the force was applied. *Curved arrows* show the direction of motion, and *thickness of the curved arrows* indicate relative amount of rotation. (Modified from Kulig PA. Assessment of lumbar spine kinematics using dynamic MRI: a proposed mechanism of sagittal plane motion induced by manual posterior-to-anterior mobilization. *J Orthop Sports Phys Ther.* 2004;34(2):60.)

with LBP who were randomly allocated to two groups: one group received a targeted manipulative thrust ($n = 29$) and the other a general manipulation thrust ($n = 31$) to the lumbar spine over three treatment sessions. Thrust was either localized to a clinician-defined symptomatic spinal level or an equal force was applied through the whole lumbosacral region using a similar side-lying lumbar rotation thrust manipulation technique. Repeated measures of analysis of covariance revealed no between-group differences in self-reported pain or pressure pain thresholds for the lumbar muscles studied, but there was a larger surface EMG reflex response in the targeted thrust manipulation group.

Chiradejnant et al.[169] completed an RCT to determine the immediate effects on pain level and AROM of patients with LBP treated with a PA lumbar mobilization technique either at the therapist-selected level or at a randomly selected level. The study found no difference in short-term outcomes between these two groups, and both groups reported improvements in pain level and lumbar ROM. Further data analysis revealed better outcomes in patients who received the mobilization technique to the lower lumbar levels, which will tend to be stiffer, compared with the upper lumbar levels. The results of this study confirm that lumbar mobilization treatment has an immediate effect on relief of pain but also suggest that the specific technique used may not be important.[169] The results of the study of Chiradejnant et al.[169] are not surprising after a review of the Kulig, Landel, and Powers[166] MRI study. The results should only be interpreted for the PA mobilization technique, which has shown with MRI studies to move multiple levels, and the PA lumbar mobilization technique should be considered a general lumbar mobilization/manipulation technique.

Haas et al.[170] found a similar result in comparison with the short-term effects of cervical spine manipulations that were randomly selected versus those techniques that were selected because of results of cervical PIVM testing. Both groups of patients showed same-day reduction in pain and stiffness, but no difference in results could be attributed to the results of PIVM testing.[170] Long-term effects of a random approach to manipulation technique selection have not been studied. The data suggest that pain modulation may not be limited to mechanisms associated with manipulation of joints with restricted motion. In addition, there is evidence of systemic and regional hypoalgesia resulting from a variety of spinal manipulation techniques, which is presented in greater detail in the neurophysiologic effects of manipulation section of this chapter.

A third argument against the use of a biomechanical model is that evidence suggests that manipulation techniques are not segment specific.[162] Studies have investigated the accuracy and precision of spinal thrust manipulation techniques as determined by location of audible joint sounds. Ross, Bereznick, and McGill[171] investigated the accuracy of thrust manipulation directed at the lumbar and thoracic spine with skin sensors for detection of the audible joint sounds, and engineering principles were used to determine the distance of the audible

joint sound from the targeted spinal segment. The results showed that thoracic spine thrust manipulation was accurate (i.e., audible joint sound occurred at the targeted segment) 53% of the time and that lumbar spine thrust manipulation was accurate 46% of the time.[171] Most of the thrust manipulations resulted in multiple audible joint sounds, which usually included the targeted segment, but the authors included the multiple audible joint sound techniques in their calculations as being not segment specific.[171] In fact, other studies have found the production of multiple joint sounds (3–5) with a thrust manipulation is more the norm than the exception.[172,173] This study assumes that an audible joint sound is vital to localization of force and success of thrust manipulation. Neither premise has been proven. In fact, multiple studies[113,156–158] have shown that the beneficial effects of thrust manipulation have little to do with production of an audible joint sound during the manipulation. In addition, multiple techniques are typically used during any one treatment session, which further increases the odds of manipulating the targeted segment.

In summary, preliminary evidence shows that manual therapists are unable to be as specific with segmental manual therapy assessment and manipulation techniques as they have purported to be in the past, especially in the lumbar spine. As manual therapy procedures are taught and practiced clinically, consideration of these limitations must be considered. However, the refinement of manual therapy skill and the application of successful techniques to produce favorable outcomes are dependent on efforts to strive to be as specific as possible. Undue claims of supernatural palpation skills are unwarranted; but as the evidence emerges to guide clinical practice, the identification of patients who will benefit from manipulation continues to be dependent on skillful manual examination and manipulation procedures.[174–176]

There is preliminary evidence that manual therapy treatment of symptomatic, stiff spinal segments can result in enhanced gains in mobility and pain reduction,[34–37] but there is a lack of technology available to reliability measure segmental spinal stiffness throughout the spine. Fritz, Whitman, and Childs[176] showed a correlation between patients who had passive lumbar hypomobility with central posterior to anterior PAIVM testing and the patients who responded favorably to spinal thrust manipulation. In other words, patients with lumbar mobility deficits are more likely to respond favorably to spinal thrust manipulation. In addition, a strong correlation for a positive response to a spinal stabilization exercise program was correlated with hypermobility noted with central PA PAIVM testing of the lumbar spine. This correlation provides further evidence for an impairment-based approach and validates the use of PA PAIVM testing as an important component of a physical therapist examination scheme to determine the most effective intervention for spinal disorders.[176]

Clinical reasoning in musculoskeletal and manual physical therapy relies on an evidence-informed approach combined with consideration of patient preferences and the clinician's experience and pattern recognition. Research evidence supports the effectiveness of treatment of spinal disorders by subgrouping patients based on identification of key physical impairments, patient characteristics, and symptoms. Use of a biomechanical impairment-based approach is the foundation of physical therapy treatment of musculoskeletal disorders and the specific interventions that include education, exercises, and manual therapy techniques must be tailored to meet each individual patient's specific needs. An impairment approach can guide clinical decision making where specific physical impairments (such as joint mobility deficits, joint hypermobility, muscle weakness, or tightness) are identified through clinical examination and appropriate interventions are administered based on the examination findings. When examination reveals impairments, such as a heightened level of fear and anxiety or signs of central sensitization, patient education should focus on pain science education, coping, and self-treatment strategies with active exercise. If manual therapy is used in these situations, overemphasis on a biomechanical explanation of the patient's condition may be detrimental to positive outcomes as discussed earlier in this chapter.

This textbook presents the evidence for clinical reasoning that includes a biomechanical impairment-based approach in the assessment and treatment of spinal disorders. Impairment-based classifications are presented to assist in management of common signs and symptoms. Likewise, the Orthopaedic Academy of the APTA has linked their clinical practice guidelines for LBP and neck pain to the World Health Organization's International Classification of Functioning, Disability, and Health, which advocates use of impairment-based classifications for management of musculoskeletal disorders.[23,177,178]

Adverse Effects, Safety, and Contraindications With Spinal Manipulation

Adverse events following a spinal manipulation procedure are extremely rare, but they can occur, and therapists must be vigilant to assure safety with application of proper technique and screening patients with a comprehensive examination for contraindications and precautions to manipulation. Adverse events have been defined as the sequalae following an intervention that result in medium to severe symptoms, and of a nature that is serious, distressing, and unacceptable to the patient and requires treatment.[179] Unwanted side effects of interventions, such as manipulation, are more common and are defined as short term, mild in nature, nonserious, transient, and reversible consequences of treatment, such as increase in pain, headache, discomfort, and fatigue.[179]

Lumbar Spine

Serious or severe adverse events of lumbar spinal manipulation are extremely rare.[180] The most serious potential adverse event from lumbar manipulation is development of cauda equina syndrome. Cauda equina syndrome is a medical emergency that should be treated surgically as soon as possible for decompression of the cauda equina. The signs and symptoms of cauda equina syndrome may include urinary retention, fecal incontinence, and widespread neurologic signs and symptoms in the lower extremities that may include gait abnormality, saddle area numbness, and a lax anal sphincter.[181]

Haldeman and Rubenstein[182] reviewed the literature in a 77-year period and could only find 10 reports of cauda equina syndrome after lumbar manipulation. The risk of cauda equina syndrome from lumbar manipulation has been estimated to be less than one in 100 million manipulations.[183,184] This level of risk of serious harm can be put into perspective relative to other common interventions for LBP. With use of nonsteroidal antiinflammatory drugs (NSAIDs), the chance of development of serious gastrointestinal (GI) bleeding as a consequence is 1% to 3%; 7600 deaths and 76,000 hospitalizations annually in the United States are attributable to NSAIDs. If NSAIDs are used for more than 4 weeks, the chance of development of a GI bleed is 1/1000.[185–187] Compared with exercise, spinal manipulation is safer as well, with a risk of sudden death from exercise estimated to be 1:1.5 million episodes of vigorous physical exertion.[188] The risk of a serious complication of lumbar spinal manipulation compares favorably with other common interventions used to treat LBP.

Minor short-lived side effects of lumbar manipulation are more common. Senstad, Leboeuf-Yde, and Borchgrevink[184] surveyed 1058 patients seen for 4712 treatment sessions by chiropractors in Norway, and 75% of all treatments included thrust manipulation to the lumbar spine. No severe complications were noted, but 55% reported at least one minor side effect. The most common side effects included local discomfort (53%), headache (12%), fatigue (11%), and radiating discomfort (10%). Reactions were mild or moderate in 85% of the cases. Some 64% of the reactions appeared within 4 hours of treatment, and 74% had disappeared within 24 hours. Uncommon reactions were dizziness, nausea, hot skin, or "other" symptoms, each accounting for 5% or less of the reactions.[162] Symptoms that began later than the day of or the day after treatment or symptoms that caused reduced activities of daily living were unusual.[184]

Leboeuf-Yde et al.[189] surveyed 625 patients treated with 1856 spinal manipulations by chiropractors in Sweden. No severe complications or injuries were noted, but 44% reported at least one side effect, such as local discomfort, fatigue, or headache. The symptoms resolved in less than 48 hours in 81% of the cases.[189] The two studies on minor side effects of manipulation both surveyed patients who were treated with chiropractic manipulation. Similar data have not been collected on other practitioners, such as physical therapists who regularly practice spinal manipulation.

Thoracic Spine

There is very little in the research literature on the safety of thrust joint manipulation applied to the thoracic spine. Puentedura and O'Grady[179] completed a systematic review of documented case reports in the literature describing patients who had experienced severe adverse events after receiving a thoracic spine thrust manipulation. Case reports published in peer-reviewed journals were searched from dates January 1950 to February 2015.[179] Ten cases, reported in seven case reports, were identified and involved females (eight) more than males (two), with mean age of 43.5 years (standard deviation [SD] = 18.73, range = 17–71).[179] The most frequent adverse event reported was injury (mechanical or vascular) to the spinal cord (7/10), with pneumothorax and hematothorax (2/10), and cerebral spinal fluid leak secondary to dural sleeve injury (1/10).[179] The most common postmanipulation symptoms described were progressive weakness/paresthesia in the lower extremities (n = 7), thoracic pain (n = 6), nausea (n = 2), and single incidences of shortness of breath/dyspnea at rest, neck stiffness, photophobia, and severe headache relieved by lying supine.[179] Chiropractors were the practitioner in seven of 10 of the cases with one each case for an osteopath, lay person, and physical therapist.[179] The authors concluded that serious adverse events can occur in the thoracic spine as a result of spinal manipulation including trauma to the spinal cord and pneumothorax suggesting that excessive peak forces were likely applied to the thoracic spine in these cases of adverse events.

Thrust joint manipulation techniques to the thoracic spine have been shown to involve greater maximum peak loads compared with lumbar techniques.[190] In this study, maximum peak load through the thoracic spine ranged from 212.30 N to 562.68 N recorded during a PA thrust manipulation technique, and the forces ranged from 105.84 N to 441.11 N for side-lying lumbar rotation manipulation technique.[190] Sran et al.[191] conducted a biomechanical study to quantify the failure load of mid-thoracic vertebral spinous process under PA load and found a mean in vitro failure load of 479 N (range was 200–728 N). Sran et al.[191] found in vivo applied loads with a physiotherapist performing PA nonthrust mobilization techniques to range from 106 to 223 N with a mean of 145 N. There is overlap between the higher end of the range of forces potentially used for both nonthrust and thrust PA mid-thoracic manipulation techniques and the lower end of the range of forces required to fracture a thoracic spinous process.

To assure patient safety and minimize potential side effects, clinicians must attempt to minimize peak forces in their technique application with thoracic manipulation techniques, closely monitor patient response to force application, and screen for contraindications.

Cervical Spine

Cervical spine manipulation techniques pose a risk of side effects and adverse events that range from mild soreness to severe neurovascular injury. Side effects from cervical spine manipulation may include temporary increase in neck pain, radiating arm pain, headache, dizziness, impaired vision, or ringing in the ears.[192] Hurwitz et al.[192] surveyed 280 participants in a chiropractic cervical spine manipulation clinical trial 2 weeks after the trial was started, and 25% of the participants reported increased neck pain or stiffness/soreness that most commonly lasted less than 24 hours after the manipulation. Patients who received nonthrust mobilization techniques reported fewer side effects.[192] Participants with histories of the conditions in Box 3.3 were more likely than others to report side effects, such as discomfort with the chiropractic manipulation.[192]

Based on these results, Hurwitz et al.[192] suggest that nonthrust mobilization techniques may be preferable when the patient has high levels of pain and disability associated with an acute neck pain episode. Cagnie et al.[193] surveyed 465 patients after their first visit with one of 59 manipulative physical therapists, and 60% reported at least one postmanipulation side effect. The most common side effects were headache (19%), stiffness (19.5%), local discomfort (15.2%), radiating discomfort (12.1%), and fatigue (12.1%). Most of these reactions began within 4 hours and generally disappeared within 24 hours. Women were more likely to report side effects than were men. Use of upper cervical manipulations and use of medication, gender, and age were independent predictors of headache after manipulation. Upper cervical spine manipulation was 3.17 times more likely to cause headache than manipulation of the lower cervical spine, and for every 1-year increase in age, a 2.4% decrease was seen in risk of headache after manipulation.[193]

Although minor temporary side effects to cervical spine mobilization/manipulation are fairly common, catastrophic adverse events from cervical mobilization/manipulation are extremely rare. The most catastrophic adverse event is vertebral basilar or internal carotid artery dissection that may lead to vertebrobasilar insufficiency (VBI), stroke, or even death. VBI is a condition characterized by occlusion or injury to the vertebral artery that causes loss of blood flow to the hindbrain. The vertebrobasilar system provides 10% to 20% of the blood supply to the brain and branches to many vital neural structures, including the brainstem, cerebellum, spinal cord, cranial nerves III to XII and their nuclei, and portions of the cerebral cortex.[194]

VBI may cause dizziness, vertigo, headaches, diplopia, blindness, ataxia, lightheadedness, nausea, or numbness to the

---

BOX 3.3	Factors That Affect Increased Likelihood of Side Effects to Cervical Spine Thrust Manipulation

- History of neck trauma
- Pain less than 1 year
- Worsening of pain since onset
- Pain ratings of 8+ on a 0 to 10 scale
- Neck Disability Index scores of 16 or more
- Moderate or severe headache
- Nausea during the past month
- Lack of confidence in the treatment

(Data from Hurwitz EL, Morgenstern H, Vassilaki M, et al. Frequency and clinical predictors of adverse reactions to chiropractic care in the UCLA neck pain study. *Spine*. 2005;30(13):1477-1484.)

face. It could also result in slurred speech, nystagmus, or blurred vision. More severe cases of VBI can present as a cerebrovascular accident and even on occasion can cause death. The signs of VBI complications commonly reported include dizziness, diplopia, dysphagia, drop attacks, difficulty in swallowing, and nausea.[195]

The vertebral artery is believed to be particularly susceptible to injury at the atlas because of its orientation and position at this mobile spinal level. Vigorous rotation of the neck is thought to potentially "kink" the vertebral artery along its course, which could cause dissection of the artery or trauma that may cause formation of a blood clot.[196] End range and forceful cervical spine rotation forces, especially when combined with cervical extension, have been implicated as the most likely source of injury to this portion of the vertebral artery.[197] Also important to note is that a patient with a vertebral artery dissection may initially have only a symptom of neck pain.[198,199]

DiFabio[200] completed an extensive review of the literature and found reports in the literature of 177 patients (from 1925 to 1997) with adverse events to manipulation. The primary diagnosis was arterial dissection/spasm and brainstem lesions, and 32 cases (18%) resulted in death.[200] Physical therapists were involved in less than 2% of the cases, and no deaths were attributed to cervical spine manipulation provided by physical therapists.[200] The type of manipulation was not described in 46% of the cases, but the largest percentage of cases in which the technique was reported included rotation (23%).[200] Only 10% of the cases reported that the injury occurred during the first manipulation.[200]

Puentedura et al.[201] identified 134 reports of severe adverse events after a cervical spine thrust manipulation documented in the literature between 1950 and 2010. After further analysis of the case reports to determine whether there were appropriate indications for the manipulation and whether the adverse event was preventable because of identification of red flags and clinical reasoning, the authors concluded that 44.8% of the cases were preventable, 10.4% were unpreventable, and 44.8% were unknown because of lack of available information in the case report.[123,201] The cervical spine manipulations were performed for appropriate reasons in 80.6% of the cases. Death occurred in 5.2% of the cases either because of arterial dissection or cerebrovascular accident. The most common preexisting serious pathologies for serious adverse events in this review were bony pathologies (70%), including severe osteoporosis and rheumatoid arthritis.[179] These conditions are contraindications to cervical spine manipulation, and some are identifiable through a detailed patient interview and clinical examination.[179] Therefore with proper clinical reasoning and screening for red flags, 44.8% of these cases of severe adverse events could have been prevented, but 10.8% of the cases were unpreventable, which suggests that some inherent risk exists even after a thorough examination and proper clinical reasoning.[201]

Kerry et al.[202] suggests that both the internal carotid artery and vertebral artery should be considered in the risk assessment of treating patients with neck pain because the arterial hemodynamics of the neck as a whole involve both the vertebral artery and internal carotid artery. Blood flow of the neck vessels generally shows reduction in vertebral artery blood flow with end-range cervical rotation and reduction of internal carotid blood flow with end-range cervical extension. Normal hemodynamics occur when the internal carotid blood flow can compensate for reduction in vertebral artery blood flow with rotation and vice versa when blood flow is reduced in the carotids with cervical extension. The blood flow in the vertebral artery and internal carotid artery systems is intricately linked via the Circle of Willis; therefore both vertebral artery and internal carotid artery blood flow and pathologic conditions should be considered in pretreatment risk assessment.[202]

A case control study ($n = 818$) by Cassidy et al.[203] found a comparable level of risk of vertebral basilar artery stroke for patients with headache and neck pain following a visit with a chiropractor for cervical thrust manipulation as compared with a visit to a primary medical physician. The underlying hypothesis is that patients present with existing or impending vascular pathology that may subsequently be aggravated by treatment.[203] This suggests that manual therapy does not result in vascular pathology in those who are otherwise "healthy" and biomechanical studies in healthy individuals suggest that if manual therapy of the neck is undertaken in a combination of mid-range positions, it does not generate sufficient vessel stress or hemodynamic changes to cause a dissection event.[204–207]

Vascular pathology of the neck occurs when there is dissection or clotting of one of more of these vessels and interruption of the normal hemodynamics.[145] Dissections of the vertebral and internal carotid arteries arise from a tear of the inner wall of the vessel.[208] Blood under arterial pressure can then enter the deeper layers of the vessel to form an intramural hematoma that will alter blood flow.[208] This alteration in blood flow may trigger the clotting cascade or an embolus to break off that eventually could move to the brain causing an ischemic stroke. This process may take several days to fully emerge after the initial traumatic event.[208] Infections in the region, for instance of the throat, can also weaken the vessel making this process more likely to occur.[208] Trauma to cervical blood vessels is generally classified as either dissection resulting from direct trauma to the vessel or localized thrombogenesis and embolus formation in response to endothelial damage.[202] Either pathologic state may lead to stroke. Arterial dissection may occur after trivial trauma to the vessel or spontaneously. This could also be related to preexisting, congenital weakness of the vessel wall or acquired vascular pathologic conditions, such as atherosclerosis.[202]

Atherosclerosis is an inflammatory process associated with a number of factors, including hypertension, hypercholesterolemia, hyperlipidemia, diabetes mellitus, infections, and smoking.[209] Risk factors for atherosclerosis are often present in older people and atherosclerosis could lead to thrombotic stroke, which is typically a disease of the elderly.[210] Because of concern of the potential for a nondissection event where a manipulation might break loose a plaque association with atherosclerosis, in older people, it is important to address all the atherosclerosis related factors in the patient interview per Table 3.7 that outlines the risk factors of a nondissection event. These risk factors might be a contraindication for manipulation, especially if not medically managed appropriately.[211]

The exact risk of serious complications from cervical spine manipulation is not known. Rivett and Milburn[212] reported that the incidence rate of severe neurovascular compromise was estimated to be within a wide range of 1:50,000 manipulations to 1:5 million manipulations. Other estimates of risk of VBI from cervical spine manipulation have been stated as being six in 10 million manipulations or 0.00006%,[197,213] and the risk of death has been stated as three in 10 million manipulations.[201] Haldeman, Kohlbeck, and McGregor[197] found 367 cases of vertebral artery dissection or occlusion reported in the literature between 1966 and 1993 regardless of the mechanism of injury and reported that 43% of these cases were the result of spontaneous events (such as standing up from a nap), 31% were from cervical spine manipulation, 16% were from trivial trauma (such as a sudden head movement), and 10% were from major trauma (such as a motor vehicle accident). Haldeman and Rubinstein[182] reviewed 64 cases of VBI (two deaths) after cervical spine manipulation and were unable to identify risk factors in the patient's history or physical examination that could predict the likelihood of a VBI event. Haldeman, Kohlbeck, and McGregor[197] concluded that vertebral artery dissection should be considered a rare, random, and unpredictable complication associated with activities, such as neck movement, trauma, and manipulation.

The level of risk of serious injury from cervical spine manipulation compared with serious complications from other interventions commonly used to treat neck pain is very low. For instance, the likelihood of a serious GI bleed from NSAIDs is one per 1000 versus six per 10 million cervical manipulations.[196] The death rate for NSAID-associated GI problems is estimated at 0.04% per year among patients with osteoarthritis who receive NSAIDs, with 3200 deaths per year. Likewise, the risk of complication after cervical surgery is 16 per 1000.[213] Therefore if the level of risk is put in this context, the risk associated with cervical manipulation is extremely low and the potential for successful outcomes is fairly high.

In light of the lack of certainty in prediction of risk associated with manual therapy treatment the cervical spine, the IFOMPT developed a framework for examination of the cervical region for potential vascular pathologies of the neck before orthopedic manual physical therapy interventions with an updated framework under review.[214] The premise of this framework is that because the determination of the exact risk is impossible to predict for each individual patient, a risk/benefit analysis and sound clinical reasoning framework must be used to minimize risk and maximize benefit.[214] The adverse events are very rare, and clinicians cannot rely on the results of just one test or measure but instead should consider the patient's medical history and cardiovascular and neurologic risk factors for vascular pathologies of the neck and upper cervical structural instability; and they must consider signs, symptoms, and risk factors for presentation of internal carotid disease, vertebrobasilar artery disease, and upper cervical structural instability before initiating treatment of the neck that might involve end-range active or passive movements. Hutting et al.[211] further illustrates the clinical reasoning for risk assessment before cervical manual therapy. There are three important steps in the clinical reasoning process: (1) identify a possible vasculogenic contribution or other serious pathology; (2) determine if there is an indication or contraindication for mobilization/manipulation; and (3) assess the presence of any potential risk factors associated with potential serious adverse events which are reported to occur after cervical spine mobilization/manipulation.[211]

Headache and neck pain are common early presenting symptoms of patients with vascular pathologies of the neck (Figs. 3.15 and 3.16). It is critical for therapists to identify a cervical artery dissection in progress and susceptible individuals.[208] Because patients may present to a therapist's clinic with early signs and symptoms of a vascular pathology of the neck that have yet to be detected,[215] therapists must consider these signs and symptoms in the assessment of patients with neck pain with or without headaches (Figs. 3.15 and 3.16) and maintain a high level of suspicion that the cause of the patient's neck pain and headache could be vascular. Consideration of the cervical arterial system, together with the range of vascular pathologic conditions apparent within this system, may enhance the clinician's reasoning process. Subjectively, patients may report a different character of neck pain and headache than their typical pain and may use descriptors, such as pulsating or throbbing, to describe the nature of the symptoms.[216]

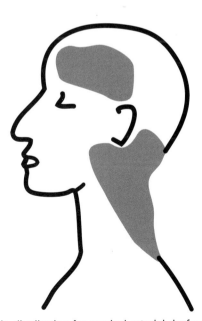

FIG. 3.15 Pain distribution for cervical arterial dysfunction. Typical pain distribution relating to dissection of internal carotid artery; ipsilateral front-temporal headache and upper cervical/midcervical pain. (Reprinted from Kerry R, Taylor AJ. Cervical artery dysfunction assessment and manual therapy, *Man Ther.* 2006;11(4):243-253, with permission from Elsevier.)

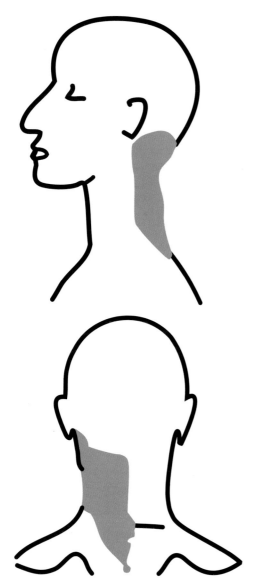

FIG. 3.16 Typical pain distribution relating to extracranial vertebral artery dissection: ipsilateral posterior upper cervical pain and occipital headache. (Reprinted from Kerry R, Taylor AJ. Cervical artery dysfunction assessment and manual therapy, *Man Ther.* 2006;11(4):243-253, with permission from Elsevier.)

TABLE 3.2   Symptoms of a Dissection Vascular Event

SYMPTOMS—IN ORDER OF MOST-TO-LEAST COMMON	DISSECTION VASCULAR EVENT %
Headache	81
Neck pain	57–80
Visual disturbance	34
Paresthesia (upper limb)	34
Dizziness	32
Paresthesia (face)	30
Paresthesia (lower limb)	19

(Data from Thomas LC, Rivett DA, Attia JR, et al. Risk factors and clinical features of craniocervical arterial dissection. *Man Ther.* 2011;16(4):351-356; Kranenburg HAR, Tyer R, Schmitt M, et al. Effects of head and neck positions on blood flow in the vertebral, internal carotid, and intracranial arteries: a systematic review. *J Orthop Sports Phys Ther.* 2019;49(10):688-697; and modified from Rushton A, Carlesso LC, Flynn T, et al. International Framework for Examination of the Cervical Region for potential of vascular pathologies of the neck prior to Orthopaedic Manual Therapy Intervention: International IFOMPT Cervical Framework, 2020.)

TABLE 3.3   Signs of Internal Carotid Artery Dissection

SIGNS OF INTERNAL CAROTID ARTERY DISSECTION— IN ORDER OF MOST-TO-LEAST COMMON	ICA DISSECTION %
Ptosis (drooping eyelid)	60–80
Weakness (upper limb)	65
Facial palsy	60
Weakness (lower limb)	50
Dysphasia/dysarthria/aphasia	45
Unsteadiness/ataxia	40
Nausea/vomiting	30
Drowsiness	20
Loss of consciousness	20
Confusion	15
Dysphagia	0.5

(Tables are based on retrospective and prospective study data from Thomas et al. (Thomas JS, France CR. Pain-related fear is associated with avoidance of spinal motion during recovery from low back pain. *Spine* 2007;32(16):E460-E466; Thomas L. Cervical arterial dissection: an overview and implications for manipulative therapy practice. *Man Ther.* 2016;21:2-9; Thomas LC, Rivett DA, Attia JR, et al. Risk factors and clinical features of craniocervical arterial dissection. *Man Ther.* 2011;16(4):351-356; Thomas LC, Makaroff AP, Oldmeadow C, et al. Seasonal variation in cervical artery dissection in the Hunter New England region, New South Wales, Australia: a retrospective cohort study. *Musculoskelet Sci Pract.* 2017;27:106-111; Rubenstein et al. (Rubinstein SM, Peerdeman SM, Van Tulder MW, et al. A systematic review of the risk factors for cervical artery dissection. *Stroke.* 2005;36(7):1575-1580); and contemporary reviews (Selwaness M, van den Bouwhuijsen Q.J, Verwoert G.C, et al. Blood pressure parameters and carotid intraplaque hemorrhage as measured by magnetic resonance imaging: The Rotterdam Study. *Hypertension.* 2013;61(1):76-81. https://pubmed.ncbi.nlm.nih.gov/23213192/; Chauhan G, Debette S. Genetic risk factors for ischemic and hemorrhagic stroke. *Curr Cardiol Rep.* 2016;18(12):124 https://pubmed.ncbi.nlm.nih.gov/27796860/; Isabel C, Calvet D, Mas JL. Stroke prevention. *La Presse Med.* 2016;45(12):e457-e471. https://pubmed.ncbi.nlm.nih.gov/27816341/; Selwaness M, Hameeteman R, Van't Klooster R, et al. Determinants of carotid atherosclerotic plaque burden in a stroke-free population. *Atherosclerosis.* 2016;255:186-192. https://pubmed.ncbi.nlm.nih.gov/27806835/); and modified from Rushton A, Carlesso LC, Flynn T, et al. International Framework for Examination of the Cervical Region for potential of vascular pathologies of the neck prior to Orthopaedic Manual Therapy Intervention: International IFOMPT Cervical Framework, 2020.)

Suspicion of vascular pathology of the neck is heightened with presentation of acute/recent onset of unusual moderate/severe neck pain or headache with recent exposure to minor trauma or infection in conjunction with any ischemic features, even if transient and subtle.[208] Therefore much of the clinical reasoning can take place with taking a thorough patient interview so that when a patient presents with potential symptoms of vascular pathology of the neck, the therapist should ask follow-up questions to identify signs of ischemia, such as the five Ds (dizziness, diplopia, dysarthria, dysphagia, drop attacks), and other neurologic symptoms, such as limb paresthesia or weakness, or Horner syndrome.[208] See Tables 3.2 through 3.8 for reported risk factors, signs and symptoms for dissection and nondissection events as developed by the

TABLE 3.4 Signs of Vertebral Basilar Artery Dissection	
SIGNS OF VERTEBRAL BASILAR ARTERY DISSECTION—IN ORDER OF MOST-TO-LEAST COMMON	**VERTEBRAL BASILAR ARTERY DISSECTION %**
Unsteadiness/ataxia	67
Dysphasia/dysarthria/aphasia	44
Weakness (lower limb)	41
Weakness (upper limb)	33
Dysphagia	26
Nausea/vomiting	26
Facial palsy	22
Dizziness/disequilibrium	20
Ptosis	19
Loss of consciousness	15
Confusion	7
Drowsiness	4

(Retrospective and prospective study data from Thomas JS, France CR. Pain-related fear is associated with avoidance of spinal motion during recovery from low back pain. *Spine* 2007;32(16):E460-E466; Thomas L. Cervical arterial dissection: an overview and implications for manipulative therapy practice. *Man Ther.* 2016;21:2-9; Thomas LC, Rivett DA, Attia JR, et al. Risk factors and clinical features of craniocervical arterial dissection. *Man Ther.* 2011;16(4):351-356; Thomas LC, Makaroff AP, Oldmeadow C, et al. Seasonal variation in cervical artery dissection in the Hunter New England region, New South Wales, Australia: a retrospective cohort study. *Musculoskelet Sci Pract.* 2017;27:106-111; Rubinstein SM, Peerdeman SM, Van Tulder MW, et al. A systematic review of the risk factors for cervical artery dissection. *Stroke.* 2005;36(7):1575-1580; and modified from Rushton A, Carlesso LC, Flynn T, et al. International Framework for Examination of the Cervical Region for potential of vascular pathologies of the neck prior to Orthopaedic Manual Therapy Intervention: International IFOMPT Cervical Framework, 2020.)

TABLE 3.5 Symptoms for Nondissection Vascular Event of the Neck	
SYMPTOMS FOR NONDISSECTION VASCULAR EVENTS OF THE NECK—IN ORDER OF MOST-TO-LEAST COMMON	**NONDISSECTION VASCULAR EVENT %**
Headache	51
Paresthesia (upper limb)	47
Paresthesia (lower limb)	33
Visual disturbance	28
Paresthesia (face)	19
Neck pain	14
Dizziness	7

(Data from Thomas LC, Rivett DA, Attia JR, et al. Risk factors and clinical features of craniocervical arterial dissection. *Man Ther.* 2011;16(4):351-356; Kranenburg HAR, Tyer R, Schmitt M, et al. Effects of head and neck positions on blood flow in the vertebral, internal carotid, and intracranial arteries: a systematic review. *J Orthop Sports Phys Ther.* 2019;49(10):688-697; and modified from Rushton A, Carlesso LC, Flynn T, et al. International Framework for Examination of the Cervical Region show for potential of vascular pathologies of the neck prior to Orthopaedic Manual Therapy Intervention: International IFOMPT Cervical Framework, 2020.)

TABLE 3.6 Signs of Nondissection Vascular Event of the Neck	
SIGNS OF NONDISSECTION VASCULAR EVENTS OF THE NECK—IN ORDER OF MOST-TO-LEAST COMMON	**NONDISSECTION VASCULAR EVENT %**
Weakness (upper limb)	74
Dysphasia/dysarthria/aphasia	70
Weakness (lower limb)	60
Ptosis	5–50
Facial palsy	47
Unsteadiness/ataxia	35
Confusion	14
Nausea/vomiting	14
Dysphagia	5
Loss of consciousness	5
Drowsiness	2

Data from Thomas LC, Rivett DA, Attia JR, et al. Risk factors and clinical features of craniocervical arterial dissection. *Man Ther.* 2011;16(4):351-356; Kranenburg HAR, Tyer R, Schmitt M, et al. Effects of head and neck positions on blood flow in the vertebral, internal carotid, and intracranial arteries: a systematic review. *J Orthop Sports Phys Ther.* 2019;49(10):688-697; and modified from Rushton A, Carlesso LC, Flynn T, et al. International Framework for Examination of the Cervical Region for potential of vascular pathologies of the neck prior to Orthopaedic Manual Therapy Intervention: International IFOMPT Cervical Framework, 2020.

TABLE 3.7 Risk Factors for Nondissection Vascular Pathology of the Neck	
RISK FACTORS FOR NONDISSECTION VASCULAR PATHOLOGY OF THE NECK EVENTS—IN ORDER OF MOST-TO-LEAST COMMON	**NONDISSECTION EVENT (%)**
Current or past smoker	65–74
Hypertension	53–74
High cholesterol	53
Migraine	19
Vascular anomaly	16
Family history of stroke	14
Oral contraception	9
Recent infection	9
Recent trauma (mild-moderate, which may include recent orthopaedic manual therapy)	7

(From Thomas JS, France CR. Pain-related fear is associated with avoidance of spinal motion during recovery from low back pain. *Spine* 2007;32(16):E460-E466; Thomas L. Cervical arterial dissection: an overview and implications for manipulative therapy practice. *Man Ther.* 2016;21:2-9; Thomas LC, Rivett DA, Attia JR, et al. Risk factors and clinical features of craniocervical arterial dissection. *Man Ther.* 2011;16(4):351-356; Thomas LC, Makaroff AP, Oldmeadow C, et al. Seasonal variation in cervical artery dissection in the Hunter New England region, New South Wales, Australia: a retrospective cohort study. *Musculoskelet Sci Pract.* 2017;27:106-111; Rubinstein SM, Peerdeman SM, Van Tulder MW, et al. A systematic review of the risk factors for cervical artery dissection. *Stroke.* 2005;36(7):1575-1580; and modified from Rushton A, Carlesso LC, Flynn T, et al. International Framework for Examination of the Cervical Region for potential of vascular pathologies of the neck prior to Orthopaedic Manual Therapy Intervention: International IFOMPT Cervical Framework, 2020.)

TABLE 3.8 Risk Factors for Dissection Vascular Pathology of the Neck Events	
RISK FACTORS FOR DISSECTION VASCULAR PATHOLOGY OF THE NECK EVENTS—IN ORDER OF MOST-TO-LEAST COMMON	**DISSECTION EVENT (%)**
Recent trauma (mild-moderate, which may include recent orthopaedic manual therapy)	40–64
Vascular anomaly	39
Current or past smoker	30
Migraine	23
High cholesterol	23
Recent infection	22
Hypertension	19
Oral contraception	11
Family history of stroke	9

(From Thomas JS, France CR. Pain-related fear is associated with avoidance of spinal motion during recovery from low back pain. *Spine* 2007;32(16):E460-E466; Thomas L. Cervical arterial dissection: an overview and implications for manipulative therapy practice. *Man Ther.* 2016;21:2-9; Thomas LC, Rivett DA, Attia JR, et al. Risk factors and clinical features of craniocervical arterial dissection. *Man Ther.* 2011;16(4):351-356; Thomas LC, Makaroff AP, Oldmeadow C, et al. Seasonal variation in cervical artery dissection in the Hunter New England region, New South Wales, Australia: a retrospective cohort study. *Musculoskelet Sci Pract.* 2017;27:106-111; Rubinstein SM, Peerdeman SM, Van Tulder MW, et al. A systematic review of the risk factors for cervical artery dissection. *Stroke.* 2005;36(7):1575-1580; and modified from Rushton A, Carlesso LC, Flynn T, et al. International Framework for Examination of the Cervical Region for potential of vascular pathologies of the neck prior to Orthopaedic Manual Therapy Intervention: International IFOMPT Cervical Framework, 2020.)

IFOMPT vascular pathology of the neck workgroup. These tables illustrate a collation of the frequency of symptoms and signs reported in the literature from multiple studies investigating reports of both dissection and nondissection events. The clinical profile of patients with vascular pathology of the neck is variable and the information in these tables is intended to assist the clinician in detecting a clinical presentation that supports the vascular pathology hypothesis enough to potentially warrant referral for further vascular diagnostic testing. Once the signs and symptoms for vascular pathology of the neck have been screened, risk factors for potential development of future vascular pathologic conditions should be considered from the framework (Tables 3.7–3.8).

With screening examination procedures designed to occlude the vertebral artery test for potential risk of VBI, clinicians must recognize the strong possibility of a false-negative finding from the test. Cote et al.[217] showed that the extension-rotation test has a sensitivity of approximately zero, which indicates a high likelihood of false-negative results from this commonly performed screening examination procedure (see Ch. 6). In a systematic review that included four studies, Hutting et al.[218] concluded that the data on diagnostic accuracy indicate that this premanipulative test is not a valid premanipulative screening procedure. The IFOMPT work-

group on vascular pathology of the neck recommends not to include this type of testing in the clinical reasoning framework for screening for vascular pathology of the neck before cervical spinal manual therapy treatment.[214]

The physical examination should be individualized to each patient's presentation and should include assessment of blood pressure. Hypertension is considered a risk factor for carotid and vertebral artery disease associated with athrosclerosis especially in an older population[211,214] (Fig. 3.17). In addition, an increase in blood pressure may be related to acute arterial trauma.[219] Cardiovascular risk factors and hypertension seem to be less of a risk factor in younger patients (<38 years of age) who have experienced vascular pathology of the neck, so routine assessment of blood pressure in younger people may not be particularly useful for therapists when attempting to determine the risks of serious adverse events.[220,221] However, in older patients (>60 years of age), measuring blood pressure should always be included in the examination and factored in as a risk factor for potential vascular pathology of the neck because hypertension is a recognized risk factor for both stroke and cardiovascular disease.[221–223]

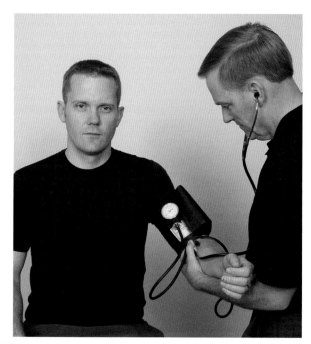

FIG. 3.17 Assessment of blood pressure is an important component of the vascular screening examination recommended before manual therapy or exercise treatment procedures of the cervical spine. Hypertension and neck pain are only two of the many factors that influence the decision on probability of vascular pathology. There is a positive correlation between increased systolic and diastolic pressure and risk of stroke; so the higher the pressure, the greater the risk. This would mean that a patient with 190 mm Hg/100 mm Hg is at greater risk than a patient with 160 mm Hg/95 mm Hg. Thus the risk is different even though they are both hypertensive and the relative risk from this one finding needs be considered along with the patient's other risk factors.

Younger people (<45 years of age) seem to have an increased risk to develop a craniocervical artery dissection, as opposed to older people with multiple cardiovascular risk factors for atherosclerosis.[203,207,223,224] A review of 134 case reports of serious adverse events after cervical spine manipulation showed that the mean age was 44 (range 23–86) years, and only 26.1% were older than 50 years.[179] In this review, vascular pathologies as a preexisting condition accounted for only 13.3% the people having a serious adverse event after cervical spine manipulation.[179] Another group of researchers found that cardiovascular risk factors commonly associated with stroke were not strongly represented in the dissection group as compared with the nondissection controls, and there was a mean of 1.4 cardiovascular risk factors per dissection, compared with 3.2 in the nondissection group.[225] In general, there seems to be a strong association for risk factors with a genetic component, while there is only a weak association for environmental factors, except for trivial head or neck trauma.[212,220,224,225]

One of the primary physical assessments used to evaluate for carotid artery stenosis because of arthrosclerosis is auscultation for the presence of a carotid bruit. A carotid bruit is a low-pitched, unintended vascular sound heard over the bifurcation of the common carotid artery into the internal and external carotid arteries.[226] A carotid bruit is the result of blood flow turbulence immediately distal to an atherosclerotic area of arterial narrowing. Portions of the plaque can embolize and move cranially from the proximal internal carotid artery causing either a transient ischemic attack or stroke. The Framingham study reported an age-adjusted, 2.6 times greater incidence of stroke in patients with a bruit compared with those without a bruit.[227] For guidance in assessment for a carotid bruit, see Fig. 3.18. Auscultating a carotid bruit increases the potential for the existence of a significant atherosclerotic lesion, but absence of a bruit (especially in patients with atherosclerotic risk factors) does not rule out carotid stenosis.[228] A carotid bruit, if present, also cannot predict the severity of carotid artery stenosis. Further diagnostic testing via duplex ultrasonography is appropriate to evaluate the extent of atherosclerotic disease in an asymptomatic patient with a carotid bruit.[228]

Because an enlarged carotid artery may compress the lower cranial nerves,[212] a cranial nerve examination (Table 3.9) should also be included in the screening for vascular pathology of the neck.[226] Cranial-nerve palsies are rare, representing less than 7% of cervical arterial dissection cases in large hospital-based series.[229] The hypoglossal (II) nerve is the most commonly affected, followed by the IXth and Xth cranial nerves, which are anatomically close in proximity to the carotid artery in its trajectory.[230] Therefore a cranial nerve examination that includes assessment of motor control of the tongue (XII), swallowing (IX), and speech phonation (X) should be included in the examination of patients with neck pain and headaches, especially following trauma and/or infection (Fig. 3.19).

Patients with upper cervical structural instability caused by boney or ligamentous compromise of the upper cervical anatomic structures, such as a fractured dens of C2 or compromise

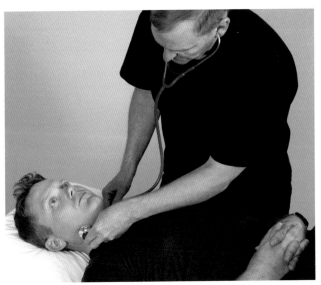

FIG. 3.18 Assessment for a carotid bruit. When assessing for a carotid bruit, it is important to understand carotid anatomy. The common carotid arteries run upward and backward on either side of the neck, from the sternoclavicular joint to the upper border of the thyroid cartilage, where each divides into the external and internal carotid arteries. The patient may be in either a seated or lying position and in a quiet room to minimize extraneous noise. The patient's head should be rotated slightly away from the side being examined. The area to be auscultated is located from the upper border of the thyroid cartilage to below the angle of the mandible. The targeted area is bound superiorly by the angle of the mandible, inferiorly by the upper border of the thyroid cartilage, and posteriorly by the sternocleidomastoid muscle. To auscultate the right carotid artery, position the bell of the stethoscope at the right upper border of the thyroid cartilage and have the patient hold his or her breath for approximately 15 seconds. Breath holding eliminates any lung or /upper airway sounds that may mask a bruit. Apply only enough pressure on the bell to ensure good contact with the skin. While listening, move the stethoscope up the right side of the neck to just below the angle of the mandible, taking note of the pulse and assessing for the presence of a bruit. Repeat the process on the opposite carotid. (From Rich K. Carotid Bruit: a review. *J Vasc Nurs.* 2015;33(1):26-27.)

of the alar or transverse ligament, will present with severe neck pain and muscle guarding, which may also be associated with neurovascular compromise[3] (Box 3.4). Therefore screening for upper cervical structural instability is recommended when risk factors for upper cervical structural instability are present.[214,231] Active and passive upper cervical mobility assessment and upper cervical ligamentous stability tests can potentially be performed to evaluate for signs of instability. Signs of structural instability with upper cervical ligamentous stability tests may include increase in motion or empty end feel, reproduction of symptoms of instability (such as paresthesia in the face or extremities), and production of lateral nystagmus and nausea with neck movements.[214] For each individual patient, the therapist needs to decide the value of upper cervical instability testing by evaluating the risks and benefits of the specific test procedure. In a systematic review, Hutting et al.[221] pooled data

TABLE 3.9	Evaluating the Cranial Nerves			
NERVES	**FUNCTION**	**LOCATION**	**TESTS**	**SIGNIFICANT FINDINGS**
I Olfactory	Smell	Olfactory bulb and tract	Odor recognition (unilaterally)	Lack of odor perception on one or both sides
II Optic	Vision	Optic nerve, chiasm, and tracts	Visual acuity; peripheral vision; pupillary light reflex	Reduced vision
III Oculomotor	Eye movement; pupil contraction and accommodation; eyelid elevation	Midbrain	Extraocular eye movements; pupillary light reflex	Impairment of one or more eye movements or disconjugate gaze, pupillary dilation; ptosis
IV Trochlear	Eye movement	Midbrain	Extraocular eye movements	Impairment of one or more eye movements or disconjugate gaze
V Trigeminal	Facial sensation; muscles of mastication	Pons	Sensation above eye, between eye and mouth, below mouth to angle of jaw; palpation of contraction of masseter and temporalis muscles	Reduced sensation in one or more divisions of the fifth nerve; impaired jaw reflex; reduced strength in masseter and temporalis muscles
VI Abducens	Ocular movement	Pons	Extraocular eye movements	Reduced eye abduction
VII Facial	Facial expression; secretions; taste; visceral and cutaneous sensibility	Pons	Facial expression; taste of anterior two-thirds of tongue	Weakness of upper or lower face or eye closure; reduced taste perception (salty, sweet, bitter, and sour)
VIII Acoustic	Hearing; equilibrium	Pons	Auditory and vestibular	Reduced hearing; impaired balance
IX Glossopha-ryngeal	Taste; glandular secretions; swallowing; visceral sensibility (pharynx, tongue, and tonsils)	Medulla	Gag reflex; speech (phonation); swallowing	Impaired reflex; dysarthria; dysphagia
X Vagus	Involuntary muscle and gland control (pharynx, larynx, trachea, bronchi, lungs, digestive tract, and heart); swallowing and phonation; visceral and cutaneous sensibility; taste	Medulla	Phonation; coughing, gag reflex	Hoarseness; weak cough; impaired reflex
XI Accessory	Movement of head and shoulders	Cervical	Resisted head; shoulder shrug	Weakness of trapezius and sterno-cleidomastoid
XII Hypoglossal	Movement of tongue	Medulla	Tongue protrusion	Deviation, atrophy, or fasciculations of tongue

(Modified from Boissonnault WG. *Primary Care for the Physical Therapist: Examination and Triage*, ed 2. St. Louis: Elsevier/Saunders; 2011.)

from three studies and reported that specificity was adequate to rule in instability, but sensitivity was inadequate to rule out instability making procedures, such as the Sharp-Purser test, an inadequate screening tool based on the current data.[221] When upper cervical structural instability is suspected, the patient should be referred for diagnostic imaging and orthopaedic medicosurgical management.

The following risk factors are associated with the potential for bony or ligamentous compromise of the upper cervical spine:[232]

- History of trauma (e.g., whiplash and rugby neck injury)
- Throat infection
- Congenital collagenous compromise (e.g., Down, Ehlers-Danlos, Grisel, and Morquio syndromes)

- Inflammatory arthritides (e.g., rheumatoid arthritis and ankylosing spondylitis)
- Recent neck/head/dental surgery

Signs and symptoms of upper cervical structural instability are presented in Box 3.4 and when present, further medical assessment and imaging are likely indicated especially following trauma.

Once the potential for serious vascular pathology of the neck and other contraindications to manual therapy have been assessed and indications for cervical manual therapy have been determined, the risk/benefit ratio should be incorporated into the clinical reasoning.[214] The risk of neurovascular compromise from a treatment procedure must be weighed against the potential for benefit from the procedure before considering

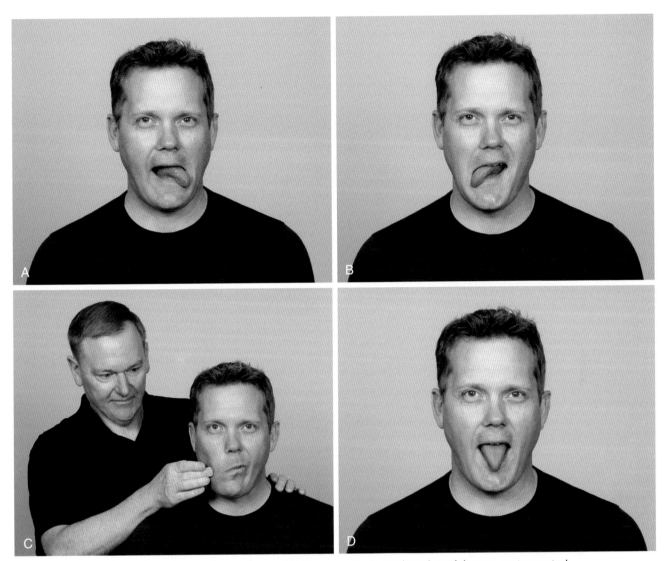

FIG. 3.19 Assessment of cranial nerve XII. To assess the hypoglossal cranial nerve, motor control of the tongue is evaluated including **D** protrusion and **A** and **B** lateral deviation of the tongue. The tongue strength can also be assessed with having the patient press their tongue into their cheek while the therapist applies resistance **C**. If motor control of the tongue is lost, the tongue will tend to deviate to the unaffected side with protrusion and atrophy may be noted on the affected side.

proceeding with the intervention. The typical clinical presentations that would suggest an indication for cervical manipulation include: a primary complaint of neck pain; a problem that is mechanical in nature and fits with a biomechanical pattern that is regular and recognizable; limited ROM (direction specific); pain that has clear mechanical aggravating and easing positions or movements; and local provocation tests that produce recognizable symptoms.[233]

If the risk is low and the potential for benefit is high based on the patient's signs and symptoms and considering the evidence for positive outcomes of the procedure, then the clinician should move forward with the intervention. However, if the risk is high and potential for benefit is low, manual therapy treatment should not be provided and the patient should be referred for further medical diagnostic testing and management. When

there is moderate risk and moderate potential benefit, treatment can proceed as long as the risk factors are being properly managed and monitored.

Ongoing patient assessment is needed throughout cervical spine manipulation technique application. This assessment should include holding the manipulation position (10 seconds) before application of the thrust while monitoring for nystagmus, slurred speech, nausea, or dizziness. If the patient tolerates the neck position well, the technique can be used. If the patient does not tolerate it well or is apprehensive about the use of manipulation, other procedures should be used. In addition, safety should be built into technique selection and application for all patients. Haldeman, Kohlbeck, and McGregor[197] reported that 84% of the 115 cases of vertebral artery injury from manipulation involved end-range cervical

BOX 3.4	Symptoms and Signs of Cervical Structural Instability

- Neck and head pain
- Feeling of instability
- Cervical muscle hyperactivity
- Constant support needed for head
- Worsening symptoms
- Facial paresthesia, reproduced by active or passive neck movements
- Overt loss of balance in relation to head movements
- Bilateral or quadrilateral limb paresthesia, either constant or reproduced by neck movements
- Nystagmus produced by active or passive neck movements
  - Feeling of lump in the throat
  - Metallic taste in mouth (Cranial nerve VII)
  - Arm and leg weakness
  - Lack of coordination bilaterally

(Modified from Gibbons P, Tehan P. *Manipulation of the spine, thorax and pelvis: an osteopathic perspective*, ed 2. London: Churchill Livingstone; 2005; and Rushton A, Rivett D, Carlesso L, et al. International framework for examination of the cervical region for potential of cervical arterial dysfunction prior to orthopaedic manual therapy intervention. *Man Ther.* 2014;19:222-228.)

BOX 3.5	Red Flags

The following are considered red flags that should heighten a therapist's level of suspicion of the potential for serious pathology:

- Significant trauma
- Weight loss
- History of cancer
- Fever
- Intravenous drug use
- Steroid use
- Patient age >50 years
- Severe unremitting nighttime pain
- Pain that worsens on lying down

(Modified from Kendall NAS, Linton SJ, Main CJ. *Guide to Assessing Psychosocial Yellow Flags in Acute Low Back Pain: Risk Factors for Long-Term Disability and Work Loss*. Wellington, New Zealand:Accident Rehabilitation and Compensation Insurance Corporation of New Zealand and the National Health Committee; 2002.)

BOX 3.6	Absolute Contraindications to Manipulation

- Lack of indications
- Poor integrity of ligamentous or bony structures from recent injury or disease process
- Unstable fracture
- Bone tumors
- Infectious disease
- Osteomyelitis
- Upper cervical instability
- Cervical arterial dysfunction
- Multilevel nerve root pathology
- Worsening neurologic function
- Unremitting, severe, nonmechanical pain
- Unremitting night pain
- Upper motor neuron lesions
- Spinal cord damageLack of skill of the clinician
- Lack of consent from the patient

rotation as a component of the technique. Use of multiple planes of movement can assist in finding a manipulative barrier for an effective technique while avoiding end-range rotation with the manipulation procedure. Also maintenance of slight cervical spine forward bending with application of cervical manipulation may facilitate safety by avoiding extremes of cervical extension. Thoracic spine manipulation techniques can also be used to relieve cervical spine pain,[234] and thoracic manipulation is generally safe. A trial of more gentle nonthrust cervical manipulation techniques is wise, especially in patients with risk factors for adverse reactions to thrust manipulation, including a history of trauma, higher pain scores (8+), higher NDI scores (>30%), female gender, and treatment of the upper cervical spine. Use of the gentlest forces to the cervical spine to accomplish the therapy goals can assist in patient comfort and safety. It is recommended that the clinician always uses the least amount of force in the manual therapy techniques that can accomplish the therapeutic goal of enhanced movement and reduced pain, and no replacement exists for ongoing assessment of the patient as manual physical therapy techniques are used to ensure a safe patient response.

In summary, severe adverse effects to mobilization/manipulation of the cervical spine are extremely rare. Thorough ongoing patient assessment is necessary to identify signs of vascular pathologies of the neck or upper cervical structural instability throughout the examination and treatment sessions, and thrust manipulation techniques to the cervical spine must not be used when positive signs of vascular pathologies of the neck or upper cervical structural instability are noted during the screening examination or treatment session. When in doubt or if the patient is apprehensive about the use of thrust manipulation, therapy should start with the gentler cervical spine techniques, and the therapist can also use thoracic manipulation techniques to assist in the treatment of neck pain.

Contraindications

Contraindications to spinal manipulation can be separated into two categories: relative and absolute. The first contraindication to consider is a lack of indications. If other interventions have evidence of greater effectiveness for a particular disorder, manipulation should not be used. In addition, the patient must be screened for red flags per the discussion in chapter 2 and see Box 3.5. The absolute contraindications involve a situation in which the forces to be used for the manipulation are likely to cause harm regardless of modification in technique (Box 3.6). Relative contraindications or precautions are situations in which the potential exists for harm with manipulation but with adequate technique modification, skill, and special care, the technique may still be effective and cause no harm (Box 3.7).

GUIDING PRINCIPLES OF MANIPULATION PERFORMANCE

The patient must be positioned in a relaxed supported position. The therapist must learn to effectively use his or her entire body

BOX 3.7	Relative Contraindications/Precautions to Manipulation

- Minor osteoporosis/osteopenia
- Herniated disc with radiculopathy
- Signs of spinal instability and ligamentous laxity
- Rheumatoid arthritis with upper cervical instability
- Pregnancy
- Local infection
- Inflammatory disease
- Active cancer
- History of cancer
- Long-term steroid use
- Systemically unwell
- Hypermobility syndromes
- Connective tissue disease
- First sudden episode before age 18 or after age 55 years
- Cervical anomalies
- Throat infections in children
- Recent manipulation by another health professional
- No change or worsening of symptoms after multiple manipulations
- Pain with a psychologic overlay
- Adverse reaction to a previous manipulation
- Vertigo
- Systemic infections

to most effectively manipulate the spine. A diagonal stance position is usually most beneficial to create a stable base of support, and the therapist must use an athletic stance (like a baseball player uses to hit a baseball or a tennis player uses to react to the direction of the ball) with the knees and hips slightly flexed, the spine in neutral, and the weight forward on the balls of the feet. The touch must be a firm professional contact that shows the patient competence and caring. The forearms, when appropriate, should be positioned in line with the direction of the manipulation force to be applied. With application of the manipulation forces, a firm stable trunk should be created through active engagement of the spinal and scapular muscles. The fingers/hands should be as relaxed and supple as possible for patient comfort.

For a thrust manipulation, the tissue slack of the joint and surrounding soft tissues is taken up with the primary and secondary levers. A primary lever is used to first begin the application of the force, followed by further slack taken up with use of secondary levers; the final manipulation force is through the primary lever. The application of multiple vectors or levers of force used in a spinal manipulation follows the same basic principles regardless of the technique used. Once the therapist and patient positions are attained, the therapist should begin with application of the primary vector (force plus direction) to take up part of the tissue slack. Secondary vectors are then used to further take up tissue slack to create a firm joint barrier. As each secondary force vector is applied, the primary vector is retested to determine whether a firm joint barrier (end feel) has been reached. Once a firm joint barrier has been attained, the primary force vector (or lever) is applied with a manipulative force to create a treatment effect.

The advantage of use of multiple vectors or levers of force with a thrust manipulation is that a tissue tension barrier can be attained against which to stretch a joint without a forceful end ROM position of the targeted joint. This is thought to provide a safer technique, especially in avoiding end-range rotation of the cervical spine, which has been implicated as a risk factor for injury to vertebral artery with cervical spine thrust manipulations. The use of multiple lever arms/directions of force creates a firm end feel or barrier at which point the primary technique lever is used to induce the final manipulative thrust. Many of the oscillatory techniques do not use a great deal of locking with multiple levers of motion but instead use only one direction of force to induce the motion, which would tend to make the technique less specific to a targeted spinal segment. With the thrust techniques, creation of a firm end barrier is necessary for effective manipulation of the targeted spinal segment.

Patients need to be encouraged to relax throughout the manipulation procedure. If a patient is actively resisting the premanipulation positioning, a less vigorous technique is best to use to gain greater confidence from the patient, or an isometric manipulation technique can be used. For an isometric manipulation technique or MET, the patient is positioned at a joint barrier, and then light manual pressure is applied as the patient actively resists the movement to create an isometric contraction of the agonistic muscles for the desired motion. After a 10-second hold, the tissue slack is taken up with passive or active moving of the spine further into the desired ROM. The barrier could be a sense of tissue resistance or pain. At this new barrier or just short of the painful barrier, another 10-second agonist isometric contraction is completed. The sequence is repeated 3 to 4 times, after which the motion is reassessed. If gains are made, this treatment may be enough at that segment for the treatment session; or if joint stiffness is still evident, the segment may be further manipulated.

Before mobilization/manipulation, warming of the tissues and body through exercise is advisable. Often a general warm-up is used, such as an upper body ergometer, NuStep (NuStep Inc., Ann Arbor, MI), elliptical machine, or treadmill. The warm-up is followed by specific exercises that target the impaired region, such as cervical or lumbar motor control or mobility exercises or shoulder girdle elastic band exercises. Beginning a treatment session with exercise also emphasizes to the patient the importance of the home exercise program and allows the therapist to reassess the patient by observing movement patterns and ROM with the exercises. Key impairment findings should be reexamined before application of the manual therapy techniques. At this point, manual therapy techniques can be applied to the impaired regions and might include, in the case of a patient with primary LBP symptoms, manipulation of the hip joints, lumbopelvic region, lumbar spine, or thoracic spine.

Immediately after the manipulation procedures, key findings should be reassessed, such as muscle tissue tone and active or passive motion testing, to determine whether the patient had a positive effect from the manipulation. Additional exercise or functional activities should be completed after the manipulation to further assess the patient's progress, to provide further education on movement pattern training or home exercise programs, and to move into the greater and more comfortable ranges of motion created with the manual therapy procedures.

TEACHING STRATEGIES FOR THE PSYCHOMOTOR COMPONENTS OF MANIPULATION

In the past, physical therapist educators have argued that only experienced physical therapists are qualified to learn high-velocity thrust manipulation.[175] However, Cohen et al.[235] showed that skilled performance of a spinal manipulation technique, as quantified with a force plate device, was no different for a group of experienced chiropractors compared with a group of newly trained chiropractic students. However, 12 of the 15 experienced chiropractors admitted to not using the manipulation technique that was tested on a regular basis even though they were previously trained in the technique. This study suggests that with training and practice, a novice practitioner can have an equal level of skill in performance of a spinal manipulation procedure as an experienced manipulator. The key to further skill enhancement for both the novice and the experienced practitioners is further practice and feedback. Flynn, Fritz, and Wainner[236] further illustrated how well physical therapy students could do with training in manipulation by reporting on the successful clinical outcomes of final-year physical therapy students who used an evidence-based approach to show successful patient outcomes with use of manipulation and therapeutic exercise for patients with symptoms of LBP. The physical therapy students showed practice patterns more in line with clinical practice guidelines than past surveys of practicing physical therapists.[236]

There are three stages of learning motor skills, such as manipulation. First is the cognitive stage, in which the learner is new at a task and the primary concern is to understand what is to be done, how the performance is to be assessed, and how best to attempt the first few trials.[237] Much cognitive activity is needed to determine appropriate strategies, but with practice the performance rapidly improves. The second phase is the associative phase, in which the individual has determined the most effective way of doing the task and begins to make more subtle adjustments in how the skill is performed.[237] Performance improvements are subtler, but gradual changes in performance make the task more effective. The last stage is the autonomous phase, in which the skill has become automatic.[237] At this phase, the learner can perform the task at a high level without much thought and can concurrently perform other tasks if needed.[166] For students to develop enough confidence in manipulation technique performance to use them on a regular basis in a clinical situation after graduation, they likely need to develop the skill to at least the associative phase.

Mann, Patriquin, and Johnson[238] reported on the use of the mastery learning technique to instruct osteopathic students in the performance of a shoulder manipulation procedure. The four key components of mastery learning are as follows: first, clear specification of desired learning outcomes; second, careful development of detailed learning materials that closely match the learning objectives; third, self-paced learning that may include independent study and group-based methods so that the student studies and practices until confident of meeting the criteria specified in the objectives; and fourth, multiple opportunities to demonstrate achievement of the learning objectives with individualized corrective feedback.[238] A total of 90 second-year osteopathic students were given a handout and asked to view a videotape of a shoulder manipulation technique.[238] They were given 2 days to practice the shoulder manipulation procedure and then set up an appointment with an instructor to demonstrate the technique and receive feedback. No penalty was applied for students who needed corrective feedback, but after the feedback, the students were requested to demonstrate the technique correctly. Only four students were required to repeat the technique, and their errors were easily corrected after the feedback session.[238] The authors commented that student anxiety was less because students were given more than one opportunity to demonstrate the technique correctly. Students reported that they practiced on average 67 minutes with a range of 5 minutes to 4 hours. Positive student feedback was received regarding this method of teaching; however, a retest was never performed to determine retention of the manipulative procedure, nor was this learning method compared with other traditional means of teaching manipulation.[238]

Watson[239] completed a pilot study that used a similar method of instruction of a thoracic spinal thrust manipulation technique with physical therapy students. In this study, 23 students were divided into three groups. All students received training in a thoracic spinal manipulation technique. Group 1 ($n = 8$) was trained by an instructor who gave delayed (summary) verbal feedback after a practice session. Group 2 ($n = 8$) received training via videotape observation with no instructor feedback, and group 3 ($n = 7$) was trained by an instructor who gave concurrent verbal feedback while the students practiced.[239] The students were then asked to train 10 minutes per day for 1 week, after which time they were graded on performance of the technique. Next, the students were asked to refrain from practice and to return 1 week later for retention testing. No difference was seen in acquisition of the motor skill at the first testing session between the three teaching methods, but group 3 showed significantly better retention of the skill when tested 1 week later compared with the other two groups.[239] Although Watson's study is somewhat inconclusive because of the small sample size, it provides some initial data to illustrate the importance of qualitative concurrent performance feedback in skill retention. Also of interest is that the results of the initial level of performance were the same regardless of whether the technique was demonstrated via videotape or in person, but the primary factor that influenced retention was the quality and quantity of the feedback.

In the motor learning literature, practice and feedback have been recognized as the two most important factors in learning motor skills. First, a student must be motivated to learn a task. For facilitation of motivation, Schmidt[237] suggests taking the time to make the task seem important and setting goals. Next, the learner must be provided with an image of the task, which can be done with instructions, demonstrations, videos, and other means. The instruction can begin to develop the student's "error detection mechanism" and the dos and don'ts of the task.[237] Further research is needed to investigate the optimal amount of instructions to give at one time, but Schmidt recommends starting with the most essential elements of the task, followed by more instruction and feedback as the student starts to practice and refine the task.[237] However, for complex tasks, instructions alone are crude and inadequate. Demonstration enhances performance compared with just verbal instruction, and a second demonstration during the practice session further enhances learning.[237]

Once the task is instructed and demonstrated, the student must practice. Variability in practice tends to allow students to learn the task more effectively and allows them to perform a new version of the task with less error than if the practice was more constant.[237] Therefore students should be encouraged to practice manipulation techniques for multiple regions of the spine during one practice session to be challenged in discussing and manipulating the varying spinal mechanics of each region of the spine. This practice should facilitate greater retention and skill acquisition, but further research is needed in this area. The two most important variables in practice are the amount of practice attempts and the knowledge of results (i.e., feedback).

Knowledge of results (KR) refers to the information about the success in performance of the task that the performer receives after the trial has been completed, and it serves as a basis for corrections on the next trial, leading to more effective performance as the trial continues.[237] Although more practice trials tend to result in greater learning, without knowledge of success in the task, as practice continues, learning may be drastically reduced (or nonexistent) even though many practice trials are provided.[237] Students should be given basic guidelines of self-assessment measures to be used in manual therapy, such as proper body mechanics, forearm alignment, and use of a diagonal stance. Students should also seek feedback from classmates and instructors regarding depth and comfort of pressure application.

KR can facilitate motivation to practice, provide guidance to the practice session, and assist with better goal setting, which causes the performer to set higher performing goals, but these effects may disappear as soon as KR is removed.[236] Decreasing the relative frequency of KR by increasing frequency of no KR aids long-term retention of the task.[236] Relative frequency of KR should be high in initial practice, when guidance and motivation are critical, but the instructor should systematically decrease frequency of KR as the performer becomes more proficient.[236] Therefore initially the instructor and classmates should provide a good deal of feedback, but as practice continues, the student needs to develop intrinsic means to monitor performance and to self-correct to perform successfully in future clinical setting.

An underappreciated function of feedback in the motor learning literature has been its influence on the performer's motivational state.[240] More effective learning has been demonstrated in a series of studies providing learners with feedback after "good" trials rather than after their "poor" trials.[241-245] In these studies, feedback about task performance was given after blocks of trials, but it was provided for only half of the trials in each block. The participants were given feedback about either their most or least accurate trials in the block. Groups that received feedback on the more accurate trials demonstrated more effective learning on retention tests which demonstrates that feedback emphasizing successful performance, while ignoring less successful attempts, benefited learning.[240] Feedback after good trials has also been found to increase perceptions of competence[241,245,246] and self-efficacy.[241,244] The reinforcement that a student is doing well and is developing confidence in being able to perform well in the future creates a condition consistent with optimal performance and learning.[240]

Guidance is useful for skill acquisition, but some loss of long-term learning effect occurs as a result of loss of trial and error and the self-corrections that facilitate learning.[237] Guidance is, however, helpful to prevent injury with potentially dangerous motor skills like certain maneuvers in gymnastics, but the student must eventually practice the task without guidance to fully develop the skill.[237] With more complex manipulation procedures (such as, lumbar rotation manipulation), verbal step-by-step instructions to the class are often helpful to talk the students safely through the procedure during the first attempt. For facilitation of learning, students must be allowed to progress to further practice without verbal cueing. However, feedback on performance errors are needed to enhance the skill performance.

Knowledge of performance (KP) is the feedback instructors typically give students regarding correction of improper movement patterns rather than just outcome of movement in the environment.[237] KP has been studied with videotape replays; and in general, the benefit of this type of feedback is best if the instructor can cue the learner to focus on specific aspects of the task. A more general viewing can provide too much extra information that may not enhance performance.[237] KP feedback can be provided verbally during a performance by a coach or instructor who is knowledgeable of the procedure. Detailed analysis of movement patterns of skilled individuals can also facilitate training programs.[237] A skilled manual therapy instructor can observe the student's performance and provide feedback to instantly enhance the student's performance of the technique. In contrast, KR is often provided in manual therapy by the patient's response to the treatment, such as favorable reassessment results like increased ROM.

Despite the evidence supporting the importance of feedback for motor skill learning, the quality and quantity of feedback provided to physical therapy students learning new manual therapy techniques are often lacking. In many academic laboratory sessions, the instructor demonstrates a technique and the students practice the techniques on each other as the instructor walks through the room to provide feedback. However, because the student/faculty ratios are typically 15:1 (SD = 4.9),[247] the instructors are not able to provide feedback for most of the students for each technique. Most instructors are hopeful that the students provide each other with quality feedback. However, Petty and Cheek[248] found that even postgraduate students participating in a manual therapy residency program provided inconsistent and unreliable feedback to classmates while learning manual therapy procedures. Petty and Cheek[248] point out that one factor that likely contributes to the poor reliability commonly associated with PIVM testing procedures is inadequate learning of the skills. The cause of the inadequate learning of manual therapy procedures may be inadequate teaching, practice, and feedback that are necessary for complex skill acquisition and retention.

Keating and Bach[249] used a bathroom scale to train a group of six postgraduate manual therapy residency students to produce a specific level of PA force and compared this group's ability to reproduce these forces on a subject's lumbar spine with a similar group of manual therapy residents who did not participate in the bathroom scale training. The trained group was able to be more specific with force application for PA force application in the lumbar spine compared with the control group.[249] This study shows that if the therapist is given specific KR (i.e., feedback), skill level improves.[249]

Lee and Refshauge[250] used a similar force plate treatment table device to provide concurrent quantitative feedback to a group of 31 physical therapy students who were taught a grade II mobilization technique at the third lumbar vertebral level. A second group of 22 students were in the control group and were taught the same procedures in the traditional manner. After training with this device, the students' forces were compared with the "ideal forces" as applied by the expert instructor. The accuracy and consistency of force application of the experimental group was greater than that of the control group.[250] If this type of device were more readily available, mobilization/manipulation skill acquisition might be enhanced. However, this force plate device does not provide the student with feedback regarding tissue tension, resistance, or end feel. Therefore this device cannot replace the type of qualitative feedback that a skilled clinical instructor can provide a student in a clinical setting.

Triano et al.[251] used an electromechanical training aid (Dynadjust) at different stages (year 2 and year 4 of a chiropractic education program) of training to simulate performance of a thrust manipulation for a side-lying lumbar rotation technique. Learners were assigned to either the aid group or the no aid group. Independent assessment of skill was evaluated before and after 6 weeks by means of recording force time profiles of high-velocity, low-amplitude performance. Repeated measures analysis of variance (ANOVA) evaluated change scores in the force amplitude and rate of rise in force. Use of the aid was not associated with any measurable gains for participants when used in year 2. However, later participation in year 4 demonstrated enhanced development in rate of rise for force and for peak force, which suggests that this type of feedback was more effective at refining a high velocity thrust motor skill once the students had reached a higher level of autonomous performance of the technique.[251]

Further research is needed in development of training tools to assist therapists to learn to more effectively and accurately grade PIVM and end feel resistance and to more consistently apply safe, therapeutic levels of force.

The research suggests that manual skills can be learned and retained more effectively if concurrent qualitative and quantitative feedback is provided. Positive feedback that highlights successful performance of manual techniques can also promote a positive learning environment and enhance learner confidence for future performance of the motor skill. If an instructor must provide all the feedback, small student/faculty ratios are needed to provide the necessary feedback and an extra laboratory practice sessions are needed with instructors present to provide quality feedback.

REFERENCES

1. American Physical Therapy Association (APTA). Guide to physical therapist practice, ed 2. *Phys Ther.* 2001;81:9-746.
2. American Physical Therapy Association (APTA). *Manipulation Education Committee.* Manipulation education manual for physical therapist professional degree programs. Alexandria, VA: APTA; 2004.
3. Rushton A, Beeton K, Landendoen J, et al. *International Federation of Orthopaedic Manipulative Physical Therapists Educational Standards in Orthopaedic Manipulative Therapy. Part A: Educational Standards 2016: glossary of terms.* Available at www.IFOMPT.com. Accessed November 17, 2019.
4. Mintken PE, DeRosa C, Little T. Moving past sleight of hand. *J Orthop Sports Phys Ther.* 2010;40(5):253-255.
5. Mintken PE, Derosa C, Little T, et al. A model for standardizing manipulation terminology in physical therapy practice. *J Man Manip Ther.* 2008;16:50-56.
6. Maitland G. *Vertebral manipulation*, ed 5. London: Butterworth; 1986.
7. Paris SV. *Introduction to spinal evaluation and manipulation.* Atlanta: Institute Press; 1986.
8. Goodridge JP. Muscle energy technique: definition, explanation, methods of procedure. *J Am Osteopath Assoc.* 1981;81(4):249-254.
9. Knott M, Voss D. *Proprioceptive neuromuscular facilitation*, ed 2. New York: Harper and Row; 1968.
10. Vicenzino B, Hing W, Rivett D, et al. *Mobilisation with movement.* Edinburgh: Churchill Livingstone/Elsevier; 2011.

11. Mulligan BR. *Manual therapy: NAGS SNAGS MWMS*, etc, ed 5. Minneapolis: Orthopedic Physical Therapy Products; 2004.

12. Sackett DL, Straus SE, Richardson WS, et al. *Evidence-based medicine: how to practice and teach EBM*, ed 2. Edinburgh: Churchill Livingstone; 2000.

13. Bigos S, Bowyer O, Braen G. *Acute low back problems in adults: clinical practice guideline no.* 14; Agency for Health Care Policy and Research (AHCPR) Publication No. 95–0642. Rockville, MD: Public Health Service, US Department of Health and Human Services; 1994.

14. Department of Defense/Veterans Administration (DOD/VA). *Guidelines*, 1999. Available at www.cs.amedd.army.mil/qmo/lbpfr.htm.

15. Hutchinson A, Waddell G, Feder G, et al. *Clinical guidelines for the management of acute low back pain*. London: Royal College of General Practitioners; 1996.

16. Koes BW, van Tulder M, Lin CWC, et al. An updated overview of clinical guidelines for the management of non-specific low back pain in primary care. *Eur Spine J*. 2010;19(12):2075-2094.

17. Rubinstein SM, de Zoete AM, van Middelkoop M, et al. Benefits and harms of spinal manipulative therapy for the treatment of chronic low back pain: systematic review and meta-analysis of randomized controlled trials. *BMJ*. 2019;364:1689.

18. Paige NM, Make-Lye IM, Booth MS, et al. Association of Spinal Manipulative Therapy with clinical benefit and harm for acute low back pain: systematic review and meta-analysis. *JAMA*. 2017;317(14):1451-1460.

19. Delitto A, George SZ, Van Dillen L, et al. Low back pain: clinical practice guidelines linked to the international classification of functioning, disability, health from the orthopaedic section of the American Physical Therapy Association. *J Orthop Sports Phys Ther*. 2012;42(4):A1-A57.

20. Gross AR, Hoving JL, Haines TA, et al. A Cochrane review of manipulation and mobilization for mechanical neck disorders. *Spine*. 2004;29(14):1541-1548.

21. Gross A, Miller J, D'Sylva J, et al. Manipulation or mobilization for neck pain: a Cochrane review. *Man Ther*. 2010;15(4):315-333.

22. Sutton DA, Cote P, Wong JL, et al. In multimodal care effective for the management of patients with whiplash-associated disorders or neck pain and associated disorder? A systematic review by the Ontario Protocol for Traffic Injury Management (OPTIMa) Collaboration. *Spine J*. 2016;16:1541-1565.

23. Blanpied PR, Gross AR, Elliott JM, et al. Neck pain: revision 2017, Clinical Practice Guidelines linked to the international classification of functioning, disability and health from the Orthopaedic Section of the American Physical Therapy Association. *J Orthop Sports Phys Ther*. 2017;47(7):A1-A83.

24. Mirtz TA, Morgan L, Wyatt LH, et al. An epidemiological examination of the subluxation construct using Hill's criteria of causation. *Chiropr Osteopat*. 2009;17(13):1-7.

25. Schmid A, Brunner F, Wright A, et al. Paradigm shift in manual therapy? Evidence for a central nervous system component in the response to passive cervical joint mobilization. Systematic review. *Man Ther*. 2008;13:387-396.

26. Bialosky JE, Bishop MD, Price DD, et al. The mechanisms of manual therapy in the treatment of musculoskeletal pain: a comprehensive model. *Man Ther*. 2009;14(5):531-538.

27. Paris SV. Spinal manipulative therapy. *Clin Orthop Related Res*. 1983;179:55-61.

28. Nansel D, Jansen R, Cremata E. Effects of cervical adjustment on lateral-flexion passive end-range asymmetry and on blood pressure, heart rate and plasma catecholamine levels. *J Manipulative Physiol Ther*. 1991;14(8):450-456.

29. Suter E, McMorland G. Decrease in elbow flexor inhibition after cervical spine manipulation in patients with chronic neck pain. *Clin Biomech*. 2002;17(7):541-544.

30. Cassidy JD, Lopes AA, Yong-Hing K. The immediate effect of manipulation versus mobilization on pain and range of motion in cervical spine: a randomized controlled trial. *J Manipulative Physiol Ther*. 1992;15(9):570-575.

31. Gavin D. The effect of joint manipulation techniques on active arrange of motion in the mid-thoracic spine of asymptomatic subjects. *J Man Manipulative Ther*. 1999;7:114-122.

32. Campbell BD, Snodgrass SJ. The effects of thoracic manipulation on posteroanterior spinal stiffness. *J Orthop Sports Phys Ther*. 2010;40(11):685-693.

33. Sims-Williams H, Jayson MI, Yong SM, et al. Controlled trial of mobilization and manipulation for patients with low back pain in general practice. *Br Med J*. 1978;2(6148):1338-1340.

34. Shum GL, Tsung BY, Lee RY. The immediate effect of postero-anterior mobilization on reducing back pain and the stiffness of the lumbar spine. *Arch Phys Med Rehabil*. 2013;94:673-679.

35. Powers CM, Beneck GJ, Kulig K, et al. Effects of a single session of posterior-to-anterior spinal mobilization and press-up exercise on pain response and lumbar spine extension in people with non-specific low back pain. *Phys Ther*. 2008;88:485-493.

36. Tuttle N, Barrett R, Laakso L. Postero-anterior movements of the cervical spine: repeatability of force displacement curves. *Man Ther*. 2008;13:341-348.

37. Tuttle N, Barrett R, Laakso L. Relation between changes in posterioanterior stiffness and active range of movement of the cervical spine following manual therapy treatment. *Spine*. 2008;33(19):E673-E679.

38. Snodgrass SJ, Rivett DA, Sterling M, et al. Dose optimization for spinal treatment effectiveness: a randomized controlled trial investigating the effects of high and low mobilization forces in patients with neck pain. *J Orthop Sports Phys Ther*. 2014;44(3):141-152.

39. Schenk RJ, MacDiarmid A, Rousselle J. The effects of muscle energy technique on lumbar range of motion. *J Man Manipulative Ther*. 1997;5(4):179-183.

40. Schenk RJ, Adelman K, Rousselle J. The effects of muscle energy technique on cervical range of motion. *J Man Manipulative Ther*. 1994;2(4):149-155.

41. Lenehan KL, Fryer G, McLaughlin P. The effect of muscle energy technique on gross trunk range of motion. *J Osteopath Med*. 2003;6(1):13-18.

42. Frankel VH, Norkin M. *Basic Biomechanics of the Skeletal System*. Philadelphia: Lea & Febiger; 1980.

43. Woo S, Matthews J, Akeson WH, et al. *Connective tissue response to immobility. Arthritis Rheum*. 1975;18(3):257-264.

44. Taylor DC, Dalton JD, Seaber AV, et al. Viscoelastic properties of muscle tendon units. the biomechanical effects of stretching. *Am J Sports Med*. 1990;18(3):211-220.

45. Warren CG, Lehmann JF, Koblanski JN. Elongation of rat tail tendon: effect of load and temperature. *Arch Phys Med Rehabil*. 1971;52(10):465-474.

46. Warren CG, Lehmann JF, Koblanski JN. Heat and stretch procedures: an evaluation using rat tail tendon. *Arch Phys Med Rehabil*. 1976;57(3):122-126.

47. Nachemson AL, Evans JH. Some mechanical properties of the third human lumbar interlaminar ligament. *J Biomech.* 1968;1(3): 211-220.

48. Tipton CM, Matthes RD, Maynard JA, et al. The influence of physical activity on ligaments and tendons. *Med Sci Sports.* 1975;7(3):165-175.

49. Cummings GS, Crutchfield CA, Barnes MR. *Orthopedic Physical Therapy Series Volume I: Soft Tissue Changes in Contractures*, ed 2. Atlanta: Stokesville Publishing; 1983.

50. Baur PS, Parks DH, Hudson JD. Epithelial mediated wound contraction in experimental wounds: the purse-string effect. *J Trauma.* 1984;24(8):713-721.

51. Hertling D, Kessler RM. *Management of Common Musculoskeletal Disorders: Physical Therapy Principles and Methods*, ed 3. Philadelphia: Lippincott Williams and Wilkins; 1996.

52. Gainsbury JM. High-velocity thrust and pathophysiology of segmental dysfunction. In: Glaswo EF, Twomey LT, Scull ER, et al., eds. *Aspects of Manipulative Therapy*, ed 2. New York: Churchill Livingstone; 1985.

53. Lewitt K. *Manipulative Therapy in Rehabilitation of the Local Motor System*. Boston: Butterworth; 1985.

54. Edmond SL. *Joint Mobilization/Manipulation Extremity and Spinal Techniques*, ed 2. St. Louis: Mosby; 2008.

55. Bogduk N, Engel R. The menisci of the lumbar zygapophyseal joints: a review of their anatomy and clinical significance. *Spine.* 1984;9(5):454-460.

56. Engel R, Bogduk N. The menisci of the lumbar zygapophysial joints. *J Anat.* 1982;135:795-809.

57. Tullberg T, Blomberg S, Branth B, et al. Manipulation does not alter the position of the sacroiliac joint: a roentgen stereophoto-prammetric analysis. *Spine.* 1998;23(10):1124-1128.

58. Bialosky JE, Beneciuk JM, Bishop MD, et al. Unraveling the mechanisms of manual therapy: modeling an approach. *J Orthop Sports Phys Ther.* 2018;48(1):8-18.

59. Thomas JS, France CR. Pain-related fear is associated with avoidance of spinal motion during recovery from low back pain. *Spine.* 2007;32(16):E460-E466.

60. Bialosky JE, Bishop MD, Robinson ME, et al. Spinal manipulative therapy has an immediate effect on thermal pain sensitivity in people with low back pain: a randomized controlled trial. *Phys Ther.* 2009;89(12):1292-1303.

61. George SZ, Bishop MD, Bialosky JE, et al. Immediate effects of spinal manipulation on thermal pain sensitivity: an experimental study. *BMC Musculoskeletal Disord.* 2006;7:68.

62. Coronado RA, Gay CW, Bialosky JE, et al. Changes in pain sensitivity following spinal manipulation: a systematic review and meta-analysis. *J Electromyogr Kinesiol.* 2012;22:752-767.

63. Bishop MD, Beneciuk JM, George SZ. Immediate reduction in temporal sensory summation after thoracic spinal manipulation. *Spine J.* 2011;11(5):440-446.

64. Lascurain-Aguirrebena I, Newham D, Critchley DJ. Mechanism of action of spinal mobilizations: a systematic review. *Spine (Phila Pa 1976).* 2016;41:159-172.

65. Groen GJ, Baljet B, Drukker J. Nerve and nerve plexuses of the human vertebral column. *Am J Anat.* 1990;188:282-296.

66. McLain RF. Mechanoreceptor endings in human cervical facet joints. *Spine.* 1994;19:495-501.

67. Amonoo-Kuofi HS. The number and distribution of muscle spindles in human intrinsic postvertebral muscles. *J Anat.* 1982; 135:585-599.

68. Richmond FJR, Bakker DA. Anatomical organization and sensory receptor content of soft tissues surrounding upper cervical vertebrae in the cat. *J Neurophysiol.* 1982;48:49-61.

69. McLain RF, Pickar JG. Mechanoreceptor endings in human thoracic and lumbar facet joints, *Spine.* 1998;23:168-173.

70. Wyke B. The neurology of joints: a review of general principles. *Clinics Rheum Dis.* 1981;7(1):223-239.

71. Bolton PS. The somatosensory system of the neck and its effect on the central nervous system. *J Manipulative Physiol Ther.* 1998;21:553-563.

72. Souvils T, Vicenzino B, Wright A. Neurophysiological effects of spinal manual therapy. In: Boyling JD, Jull G, editors. *Grieve's Modern Manual Therapy: the Vertebral Column.* Edinburgh: Churchill Livingstone; 2004.

73. Lundy-Ekman L. *Neuroscience fundamentals for rehabilitation*, ed 5. Elsevier; 2018.

74. Cannon JT, Prieto GJ, Lee A, et al. Evidence for opioid and non-opioid forms of stimulation produced analgesia in the rat. *Brain Res.* 1982;243:315-321.

75. Hosobuchi Y, Adams JE, Linchitz R. Pain relief by electrical stimulation of the central gray matter in human an its reversal by naloxone. *Science.* 1977;197:183-186.

76. Reynolds DV. Surgery in the rat during electrical analgesia induced by focal brain stimulations. *Science.* 1969;164:444-445.

77. Fanselow MS. The midbrain periaqueductal gray as a coordinator of action in response to fear and anxiety. In: Depaulis A, Bandler R, editors. *The Midbrain Periaqueductal Gray Matter.* New York: Plenum Press; 1991.

78. Lovick TA. Interactions between descending pathways from dorsal and ventrolateral periaqueductal gray matter in rats. In: Depaulis A, Bandler R, editors. *The Midbrain Periaqueductal Gray Matter.* New York: Plenum Press; 1991.

79. Morgan MM. Differences in antinociception evoked from dorsal and ventral regions of the caudal periaqueductal gray matter. In: Depaulis A, Bandler R, editors. *The Midbrain Periaqueductal Gray Matter.* New York: Plenum Press; 1991.

80. Yezierski RP. Somatosensory input to the periaqueductal gray: a spinal relay to a descending control center. In: Depaulis A, Bandler R, editors. *The Midbrain Periaqueductal Gray Matter.* New York: Plenum Press; 1991.

81. Wright A. Hypoalgesic post-manipulative therapy: a review of a potential neurophysiological mechanism. *Man Ther.* 1995;1:11-16.

82. Bialosky JE, George SZ, Horn ME, et al. Spinal manipulative therapy-specific changes in pain sensitivity in individuals with low back pain (NCT01168999). *J Pain.* 2014;15(2):136-148.

83. Bialosky JE, Bishop MD, Robinson ME, et al. The influence of expectation on spinal manipulation induced hypoalgesia: an experimental study in normal subjects. *BMC Musculoskelet Disord.* 2008;9:19.

84. Sterling M, Jull G, Wright A. Cervical mobilization: concurrent effects on pain, sympathetic nervous system activity and motor activity. *Man Ther.* 2001;6:72-81.

85. La Touche R, Paris-Alemany A, Mannheimer JS, et al. Does mobilization of the upper cervical spine affect pain sensitivity and autonomic nervous system function in patients with cervico-craniofacial pain? A randomized-controlled trial. *Clin J Pain.* 2013;29:205-215.

86. Peterson NP, Vicenzino B, Wright A. The effects of a cervical mobilization technique on sympathetic outflow to the upper limb in normal subjects. *Physiother Theory Pract.* 1993;9:149-156.

87. Vicenzino B, Guschlag F, Collins D, et al. An investigation of the effects of spinal manual therapy on forequarter pressure and thermal pain thresholds and sympathetic nervous system activity in asymptomatic subjects. In: Shakclock M, ed. *Moving in on Pain.* Melbourne: Butterworth Heinemann; 1995.

88. McGuiness J, Vicenzino B, Wright A. The influence of a cervical mobilization technique on respiratory and cardiovascular function. *Man Ther.* 1997;2:216-220.

89. Vicenzino B, Cartwright T, Collins D, et al. Cardiovascular and respiratory changes produced by lateral glide mobilization of the cervical spine. *Man Ther.* 1998;3:67-71.

90. Vicenzino B, Collins D, Wright A. The initial effects of cervical spine manipulative physiotherapy on pain and dysfunction in lateral epicondylalgia. *Pain.* 1996;68:69-74.

91. Marks M, Schottker-Koniger T, Probst A. Efficacy of cervical spine mobilization versus peripheral nerve slider techniques in cervico- brachial pain syndrome: a randomized clinical trial. *J Phys Ther.* 2011;4:9-17.

92. Cleland JA, Whitman JM, Fritz JM. Effectiveness of manual physical therapy to the cervical spine in the management of lateral epicondylalgia: a retrospective analysis. *J Orthop Sports Phys Ther.* 2004;34:713-724.

93. Jowsey P, Perry J. Sympathetic nervous system effects in the hands following a grade III postero-anterior rotatory mobilization technique applied to T4: a randomized, placebo-controlled trial. *Man Ther.* 2010;15:248-253.

94. Perry J, Green A. An investigation into the effects of a unilaterally applied lumbar mobilization technique on peripheral sympathetic nervous system activity in the lower limbs. *Man Ther.* 2008;13:492-499.

95. Randoll C, Normandin VG, Tessier J, et al. The mechanism of back pain relief by spinal manipulation relies on decreased temporal summation of pain. *Neuroscience.* 2017;349:220-228.

96. Willet E, Hebron C, Krouwel O. The effects of different rates of lumbar mobilizations on pressure pain thresholds in asymptomatic subjects. *Man Ther.* 2010;15:173-178.

97. Sparks C, Cleland JA, Elliott JM, et al. Using functional magnetic resonance imaging to determine if cerebral hemodynamic responses to pain change following thoracic spine thrust manipulation in healthy individuals. *J Orthop Sports Phys Ther.* 2013;43(5):340-348.

98. Wirth B, Gassner A, de Bruin ED, et al. Neurophysiological effects of high velocity and low amplitude spinal manipulation in symptomatic and asymptomatic humans. *Spine (Phila Pa 1976).* 2019;44(15):e914-e926.

99. Kovanur-Sampath K, Mani R, Cotter J, et al. Changes in biochemical markers following spinal manipulation-systematic review and meta-analysis. *Musculoskelet Sci Pract.* 2017;29:120-131.

100. Vernon HT, Dhami MSI, Howley TP, et al. Spinal manipulation and beta-endorphin: a controlled study of the effects of a spinal manipulation on plasma beta-endorphin levels in normal males. *J Manipulative Physiol Ther.* 1986;9(2):115-123.

101. Christian GH, Stanton GJ, Sissons D, et al. Immunoreactive ACTH, beta-endorphin, and cortisol levels in plasma following spinal manipulative therapy. *Spine.* 1988;13:141-147.

102. Sanders GE, Reinnert O, Tepe R, et al. Chiropractic adjustive manipulation on subjects with acute low back pain: visual analog scores and plasma beta-endorphin levels. *J Manipulative Physiol Ther.* 1990;13:391-395.

103. Zusman M, Edwards B, Donaghy A. Investigation of a proposed mechanism for the relief of spinal pain with passive joint movement. *J Manual Med.* 1989;4:58-61.

104. Vicenzino B, O'Callaghan J, Felicity K, et al. *No Influence of Naloxone on the Initial Hypalgesic Effect of Spinal Manual Therapy.* Vienna: Ninth World Congress on Pain; 2000.

105. Sykba DA, Radhakrishnana R, Rohlwing JJ, et al. Joint manipulation reduces hyperalgesia by activation of monoamine receptors by not opioid or GAGA receptors in the spinal cord. *Pain.* 2003;106:159-168.

106. Beaulieu JE. Developing a stretching program. *Phys Sports Med.* 1981;9(11):59-65.

107. Levine MG, Kabat H, Knott M, et al. Relaxation of spasticity by physiological technics. *Arch Phys Med Rehabil.* 1954;35:214-223.

108. Greenman P. *Principles of Manual Medicine.* Baltimore: Williams and Wilkins; 1989.

109. Pecos-Martin D, de Melo Aroeira AE, Silva V, et al. Immediate effects of thoracic spinal mobilization on erector spinae muscle activity and pain in patients with thoracic spine pain: a preliminary randomized controlled trial. *Physiotherapy.* 2017;103:90-97.

110. Shambaugh P. Changes in electrical activity in muscles resulting from chiropractic adjustment: a pilot study. *J Manipulative Physiol Ther.* 1987;10:300-304.

111. Fisk JW. A controlled trial of manipulation in a selected group of patients with low back pain favoring one side. *N Z Med J.* 1979;90:228-291.

112. Dishman JD, Cunningham BM, Burke J. Comparison of tibial nerve H-reflex excitability after cervical and lumbar spine manipulation. *J Manipulative Physiol Ther.* 2002;25:318-325.

113. Dunning J, Rushton A. The effects of cervical high-velocity low-amplitude thrust manipulation on resting electromyographic activity of the biceps brachii muscle. *Man Ther.* 2009;14:508-513.

114. Liebler EJ, Tufano-Coors L, Douris P, et al. The effect of thoracic spine mobilization on lower trapezius strength testing. *J Man Manipulative Ther.* 1986;9:207-212.

115. Cleland J, Selleck B, Stowell T, et al. Short-term effects of thoracic manipulation on lower trapezius muscle strength. *J Man Manipulative Ther.* 2004;12(2):82-90.

116. Suter E, McMorland G, Herzog W, et al. Decrease in quadriceps inhibition after sacroiliac joint manipulation in patients with anterior knee pain. *J Manipulative Physiol Ther.* 1999;22:149-153.

117. Keller TS, Colloca CJ. Mechanical force spinal manipulation increases trunk muscle strength assessed by electromyography: a comparative clinical trial. *J Manipulative Physiol Ther.* 2000;23:585-595.

118. Brenner AK, Gill NW, Buscema CJ, et al. Improved activation of lumbar multifidus following spinal manipulation: a case report applying rehabilitative ultrasound imaging. *J Orthop Sports Phys Ther.* 2007;37(10):613-619.

119. Bicalho E, Setti JAP, Macagnan J, et al. Immediate effects of a high-velocity spine manipulation in paraspinal muscles activity of nonspecific chronic low-back pain subjects. *Man Ther.* 2010;15:469-475.

120. Jamison JR, McEwen AP, Thomas SJ. Chiropractic adjustment in the management of visceral conditions: a critical appraisal. *J Manipulative Physiol Ther.* 1992;15:171-180.

121. Williams NH, Hendry M, Lewis R, et al. Psychological response in spinal manipulation (PRIMS): a systematic review of psychological outcomes in randomized controlled trials. *Complement Ther Med.* 2007;15(4):271-283.

122. Bishop MD, Mintken P, Bialosky JE, et al. Patient expectations of benefit from interventions for neck pain and resulting influence on outcomes. *J Orthop Sports Phys Ther.* 2013;43(7):457-465.

123. Puentedura EJ, Cleland JA, Landers MR, et al. Development of a clinical prediction rule to identify patients with neck pain likely to benefit from thrust joint manipulation to the cervical spine. *J Orthop Sports Phys Ther.* 2012;42(7):577-592.

124. George SZ, Robinson ME. Dynamic nature of the placebo response (guest editorial). *J Orthop Sports Phys Ther.* 2010;40(8):452-454.

125. Bialosky JE, Bishop MD, Robinson ME, et al. The influence of expectation on spinal manipulation induced hypoalgesia: an experimental study in normal subjects. *BMC Musculoskelet Disord.* 2008;9:19.

126. Koshi EB, Short CA. Placebo theory and its implications for research and clinical practice: a review of the recent literature. *Pain Pract.* 2007;7:4-20.

127. Setchell J, Costa N, Ferreira M, et al. Individuals' explanations for their persistent or recurrent low back pain: a cross-sectional survey. *BMC Musculoskelet Disord.* 2017;18:466.

128. Stewart M, Loftus S. Sticks and stones: the impact of language in musculoskeletal rehabilitation. *J Orthop Sports Phys Ther.* 2018;48(7):519-522.

129. Fritz JM, Brennan GP, Hunter SJ. Physical therapy or advanced imaging as first management strategy. *Health Serv Res.* 2015;50:1927-1940.

130. Brinjikji W, Luetmer PH, Comstock B, et al. Systematic literature review of imaging features of spinal degeneration in asymptomatic populations. *AJNR Am J Neuroradiol.* 2014;36:811-816.

131. Bialosky JE, Bishop MD, Robinson ME, et al. The influence of expectation on spinal manipulation induced hypoalgesia: an experimental study in normal subjects. *BMC Musculoskelet Disord.* 2008;9:19.

132. Foster NE, Anema JR, Cherkin D, et al. Low back pain 2: prevention and treatment of low back pain: evidence, challenges, and promising directions. *Lancet.* 2018;391:2368-2383.

133. Lluch Girbés E, Meeus M, Baert I, et al. Balancing "hands-on" with "hands-off" physical therapy interventions for the treatment of central sensitization pain in osteoarthritis. *Man Ther.* 2015;20:349-352.

134. Nicholas MK, George SZ. Psychologically informed interventions for low back pain: an update for physical therapists. *Phys Ther.* 2011;91:765-776.

135. Mayer TG, Neblett R, Cohen H, et al. The development and psychometric validation of the central sensitization inventory. *Pain Pract.* 2012;12:276-285.

136. Neblett R, Cohen H, Choi Y, et al. The central sensitization inventory (CSI): establishing clinically significant values for identifying central sensitivity syndromes in an outpatient chronic pain sample. *J Pain.* 2013;14(5):438-445.

137. Hill JC, Whitehurst DGT, Lewis M, et al. Comparison of stratified primary care management for low back pain with current best practice (STarT Back): a randomized controlled trial. *Lancet.* 2011;378:1560-1571.

138. Louw A, Diener I, Butler D, et al. The Effect of neuroscience education on pain, disability, anxiety, and stress in chronic musculoskeletal pain. Systematic Review. *Arch Phys Med Rehabil.* 2011;92:2041-2056.

139. Nijs J, Wijma AJ, Willaert W, et al. Integrating motivational interviewing in pain neuroscience education for people with chronic pain: a practical guide for clinicians: motivational interviewing plus explaining pain. *Phys Ther.* 2020;100:846-859.

140. Louw A, Zimney K, Puentedura EJ, et al. The efficacy of pain neuroscience education on musculoskeletal pain: a systematic review of the literature. *Physiother Theory Pract.* 2016;32:332-355.

141. Watson JA, Ryan CG, Cooper L, et al. Pain neuroscience education for adults with chronic musculoskeletal pain: a mixed-methods systematic review and meta-analysis. *J Pain.* 2019;20(10):1140.e1-1140.e22.

142. Louw A, Puentedura E, Schmidt S, et al. *Integrating Manual Therapy and Pain Neuroscience.* Minneapolis, MN: USA:OPTP; 2019.

143. Woolf CJ, Mannion RJ. Neuropathic pain: aetiology, symptoms, mechanisms, and management. *Lancet.* 1999;353(9168):1959-1964.

144. Devor M, Govrin-Lippman R, Angelides K. Na+ channel immunolocalization in peripheral mammalian axons and changes following nerve injury and neuroma formation. *J Neurosci.* 1993;13:1976-1992.

145. Latremoliere A, Woolf CJ. Central sensitization: a generator of pain hypersensitivity by central neural plasticity. *J Pain.* 2009;10(9):895-926.

146. Woolf CJ. Pain. *Neurobiol Dis.* 2000;7(5):504-510.

147. Louw A, Farrell K, Wettach L, et al. Immediate effects of sensory discrimination for chronic low back pain: a case series. *N Z J Physiother.* 2015;43(2):58-63.

148. Nijs J, van Wilgen CP, Van Oosterwijck J, et al. How to explain central sensitization to patients with unexplained chronic musculoskeletal pain: practice guidelines. *Man Ther.* 2011;16:413-418.

149. Butler D, Moseley GL. *Explain Pain.* Adelaide: NOI Group Publishing; 2003.

150. Malfliet A, Kregel J, Meeus M, et al. Clinical Trial Protocol, Applying contemporary neuroscience in exercise interventions for chronic spinal pain: treatment protocol. *Braz J Phys Ther.* 2017;21(5):378-387.

151. Moseley GL, Nicholas MK, Hodges PW. A randomized controlled trial of intensive neurophysiology education in chronic low back pain. *Clin J Pain.* 2004;20:324-330.

152. Moseley GL. Whole of Community pain education for back pain. Why does first-line care get almost no attention and what exactly are we waiting for? *Br J Sports Med.* 2019;53(10):588-589.

153. Roston JB, Haines RW. Cracking in the metacarpophalangeal joint. *Anatomy.* 1947;81(2):166-173.

154. Unsworth A, Dowson D, Wright V. Cracking joints: a bioengineering study of cavitation in the metacarpophalangeal joint. *Ann Rheum Dis.* 1971;30:348-357.

155. Kawchuk GN, Fryer J, Jaremko JL, et al. Real-time visualization of joint cavitation. *PLoS One.* 2015;10(4):e01194705.

156. Flynn TW, Fritz JM, Wainner RS, et al. The audible pop is not necessary for successful spinal high-velocity thrust manipulation in individuals with low back pain. *Arch Phys Med Rehabil.* 2003;84:1057-1060.

157. Bialosky JE, Bishop MD, Robinson ME, et al. The relationship of the audible pop to hypoalgesia associated with high-velocity, low-amplitude thrust manipulation: a secondary analysis of an experimental study in pain-free participants. *J Manipulative Physiol Ther.* 2010;33:117-124.

158. Silevis R, Cleland J. Immediate effects of the audible pop from a thoracic spine thrust manipulation on the autonomic nervous system and pain: a secondary analysis of a randomized clinical trial. *J Manipulative Physiol Ther.* 2011;34:37-45.

159. Doody C, McAteer M. Clinical reasoning of expert and novice physiotherapists in an outpatient orthopaedic setting. *Physiotherapy.* 2002;88:258-268.

160. Hahne AJ, Keating JL, Wilson SC. Do within-session changes in pain intensity and range of motion predict between-session changes in patients with low back pain? *Aust J Physiother.* 2004;50:17-23.

161. Cook CE, Showalter C, Kabbaz V, et al. Can a within/between session change in pain during reassessment predict outcome using a manual therapy intervention in patients with mechanical low back pain? *Man Ther.* 2012;17(4):325-329.

162. Cleland JA, Childs JD. Does the manual therapy technique matter? *Orthop Division Rev.* 2005;18(3)27-28.

163. Farrell JP, Twomey LT. Acute low back pain: comparison of two conservative treatment approaches. *Med J Aust.* 1982;1:160-164.

164. Hoving JL, Koes BW, de Vet HCW, et al. Manual therapy, physical therapy, or continued care by a general practitioner for patients with neck pain: a randomized controlled trial. *Ann Intern Med.* 2002;136:713-722.

165. Jull G, Trott P, Potter H, et al. A randomized controlled trial of physiotherapy management for cervicogenic headache. *Spine.* 2002;27:1835-1843.

166. Kulig K, Landel RF, Powers CM. Using dynamic MRI: a proposed mechanism of sagittal plane motion induced by manual posterior-to-anterior mobilization. *J Orthop Sports Phys Ther.* 2004;34(2):61-64.

167. Tuttle N, Hazle C. Spinal PA movements behave 'as if' there are limitations of local segmental mobility and are large enough to be perceivable by manual palpation: a synthesis of the literature. *Musculoskelet Sci Pract.* 2018;36:25-31.

168. McCarthy CJ,,Ä®Potter L, Oldham JA. Comparing targeted thrust manipulation with general thrust manipulation in patients with low back pain. A general approach is as effective as a specific one. A randomized controlled trial. *BMJ Open Sport Exerc Med.* 2019;5:e000514.

169. Chiradejnant A, Maher CG, Latimer J, et al. Efficacy of "therapist-selected" versus "randomly selected" mobilization techniques for the treatment of low back pain: a randomized controlled trial. *Aust J Physiother.* 2003;49:223-241.

170. Haas M, Groupp E, Panzer D, et al. Efficacy of cervical endplay assessment as an indicator for spinal manipulation. *Spine.* 2003;28(11):1091-1096.

171. Ross JK, Bereznick DE, McGill SM. Determining cavitation location during lumbar and thoracic spinal manipulation: is spinal manipulation accurate and specific? *Spine.* 2004;29(13):1452-1457.

172. Dunning J, Mourad F, Barbero M, et al. Bilateral and multiple cavitation sounds during upper cervical thrust manipulation. *BMC Musculoskelet Disord.* 2013;14:24.

173. Dunning J, Mourad F, Zingoni A, et al. Cavitation sounds during cervicothoracic spinal manipulation. *Int J Sports Phys Ther.* 2017;12(4):642-654.

174. Childs JD, Fritz JM, Flynn TW, et al. A clinical prediction rule to identify patients with low back pain most likely to benefit from spinal manipulation: a validation study. *Ann Intern Med.* 2004;141:920-928.

175. Flynn TW. Move it and move on. *J Orthop Sports Phys Ther.* 2002;32(5):192-193.

176. Fritz J, Whitman JM, Childs JD. Lumbar spine segmental mobility assessment: an examination of validity for determining intervention strategies in patients with low back pain. *Arch Phys Med Rehabil.* 2005;86:1745-1752.

177. Delitto A, George SZ, Van Dillen L, et al. Low back pain: clinical practice guidelines linked to the international classification of functioning, disability, health from the orthopaedic section of the American Physical Therapy Association. *J Orthop Sports Phys Ther.* 2012;42(4):A1-A57.

178. Childs JD, Cleland JA, Elliott JM, et al. Neck pain: clinical practice guidelines linked to the international classification of functioning, disability, and health from the orthopaedic section of the American Physical Therapy Association. *J Orthop Sports Phys Ther.* 2008;38(9):A1-A34.

179. Puentedura EJ, O'Grady WH. Safety of thrust joint manipulation in the thoracic spine: a systematic review. *J Man Manip Ther.* 2015;23(3):154-161.

180. Bronfort G, Haas M, Evans RL, et al. Efficacy of spinal manipulation and mobilization for low back pain and neck pain: a systematic review and best evidence synthesis. *Spine J.* 2004;4(3):335-356.

181. Danish Institute for Health Technology Assessment. *Low back pain: frequency,* management and prevention from a health technology perspective. Copenhagen, Denmark: National Board of Health. Available at www.gacguidelines.ca/article.pl?sid02/07/05/2022215.

182. Haldeman S, Rubinstein SM. Cauda equina syndrome in patients undergoing manipulation of the lumbar spine. *Spine.* 1992;17(12):1469-1473.

183. Assendelft WJ, Bouter LM, Knipschild PG. Complications of spinal manipulation: a comprehensive review of the literature. *J Fam Pract.* 1996;42(5):475-480.

184. Senstad O, Leboeuf-Yde C, Borchgrevink C. Frequency and characteristics of side effects of spinal manipulative therapy. *Spine.* 1997;22(4):435-441.

185. Hungin AP, Kean WF. Nonsteroidal anti-inflammatory drugs: overused or underused in osteoarthritis? *Am J Med.* 2001; 110(1A):8S-11S.

186. Tamblyn R, Berkson L, Dauphinee WD, et al. Unnecessary prescribing of NSAIDS and the management of NSAID-related gastropathy in medical practice. *Ann Intern Med.* 1997;127(6): 429-438.

187. Tannenbaum H, Davis P, Russell AS, et al. An evidence-based approach to prescribing NSAIDs in musculoskeletal disease: a Canadian consensus: Canadian NSAID consensus participants. *CMAJ.* 1996;155(1):77-88.

188. Albert CM, Mittleman MA, Chae CU, et al. Triggering of sudden death from cardiac causes by vigorous exertion. *N Engl J Med.* 2000;343(19):1355-1361.

189. Leboeuf-Yde C, Hennius B, Rudberg E, et al. Side effects of chiropractic treatment: a prospective study. *J Manipulative Physiol Ther.* 1997;20(8):511-515.

190. Gudavalli MR. Instantaneous rate of loading during manual high-velocity, low-amplitude spinal manipulations. *J Manipulative Physiol Ther.* 2014;37(5):294-299.

191. Sran MM, Khan KM, Zhu Q, et al. Failure characteristics of the thoracic spine with a posteroanterior load: investigating the safety of spinal mobilization. *Spine (Phila Pa 1976).* 2004; 29(21):2382-2388.

192. Hurwitz EL, Morgenstern H, Vassilaki M, et al. Frequency and clinical predictors of adverse reactions to chiropractic care in the UCLA neck pain study. *Spine.* 2005;30(13):1477-1484.

193. Cagnie B, Vinck E, Beernaert A, et al. How common are side effects of spinal manipulation and can these side effects be predicted? *Man Ther.* 2004;9:151-156.

194. Rivett DA. The vertebral artery and vertebrobasilar insufficiency. In: Bouling JD, Jull GA, editors. *Greive's Modern Manual Therapy, the Vertebral Column,* ed 3. London: Churchill Livingstone.

195. Magarey ME, Rebbeck T, Coughlan B, et al. Pre-manipulative testing of the cervical spine review, revision and new clinical guidelines. *Man Ther.* 2004;9:95-108.

196. Daubs V, Lauretti WJ. A risk assessment of cervical manipulation versus NSAIDs for the treatment of neck pain. *J Manipulative Physiol Ther.* 1995;18(8):530-535.

197. Haldeman S, Kohlbeck FJ, McGregor M. Risk factors and precipitating neck movements causing vertebrobasilar artery dissection after cervical trauma and spinal manipulation. *Spine.* 1999;24:785-794.

198. Krespi Y, Mahmu EG, Coban O, et al. Vertebral artery dissection presenting with isolated neck pain. *J Neuroimaging.* 2002; 12(2):179-182.

199. Thiel H, Rix G. Is it time to stop functional pre-manipulation testing of the cervical spine? *Man Ther.* 2005;10:154-158.

200. DiFabio RP. Manipulation of the cervical spine: risks and benefits. *Phys Ther.* 1999;79(1):50-65.

201. Puentedura EJ, March J, Anders J, et al. Safety of cervical spine manipulation: are adverse events preventable and are manipulations being performed appropriately? A review of 134 reports. *J Man Manipulative Ther.* 2012;20(2):66-74.

202. Kerry R, Taylor AJ, Mitchell JM, et al. Cervical arterial dysfunction and manual therapy: a critical literature review to inform professional practice. *Man Ther.* 2008;13(4):278-288.

203. Cassidy J, Boyle E, Cote P, et al. Risk of vertebrobasilar stroke and chiropractic care. *Spine.* 2008;33:S176-S183.

204. Symons BP, Leonard T, Herzog W. Internal forces sustained by the vertebral artery during spinal manipulative therapy. *J Manipulative Physiol Ther.* 2002;25(8):504-510.

205. Symons B, Wuest S, Leonard T, et al. Biomechanical characterization of cervical spinal manipulation in living subjects and cadavers. *J Electromyogr Kinesiol.* 2012;22(5):747-751.

206. Herzog W, Leonard TR, Symons B, et al. Vertebral artery strains during high-speed, low amplitude cervical spinal manipulation. *J Electromyogr Kinesiol.* 2012;22(5):740-746.

207. Kranenburg HAR, Tyer R, Schmitt M, et al. Effects of head and neck positions on blood flow in the vertebral, internal carotid, and intracranial arteries: a systematic review. *J Orthop Sports Phys Ther.* 2019;49(10):688-697.

208. Thomas L. Cervical arterial dissection: an overview and implications for manipulative therapy practice. *Man Ther.* 2016; 21:2-9.

209. Taylor AJ, Kerry R. A systems-based approach to risk assessment of the cervical spine prior to manual therapy. *Int J Osteopath Med.* 2010;13(3):85-93.

210. Debette S, Leys D. Cervical-artery dissections: predisposing factors, diagnosis, and outcomes. *Lancet Neurol.* 2009;8:668-678.

211. Hutting N, Kerry R, Coppieters MW, Scholten-Peeters GGM. Considerations to improve the safety of cervical spine manual therapy. *Musculoskelet Sci Pract.* 2018;33:41-45.

212. Rivett DA, Milburn P. A prospective study of complications of cervical spine manipulation. *J Man Manipulative Ther.* 1996;4:166-170.

213. Hurwitz EL, Aker PD, Adams AH, et al. Manipulation and mobilization of the cervical spine: a systematic review of the literature. *Spine.* 1996;21:1746-1760.

214. Rushton A, Carlesso LC, Flynn T, et al. International Framework for Examination of the Cervical Region for potential of vascular pathologies of the neck prior to Orthopaedic Manual Therapy Intervention: International IFOMPT Cervical Framework, 2020.

215. Murphy DR. Current understanding of the relationship between cervical manipulation and stroke: what does it mean for the chiropractic profession? *Chiropr Osteop.* 2010;18(22):1-9.

216. Kerry R, Taylor AJ. Cervical arterial dysfunction: knowledge and reasoning for manual physical therapists. *J Orthop Sports Phys Ther.* 2009;39(5):378-387.

217. Cote P, Kreitz BG, Cassidy JD, et al. The validity of the extension-rotation test as a clinical screening procedure before neck manipulation: a secondary analysis. *J Manipulative Physiol Ther.* 1996;19:159-164.

218. Hutting N, Scholten-Peeters GGM, Vijverman V, et al. Diagnostic accuracy of premanipulative vertebrobasilar insufficiency tests: a systematic review. *Man Ther.* 2013;18(3):177-182.

219. Arnold M, Bousser MG, Fahrni G, et al. Vertebral artery dissection: presenting findings and predictors of outcome. *Stroke.* 2006;37(10):2499-2503.

220. Thomas LC, Rivett DA, Attia JR, et al. Risk factors and clinical features of craniocervical arterial dissection. *Man Ther.* 2011; 16(4):351-356.

221. Hutting N, Scholten-Peeters GGM, Vijverman V, et al. Diagnostic accuracy of upper cervical spine instability tests: a systematic review. *Phys Ther.* 2013;93:1686-1695.

222. Taylor AJ, Kerry R. Vascular profiling: Should manual therapists take blood pressure? *Man Ther.* 2013;18(4):351-353.

223. Traenka C, Dougoud D, Simonetti BG, CADISP-Plus Study Group, et al. Cervical artery dissection in patients ≥60 years: often painless, few mechanical triggers. *Neurology.* 2017;88(14): 1313-1320.

224. Rubinstein SM, Peerdeman SM, Van Tulder MW, et al. A systematic review of the risk factors for cervical artery dissection. *Stroke.* 2005;36(7):1575-1580.

225. Thomas LC, Makaroff AP, Oldmeadow C, et al. Seasonal variation in cervical artery dissection in the Hunter New England region, New South Wales, Australia: a retrospective cohort study. *Musculoskelet Sci Pract.* 2017;27:106-111.

226. Boissonnault WG. *Primary Care for the Physical Therapist: Examination and Triage.* St. Louis Elsevier Saunders; 2005.

227. Wolf P, Kannel WB, Sorlie P. Asymptomatic carotid bruit and risk of stroke, the Farmingham study. *JAMA.* 1981;245: 1442-1445.

228. Rich K. Carotid Bruit: a review. *J Vasc Nurs.* 2015;33(1):26-27.

229. Arnold M, Kappeler L, Georgiadis D, et al. Gender differences in spontaneous cervical artery dissection. *Neurology.* 2006;67: 1050-1052.

230. Sturzenegger M, Huber P. Cranial nerve palsies in spontaneous carotid artery dissection. *J Neurol Neurosurg Psychiatry.* 1993; 56:1191-1199.

231. Gibbons P, Tehan P. *Manipulation of the Spine*, Thorax and Pelvis: an Osteopathic Perspective, ed 2. London: Churchill Livingstone.

232. Cook C, Brismee JM, Fleming R, et al. Identifiers suggestive of clinical cervical spine instability: a Delphi study of physical therapists. *Phys Ther*. 2005;85(9):895-906.

233. Dewitte V, Beernaert A, Vanthillo B, et al. Articular dysfunction patterns in patients with mechanical neck pain: a clinical algorithm to guide specific mobilization and manipulation techniques. *Man Ther*. 2014;19(1):2-9.

234. Cleland JA, Childs JD, Fritz JM, et al. Development of a clinical prediction rule for guiding treatment of a subgroup of patients with neck pain: use of thoracic spine manipulation, exercise, and patient education. *Phys Ther*. 2007;87(1):9-23.

235. Cohen E, Triano J, McGregor M, et al. Biomechanical performance of spinal manipulation therapy by newly trained vs. practicing providers: does experience transfer to unfamiliar procedures? *J Manipulative Physiol Ther*. 1995;18(6):347-352.

236. Flynn TW, Fritz JM, Wainner RS. Spinal manipulation in physical therapist professional degree education: a model for teaching and integration into clinical practice. *J Orthop Sports Phys Ther*. 2006;36(8):577-587.

237. Schmidt RA. *Motor Control and Learning*, ed 2. Champaign, IL: Human Kinetics Publishers.

238. Mann DD, Patriquin DA, Johnson DF. Increasing osteopathic manipulative treatment skills and confidence through mastery learning. *J Am Osteopath Assoc*. 2000;100(5):301-304.

239. Watson TA. Comparison of three teaching methods for learning spinal manipulation skill: a pilot study. *J Man Manipulative Ther*. 2001;9(1):48-52.

240. Wulf G, Lewthwaite R. Optimizing performance through intrinsic motivation and attention for learning: the OPTIMAL theory of motor learning. *Psychon Bull Rev*. 2016;23:1382-1414.

241. Badami R, VaezMousavi M, Wulf G, et al. Feedback about more accurate versus less accurate trials: differential effects on self-confidence and activation. *Res Q Exerc Sport*. 2012;83:196-203.

242. Chiviacowsky S, Wulf G. Feedback after good trials enhances learning. *Res Q Exerc Sport*. 2007;78:40-47.

243. Chiviacowsky S, Wulf G, Wally R, et al. KR after good trials enhances learning in older adults. *Res Q Exerc Sport*. 2009;80:663-668.

244. Saemi E, Porter JM, Ghotbi-Varzaneh A, et al. Knowledge of results after relatively good trials enhances self-efficacy and motor learning. *Psychol Sport Exerc*. 2012;13:378-382.

245. Saemi E, Wulf G, Varzaneh AG, et al. Feedback after good versus poor trials enhances motor learning in children. *Revista Brasileira de EducacÃßaÃÉo FiÃÃsica e Esporte (Brazilian J Physic Educ Sport Manag)*. 2011;25:671-679.

246. Badami R, VaezMousavi M, Wulf G, et al. Feedback after good trials enhances intrinsic motivation. *Res Q Exerc Sport*. 2011;82:360-364.

247. Bryan JM, McClune LD, Romito S, et al. Spinal mobilization curricula in professional physical therapy education programs. *J Phys Ther Educ*. 1997;11(2):11-15.

248. Petty NJ, Cheek L. Accuracy of feedback during training of passive accessory intervertebral movements. *J Man Manipulative Ther*. 2001;9(2):99-108.

249. Keating JM, Bach TM. The effect of training on physical therapists' ability to apply specified forces of palpation. *Phys Ther*. 1993;73(1):38-46.

250. Lee M, Refshauge K. Effect of feedback on learning vertebral joint mobilization skill. *Phys Ther*. 1990;70(2):97-103.

251. Triano JJ, McGregor M, Dinulos M, et al. Staging the use of teaching aids in the development of manipulation skill. *Man Ther*. 2014;19:184-189.

CHAPTER 4

Examination and Treatment of Lumbopelvic Spine Disorders

OVERVIEW

This chapter covers the kinematics of the lumbar spine, pelvis, and hips; describes common lumbopelvic spine disorders with a diagnostic classification system to guide clinical reasoning and management; and provides a detailed description of special tests, manual examination, manipulation, and exercise procedures for the lumbar spine, pelvis, and hips. Pain science education and psychologically informed management principles are integrated with the overall management approach for low back pain (LBP) disorders. Video clips of the majority of the examination and manual therapy procedures are also included.

OBJECTIVES

- Describe the significance and impact of lumbopelvic spine disorders.
- Describe lumbar spine, pelvic, and hip kinematics.
- Use clinical reasoning to classify lumbopelvic spine disorders based on signs and symptoms.
- Determine the most effective and perform manual therapy and therapeutic exercise interventions for lumbar spine, pelvic, and hip disorders.
- Demonstrate and interpret lumbopelvic spine and hip examination procedures.
- Describe contraindications and precautions for lumbopelvic spine mobilization/manipulation.
- Demonstrate mobilization/manipulation techniques for the lumbar spine, pelvis, and hips.
- Instruct exercises for lumbopelvic spine disorders.
- Incorporate psychologically informed education and management principles for treatment of patients with lumbopelvic disorders.

▶ *To view videos pertaining to this chapter, please visit the eBook.*

SIGNIFICANCE OF THE LOW BACK PAIN PROBLEM

As many as 80% of Americans have symptoms of LBP during their lifetime.[1,2] LBP is the leading cause of injury and disability for those younger than 45 years of age and the third most prevalent impairment for those 45 years or older.[3]

LBP is the third costliest medical condition in the United States, behind only diabetes and heart disease; and over the past 10 years, the cost of treating LBP has risen at a rate exceeded only by diabetes.[4] The prevalence of chronic LBP is about 23% with 11% to 12% of the population being disabled by LBP.[2]

From an international perspective, LBP is a leading cause of global disability, with a global point prevalence of 9.4%.[5] LBP ranked as the number-one cause of disability among 291 conditions and sixth in terms of overall burden in the 2010 Global Burden of Disease study.[5] Among Western populations, back pain is associated with a range of negative consequences, such as reduced quality of life, heightened risk of other physical health comorbidities, and greatly increased healthcare costs.[6–9] Even in low- to middle-income countries, back pain has also been associated with higher than normal prevalence of depression, anxiety, stress sensitivity, and sleep disturbances in adult populations.[10]

Lumbar spinal stenosis (LSS) is associated with substantial medical costs, with an estimated 13% to 14% of patients seeking help from a specialty physician; up to 4% of those who seek care from a general practitioner for LBP are diagnosed with LSS.[11]

In 2001, 122,316 lumbar spinal fusion procedures were performed for degenerative conditions in the United States, compared with 32,701 operations in 1990, which calculates to 61.1 operations per 100,000 adults in 2001 compared with 19.1 operations per 100,000 adults in 1990.[12] The increase is 220%.[12] The most rapid rise in fusion rates occurred for the diagnosis of degenerative disk disease. Lumbar fusion is among the most rapidly increasing of all major surgical procedures and one of the most expensive, with $4.8 billion spent on spinal fusion surgeries in 2001 in the United States.[12] A 20-fold regional variation of lumbar fusion rates is found in the United States among Medicare enrollees in 2002 and 2003, which is likely the result of a lack of scientific evidence to guide surgical decision making, financial incentives, and professional opinion.[13] In other words, the likelihood of patients with degenerative spinal conditions undergoing fusion procedures is more dependent on where they live than clinical presentation.

The rapid increase in surgical rates and the escalating costs for diagnosis and treatment of lumbar conditions have not been matched by improved outcomes and reductions in disability. On the contrary, the level of disability associated with LBP as noted with work loss, early retirement, and state benefits has escalated as cost and surgical rates have increased.[14] With advancements in technology and radiologic research, use of advanced diagnostic imaging has increased rapidly.[15,16] The use of complex diagnostic testing rose 57% in the United States from 1996 to 2002 for injured workers.[17] In contrast, among workers with LBP, early use of magnetic resonance imaging (MRI) is associated with worse health outcomes and with increased likelihood of longer duration and more severe disability.[18]

Clinicians who treat patients with LBP should also keep in mind the high prevalence of degenerative imaging findings in asymptomatic individuals. Brinjkji et al.[19] completed a systematic review of 33 articles reporting imaging findings for 3110 asymptomatic individuals and found a 30% prevalence of disk bulge prevalence in those 20 years of age that increased to 84% of those 80 years of age (Table 4.1). Disk protrusion prevalence increased from 29% of those 20 years of age to 43% of those 80 years of age.[19] These findings demonstrate that imaging findings of spine degeneration are present in high proportions of asymptomatic individuals and increase with age. Imaging-based degenerative findings are likely part of normal aging and may be unassociated with pain. Therefore imaging findings must be interpreted in the context of the patient's clinical condition.[19] In addition, in a review of 202 patients who underwent decompressive lumbar surgery, researchers were unable to find a link between the severity of LSS on MRI and the degree of pain or disability, concluding that the radiologic severity of LSS has no clear clinical correlation with pain or disability and should not be overemphasized in clinical reasoning.[20]

An evidence-based approach to management of lumbar spine disorders is needed to prevent long-term disability and to empower patients to self-manage recurrent episodes of LBP. Early access to physical therapy tends to result in faster return to physical activity and reduction of costs associated with imaging and injections.[21] Likewise, another study showed that early referral (within 14 days of the primary care consultation) to physical therapy is associated with lower overall healthcare costs and reduced risk of subsequent healthcare utilization, including advanced imaging, additional physician visits, major surgery, lumbar spine injections, and opioid medications.[22]

Many clinical practice guidelines recommend a similar approach for the assessment and management of LBP that includes use of a biopsychosocial framework to guide management with initial nonpharmacologic treatment including education that supports self-management and resumption of normal activities and exercise, and psychologic programs for those with persistent symptoms.[23] Guidelines recommend

TABLE 4.1	Magnetic Resonance Imaging Findings in Asymptomatic Subjects Sorted by Decade of Age						
	AGE (YEARS)						
IMAGE FINDING	**20**	**30**	**40**	**50**	**60**	**70**	**80**
Disk degeneration	37%	52%	68%	80%	88%	93%	96%
Disk signal loss	17%	33%	54%	73%	86%	94%	97%
Disk height loss	24%	34%	45%	56%	67%	76%	84%
Disk bulge	30%	40%	50%	60%	69%	77%	84%
Disk protrusion	29%	31%	33%	36%	38%	40%	43%
Annular fissure	19%	20%	22%	23%	25%	27%	29%
Facet degeneration	4%	9%	18%	32%	50%	69%	83%
Spondylolisthesis	3%	5%	8%	14%	23%	35%	50%

Prevalence rates estimated with a generalized linear mixed-effects model for the age-specific prevalence estimate (binomial outcome) clustering on study and adjusting for the midpoint of each reported age interval of the study.
(From Brinjkji W, Luetmer PH, Comstock B, et al. Systematic literature review of imaging features of spinal degeneration in asymptomatic populations. *AJNR Am J Neuroradiol.* 2015;36:811-816.)

prudent and limited use of medication, imaging, and surgery.[23] However, globally, gaps between evidence and practice exist with limited use of recommended first-line treatments and inappropriately high use of imaging, rest, opioids, spinal injections, and surgery.[23] High-quality Orthopaedic Manual Physical Therapy (OMPT) can be part of the answer to curbing the spiraling epidemic of increased cost and disability associated with diagnosis and treatment of LBP conditions.

Lumbopelvic Kinematics: Functional Anatomy and Mechanics

An understanding of the functional anatomy and mechanics of the lumbar spine, pelvis, and hips establishes a foundation for the nonsurgical examination and treatment of these anatomic areas. Lumbar spine active range of motion (AROM) has been reported as 60 degrees flexion, 25 degrees extension, 25 degrees left and right lateral flexion, and 30 degrees left and right rotation.[24] Troke et al.[25] established normative lumbar spine range of motion (ROM) values for 405 participants ages 16 to 90 years. The median ROM for lumbar forward bending ranged from 73 degrees for the youngest age group to 40 degrees for the oldest.[25] Backward bending ranged from 29 to 6 degrees, with a decline of 79% from the youngest age group to the oldest. Lateral flexion declined from 28 to 16 degrees, and rotation stayed consistent at 7 degrees.[25] Troke et al.[25] found little difference in the median range of lumbar motion between male and female participants across a large age spectrum (Table 4.2).

The lumbopelvic region moves in coordination with the hip joints to create a lumbopelvic rhythm with forward and backward bending. In a standing position with the knees extended, forward bending is produced with hip flexion, anterior pelvic tilt, and forward bending of the lumbar spine. The relative contribution of each to the total amount of forward bending is dependent on muscle length (e.g., hamstrings), joint mobility (e.g., hips, facet joints, and sacroiliac joints [SIJs]), and neuromuscular control. Intersegment coordination or lumbopelvic rhythm during a forward bending motion is described as smooth and continuous motion with the first third

being dominated by lumbar spine motion, the second third shared motion between the lumbar and pelvic segments, and the last third being dominated by pelvic motion.[26] The control of each segmental movement with forward bending should include a smooth gradual increase in velocity to mid-point of forward bending and then a smooth gradual decrease in velocity to the end of the forward bending motion.[26] Alterations in the sequence of lumbopelvic rhythm or disruptions in the smooth coordination of segmental acceleration/deceleration (i.e., juddering) are defined as aberrant movements, which is a common finding with functional instability (i.e., movement coordination impairment) of the lumbar spine.[26]

With forward bending of the lumbar spine, the posterior annular fibers of the intervertebral disk become taut and the anterior fibers become slack and bulge anteriorly. The nucleus pulposus of the disk is compressed anteriorly, and pressure is relieved over the posterior surface.[27] Based on computed tomography (CT) scan data, forward bending increases the size of the central canal 24 mm[2], or 11%, and backward bending decreases the size of the canal 26 mm[2], or 11%.[28] The neuroforaminal area increases 13 mm[2] (12%) in forward bending and decreases 9 mm[2] (15%) in backward bending.[28] Among the 25 motion segments studied, three compressed nerve roots were relieved with forward bending and five nerve roots were compressed with backward bending[28] (Fig. 4.1).

The layers of annular fibers have an alternating oblique orientation to allow for only half of the fibers to be on tension during rotation. Forward bending places tension through all of the posterior annular fibers, so the combination of rotation with forward bending may result in excessive strain to the posterior annular intervertebral disk fibers.[27] Nachemson[29] measured intradiscal pressure of the L3 vertebrae in various positions and found that intervertebral disk pressure was greatest with participants sitting and leaning forward 20 degrees with weights in the hands. The standing position had less intradiscal pressure than did the sitting position, and the supine position was the least loaded discal pressure position (Fig. 4.2). Nachemson's[29] work provides a basis for clinical decision making in interpretation of the symptom behaviors in patients

TABLE 4.2	Maximal and Minimal Median Ranges of Lumbar Spinal Motion Across All Subjects (Overall Age Range of Subjects, 16–90 Years)				
	MALE		**FEMALE**		
MOVEMENT	MAXIMAL (MEDIAN OF VALUES; DEGREES)	MINIMAL	MAXIMAL (MEDIAN OF VALUES; DEGREES)	MINIMAL	
Flexion	73	40	68	40	
Extension	29	7	28	6	
Right lateral flexion	28	15	27	14	
Left lateral flexion	28	16	28	18	
Right axial rotation	7	7	8	8	
Left axial rotation	7	7	6	6	

(From Troke M, Moore AP, Maillardet FJ, et al. A normative database of lumbar spine ranges of motion. *Man Ther.* 2005;10(3):198-206.)

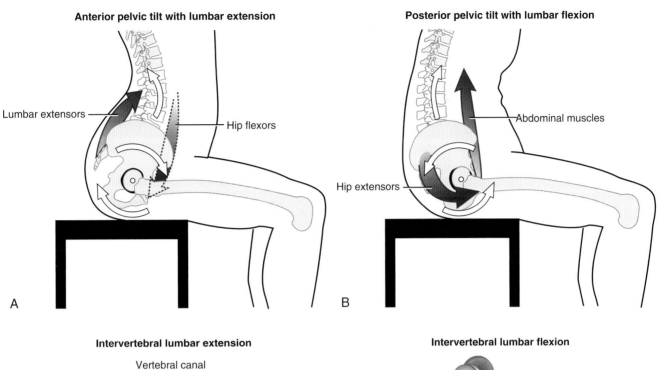

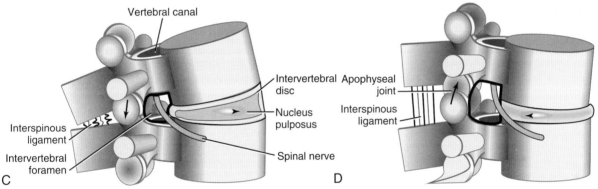

FIG. 4.1 Anterior and posterior tilt of pelvis and its effect on kinematics of lumbar spine. A and C, Anterior pelvic tilt extends lumbar spine and increases lordosis. B and D, Posterior pelvic tilt flexes lumbar spine and decreases lordosis. This action tends to shift nucleus pulposus posteriorly and increases diameter of intervertebral foramina. Muscle activity is shown in *red*. (From Neumann DA. Kinesiology of the Musculoskeletal System. St. Louis: Elsevier; 2017.)

with discogenic symptoms. For instance, if low back and leg pain symptoms are provoked with sitting and leaning forward, the likelihood of symptoms originating from a discogenic condition is increased.

The facet joints have two principal movements: translation (slide, slope, or glide) and distraction (gapping).[24] When upglide occurs from both sides simultaneously, the result is forward bending; likewise, when downglide occurs from both sides simultaneously, backward bending is the result.[30] Forward bending involves a flattening of the lumbar lordosis, especially at the upper lumbar levels,[31] and it involves a combination of anterior sagittal rotation and superior anterior translation (i.e., upglide) of the bilateral facet joints.

When upglide occurs on one side alone with downglide on the opposite side, the result is side bending (lateral flexion). Distraction occurs with axial rotation of the lumbar spine

when one facet is compressed and becomes a fulcrum and when the facet on the side of rotation is distracted[30] (Fig. 4.3). Tables 4.3 and 4.4 provide a list of the segmental lumbar forward and backward bending motions reported in the literature.[31–33] These findings are based on healthy young adult participants.

Lateral flexion and axial rotation of the lumbar spine tend to occur as coupled motions, but the exact patterns of coupling direction seem to vary from one individual to another and from one lumbar spinal level to another. With rotation, a coupled lateral flexion tends to occur to the opposite side; and this pattern is more consistent for levels L1–L2 to L3–L4 in participants without LBP. Inconsistent findings are seen with lower lumbar spinal segments with this coupling pattern. Panjabi et al.[32] found L4–L5 and L5–S1 rotation and coupled lateral flexion that occurred to the same side (Tables 4.5 and 4.6).

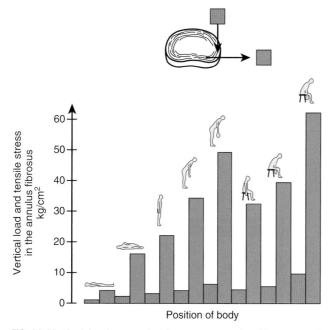

FIG. 4.2 Vertical load per unit of area on annulus fibrosus and tangential tensile stress in dorsal part of annulus fibrosus in L3 disk in participant weighing 70 kg and assuming positions schematically shown. (From Nachemson A. In vivo discometry in lumbar discs with irregular nucleograms. Some differences in stress distribution between normal and moderately degenerated discs. *Acta Orthop Scand*. 1965;36:426.)

TABLE 4.3	Lumbar Forward-Bending Segmental Range of Motion in Degrees		
LEVEL	**PEARCY et al.**	**PLAMONDON et al.**	**PANJABI et al.**
L1–L2	8.0 ± 0.02	5.1 ± 0.12	5.0 ± 5.0
L2–L3	10.0 ± 10.0	8.8 ± 0.80	7.0 ± 7.0
L3–L4	12.0 ± 12.0	11.6 ± 11.6	7.3 ± 7.3
L4–L5	13.0 ± 13.0	13.1 ± 13.1	9.1 ± 9.1
L5–S1	9.0 ± 0.01	–	9.0 ± 9.0

(Modified from Pearcy MJ, Tibrewal SB. Axial rotation and lateral bending in the normal lumbar spine measured by three-dimensional radiography. *Spine*. 1984;9:582-587; Plamondon A, Gagnon M, Maurais G. Application of a stereoradiographic method for the study of intervertebral motion. *Spine* 1988;13:1027-1032; and Panjabi MM, Oxland TR, Yamamoto I, et al. Mechanical behavior of the lumbar and lumbosacral spine as shown by three-dimensional load-displacement curves *J Bone Joint Surg (Am)*. 1994;76:413-424.)

Other findings showed that in patients with chronic low back pain (CLBP), three different patterns of coupled motion may occur: either the opposite lateral flexion was coupled with axial rotation ("normal"), the same direction of lateral flexion was coupled with rotation, or no coupling lateral flexion occurred with rotation.[34] In one study, only 14% of the patients had "normal" coupling patterns of axial rotation in the opposite direction of the lateral flexion. Fifty percent showed coupled axial rotation in the same direction as the lateral flexion, and the remainder showed no rotation with lateral flexion.[34]

FIG. 4.3 Taken from videotape of fresh cadavers mounted in frame, this illustration shows hatched areas where facets are exposed. A, Neutral position with facets neatly coupled is shown. B, Forward bending is depicted and exposes some 40% of facet joint area. C, Side bending to left causes more upward slide on right facet than did forward bending. Further, angular distraction of lower pole of left facet is shown. Note also upper vertebrae in side-bending left also rotated to that side. D, Right rotation is shown, in which right facet has distracted and left facet has compressed and slid somewhat forward with vertebrae tilting into left side bending. (Modified from Paris SV. Anatomy as related to function and pain. *Orthop Clin North Am.* 1983;14(3): 475-489.)

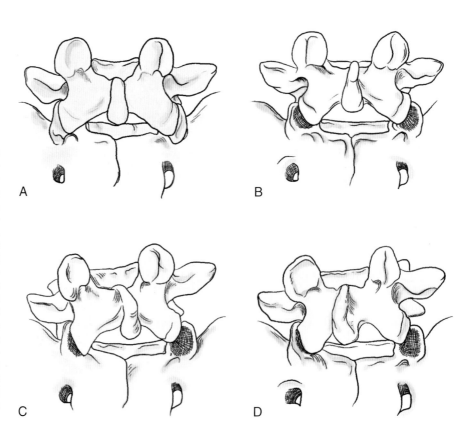

TABLE 4.4	Lumbar Backward-Bending Segmental Range of Motion in Degrees		
LEVEL	**PEARCY et al.**	**PLAMONDON et al.**	**PANJABI et al.**
L1–L2	5.0 ± 5.0	3.0 ± 3.0	4.1 ± 4.1
L2–L3	3.0 ± 3.0	3.9 ± 3.9	3.3 ± 3.3
L3–L4	1.0 ± 1.0	2.1 ± 2.1	2.6 ± 2.6
L4–L5	2.0 ± 2.0	1.2 ± 1.2	3.6 ± 3.6
L5–S1	5.0 ± 5.0	–	5.3 ± 5.3

(Modified from Pearcy MJ, Tibrewal SB. Axial rotation and lateral bending in the normal lumbar spine measured by three-dimensional radiography. *Spine.* 1984;9:582-587; Plamondon A, Gagnon M, Maurais G. Application of a stereoradiographic method for the study of intervertebral motion. *Spine* 1988;13:1027-1032; and Panjabi MM, Oxland TR, Yamamoto I, et al. Mechanical behavior of the lumbar and lumbosacral spine as shown by three-dimensional load-displacement curves *J Bone Joint Surg (Am).* 1994;76:413-424.)

TABLE 4.5	Lumbar Axial Rotation Segmental Range of Motion With Couple Lateral Flexion in Degrees			
	PEARCY et al.		**PANJABI et al.**	
LEVEL	**LEFT ROTATION**	**RIGHT LATERAL FLEXION**	**LEFT ROTATION**	**RIGHT LATERAL FLEXION**
L1–L2	1.0	3.0	2.3 ± 2.3	1.9 ± 1.9
L2–L3	1.0	3.0	1.7 ± 1.7	2.2 ± 2.2
L3–L4	2.0	3.0	2.3 ± 2.3	0.2 ± 0.2
L4–L5	2.0	2.0	1.2 ± 1.2	−1.2 ± 1.21
L5–S1	0.0	−0.0	1.0 ± 1.0	−1.0 ± 1.0

(Data compiled from Pearcy MJ, Tibrewal SB. Axial rotation and lateral bending in the normal lumbar spine measured by three-dimensional radiography. *Spine.* 1984;9:582-587; and Panjabi MM, Oxland TR, Yamamoto I, et al. Mechanical behavior of the lumbar and lumbosacral spine as shown by three-dimensional load-displacement curves *J Bone Joint Surg (Am).* 1994;76:413-424.)

TABLE 4.6	Lumbar Lateral Flexion Segmental Range of Motion With Coupled Axial Rotation in Degrees			
	PEARCY et al.		**PANJABI et al.**	
LEVEL	**RIGHT LATERAL FLEXION**	**LEFT ROTATION**	**RIGHT LATERAL FLEXION**	**LEFT ROTATION**
L1–L2	5.0	0.0	4.4 ± 4.4	0.0 ± 0.0
L2–L3	5.0	1.0	5.8 ± 5.8	1.7 ± 1.7
L3–L4	5.0	1.0	5.4 ± 5.4	0.9 ± 0.9
L4–L5	3.0	1.0	5.3 ± 5.3	1.8 ± 1.8
L5–S1	0.0	0.0	4.7 ± 4.7	1.7 ± 1.7

(Data compiled from Pearcy MJ, Tibrewal SB. Axial rotation and lateral bending in the normal lumbar spine measured by three-dimensional radiography. *Spine.* 1984;9:582-587; and Panjabi MM, Oxland TR, Yamamoto I, et al. Mechanical behavior of the lumbar and lumbosacral spine as shown by three-dimensional load-displacement curves *J Bone Joint Surg (Am).* 1994;76:413-424.)

Legaspi and Edmond[35] completed an extensive review of the literature on studies (*n* = 32) that measured lumbar segmental coupled motion and concluded that no consistent coupling pattern was seen with lumbar lateral flexion or rotation. Twenty-nine percent of the studies in which lateral flexion was the first motion performed found that, for most participants, lateral flexion and rotation were coupled to the opposite side (the classic "normal" description). However, 33% of the studies in which lateral flexion was the first motion performed found that, for most of the participants, coupling varied depending on the spinal level.[35] Some 45% of the studies in which rotation was the first motion performed found that coupling between lateral flexion and rotation was inconsistent, and another 45% of the studies found that, for most participants, coupling varied depending on the spinal level.[35]

Based on these findings, manual therapy practitioners should not rely on classical descriptions of coupling patterns for development and implementation of spinal manipulation techniques. When restoration of rotation or lateral flexion is a goal of intervention, multiple planar manipulation techniques can be used to take up tissue slack and isolate the forces to a specific spinal level, but the primary directional impairments should be addressed with the primary lever used in performance of the manipulation techniques.

The muscles of the back can be grossly divided between the global and the local muscles.[36] The global muscle system consists of large torque-producing muscles that act on the trunk and spine without directly attaching to the vertebrae. The global muscles include the rectus abdominis, external oblique, and thoracic part of the lumbar iliocostalis. The local muscle system consists of muscles that directly attach to the lumbar vertebrae and are responsible for providing segmental stability and directly controlling the lumbar segments.[36] The lumbar multifidus, psoas major, quadratus lumborum, interspinales, intertransversarii, lumbar portions of the iliocostalis and longissimus, transversus abdominis (TrA), diaphragm, and posterior fibers of the internal oblique all form part of the local muscle system[37] (Figs. 4.4 and 4.5). The local muscles, TrA, and lumbosacral multifidus tend to play a large role in the successful rehabilitation of spinal instability disorders with movement coordination impairments (Fig. 4.6).

The lumbar multifidus muscle (LMM) is bipennate in both origin and insertion. It arises from a tendinous slip from the mammillary process just lateral and inferior to the facet joint.[30] From this point, it passes upward and medially to gain a muscle origin from the upper third of the facet adjacent to its origin.[30] Two sets of these muscles then are joined together with further muscle tissue that ends in a tendinous slip that inserts into the posterior inferior aspect of the spinous process[30] (Fig. 4.7). The fascicles of the lumbar multifidus are well positioned to act as posterior sagittal rotators on the vertebrae of their origin, and the length of the spinous process provides a great mechanical advantage.[38] The multifidus is not well positioned to contribute to the posterior translation component of extension, and the multifidus has a short lever arm to assist with vertebral axial rotation. The muscles best suited for

Posterior view

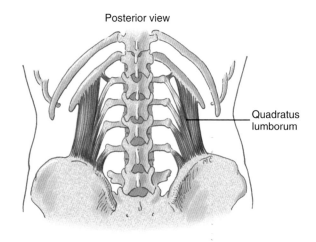

FIG. 4.4 A posterior view of the quadratus lumborum muscles. (Modified from Luttgens K, Hamilton N. *Kinesiology: Scientific Basis of Human Motion,* ed 9. Madison, WI: Brown and Benchmark; 1997.)

axial rotation are the oblique abdominal muscles, but they also at the same time produce a flexion moment.[38] The erector spinae and the multifidus have been suggested to be active during rotation to counter this flexion moment.[38] Although the multifidus has been said to be a lateral flexor of the lumbar vertebral column, it attaches too close to the axis of the movement to contribute significantly to lateral flexion.[38] Any apparent lateral flexion produced by the multifidus causes a combination of extension combined with slight contralateral axial rotation, which may be part of the reason for the more consistent upper lumbar coupled contralateral rotation motion with lateral flexion.[38] The multifidus contributes to the control of lumbar segmental motion by maintaining segmental equilibrium and development of intersegmental stiffness.[36]

Most of the structures of the lumbar spine are innervated by at least two, and usually three, segmental nerves.[30] This multiple segmental innervation may explain the variability of referred pain and pain perception reported by patients with

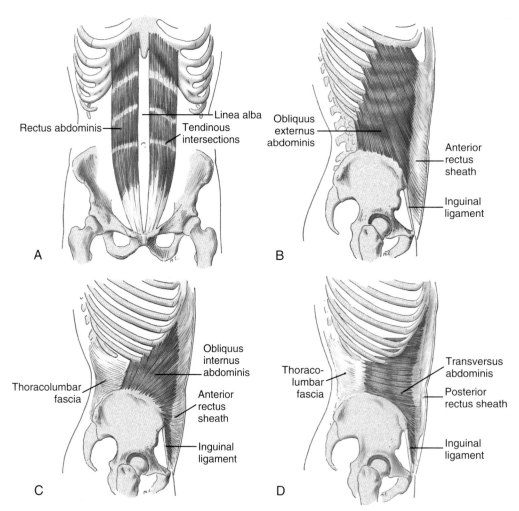

FIG. 4.5 The abdominal muscles of the anterior-lateral trunk. A, Rectus abdominis with the anterior rectus sheath removed. B, Obliquus externus abdominis. C, Obliquus internus abdominis, deep to the obliquus externus abdominis. D, Transversus abdominis, deep to other abdominal muscles. (Modified from Luttgens K, Hamilton N. *Kinesiology: Scientific Basis of Human Motion,* ed 9. Madison, WI: Brown and Benchmark; 1997.)

Posterior view

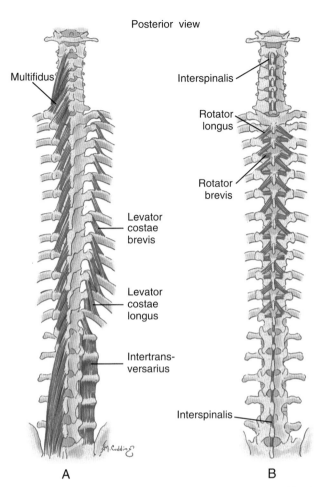

Multifidus

Interspinalis

Rotator longus

Rotator brevis

Levator costae brevis

Levator costae longus

Intertrans- versarius

Interspinalis

A   B

FIG. 4.6 A posterior view shows the deeper muscles within the transversospinal group (multifidi on entire left side of A; rotatores bilaterally in B). The muscles within the short segmental group (intertransversarius and interspinalis) are depicted in A and B, respectively. Note that intertransversarius muscles are shown for the right side of the lumbar region only. The levator costarum muscles are involved with ventilation. (Modified from Luttgens K, Hamilton N. *Kinesiology: Scientific Basis of Human Motion,* ed 9. Madison, WI: Brown and Benchmark; 1997.)

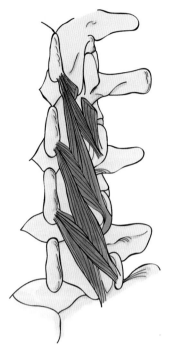

FIG. 4.7 Multifidus complex, which is difficult to illustrate, has both bipennate origin and bipennate insertion. Fiber orientation is shown. (From Paris SV. Anatomy as related to function and pain. *Orthop Clin North Am.* 1983;14(3):475-489.)

lumbopelvic disorders.[30] Clinically, the result is that clinicians cannot diagnose a specific anatomic structure as the primary cause of the patient's symptoms purely on the patient's report of pain location.

Pelvic Mechanics

Analysis of motion of the pelvis is difficult to measure with functional radiography because of the oblique orientation of the SIJs and the lack of definitive horizontal or vertical landmarks to use for motion measurement purposes. Strruresson, Selvik, and Uden[39] inserted four steel balls into the posterior aspect of the pelvis on 21 women and four men volunteers to study the motion of the pelvis with roentgen stereophotogrammetric analysis.[39] The x-ray tubes were oriented at oblique angles to the participant to capture radiographs of the participant in multiple positions. The pelvic motion measured with this technique was a mean of 0.5 mm translation and 1 to

2 degrees rotation.[39] The mean errors for rotation and translation were 0.1 to 0.2 degrees and 0.1 mm, respectively.[39]

The typical mean values of sacroiliac motion fall within the range of 0.2 to 2 degrees for anterior and posterior rotation and the range of 1 to 2 mm for translation.[40] Movements of the SIJ are primarily in the sagittal plane and primarily occur as a result of compression force of the articular cartilage and slight movement of the joint surfaces.[40] Terms commonly used to describe the motion of SIJs include *nutation, counternutation,* and *anterior/posterior rotation.* Nutation (meaning "to nod") is defined as the anterior tilt of the base (top) of the sacrum relative to the ilium and is also called sacral flexion.[40] Counternutation or sacral extension is the reverse motion, defined as the posterior tilt of the base of the sacrum relative to the ilium (Fig. 4.8).

Anterior rotation refers to the forward movement of the iliac crest and the backward movement of the ischial tuberosity in relation to the sacrum. Posterior rotation is the backward movement of the iliac crest and the forward movement of the ischial tuberosity in relation to the sacrum. Anterior rotation of the ilium tends to occur with end-range hip extension, and posterior rotation tends to occur with end-range hip flexion. The iliac crest of the ilium tends to move superiorly as it rotates anteriorly and move inferiorly as it rotates posteriorly.

In a young person, the joint surfaces of the SIJ are relatively flat; but with increasing age, they develop a series of peaks and troughs that interdigitate with each other.[41] These anatomic changes increase the joint's resistance to shearing movements by a mechanism termed *form closure.*[42] In theory, if two

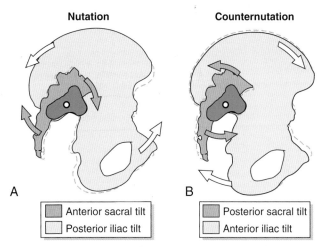

FIG. 4.8 Kinematics at sacroiliac joint. A, Nutation. B, Counternutation. Axis rotation for sagittal plane movement is indicated with *small circle*. (Modified from Neumann DA. *Kinesiology of the Musculoskeletal System.* St. Louis: Elsevier; 2017.)

opposing peaks catch on each other, the joint could become "locked" or "displaced" and require manipulation to restore the normal motion and position of the pelvis. Valid clinical measures for detection and measurement of the presence of a displaced SIJ have yet to be developed.

SIJ stability can be enhanced by muscle action. TrA contractions have been shown to enhance SIJ stability,[43] and in theory, tension generated by the gluteal muscles on one side of the body can work synergistically through the thoracolumbar fascia and the contralateral latissimus dorsi to press the joint surfaces closer together and increase stability by a mechanism termed *force closure*.[42] Therefore training of the gluteal, the contralateral latissimus dorsi, and the TrA muscles can form a muscular sling to enhance stability of the SIJ when hypermobility is suspected.

Hip Mechanics

Normal lumbopelvic rhythm includes a coordinated movement of the hip, pelvis, and lumbar spine. Typical lumbopelvic rhythm consists of about 40 degrees of forward bending of the lumbar spine and 70 degrees of flexion of the hips.[40] Limited flexion of the hips, such as with tight hamstrings or a tight hip joint capsule, requires greater flexion of the thoracic and lumbar spines. Excessive hip flexion as a result of excessive length of the hamstrings requires less lumbar and thoracic forward bending for full forward bending.[40]

The hip joint allows osteokinematic motions of flexion (120 degrees), extension (20 degrees), abduction (40 degrees), adduction (25 degrees), internal rotation (35 degrees), and external rotation (45 degrees).[40] These motions may be initiated as femur on pelvis or pelvis on femur movements. The hip joint is formed by the head of the femur and the deep socket of the acetabulum of the ilium to create the classic ball-in-socket joint. The deep socket is surrounded by an extensive set of capsular ligaments, and many large forceful muscles provide the forces needed to propel and stabilize the body.[40] The

arthrokinematics tend to follow the concave-convex rules so that if the motion is initiated with the femur on the pelvis, the gliding movement at the joint tends to be in the opposite direction of the femur movement (e.g., anterior glide of femoral head with hip extension). If the motion is initiated as the pelvis moves on the fixed femur (concave on convex), the gliding motion at the joint is in the same direction of the pelvic movement.

In a sitting position with the hips flexed about 90 degrees, an anterior pelvic tilt includes flexion of the hip joint and backward bending of the lumbar spine. A posterior pelvic tilt performed in a sitting position includes a relative extension motion of the hip joint and forward bending (straightening) of the lumbar spine.[40] With a single leg weight-bearing position, abduction and adduction of the hip joint can occur with frontal plane movements of the pelvis. Horizontal plane rotation of the pelvis occurs with internal and external rotation of the hips with the leg in a weight-bearing position.

The hip joint mobility (accessory motion) and muscle length and strength of the muscles that cross the hip joint must be evaluated and treated in patients with lumbopelvic disorders. The hamstrings, hip flexors, piriformis, and iliotibial band are muscles that typically guard and tighten with dysfunctions in the region (Fig. 4.9). The gluteal muscles (especially the gluteus medius), multifidus, and TrA are commonly weak with hip and lumbopelvic dysfunctions.

DIAGNOSIS AND TREATMENT OF LUMBOPELVIC DISORDERS

Evidence-based treatment guidelines for acute LBP have been endorsed by many countries, and a review of the available guidelines found consensus in several areas.[44,45] Regarding diagnosis, agreement exists that diagnostic triage is indicated to differentiate nonspecific LBP, radicular syndrome, and specific pathologic conditions. In addition, the history taking and physical examination must strive to identify red flags and screen the neurologic system. Radiographic examinations should not be used for the initial diagnosis of acute LBP conditions in the absence of red flags, and psychosocial factors should be assessed and considered as a component of a conservative approach.[44]

The guidelines also provide common recommendations for treatment for acute LBP, including early and gradual activation of patients, the discouragement of prescribed bed rest, and the recognition of psychosocial factors as risk factors for chronicity.[45] For CLBP, the guidelines consistently recommended interventions that included supervised exercises, cognitive-behavioral therapy, and multidisciplinary treatment.[45] Most of the guidelines recommend spinal manipulation for acute and chronic LBP, but there are a few guidelines that do not make this recommendation.[45] A recent review of international LBP clinical practice guidelines recommends self-management, physical and psychologic therapies, and to place less emphasis on pharmacologic and surgical treatments, and routine use of imaging is not recommended in the absence of red flags.[23]

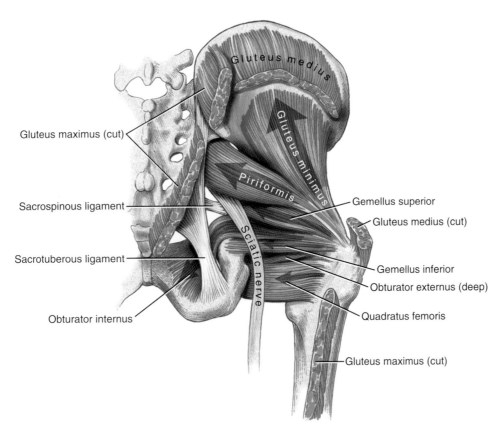

FIG. 4.9 Deep muscles of the posterior and lateral hip region. The gluteus medius and the gluteus maximus are cut to expose deeper muscles. (From Neumann DA. *Kinesiology of the Musculoskeletal System.* St Louis: Elsevier; 2017.)

A European guideline provided the following recommendations for the treatment of CLBP: cognitive behavior therapy, supervised exercise therapy, brief educational interventions, and multidisciplinary (biopsychosocial) treatment, with short-term use of nonsteroidal antiinflammatory drugs and weak opioids.[46] Additional treatments to be considered include back schools and short courses of manipulation and mobilization, antidepressants, and muscle relaxants.[46] Passive treatments, such as therapeutic ultrasound and diathermy, and invasive surgical procedures are not recommended for nonspecific LBP.[46] A significant note is that the recommendations of most evidence-based treatment guidelines for both acute and chronic LBP include patient education, manipulation, and exercise, the primary interventions provided by physical therapists.

Lumbopelvic disorders are not a homogeneous group of conditions, and subgrouping or classification of patients with back pain has been shown to enhance treatment outcomes.[47,48] Classification of lumbopelvic disorders should adequately define the primary signs and symptoms and guide therapeutic interventions. After red flags have been screened and the patient has been determined through use of medical screening procedures to be an appropriate candidate for physical therapy, further information should be gathered to arrive at a diagnosis and impairment classification for the condition.

The LBP treatment-based classification system was first described by Delitto, Erhard, and Bowling[49] and was based on

the available evidence, common practice, and expert opinion for treatment of patients with LBP. The classification categories are named by the primary intervention to be provided, and determination of the subgroup into which the patient is categorized is based on sets of signs and symptoms and impairments identified from the examination. Over time, the classification system has been modified based on results of clinical research studies to develop clinical prediction rules (CPRs) for manipulation[50] and stabilization[51] and based on results of reliability studies[52] and randomized controlled clinical trials.[48] The specific exercise category is based on a McKenzie[53] Method for Mechanical Diagnosis and Therapy (MDT) for treatment of "derangements," with use of repeated lumbar movements, that has been refined and tested by Werneke and Hart[54,55] and Long and Donelson.[56]

The treatment-based and impairment-based classification system avoids the pitfalls of attempts to identify the pathoanatomic cause of the patient's symptoms. Although clinicians often theorize about the primary anatomic structure at fault, studies estimate that the true pathoanatomic structure causing LBP can be identified in fewer than 15% of cases.[57] This chapter provides impairment-based classifications to assist in guidance of the treatment of LBP conditions that incorporate aspects of the treatment-based classifications, as well as other resources, such as the Low Back Pain Clinical Practice Guidelines linked to the International Classification of Functioning,

Disability, and Health (ICF) from the Academy of Orthopaedic Physical Therapy (AOPT) of the American Physical Therapy Association (APTA).[58] Evidence is found of improved outcomes with patients whose treatment approach is matched versus unmatched in use of the treatment-based classification for the conservative management of acute LBP.[47] Patients who underwent matched treatments had greater short-term and long-term reductions in disability than those who underwent unmatched treatments.[47] Earlier research by Fritz, Delitto, and Erhard[59] showed significantly better outcomes from 4 weeks of classification-based physical therapy treatment compared with low-stress aerobic exercise and advice to remain active. Box 4.1 outlines the primary categories used in the impairment-based classification system for LBP that labels each classification to attempt to highlight the primary impairments to be addressed in the category.

BOX 4.1 Outline of an Impairment-Based Classification System for Low Back Pain

Lumbar Mobility Deficits
ICF Classification: Low Back Pain with Mobility Deficits
Low back with or without leg pain that does not travel beyond the knee
Limited active lumbar spine mobility
Hypomobility with passive lumbar segmental motion testing
Myofascial restrictions with muscle guarding/holding

Lumbar Spine Instability
ICF Classification: Low Back Pain with Movement Coordination Impairments: Acute, or Chronic
Low back and/or low back–related lower extremity pain that worsens with sustained positions
Lumbar hypermobility with posteroanterior segmental mobility testing
Positive prone instability test
Diminished trunk and pelvic region muscle strength, endurance, and neuromuscular control
Aberrant movements with lumbar active motion testing

Lumbar and Related Leg Pain That Centralizes with Repeated Movements
ICF Classification: Low Back Pain with Related (Referred) Lower Extremity Pain
Low back and leg pain that may travel beyond the knee
Extension syndrome
  Symptoms centralize with lumbar backward bending
  Symptoms peripheralize with lumbar forward bending
Flexion syndrome
  Symptoms centralize with lumbar forward bending
  Symptoms peripheralize with lumbar backward bending
  Imaging evidence of lumbar spinal stenosis (LSS)
  Older age (>50 years)
Lateral shift
  Visible frontal plane deviation of the shoulders relative to the pelvis
  Symptoms centralize with side-glide and backward bending

Lumbar Radiculopathy That Does Not Centralize with Repeated Movements
ICF Classification: Acute, or Chronic Low Back Pain with Radiating Pain
Low back pain with associated radiating leg pain that tends to travel beyond the knee
Lower extremity paresthesia, numbness, and weakness may be reported
No lumbar movements centralize symptoms
No directional preference noted with history or clinical examination to alleviate lower leg pain
Peripheralization of leg pain with lumbar backward bending
Positive SLR for lower leg pain at <45 degrees hip flexion

Positive crossed SLR test at <45 degrees hip flexion
Lower extremity neurologic signs (weakness, numbness, and DTRs)
Poor tolerance to weight-bearing postures (i.e., sitting or standing)
Symptoms alleviated with traction

Sacroiliac Joint-Related Pain (Pelvic Girdle Pain)
ICF Classification: Low Back Pain with Movement Coordination Impairments
ICF Classification: Low back pain with Mobility Deficits
Sacroiliac Joint-Related Pain/Arthralgia
  Pain well localized at the SIJ and surrounding tissues
  Ipsilateral muscle holding at thoracolumbar paraspinals
  Positive SIJ pain provocation tests
SIJ-Related Pain with Movement Coordination Impairments
  Lumbopelvic area dull ache on assuming a fixed posture (such as prolonged sitting) that may refer into the posterior thigh region
  Periodic episodes of acute pain
  SIJ hypermobility with passive mobility testing
  Positive SIJ pain provocation tests
  Positive Active Straight Leg Raise Test
For patients who are postpartum
  Positive P4, ASLR, and Trendelenburg tests
  Pain provocation with palpation of the long dorsal sacroiliac ligament or pubic symphysis
SIJ-Related Pain with Mobility Deficits
  Raised or lowered iliac crest (noted in both sitting and standing)
  Lumbopelvic mobility deficits (active and passive)
  Positive SIJ pain provocation tests

Chronic Low Back Pain
ICF Classification: Chronic Low Back Pain with Related Generalized Pain[58]
Low back pain and/or low back–related lower extremity pain with symptom duration of more than 3 months
Generalized pain not consistent with other impairment-based classification criteria
Presence of depression, fear-avoidance beliefs, or pain catastrophizing
Movement impairments, such as hypomobility of thoracic, lumbopelvic, and hip joints with poor neuromuscular control and coordination of spinal motions

ICF Classification: Acute or Subacute Low Back Pain with Related Cognitive or Affective Tendencies
Acute or subacute low back and/or low back–related lower extremity pain
High scores on FABQ and behavioral processes consistent with an individual who has excessive fear or anxiety

ASLR, Active straight leg raise; *DTR,* deep tendon reflex; *FABQ,* Fear-Avoidance Beliefs Questionnaire; *P4,* posterior pelvic pain provocation; *SLR,* straight leg raise.

Lumbar Mobility Deficits
ICF Classification: Low Back Pain With Mobility Deficits

Numerous independent agencies have conducted systematic reviews of the literature to develop clinical practice guidelines based on the strength of the evidence and have concluded that spinal manipulation is a safe, effective intervention for the management of acute LBP.[6,60–65] Systematic reviews and treatment guidelines have included spinal manipulation as a recommendation supported by a moderate to strong level of evidence for the treatment of not only acute LBP but also subacute and CLBP.[45,58,61,62] A systematic review and meta-analysis[66] concluded that there is moderate-quality evidence that thrust manipulation and nonthrust mobilization are safe and likely to reduce pain and improve function for patients with CLBP.

The clinical practice guideline produced by the AOPT of the APTA recommends, based on strong evidence, that clinicians should use thrust manipulation to reduce pain and disability in patients with mobility deficits and acute low back and back-related buttock or thigh pain;[58] and thrust manipulation and nonthrust mobilization can also be used to improve spine and hip mobility and reduce pain and disability in patients with subacute and chronic low back and back-related lower extremity pain.[58,63] Kuczynski et al.[63] examined the effectiveness of spinal thrust manipulations performed solely by physical therapists and reported that there is evidence to support the use of spinal thrust manipulation by physical therapists in clinical practice and that spinal thrust manipulation performed by physical therapists is a safe intervention that improves clinical outcomes for patients with LBP.[63]

The vast majority of clinical research studies that have demonstrated the effectiveness of thrust manipulation and nonthrust mobilization for treatment of LBP have used a clinical decision-making framework that incorporates an impairment-based approach.[48,59,67–72] Once red flags and contraindications to manipulation are ruled out, the therapist considers the location and behavior of the patient's symptoms along with the patient's expectations of the treatment to establish a hypothesis of which lumbar spine impairment-based classification is the best fit. Low back or buttock pain with or without pain into the thigh are typical symptoms for the LBP with mobility deficits classification.

Clinical examination findings include mobility deficits with active spinal mobility and passive intervertebral motion (PIVM) testing and pain provocation with passive accessory intervertebral motion (PAIVM) testing, which guides the therapist to determine where to focus the manipulation, what direction to move the targeted spinal segment, and with what intensity and speed of force application. Palpation findings of limited myofascial tissue extensibility, trigger points, or chemical muscle holding can guide the decision to include soft tissue mobilization techniques to the treatment plan. Soft tissue mobilization techniques are useful treatment in subacute and chronic hypomobility conditions as an adjunct to the spinal joint manipulation procedures. A continual active process of examination and reexamination is required to determine the effects of each manual therapy technique and how to modify the technique to attain the desired outcome of improvement in active and passive spinal mobility and reduction of pain with functional movements. Mobility and stretching exercises are used in follow-up to the manual therapy procedures to encourage maintenance of the mobility gained during the treatment session, and these are incorporated into a home exercise program (Box 4.3). Therefore the primary indication for use of spinal manipulation (thrust and nonthrust) is mobility deficits with concurrent pain.

A CPR for thrust manipulation for acute LBP was developed by Flynn et al.[50] and is a set of five criteria that was determined to predict successful outcomes from a lumbopelvic thrust manipulation when at least four of the five criteria were met in the patient examination findings. See Box 4.2 for an outline of CPR for thrust manipulation for acute LBP. Childs et al.[48] published a randomized controlled trial (RCT) that validated the CPR for use of thrust manipulation for acute LBP.

The study from Childs et al.[48] examined 131 patients (18–60 years of age) with acute LBP who were referred to a physical therapist. Patients were randomly assigned to receive physical therapy that included two sessions of high-velocity thrust spinal manipulation plus an exercise program (manipulation + exercise group) or an exercise program without spinal manipulation (exercise-only group).[48] During the first two sessions, patients in the manipulation + exercise group received high-velocity thrust manipulation and ROM exercise. Patients in the exercise-only group were treated with a low-stress aerobic and lumbar spine–strengthening program. Patients in both groups attended physical therapy twice during the first week and then once a week for the next 3 weeks, for a total of five sessions.[48]

The patients with positive results for the CPR for thrust manipulation and who received the thrust manipulation intervention (manipulation + exercise group) had dramatic improvements in pain and disability after 1 week and 4 weeks and sustained that improvement at the 6-month follow-up examination.[48] The patients with positive results for the CPR (at

---

BOX 4.2	Clinical Prediction Rule for Improvement With Lumbopelvic Manipulation for Acute Low Back Pain

- Duration of symptoms <16 days
- At least one hip with >35 degrees of internal rotation
- Hypomobility with lumbar posteroanterior PAIVM testing
- FABQ work subscale score <19
- No symptoms distal to the knee

FABQ, Fear-Avoidance Beliefs Questionnaire; *PAIVM*, passive accessory intervertebral movement.
(From Flynn T, Fritz J, Whitman J, et al. A clinical prediction rule for classifying patients with low back pain who demonstrate short-term improvement with spinal manipulation. *Spine.* 2002;27:2835-2843.)

least four of five findings) who received the thrust spinal manipulation had a 92% chance of a successful outcome at the end of 1 week.[48] At the 6-month follow-up examination, patients who fit the CPR but did not receive spinal manipulation showed significantly greater use of medication and healthcare services and more lost time from work because of back pain than did the manipulation group.[48] Most of the participants (72%) showed meaningful clinical improvements with lumbar spinal manipulation, which supports the rationale that patients with acute-onset LBP without signs of nerve root compression are excellent candidates for a trial of thrust manipulation.[73]

Further analysis of this study reveals that the number needed to treat with spinal thrust manipulation to prevent one additional patient from a worsening in disability at 1 week was 9.9 (95% confidence interval [CI], 4.9–65.3); this number persisted at 4 weeks.[13] The patients with LBP who were provided with exercise only were eight times more likely to have a worsening in disability after 1 week than were patients who received thrust manipulation.[13] Only 10 patients need to be treated with thrust manipulation to prevent one patient from a worsening in disability after 1 week.[13]

Fritz et al.[74] analyzed the relationship between judgments of PAIVM assessments and clinical outcomes after two different interventions, stabilization exercise alone, or thrust manipulation followed by stabilization exercises. Patients who were assessed to have lumbar hypomobility on physical examination demonstrated more significant improvements with the thrust manipulation and exercise intervention than with stabilization exercises alone. Seventy-four percent of patients with hypomobility who received thrust manipulation had a successful outcome compared with 26% of the patients with hypermobility who were treated with thrust manipulation. These findings suggest that lumbar hypomobility as detected with lumbar PAIVM testing, in the absence of contraindications, is sufficient to consider use of thrust manipulation as a component of the treatment of patients with LBP.[74]

Although a supine lumbopelvic thrust manipulation technique (Fig. 4.64) was used in the studies by Flynn et al.[50] and Childs et al.[48] to develop and validate the CPR, Cleland et al.[68] showed excellent results of treatment with a different lumbar thrust manipulation technique (side-lying lumbar rotation) (Fig. 4.65) in a case series of 12 patients who fit the lumbar manipulation CPR. Cleland et al.[71] also completed an RCT of 112 patients with LBP who fit the CPR for lumbar thrust manipulation in four clinics across the United States. The participants were randomly assigned to receive either a supine lumbopelvic thrust manipulation, a side-lying lumbar rotation thrust manipulation, or a prone central posteroanterior nonthrust (lower lumbar) mobilization for two consecutive treatment sessions followed by a mobility and stabilization exercise regimen for an additional three sessions with assessment at baseline, 1 week, 4 weeks, and 6 months. Pairwise comparisons revealed no differences between the supine lumbopelvic thrust manipulation and side-lying rotation thrust manipulation at any follow-up period. Significant differences in pain

and disability existed at each follow-up between the thrust manipulation and the nonthrust mobilization groups at 1 week and 4 weeks. There was also a significant difference in disability scores at 6 months in favor of the thrust groups.[71] These studies suggest that selection of correct patient characteristics is likely more important than selection of correct technique for successful outcomes with lumbar thrust manipulation for treatment of acute LBP.

There also appears to be a more dramatic effect for patients with acute LBP who fit the lumbar thrust manipulation CPR with the use of thrust manipulation techniques compared with the use of the nonthrust techniques. Hancock et al.[75] examined the results of a randomized trial involving 240 patients with LBP randomized to receive either active or placebo manipulation. Nonthrust mobilization techniques were used for 97% of patients in the active manipulation group.[75] The authors reported that the patients' status on the CPR for lumbar manipulation was not predictive of the clinical outcomes between the treatment groups.[75] These results, along with the results of the Cleland et al.[71] study, indicate that the CPR is not generalizable to treatment protocols that substitute nonthrust mobilization techniques for thrust manipulation techniques.

Cook et al.[72] compared the effectiveness of early use of thrust manipulation and nonthrust mobilization during the first two visits of physical therapy in a sample of 149 patients with mechanical LBP. After the first two visits, the therapist was allowed to modify manual therapy and exercise interventions based on the patient's signs and symptoms, and the patients received care over an average of 35 days. Both groups improved with the treatment, but there were no significant differences between thrust manipulation and nonthrust mobilization at the second follow-up or at discharge with any of the pain or disability outcomes. The personal preference of the physical therapist toward the effectiveness of thrust manipulation versus nonthrust mobilization was found to have a significant effect on the pain and disability outcomes of his or her patients.[72] The Cook et al. study used a pragmatic research design in which the physical therapists were given more latitude to modify the nonthrust techniques based on the patient's response to treatment than was allowed in the Cleland et al.[71] study that used a prescriptive research design which standardized the nonthrust technique as central posteroanterior nonthrust technique. In addition, the inclusion criteria for participants to qualify for treatment in the Cook et al. study was that the physical therapist had to localize and reproduce the patient's pain and produce a within-session reduction in pain or improvement in mobility using central or unilateral posteroanterior PAIVMs.[72] The authors determined that this was necessary to ensure that manual therapy interventions were appropriate for each patient included in the study.

Roenz et al.[76] carried out a systematic review and meta-analysis to determine the difference in effectiveness of nonthrust mobilization versus thrust manipulation for treatment of neck or LBP when comparing a pragmatic versus a prescriptive research design. Thirteen studies met the inclusion/exclusion criteria with eight studies fitting the prescriptive research design and five fitting the pragmatic research design. Thirteen studies with a total of 1313 participants were included in the systematic review, and 12 studies with 977 participants in the metaanalysis. For most time-points, prescriptive studies found thrust manipulation to be superior to nonthrust mobilization for both pain and disability.[76] At no time-point did the pragmatic designs find a difference between nonthrust mobilization and thrust manipulation for either pain or disability. The metaanalysis found that when the pragmatic design was used there was no difference in outcomes between nonthrust mobilization and thrust manipulation, but when a prescriptive research design was used, thrust manipulation demonstrated better outcomes than nonthrust mobilization for pain and disability.[76]

These studies demonstrate that an impairment-based approach can yield successful outcomes, and a combination of thrust and nonthrust techniques combined with specific exercises will likely yield the best outcomes. The direction, location, and force used for spinal mobilization/manipulation in the plan of care are based on detection of lumbopelvic hypomobility with active and passive mobility and end feel testing. Because active ROM testing, such as lower trunk rotation (see Fig. 2.42) is a reliable impairment measurement, it is advisable to include this test in both the pre- and posttreatment assessment of patients with LBP with mobility deficits in lower trunk rotation are noted. For instance, if left lower trunk rotation is limited with AROM testing combined with posteroanterior PAIVM restriction at the L4–L5 spinal segment and PIVM testing limitation of the left rotation at the same spinal segment, a left rotation manipulation targeting the L4–L5 spinal segment is used. After the manipulation, the active and passive motion is reassessed to determine whether a positive change occurred with the intervention, such as better freedom of motion or less pain with movement. If a nonthrust mobilization technique was used, but the desired improvement in mobility and reduction in pain was not attained, modifications in the direction, intensity, and velocity of the technique should be made to attempt to create a positive effect including consideration to use a thrust manipulation technique. Similarly, if a thrust manipulation is used initially, but the desired treatment effect is not attained, modification of the treatment to include nonthrust mobilization techniques may be indicated. Continual examination and reexamination of the patient is required to effectively modify the treatment. An exercise program that includes lumbar mobility exercises enhances the clinical outcomes after the mobilization/manipulation (Box 4.3). As symptoms subside and mobility improves, the patient may also benefit from progression of lumbar motor control (stabilization) and conditioning exercises (Box 4.4).

Psychosocial issues, such as fear-avoidance beliefs, must also be considered because of evidence that spinal stabilization exercise programs are more effective than manipulation for patients with high Fear-Avoidance Beliefs Questionnaire (FABQ) scores.[51] In addition, high scores on intake forms, such as the Central Sensitization Inventory (see Fig. 2.7) or the STarT Back Screening Tool (see Fig. 2.4), would suggest that motor control exercise combined with a psychologically informed approach that includes elements of cognitive-behavioral therapy may be more effective interventions than an emphasis on manual therapy. Providing explanations of the neurophysiology associated with pain perception and the impact that psychosocial factors, such as stress, anxiety, and depression have on pain perception can help the patient better cope with and manage LBP symptoms. Manual therapy could still be an adjunct to treatment in these situations but should not be the emphasis and care in using psychologically informed language to explain the potential positive effects of the manual therapy techniques should be used in all situations. (See "Psychologically-Informed Language and Pain Neuroscience Education" in Ch. 3)

Lumbar Spine Instability
ICF Classification: Low Back Pain With Movement Coordination Impairments

Clinical instability is defined by Panjabi[77] as the inability of the spine under physiologic loads to maintain its pattern of displacement so that no neurologic damage or irritation, no development of deformity, and no incapacitating pain occur. The total ROM of a spinal segment may be divided into the neutral zone and the elastic zone.[77,78] Motion that occurs in and around the neutral mid position of the spine is produced against minimal passive resistance (i.e., neutral zone), and motion that occurs near the end range of spinal motion is produced against increased passive resistance (i.e., elastic zone).[77,79] Clinical instability is believed to be a result of increase in the size of the neutral zone and reduction in the passive resistance to motion created in the elastic zone and can be further subdivided into structural and functional instability. The loss of neuromotor capability to control segmental movement during mid-range is defined as functional instability or a movement coordination impairment.[80] The disruption of passive stabilizers that limit the excessive segmental end ROM is defined as structural instability.[80,81] Structural instability can be diagnosed and quantified with measurement of excessive anteriorposterior translation on end range flexion extension radiographs.[81] However, there is no diagnostic standard to quantify functional instability except clinical findings, such as aberrant movements to assist in the diagnosis.[80,82,83] The aberrant movements noted with functional instability is caused by a lack of motor control, and underlying structural instability may also be a contributing factor, but not in all cases.

Panjabi[77] conceptualized the components of spinal stability into three functionally integrated subsystems of the spinal stabilizing system. According to Panjabi,[77] the stabilizing system of the spine consists of the passive, active, and neural control subsystems.

The passive subsystem consists of the vertebral bodies, facet joints and joint capsules, spinal ligaments, and passive tension from spinal muscles and tendons. The passive subsystem provides significant stabilization of the elastic zone and limits the size of the neutral zone. Also the components of the

BOX 4.3   Lumbopelvic Mobility Exercises[a]

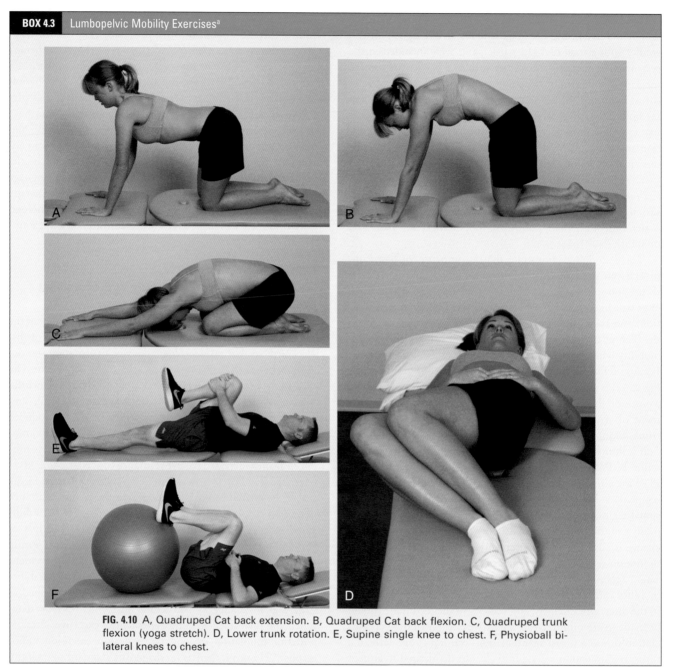

FIG. 4.10 A, Quadruped Cat back extension. B, Quadruped Cat back flexion. C, Quadruped trunk flexion (yoga stretch). D, Lower trunk rotation. E, Supine single knee to chest. F, Physioball bilateral knees to chest.

[a]After lumbopelvic manipulation, lumbopelvic mobility exercises are useful to maintain the mobility gained with the manual therapy techniques.

passive subsystem act as transducers and provide the neural control subsystem with information about vertebral position and motion.

The active subsystem, which consists of spinal muscles and tendons, generates the forces needed to stabilize the spine in response to changing loads. The active subsystem is primarily responsible for controlling the motion that occurs within the neutral zone and contributes to maintaining the size of the neutral zone. The spinal muscles also act as transducers that provide the neural control subsystem with information about the forces generated by each muscle.

Through peripheral nerves and the central nervous system, the neural control subsystem receives information from the transducers of the passive and active subsystems about vertebral position, vertebral motion, and forces generated by spinal muscles. With the information, the neural control subsystem determines the requirements for spinal stability and acts on the spinal muscles to produce the required forces.

Clinical spinal instability occurs when the neutral zone increases relative to the total ROM, the stabilizing subsystems are unable to compensate for this increase, and the quality of motion in the neutral zone becomes poor and uncontrolled.[77,78,84]

BOX 4.4 Lumbopelvic Movement Control Phase I

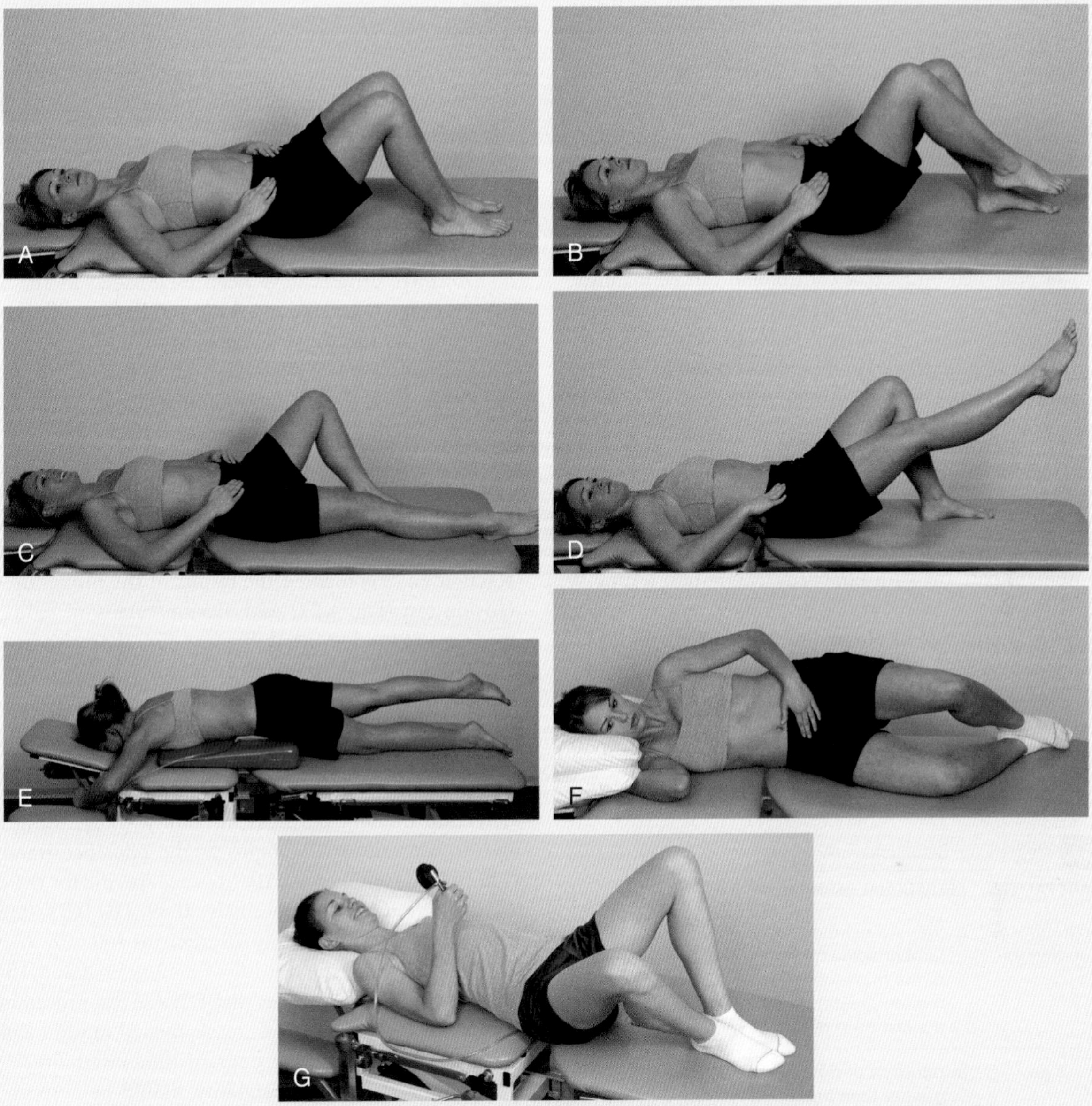

FIG. 4.11 A, Drawing in maneuver is used to isolate transversus abdominis (TrA) in hook-lying position, and tactile cues just medial to anterior superior iliac spine can facilitate isometric contractions. Work toward 10-second holds for 10 repetitions at least four times per day, and then progress to TrA isometrics in multiple positions throughout the day. B, Hook-lying marching motion with TrA contraction to control lumbopelvic spine position in neutral. C, Bent knee fall out with TrA contraction to control lumbopelvic spine position in neutral. D, Straight leg raise with TrA contraction to control lumbopelvic spine position in neutral. E, Prone over a pillow hip extension with TrA contraction to control lumbopelvic spine position in neutral. The airbag biofeedback device can be used to provide feedback on steadiness with trunk stabilization during this exercise. F, Side-lying "clamshell" hip abduction with external rotation with TrA contraction to control lumbopelvic spine position in neutral. Patient must be cued to ensure pelvis does not rotate as hip moves. B–F, Preset and sustain TrA contraction throughout leg movements. G, Bent knee fall out with airbag biofeedback for motor control training of the TrA with active hip movements.

Degeneration (especially early phases of degeneration) and mechanical injury of the spinal stabilization components are the primary causes of increases in neutral zone size.[77] Factors that contribute to degeneration or mechanical injury of the stabilizing components are poor posture, repetitive occupational trauma, acute trauma, and weakness of the local lumbar musculature.[77,85-87]

Because poor quality of motion is a key aspect of clinical functional instability, the presence of aberrant motions during active movement has been suggested by several authors to be a cardinal sign of clinical instability.[80,82,88-90] Aberrant motions are signs of poor neuromuscular control and can be manifest as either sudden accelerations or decelerations of movement, instability catch, painful arc of motion in flexion, painful arc on return from flexion, thigh climbing (Gower's sign), a reversal of lumbopelvic rhythm, shaking or juddering with spinal movements, or motions that occur outside the intended plane of movement[51,82,88,90] (Table 4.7). Physical therapists have demonstrated moderate to good interrater reliability (kappa = 0.60 with 84% agreement[91] and kappa = 0.79 with 97% agreement[83]) in their ability to agree on observations of aberrant movement patterns with lumbar active motion testing.[91] Biely et al.[92] reported excellent (kappa = 0.89) interexaminer reliability for judgments of altered lumbopelvic rhythm, but only moderate reliability for judgements of deviation from midline (kappa = 0.68) or juddering (kappa = 0.35). In addition, the prevalence of aberrant movement patterns with lumbar forward bending is greater in patients with LBP than

those without symptoms.[92] Other symptoms of clinical functional instability are general tenderness of the lumbar region, referred pain in the buttock or thigh area, paraspinal muscle guarding, and pain with sustained postures.[46,85,88,90,93-95] Also PIVM and joint play testing may reveal hypermobility and decreased passive restraints to motion at end range of PIVM (i.e., a loose end feel).[96] Imaging studies may show alterations of the components of the passive subsystem (i.e., structural causes of instability), such as ligament damage, osteophytes, vertebral fractures, disk degeneration, and vertebral displacement associated with spondylolisthesis.[77,84,86,97-99]

Objective criteria have been established in the analysis of excessive translation with end-range flexion and extension radiographs for diagnosis of spinal structural instability.[88,90,94,98,100,101] Fritz et al.[102] found that the presence of at least 53 degrees of lumbar flexion measured with a double inclinometer or a lack of hypomobility with posteroanterior PAIVM testing resulted in a positive likelihood ratio of 4.3 (95% CI, 1.8–10.6), for predicting radiographic structural instability and the positive likelihood ration was 12.8 (95% CI, 0.79–211.6) when both tests were positive. Kasai et al.[103] compared the results of the prone lumbar extension test (Fig. 4.27) with flexion/extension radiographic evidence of lumbar instability and found sensitivity of 0.84 and specificity of 0.90 with a positive likelihood ratio (+LR) of 8.84 (4.51, 17.33) and negative likelihood ratio (–LR) of 0.2 (0.1, 0.4). Abbott et al.[104] reported on the validity of the use of lumbar forward and backward bending PIVM testing and posteroanterior PAIVM testing for use in detection of lumbar spinal instability (LSI), using lumbar flexion/extension radiographs as the reference standard on 138 patients with LBP. PAIVMs were specific for the diagnosis of translation LSI (specificity 0.89, CI, 0.83–0.93), but showed poor sensitivity (0.29, CI, 0.14–0.50). A positive PAIVM test results in a +LR of 2.52 (95% CI, 1.15–5.53). This research demonstrates that PAIVM test procedures have moderate validity for detecting segmental motion abnormality but poor ability to rule out structural instability.[104] Therefore lumbar structural instability should be suspected with positive clinical examination procedures including:

- The passive lumbar extension test (Fig. 4.27) or
- Lumbar forward bending AROM greater than 53 degrees measured with the double inclinometer (Fig. 2.35) or
- Lack of lumbar hypomobility with posteroanterior PAIVM test (Fig. 4.63)

The level of suspicion of structural instability is increased when positive test results are combined, but when negative, these examination procedures cannot fully rule out structural instability with any level of certainty.[83,102,103]

Patients with LBP may present with findings of combined structural and functional instability, but in other cases, signs of functional instability may be present without evidence of a known structural instability finding.[80,83] Radiographic findings often do not correlate with symptom severity. It is also possible to have signs of structural instability with excessive translation noted on a flexion extension radiograph of an asymptomatic

TABLE 4.7	Operational Definitions of Aberrant Movement Patterns[92]
ABERRANT PATTERN	**OPERATIONAL DEFINITION**
Altered lumbo-pelvic rhythm	In forward bending, hip motion greater than lumbar spine motion during the first third of the movement and/or lumbar spine motion greater than hip motion during the last third of the movement
Gowers' sign	In return to upright, lumbar spine motion greater than hip motion during the first third of the movement and/or hip motion greater than lumbar spine motion during the last third of the movement
Deviation from sagittal plane	Return to upright stance performed by using hands to climb up the thighs, which is considered a type of altered lumbopelvic rhythm
Instability catch, shake, or judder	A sudden acceleration, stop, or deceleration; observations of a momentary quiver, vibration, or shake seen in the paravertebral muscles; or brief out-of-plane movements
Painful arc of motion	Pain, noted by the patient, that increases through a portion of the total arc of movement; a general increase in pain throughout the motion does not constitute arc

From Biely SA, Silfies SP, Smith SS, et al. Clinical observation of standing trunk movements: what do the aberrant movement patterns tell us? *J Orthop Sport Phys.* 2014;44(4):262-272.

individual, which could be explained as having lack of tissue sensitivity and adequate neuromuscular control to control the underlying instability.[80,82]

Radiographs do not yield information about the quantity or quality of motion that occurs in the neutral zone (i.e., mid-range), which limits the value of radiographic evidence in the diagnosis of functional instabilities.[88,98] Video fluoroscopy shows some promise as a means for analysis of the quality of spine motion at mid-range, but its use is still experimental for this purpose.[105] Teyhan et al.[105] developed a kinematic model with digital fluoroscopy to illustrate aberrant rates of attainment of angular and linear displacement around the mid-range postures with patients with clinical signs of instability; these patients tend to have a combination of altered segmental structural integrity, segmental stiffness, and altered neuromuscular control during lumbar spine movements. PIVM and joint play testing have diagnostic value with assessment of neutral zone size, but the tests have poor interrater reliability and only assess passive motion.[79,91,106] Because a definitive diagnostic tool for functional instability has not been established, functional instability continues to be diagnosed based on a cluster of clinical findings including history, subjective symptoms, visual analysis of active motion quality (i.e. aberrant movements), and manual examination methods.[96]

Hicks et al.[51] developed a CPR (Table 4.8) to predict the likelihood of success with use of a lumbar stabilization exercise

(LSE) program for patients with LBP. If a patient has three or more of the four variables, the +LR of success is 4.0 (95% CI, 1.6–10.0) that the patient will respond favorably to a spinal stabilization exercise program.[51] Of the four variables, age less than 41 years was the single most significant factor to predict success.[45]

The study by Hicks et al.[51] involved 8 weeks of physical therapy with instruction and monitoring of a spinal stabilization exercise program. Patients underwent reassessment after 8 weeks, and if the Oswestry Disability Index (ODI) score improved by 50%, the treatments were considered a success.[51] If six points of improvement or 49% improvement were seen, patients were considered improved; with a less than six-point reduction on the ODI, the treatments were considered a failure. The study found 18 successes, 15 failures, and 21 improved.[51] The characteristics of each group were analyzed to determine clinical findings at the initial evaluation that could predict success or failure.

The four variables that were found to predict failure of a spinal stabilization exercise program were negative prone instability test results (Fig. 4.26), absent aberrant movements, FABQ physical activity subscale score less than nine, and no hypermobility with lumbar PAIVM testing.[51] An interesting note is that patients with higher FABQ scores responded more favorably to the stabilization exercise program. This finding reinforces the importance of an active exercise-based approach for patients with high levels of fear of activity.

Rabin et al.[107] completed an RCT validation study of the LSE program CPR. The study compared LSE with a manual therapy program (lumbar thrust manipulation and nonthrust mobilization plus stretching exercises) for 105 patients with LBP who received 11 treatment sessions over 8 weeks. Patients with a positive LSE CPR experienced less disability by the end of treatment compared with patients with a negative CPR, regardless of the treatment received. Further analysis revealed that when a modified version of the CPR (mCPR) containing only the presence of aberrant movement and a positive prone instability test was used, a significant interaction with treatment was found for disability at the end of treatment.[107] Among patients with a positive mCPR, those receiving LSE experienced less disability by the end of treatment compared with those receiving manual therapy. This study was not able to fully refute or confirm the validity of the LSE CPR, but it did suggest that a modification of the CPR might be predictive of those patients who will respond favorably to an LSE program.[107] Further research is needed to validate the LSE CPR and to further assess the validity of the modified CPR. Lumbar aberrant movements continue to be supported as a clinical sign of functional instability. Therefore training of trunk muscle neuromuscular control is the primary intervention of functional instability.

Bergmark[36] divides the muscles of the trunk into two groups: local and global systems. The global muscle group includes the larger more superficial muscles, such as the erector spinae, rectus abdominis, and internal/external obliques. The primary functions of the global muscles are to transfer loads between the thoracic cage and the pelvis and to change the

TABLE 4.8	Significant Predictors (Clinical Prediction Rule) of Lumbar Stabilization Exercise Program Success and Failure (Signs of Lumbar Functional Instability)	
	VARIABLES	**ACCURACY STATISTICS**
Predictors of success	Positive prone instability test Aberrant motion present Age <41 years SLR >91	If two of the four variables are present: Sensitivity: 0.83 (0.61–0.94) Specificity: 0.56 (0.40–0.71)
Predictors of failure	Negative prone instability test Hypomobility with PAIVM testing Aberrant motion absent FABQ score ≤9 (activity scale)	If two of the four variables are present: Sensitivity: 0.85 (0.70–0.93) Specificity: 0.87 (0.62–0.96)
Modified version of the LSE CPR	Aberrant motion present Positive prone instability test	

CPR, Clinical prediction rule; *FABQ*, Fear-Avoidance Beliefs Questionnaire; *LSE*, lumbar stabilization exercise; *PAIVM*, passive accessory intervertebral motion; *SLR*, straight leg raise.
(From Hicks GE, Fritz JM, Delitto A, et al. Preliminary development of a clinical prediction rule for determining which patients with low back pain will respond to a stabilization exercise program. *Arch Phys Med Rehabil.* 2005;86:1753-1762; Rabin A, Shashua A, Pizem K, et al. A clinical prediction rule to identify patients with low back pain who are likely to experience short-term success following lumbar stabilization exercises—a randomized controlled validation study. *J Orthop Sports Phys Ther.* 2014;44(1):6-18; Teyhan DS, Flynn FW, Childs JD, et al. Arthrokinematics in a subgroup of patients likely to benefit from lumbar stabilization exercise program. *Phys Ther.* 2007;87(3):313-325.)

position of the thoracic cage in relation to the pelvis.[36] The local muscle system includes the deeper smaller muscles with direct attachments into the vertebrae. The local system is used to control the spinal curvature and to give sagittal and lateral stiffness to maintain mechanical stability of the spine.[36] Examples of the local muscles include the transverses abdominis (because of its attachment into the lumbar fascia) and the lumbar multifidi and intertransverse muscles. The quadratus lumborum is classified into both systems, with the lateral portion functioning as a global muscle and the medial portion that attaches to the lumbar transverse processes as a local muscle that stabilizes the lumbar spine in a lateral direction.[36]

In patients with functional instability or movement coordination impairments, an imbalance tends to exist between the function of the global and local muscles. The global muscles tend to be strong and overactive and in a state of muscle holding. The local muscles are weak, atrophied, and delayed in response times and coordination. The primary purpose of the early phases of a lumbopelvic motor control exercise program is to facilitate the control, strength, and coordination of the local muscles and inhibit the action of the global muscles. Manual physical therapy techniques directed to the thoracic spine may be used to inhibit the increased tone of the erector spinae (global muscles system). Motor relearning principles are used to facilitate a therapeutic exercise program designed to train the local muscle system. A motor control exercise program is actually a better term than stabilization exercise program for this approach because the ultimate goal is to more effectively and efficiently control and coordinate spinal motion rather than to stabilize spinal motion.

Electromyogram (EMG) study results have shown a delay in firing of the local lumbopelvic muscles in patients with a history of LBP compared with paired healthy participants when active upper extremity motions are performed.[108] The results of a fine-wire EMG study show that both deep and superficial fibers of the multifidus muscle are controlled differentially during movements of the arm that challenge the stability of the spine, with the superficial fibers of the multifidus acting to control spine orientation and the deep fibers controlling intersegmental motion.[109] The multifidus muscles are active in anticipation of arm movements and are active earlier for shoulder flexion than extension motions. This direction-specific activity is matched to the direction of reactive forces caused by limb movement and linked to the control of spine orientation and the displacement of the center of mass.[109] In contrast to the superficial fibers, the EMG onset of deep multifidus and TrA fibers was not altered by movement direction.[109] These deeper muscles are not affected by which direction the arm is moved. They are active through the activity regardless of direction of arm movements. Because the deep fibers are independent of reactive force direction, they may therefore control intersegmental motion and stability.[109]

Evidence also exists of excessive fat infiltration in the LMM in participants with a history of LBP.[110] Fat infiltration seems to be a late stage of muscular degeneration and can be measured in a noninvasive manner with MRI. The results of this study provide the first convincing evidence from a large population sample that fat infiltration in the LMMs is strongly associated with LBP in adults.[110] Therefore these patients lack the dynamic intersegmental motor control provided by the multifidus.

Hides, Jull, and Richardson[111] followed a control group and a group that received a spinal stabilization exercise program after a first-time episode of LBP. At the 10-week follow-up examination, atrophy of the lumbar multifidus was noted at the side and spinal level of the patient's primary pain symptom. Both groups had a return to a good functional level, but significantly higher recurrence rates of LBP episodes were noted in the control group that did not receive a spinal stabilization exercise program at the 2-year to 3-year follow-up examination.[111] During the 2-year to 3-year period after the first-time episode of LBP, the patients in the control group who did not receive the exercise program instruction were 5.9 times more likely to have recurrences of LBP than were patients in the specific exercise group and 12.4 times more likely to have a recurrence in the first year.[111] These studies support the concept that permanent motor control and physiologic muscle changes can occur after injury to the lumbar spine and that specific skilled physical therapy intervention is needed to normalize muscle function and prevent recurrence of future LBP episodes. Recovery of local muscle function appears to be a key factor in full recovery and future prevention of LBP episodes.

Hodges and Richardson[108] studied 15 patients with LBP and 15 matched control participants who performed rapid shoulder flexion, abduction, and extension while standing in response to a visual stimulus. Electromyographic activity of the abdominal muscles, lumbar multifidus, and contralateral deltoid was evaluated with fine-wire and surface electrodes.[108] The results of this study showed that shoulder movement in each direction resulted in contraction of trunk muscles before or shortly after the deltoid contraction in control participants.[108] The TrA was usually the first active muscle and was not influenced by movement direction, which supports the hypothesized role of this muscle in spinal stiffness generation.[108] Contraction of the TrA was significantly delayed in patients with LBP with all shoulder movements.[108] The delayed onset of contraction of the TrA indicates a deficit of motor control and is hypothesized to result in inefficient muscular stabilization of the spine.[108]

Hodges and Richardson[112] also showed with another fine-wire EMG study that the TrA fires in anticipation of lower extremity movements regardless of the direction of the movements, which supports the hypothesis that the TrA functions as a primary spinal stabilizer muscle. The lower fibers of the TrA with their horizontal orientation may contribute to the enhancement of the stability of the spine, either through their role in the production of intraabdominal pressure or via an increase in the tension in the thoracolumbar fascia through which these muscles are attached to the lumbar vertebrae and enhance the stiffness and stability of the spine.[112] MRI study results have confirmed that during the abdominal "drawing in" action, the TrA contracts bilaterally to form a musculofascial band that appears to tighten like a corset and improves stabilization of the lumbopelvic region.[113] The TrA muscle has also been shown to reduce sacroiliac laxity and is believed to play a significant role to enhance stability of the pelvis when functioning properly.[43]

Cross-sectional area (CSA) of the LMM and the TrA muscle can be studied with rehabilitative ultrasound imaging, which can be used to measure and compare the thickness of a muscle at rest with the thickness with an isometric contraction to quantify the motor control of the muscle. Hides et al.[114] used ultrasound imaging to measure the CSA of the lumbar multifidus in participants with CLBP and in asymptomatic participants. Patients with CLBP had significantly smaller multifidus CSAs than asymptomatic participants at the lowest two vertebral levels. The greatest asymmetry between sides was seen at the L5 vertebral level in patients with unilateral pain presentations. The smaller multifidus CSA was ipsilateral to the reported side of pain in all cases.[114] This supports the clinical assumption that exercise therapy needs to be specific and tailored to address specific localized impairments present in patients with CLBP.

Wallwork et al.[115] used ultrasound imaging techniques to measure contraction size of the multifidus muscle to compare both the CSA and the ability to voluntarily perform an isometric contraction of the multifidus muscle at four vertebral levels in 34 participants with and without CLBP. Results showed a significantly smaller CSA of the multifidus muscle for the participants in the CLBP group compared with participants from the healthy group at the L5 vertebral level and a significantly smaller percent thickness contraction for participants of the CLBP group at the same vertebral level[115] (Fig. 4.12). This result was not present at other vertebral levels. The results of this study support previous findings that the pattern of multifidus muscle atrophy in patients with CLBP is localized rather than generalized but also provides evidence of a corresponding reduced ability to voluntarily contract the atrophied muscle.[115]

Two RCTs of different subgroups of patients with LBP reported improvements in pain and function with exercise interventions that involved the "drawing in maneuver" of the lower

abdomen.[108,116] Inclusion criterion for participants in the O'Sullivan, Twomey, and Allison[116] clinical trial was radiographic evidence of spondylolysis or spondylolisthesis. Forty-four patients with these conditions were assigned randomly to two treatment groups. The first group underwent a 10-week specific exercise treatment program that involved the specific training of the deep abdominal muscles, with coactivation of the lumbar multifidus.[116] The activation of these muscles was incorporated into previously aggravating static postures and functional tasks. The control group underwent treatment as directed by the treating practitioner. After the intervention, the specific exercise group showed a statistically significant reduction in pain intensity and functional disability levels, which was maintained at a 30-month follow-up examination.[116] The control group showed no significant change in these parameters after intervention or at follow-up examination.[116] A specific exercise treatment approach appears to be more effective than other commonly prescribed conservative treatment programs in patients with chronically symptomatic spondylolysis or spondylolisthesis.

One of the goals of the early phase of a lumbopelvic movement control (stabilization) exercise program is isolation of contraction of the TrA. An EMG study has confirmed that the "inward movement of the lower abdominal wall" (i.e., abdominal drawing in maneuver) in the supine position is the most effective way to isolate a TrA contraction in isolation of the more superficial abdominal muscles (rectus abdominis, internal oblique, and external oblique).[117] In contrast, a posterior pelvic tilt and abdominal bracing procedure showed greater activity in the internal oblique muscle.[117] More lumbopelvic motion was recorded with posterior pelvic tilt, and a negative correlation was noted between movement of the spine and TrA activity.[117] In other words, greater TrA activity is produced when spinal motion is minimized.

Ultrasound imaging is increasingly being used for physical therapy research and clinical practice to assess specific motor control of the deep local trunk muscles. Koppenhaver et al.[118] reported intraclass correlation coefficient (ICC) values of 0.96 to 0.99 for intraexaminer reliability and 0.96 to 0.98 for

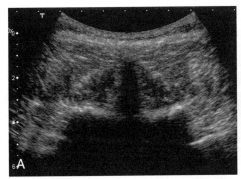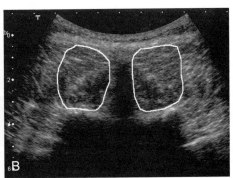

FIG. 4.12 A. Bilateral transverse ultrasound image at the L4 vertebral level, without CSA tracings. B. Bilateral transverse ultrasound image at the L4 vertebral level with CSA tracings. The CSA (in cm2) of the multifidus was measured by tracing around the muscle border with the on-screen cursor. (From Wallwork TL, Warren RS, Freke M, et al. The effect of chronic low back pain on size and contraction of the lumbar multifidus muscle. *Man Ther.* 2009;14:496-500.)

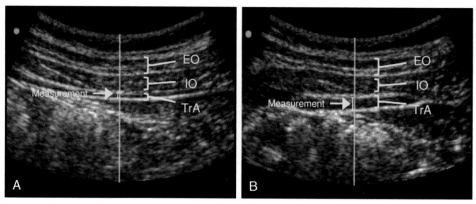

FIG. 4.13 Ultrasound images of the TrA, internal oblique (IO), and external oblique (EO) muscles (A) during rest and (B) during an ADIM. Thickness measurements were made between the superficial and deep borders of the TrA muscle. (From Koppenhaver SL, Hebert JJ, Fritz JM, et al. Reliability of rehabilitative ultrasound imaging of transversus abdominis and lumbar multifidus muscles. *Arch Phys Med Rehabil.* 2009;90:87-94.)

interexaminer reliability for thickness measurements on the TrA and lumbar multifidus muscles in patients with LBP (Fig. 4.13[118]). Teyhen et al.[119] reported that individuals with unilateral lumbopelvic pain demonstrated a smaller increase in thickness of the TrA muscle during an isometric contraction of the TrA during the abdominal drawing-in maneuver (ADIM) using ultrasound imaging both at rest and during the ADIM. However, both groups demonstrated a symmetric side-to-side change in TrA muscle thickness despite the symptomatic group having unilateral symptoms. There was no association between the side of the symptoms and reduction in the thickness of the TrA either at rest or during the ADIM.[119]

Hebert et al.[120] examined the relationship between prognostic factors associated with clinical success with a stabilization exercise program (positive prone instability test, age younger than 40 years, aberrant movements, straight leg raise [SLR] more than 91 degrees, and presence of lumbar hypermobility) and the degree of TrA and LMM activation assessed by ultrasound imaging. Significant relationships were identified between decreased LMM activation and the number of prognostic factors present.[120] A positive prone instability test and segmental hypermobility were associated with decreased LMM activation, but no significant relationships were observed between the prognostic factors and TrA muscle activation.[120] Decreased LMM activation is associated with the presence of factors predictive of clinical success with a stabilization exercise program, but this did not hold true for decreased TrA muscle activation in this study.[120] These findings provide evidence for the clinical importance of targeting the LMM for motor control exercises. Costa et al.[121] demonstrated that motor control exercise was better than placebo in patients with CLBP for improved activity and global impression of recovery. Most of the effects observed in the short term were maintained at 6- and 12-month follow-ups, but the magnitude of the effects was small.[121] The results suggest that this intervention should be considered for patients with CLBP to improve activity and global impression of recovery and to improve pain intensity in the long term.

A total of 20 volunteers with unilateral LBP were randomly assigned to cognitively activate the lumbar multifidus independently from other back muscles (skilled training) or to activate all paraspinal muscles with no attention to any specific muscles using an extension training exercise.[122] EMG activity of multifidus muscles was recorded bilaterally using intramuscular fine-wire electrodes and surface electrodes for the superficial abdominal and back muscles. Motor coordination was assessed before and immediately after training as onsets of trunk muscle EMG during rapid arm movements and as EMG amplitude at the midpoint of slow trunk flexion-extension movements. After both training programs, activation of the multifidus muscles was earlier during rapid arm movements. However, during slow trunk movements only the skilled training group demonstrated the desired increased multifidus muscle activity with reduced superficial trunk muscle EMG activity.[122] These findings show that motor coordination can be improved with skilled motor training.

Grooms et al.[123] used ultrasound imaging on patients with LBP to determine the ratio of activation of the TrA muscle during the ADIM and compared this with performance of abdominal holding as measured with the Stabilizer biofeedback airbag device (Fig. 4.11). The authors concluded that successful completion on the pressure biofeedback does not indicate high TrA activation.[123] Unsuccessful completion on pressure biofeedback may be more indicative of low TrA activation, but the correlation and likelihood coefficients indicate that the pressure test is likely of minimal value to detect TrA activation.[123] TrA activation needs to be taught by the therapist one-on-one with the patient using visualization and palpation methods to enhance the training. The biofeedback airbag device could be used as an adjunct for progression of neuromuscular lumbopelvic control exercises once the patient has mastered isolated isometric contractions of the TrA. The biofeedback airbag device provides knowledge of results feedback for holding the trunk steadier, which can enhance motor learning.

A patient is best taught a spinal movement control (stabilization) exercise program with a motor learning approach that starts with the cognitive phase of learning in which a great deal of mental concentration is needed to attain the proper muscle contraction and controlled motion.[124] Much cognitive activity is necessary to use appropriate muscle control strategies initially, but with practice, the performance rapidly improves. The movement control (stabilization) program should start with guidance, with a good deal of feedback for training in isolation of the local muscles, especially transverses abdominis and multifidus muscles, in a supported position, such as prone or supine hook lying, and with a stabilizer airbag biofeedback pressure gauge device (Box 4.4). As the patient continues to practice and feedback is provided, the patient can move into the associative phase of motor learning in which the quality of the motion and the ease of performance improve. Less mental energy is necessary. The second phase should include addition of exercises in less stable positions, such as quadruped and standing, that further challenge maintenance of a neutral spine position (Box 4.5) (Fig. 4.14). For the final phase of motor learning, autonomous, new situations and challenges need to be incorporated into the training program to make the motor control more skillful, natural, and automatic in performance. At this phase, the learner can perform the task at a high level without much thought and can concurrently perform other tasks if needed.[124] Once this phase is reached, retention of the skill is enhanced and good long-term clinical outcomes are realized. The final phase includes more dynamic movement patterns in functional planes that require control of movement of the spine combined with extremity movements in a controlled manner. For example, lunge exercises require controlled dynamic stabilization in a functional movement pattern. Use of a weighted medicine ball assists in guiding the movement pattern, and the reaching with the weighted ball toward the front lunging knee theoretically facilitates the hip gluteal muscles to eccentrically assist in control of the movement pattern (Box 4.6). Work-specific and sport-specific activities can also be incorporated in the phase III dynamic stabilization program, which might include lifting training or balance/agility activities.

Lumbar and Leg Pain That Centralizes
ICF Classification: Low Back Pain With Related (Referred) Lower Extremity Pain

McKenzie[53] describes seven types of derangements based on symptom location, response to the repeated movement examination, and presence of deformity (lateral shift or kyphotic lumbar posture). With the McKenzie Method of MDT, treatment of the derangements emphasizes that the direction of repeated movements should be governed by the centralization/peripheralization phenomena and that no repeated exercise movement or advice on positioning should be performed that causes the pain reference to peripheralize.

The clinical phenomenon known as centralization occurs during repeated lumbar movements or postures when the most distal extent of the referred or radicular pain recedes toward the lumbar midline.[125] Peripheralization is the spreading laterally or distally of the symptoms from the lumbar spine toward the foot with repeated lumbar movements or postures. McKenzie has speculated that the direction of bending that centralizes the pain precisely corresponds with the direction in which disk nuclear content has migrated to generate referred symptoms by mechanically stimulating the annulus or nerve root.[53] An MRI study demonstrated that a subgroup of patients ($n = 20$) who were classified as being good candidates for lumbar extension-based exercise and had a positive immediate response (2/10 pain reduction) following a 10-minute session of posteroanterior lumbar mobilizations and prone press ups demonstrated an increase in the diffusion of water in the middle portion of the L5S1 intervertebral disk.[126] Subjects who did not report a pain reduction of at least 2/10 did not have a change in diffusion.[126] This study provides a possible physiologic explanation for why some patients respond to these intervention and others do not, but with only 20 subjects, further research is needed to draw conclusions.

Wernecke et al.[127] define directional preference as either: (1) a specific direction of trunk movement or posture noted during the physical examination or (2) a specific aggravating or easing factor reported by the patient during the subjective history that alleviates or decreases the patient's pain, with or without the pain having changed location or increased patient's lumbar ROM. Directional preference is distinguished from centralization, which is characterized by spinal pain and referred spinal symptoms that are progressively abolished in a distal-to-proximal direction in response to therapeutic movement and positioning strategies, and it is possible for patients to have a directional preference but not meet the definition of centralization.[127] The prognosis of patients treated with a directional preference management treatment approach tends to improve when the patient can be classified with a directional preference with centralization compared with a directional preference without centralization or no directional preference at all.[127]

In a study published by Donelson et al.,[125] the repeated lumbar movements of flexion, extension, side gliding, extension in lying, flexion in lying, and flexion/rotation with overpressure in hook lying were used to make a mechanical diagnosis by a physical therapist; each patient was then given a discogram test for determination of the symptomatic disk and a CT scan for assessment of the disk integrity. This study found a high incidence rate of positive discogram results in centralizers (74%) and peripheralizers (69%). In the patients with positive discogram results, the difference between the incidence rates of disks with a competent annulus that occurred in centralizers (91%) was significantly greater than what occurred in peripheralizers (54%).[125] Donelson et al.[125] concluded that most centralizers in this population of patients with CLBP have discogenic pain with a functionally competent annulus and that peripheralizers also tend to have discogenic pain but with a higher incidence rate of outer annulus disruption.

BOX 4.5   Lumbopelvic Movement Control Phase II

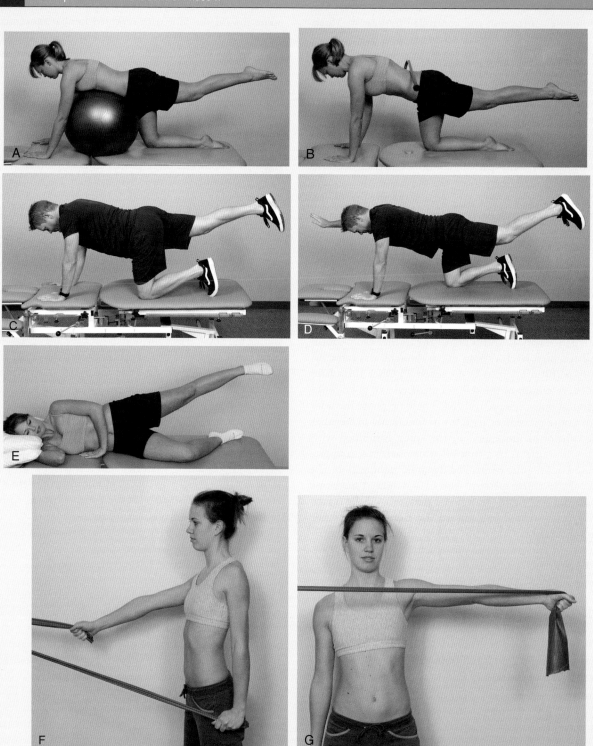

FIG. 4.14 A, All fours position over a physioball leg lift with transversus abdominis (TrA) contraction to control lumbopelvic spine position in neutral. B, All fours position leg lift with TrA contraction to control lumbopelvic spine position in neutral. A cane can be positioned on the lumbar spine to provide feedback regarding how well patient maintains a stabile lumbopelvic position. C, All fours position leg lift. D, All fours position contralateral arm and leg lift. E, Side-lying hip abduction with TrA contraction to control lumbopelvic spine position in neutral. Patient must be cued to ensure pelvis does not rotate as hip moves. A–E, Preset and sustain TrA contraction throughout leg movements. F, Theraband shoulder extension with diagonal stance and lumbopelvic movement control. G, Theraband shoulder horizontal abduction with athletic stance and lumbopelvic movement control.

BOX 4.5 Lumbopelvic Movement Control Phase II—cont'd

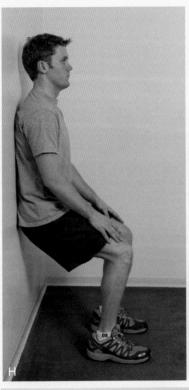

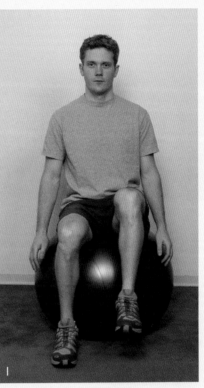

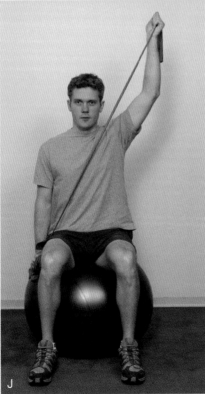

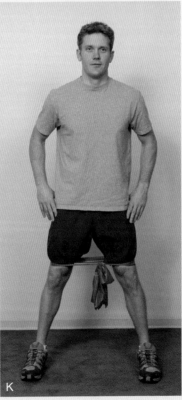

FIG. 4.14, cont'd H, Wall slide. I, Sit on physioball and march as controlling a neutral lumbopelvic position. Use caution with lumbar radiculopathy conditions that may peripheralize in sitting. J, Theraband diagonal shoulder flexion as patient stabilizes a neutral lumbopelvic position. Use caution with lumbar radiculopathy conditions that may peripheralize in sitting. K, Theraband resisted side stepping as patient controls a neutral lumbopelvic position. Continue in both directions until fatigue is noted in hip abductor muscles.

Continued

BOX 4.5 Lumbopelvic Movement Control Phase II—cont'd

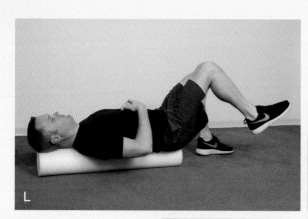

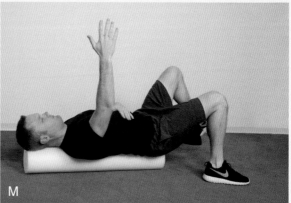

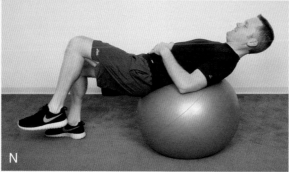

FIG. 4.14, cont'd L, Marching with stabilization on a foam roller. M, Shoulder flexion with dynamic movement control on a foam roller. N, Marching with dynamic stabilization supine on a physioball.

BOX 4.6 Lumbopelvic Movement Control Phase III

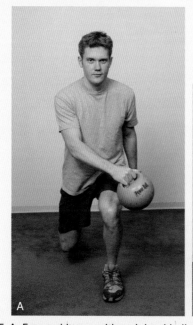

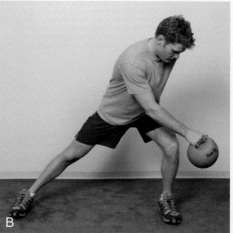

FIG. 4.15 A, Forward lunge with weighted ball reach to knee. B, Lateral lunge with weighted ball reach to knee. A and B, Spinal movement is a controlled manner into rotation and forward bending as arm reaches to knee, but a hinging flexion motion is emphasized at hips to facilitate bending that occurs with this motion.

BOX 4.6 Lumbopelvic Movement Control Phase III—cont'd

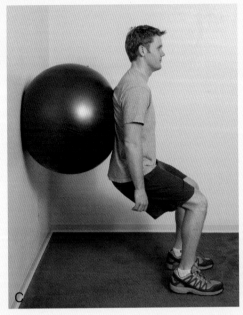

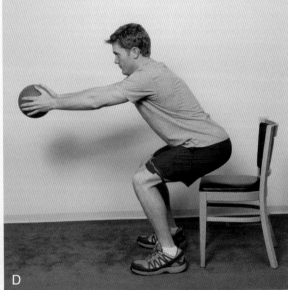

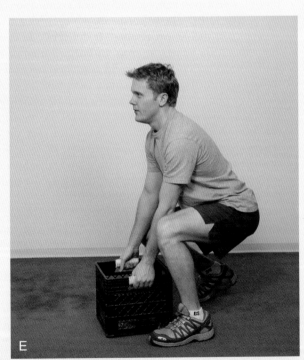

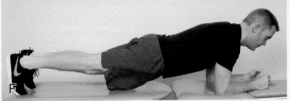

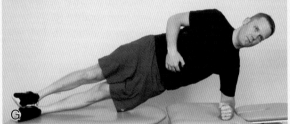

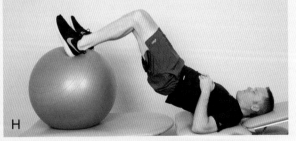

FIG. 4.15, cont'd C, Wall slide squat with physioball. D, Sit squat with hip hinging and reach to facilitate gluteal action. The knees are pressed apart against TheraBand resistance to further facilitate gluteus medius muscle action. E, Lifting training with weighted crate and diagonal movement pattern while dynamic lumbopelvic stabilization is maintained. F, Front plank. G, Side plank. F and G, Hold position as stabilize spine in neutral position. H, Bridge on physioball with stabilization. This can be done with the ball held stationary or it could be progressed to roll the ball while in the bridging position.

Although a high percentage of these patients with CLBP had positive discogenic findings, a significant number of patients was still found without positive discogram results and symptoms that either centralized (26%) or peripheralized (31%), which means that the discogenic theory cannot explain all these cases and the repeated movement examination and treatment concepts potentially affect more anatomic structures than just the intervertebral disk. However, when the disk is the source of the pain, the repeated movement treatment concepts tend to be more effective when the annular fibers remain intact.

Werneke and Hart[54] reported on the repeated movement examination findings of 223 patients with LBP and followed up with these patients 1 year after the initial examination. Classification in the noncentralization group at intake was a predictor of those who did not return to work, who continued to report pain symptoms, who had extended activity interference or downtime at home, and who continued to use healthcare resources at the 1-year follow-up examination.[54] Centralization appears to identify a subgroup of spinal patients who have a good prognosis for response to conservative treatment.[128]

Regardless of the validity of the pathoanatomic explanation for the MDT repeated movement examination and treatment regime, these treatment principles can improve patient outcomes. In a study by Long and Donelson,[56] exercise prescription based on directional preference showed better outcomes than comparison groups that performed exercises away from an identified directional preference. In a systematic review of RCTs that used a directional preference management approach for LBP, five high-quality RCTs were identified that demonstrated moderate evidence that directional preference management was more effective than a number of comparison treatments for pain, function, and work participation at short-term and intermediate-term follow-ups when directional preference management was applied to patients with LBP who demonstrated a directional preference during an initial examination.[129] Several studies have compared a directional preference management program to other physical therapy interventions, such as spinal stabilization exercises[130] or spinal manipulation[131–133] for patients with subacute or CLBP, and have found improvements in pain and function with both groups but no significant difference between the two groups. In contrast, Browder et al.[134] completed an RCT on 48 participants with LBP and symptoms distal to the buttocks that fit the additional inclusion criteria of directional preference and centralization with lumbar extension movements. These patients were randomly assigned to either receive an extension-oriented treatment approach (*n* = 26) or a strengthening exercise program (*n* = 22) for eight physical therapy sessions in addition to a home exercise program. The extension-oriented treatment approach included instruction in extension exercises and sustained positions that centralized symptoms, use of posteroanterior nonthrust mobilizations of the lumbar spine, and education to avoid sitting for greater than 30 minutes at a time. Participants in the strengthening group were instructed in a LSE program but did not receive further education or manual therapy interventions. Participants in the extension-oriented treatment approach group experienced greater improvements in disability compared with participants who received trunk strengthening exercises at 1-week, 4-week, and 6-month follow-up assessments.[134] This study offers support for the use of directional preference management in patients with LBP who demonstrate a directional preference and centralization with lumbar extension. Therefore the key to attaining the greatest success with a directional preference management program is to complete a comprehensive examination and provide directional preference exercises, nonthrust mobilizations, and education to the subgroup of patients who fit the diagnostic criteria (Box 4.1).

Riddle and Rothstein[135] evaluated the reliability of the McKenzie examination system when used by novice practitioners and found poor interrater reliability for the placement of patients into one of the three syndromes (kappa = 0.26), and they reported the primary source of error was in the therapists' ability to judge centralization versus peripheralization in the patients they examined. In contrast, Fritz reported excellent interrater reliability for physical therapists (kappa = 0.823) and physical therapist students (kappa = 0.763) in interpretation of videotaped repeated movement examinations of patients with LBP.[44] The videotape examination eliminates the variability in the patient response at different points in time and allowed the testers to focus on interpretation of the examination procedures. This study also illustrates that newly trained student therapists can attain acceptable levels of reliability without undergoing extensive training regimens. In a systematic review of reliability of the MDT examination and classification system, the authors concluded that the MDT system appears to have acceptable interrater reliability for classifying patients with back pain into main and subsyndromes when applied by therapists who have completed the credentialing examination, but unacceptable reliability in other therapists.[136] See Table 4.9 for outline of the MDT repeated movement examination scheme. Box 4.7 outlines the extension progression used in the MDT approach when extension centralizes the patient's symptoms.

In summary, in the subgroup of patients with LBP who demonstrate a directional preference for specific directional exercises, incorporation of these exercises in the treatment approach tends to yield positive clinical outcomes. The directional preference exercises should be augmented with manual therapy techniques and instruction in positioning that reinforces the patient's directional preference and centralization. Once symptomatic improvement is achieved, these patients may benefit from general conditioning, spinal mobility (in all directions), and movement control/strengthening programs to restore function and prevent future episodes of LBP. Patients with leg pain that peripheralizes tend to have a poorer prognosis for conservative management; these patients may be candidates for activity modification, motor control exercise, and spinal traction. Speculation exists that the patients with a

TABLE 4.9	Test Movements Used in a McKenzie Active Range of Motion Examination
MOVEMENT	**DEFINITION**
Side bending in standing	Patient is standing; examiner asks patient to bend in frontal plane to right or left as far as possible and then return to starting position
Flexion in standing	Patient is standing; examiner asks patient to bend forward as far as possible without flexing knees and then return to starting position
Repeated flexion in standing	Flexion in standing movement is repeated 10 times
Extension in standing	Patient is standing; examiner asks patient to bend backward as far as possible without flexing knees and then return to starting position
Repeated extension in standing	Extension in standing movement is repeated 10 times
Sustained extension in standing	Extension in standing movement is maintained for 30 seconds before returning to starting position
Pelvic translocation in standing	Patient is standing; examiner passively shifts patient's pelvis in frontal plane while stabilizing shoulders and then returns patient to starting position
Extension in prone	Patient is prone; examiner asks patient to press up by placing hands on examining surface and extending elbows while keeping pelvis flat on the surface and then return to starting position
Sustained extension in prone	Extension in prone movement is maintained for 30 seconds before returning to starting position
Sustained extension with pelvic translocation in prone	Patient is prone; examiner passively shifts patient's pelvis in frontal plane. Patient is asked to perform translocation in prone and prop up on elbows with pelvis flat on examining surface. This position is maintained for 30 seconds before returning to starting position
Repeated flexion in sitting	Patient is sitting; examiner asks patient to bend forward as far as possible and then return to starting position. This movement is repeated 10 times
Flexion in quadruped	Patient is in quadruped position; examiner asks patient to rock backward approximating heels to buttocks and then return to starting position
Repeated flexion in quadruped	Flexion in quadruped movement is repeated 10 times.

(From Fritz JM, Delitto A, Vignovic M, et al. Interrater reliability of judgments of the centralization phenomenon and status change during movement testing in patients with low back pain. *Arch Phys Med Rehabil.* 2000;81:57-61.)

directional preference toward lumbar extension (repeated backward bending) may have a symptomatic intervertebral disk with an intact annulus and that patients with a directional preference toward spinal flexion may have underlying spinal stenosis.

Lumbar Spinal Stenosis (Flexion Syndrome)
ICF Classification: Low Back Pain With Related Lower Extremity Pain

LSS is a common degenerative condition in the elderly and is associated with narrowing of the spinal canal or nerve root canals caused by degenerative arthritic changes of the facet joints and intervertebral disks; it is often associated with CLBP and leg symptoms. The leg symptoms are thought to result from compression on the vertebral venous plexus from multilevel stenosis that creates venous pooling and congestion and leads to ischemic pain and fatigue in the lower extremities during walking.[137] Spinal extension is commonly limited. Sitting or assuming a spinal flexion (forward bent) position often alleviates the leg symptoms. This clinical syndrome is termed *neurogenic claudication* and has been defined as pain, paresthesia, and cramping of the lower extremities brought on by walking and relieved by sitting.[137]

Pain in the legs brought on by walking and relieved by sitting in the elderly can be the result of several other conditions, such as osteoarthritis of the hips or knees or vascular or intermittent claudication from peripheral vascular disease, that must be screened before a diagnosis of spinal stenosis can be made.[137] The spinal canal is further narrowed in a lordotic posture and tends to widen in a more flexed posture, which explains the postural dependency exhibited by patients with spinal stenosis with neurogenic claudication.

The two-stage treadmill test is a clinical procedure that can be used to assist in the differentiation between neurogenic and vascular claudication. The neurogenic claudication should be more affected by the position of the spine during the lower extremity exertion. The vascular claudication should only be affected by the level of lower extremity exertion and the demands of blood flow to the lower extremity muscles.

The two-stage treadmill test is performed with the patient walking on a level treadmill for up to 10 minutes, followed by a 10-minute rest period in sitting and then another bout of walking on the treadmill set at a 15-degree incline for up to 10 minutes. The speed is set at 1 mile per hour and then adjusted to a comfortable pace for the patient. The patient is asked to report any symptoms increased beyond the baseline

BOX 4.7 McKenzie Prone Extension Exercise Sequence

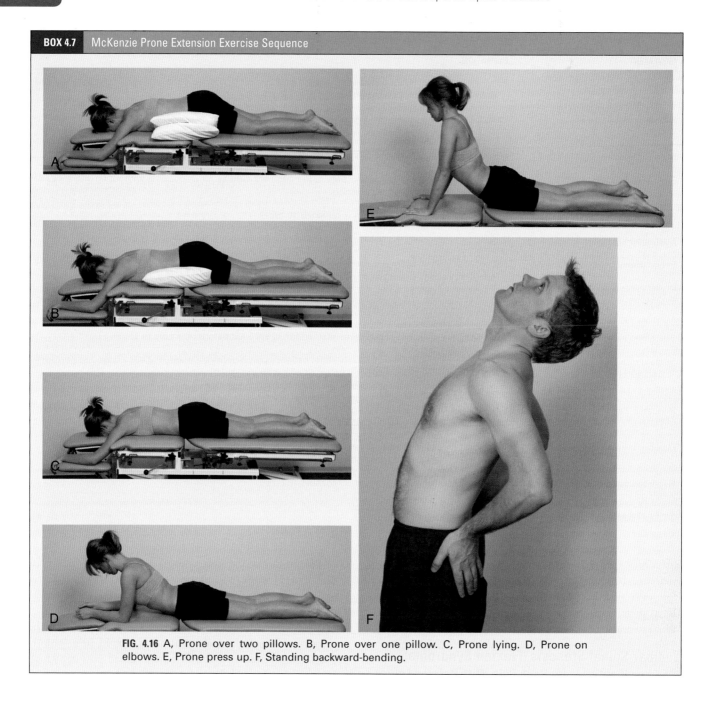

FIG. 4.16 A, Prone over two pillows. B, Prone over one pillow. C, Prone lying. D, Prone on elbows. E, Prone press up. F, Standing backward-bending.

level and given the opportunity to stop the test before 10 minutes if symptoms become intense. A positive test result for neurogenic claudication is demonstration of a greater tolerance for walking in the inclined position, which places the lumbar spine in a more flexed (forward bent) position.

Fritz et al.[137] found a high specificity (92.3%) for correlation with LSS for patients with positive test results for the two-stage treadmill test, but the sensitivity was low (50%). Fritz et al.[137] also found that the most accurate diagnosis of spinal stenosis occurred with variables based on time to onset of symptoms and recovery time, which identified 20 of 26 stenotic participants (sensitivity, 76.9%) and correctly classified 18 of 19 nonstenotic participants (specificity, 94.7%).

Participants with a prolonged recovery time after level walking and an earlier onset of symptoms with level walking were 14.5 times more likely to be stenotic than nonstenotic (+LR, 14.51).[137] In addition, the ranking of sitting as the best posture showed a significant association with the stenosis diagnosis.[137] A three-stage Delphi study of 279 clinicians from 29 countries developed consensus on seven history items that can be used to help diagnose LSS including:

- Leg or buttock pain while walking
- Flex forward to relieve symptoms
- Feel relief when using a shopping cart or bicycle
- Motor or sensory disturbance while walking
- Normal and symmetric foot pulses

- Lower extremity weakness
- LBP[138]

A flexion-based exercise physical therapy program has been shown to result in positive outcomes in the conservative management of LSS in older adults (Box 4.3).[67] Whitman et al.[67] compared the long-term effects of two physical therapy programs and showed positive effects with both the groups that received 6 weeks of physical therapy consisting of a flexion-based exercise program with a progressive walking program and even better results in the group that received manual physical therapy interventions to the hip, lumbopelvic, and thoracic spine (thrust manipulation and nonthrust mobilization techniques) combined with a progressive exercise and unweighted treadmill walking program (Fig. 4.17). At 6-week, 1-year, and long-term (29-month) follow-up examinations, both groups showed positive outcomes, but the manual physical therapy group perception of recovery was even better (79% vs. 41% at 6 weeks) at each follow-up period.[67] Nearly 25% of the patients in this clinical trial were classified as having severe spinal stenosis at multiple levels, and 55% of the patients had bilateral leg pain.[67] These results illustrate the importance of exhausting a nonsurgical approach in spite of MRI and radiographic evidence of severe degenerative spinal changes. The study also shows the importance of combining manual physical therapy with an active exercise program to maximize outcomes for patients with more chronic conditions. The manual physical therapy interventions in the Whitman et al.[67] study were provided by physical therapists with specialty training in manual therapy (Fellows of the American Academy of Orthopaedic Manual Physical Therapists [AAOMPT]), and the specific interventions and exercises were selected to address the specific impairment findings in mobility, flexibility, and strength throughout the spine and lower extremities (i.e., an impairment approach). Special attention should be paid to the hip joint in this patient population for signs of joint mobility limitation, muscle length limitations (especially hip flexors), and signs of weakness (commonly the gluteus medius). Correction of the hip dysfunctions with manual therapy techniques, stretching, and specific exercise programs can assist in positive clinical outcomes.[139]

Lurie[140] compared decompressive laminectomy surgery versus nonoperative care in an observational cohort study and found a slight advantage in pain and disability for the surgical group for the first 4 years, but the nonoperative group did just as well at a longer-term follow-up at 6 to 8 years. The nonoperative care was not standardized and included a variable amount of nonsurgical interventions, such as medication, injections, and physical therapy. Delitto et al.[141] conducted an RCT with patients with LSS that were surgical candidates and consented to surgery who demonstrated similar long-term functional gains when provided surgical decompression compared with an evidence-based physical therapy regimen consisting of lumbar flexion exercise, education, and lower extremity strengthening. Although proportions of successes were similar with both groups, there were also similar proportions of patients who did not achieve a clinically meaningful level of improvement between the two groups at the 2-year follow-up.[141]

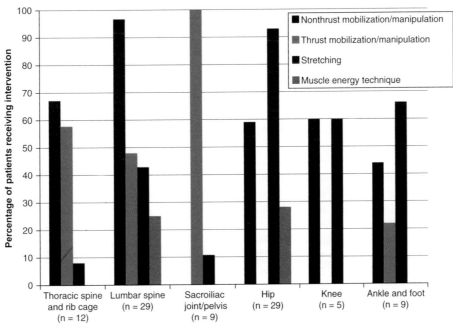

FIG. 4.17 Manual therapy interventions and regions treated in randomized controlled trial (RCT). (From Whitman JM, Flynn TW, Childs JD, et al. A comparison between two physical therapy treatment programs for patients with lumbar spinal stenosis. *Spine.* 2006;31(22):2541-2549; Backstrom KM, Whitman JM, Flynn TW. Lumbar spinal stenosis—diagnosis and management of the aging spine. *Man Ther.* 2011;16:308-317.)

Among Medicare recipients in the United States between 2002 and 2007, the frequency of complex fusion procedures for spinal stenosis increased 15-fold, whereas the frequency of decompression surgery and simple fusions decreased slightly.[142] Complex multilevel lumbar fusion surgeries are associated with increased risk of major life-threatening complications (5.6%), 30-day rehospitalization (13%), and resource use (US $80,888 average per complex fusion) compared with simple fusion and decompression surgeries.[142] Life-threatening complications occur in 3.1% of patients undergoing lumbar surgery and include cardiopulmonary resuscitation, repeat endotracheal intubation and mechanical ventilation, cardiorespiratory arrest, acute myocardial infarction, pneumonias, pulmonary embolism, and stroke.[142] In a subanalysis of the Spine Patient Outcomes Research Trial, the researchers concluded that early trends favored surgical outcomes for patients with LSS, but the positive effects declined over time.[143] The authors recommended that those patients without scoliosis or degenerative spondylolisthesis can be managed adequately nonoperatively regardless of the number of spinal levels that appeared stenotic.[143] Patients with single-level degenerative spondylolisthesis do better surgically when the stenosis is limited to the level of the slip compared with patients with additional levels of stenosis.[143] Much of the comparative conservative care used in spine surgical research lacks quality, comprehensive physical therapy.[144] The patient who makes the decision to undergo surgery should be adequately informed to weigh the risks of surgery and the long-term outcomes against his or her disability.[144] In a prospective multicenter cohort study, no correlations could be found between relevant MRI parameter findings and the severity of the pain in patients diagnosed with LSS.[145] Weber et al.[20] reported that even in patients who underwent decompressive surgery for LSS, radiographic severity of stenosis was not associated with preoperative disability and pain, or clinical outcomes 1 year after surgery. The results of these studies make it clear that the severity of LSS noted on MRI should not be overemphasized in the clinical reasoning regarding patient management of LSS.

In light of the cost and the potential for serious complications associated with complex lumbar fusion procedures, a nonsurgical impairment-based physical therapy approach should be fully used. The management approach for patients with LSS should include patient education, manual physical therapy, mobility and strengthening exercises, and aerobic conditioning.[144] The manual physical therapy should include an impairment-based approach to improve mobility of the thoracic, lumbar, pelvic, and hip regions that include thrust manipulation and nonthrust mobilization, soft tissue mobilization, and manual stretching procedures. Combining nerve mobilization procedures with manipulation and exercise has also been shown to be effective in treating LSS.[146] A flexion bias directional preference management is used for the patient education, mobility and strengthening exercises, and aerobic conditioning. The aerobic conditioning could include unweighted treadmill walking, incline treadmill walking, recumbent stepper, or use of a stationary bicycle.[144,147] Lower extremity

strengthening is recommended along with the core strengthening to enhance the patient's functional mobility.

Patients with chronic LBP may also have balance impairments that should be addressed with strengthening, mobility, and balance exercises and training.[148,149] A recent RCT demonstrated that balance exercises combined with flexibility exercises were more effective than a combination of strength and flexibility exercises in reducing disability and improving the physical component of quality of life in patients with CLBP.[149]

Lumbar Radiculopathy That Does not Centralize
ICF Classification: Low Back Pain With Radiating Pain

The clinical decisions of how to manage patients with lumbar radiculopathy that does not centralize with repeated movements creates a clinical challenge for physical therapists and physicians. Radiculopathy is an example of neuropathic pain, and patients will present with leg pain traveling distal to the knee with signs of neurosensitivity, such as a positive SLR test. Saal and Saal[150] showed excellent clinical outcomes in 90% of the patients who met the typical criteria for surgery of a herniated nucleus pulposus (HNP), including SLR less than 60 degrees, CT scan results that showed a HNP, and positive EMG results with evidence of radiculopathy. These patients underwent treatment with an active stabilization and conditioning exercise and ergonomic program and attained excellent results with avoidance of surgery.[150]

Likewise, Weber[151] randomly divided 126 patients into two groups of patients who met similar criteria for lumbar laminectomy surgery for HNP, with one group receiving the surgery and the other group treated nonsurgically with an exercise and ergonomic "back school" treatment program. Weber followed both groups for 10 years and found at 1 year that the patients who received surgical treatment showed a better result than the nonsurgical group.[108] At the 4-year and 10-year follow-up examinations, no significant difference was found between the surgical and nonsurgical groups.[151]

In another study that compared surgical and nonsurgical management of lumbar disk protrusion with radiculopathy, Thomas et al.[152] found no difference in pain, disability, or functional levels between surgical and nonsurgical groups at both a 6-month and a 12-month follow-up examination. These studies show that, in the absence of bowel/bladder dysfunction or progressive motor deficits, nonsurgical interventions should be exhausted before surgery is considered in treatment of lumbar HNP and that nonsurgical care should include physical therapy with an emphasis on an active exercise and conditioning program.

Lumbar traction is another commonly used treatment method for this type of condition that can assist in pain relief and allow progression to an exercise program. Lumbar traction can be used in either a prone or a supine position. The flexed position tends to open the neuroforamen and stretch the posterior elements of the spine. Traction in the prone position with a normal amount of lordosis tends to unload the intervertebral disk more effectively.[153] The typical protocol for traction is use of a force equal to 50% of the patient's body weight and use of an intermittent force pattern of 20 to 30 seconds on and 10 to 15 seconds off, for a total duration of 15 minutes.[153] Positive clinical outcomes have recently been shown with use of a lumbar traction protocol that included static traction in the prone position for 12 minutes applied at a force equal to 40% to 60% of the patient's body weight.[154] Variations in the traction setup can also be made to provide a unilateral pull and to vary the patient position into side bending or flexion/extension to begin the traction in a position of patient comfort. With subsequent treatments, the traction position is gradually brought back into a more neutral spine position based on the patient's response to the treatment. Boxes 4.8 to 4.10 provide further information on the use of lumbar traction. Box 4.11 provides examples of lumbar traction patient setups.

BOX 4.8	Proposed Theoretical Effects of Spinal Traction

- Widens the intervertebral foramina
- Temporarily reduces the size of a disk herniation/protrusion
- Creates a negative pressure in the disk to "suck back" a protrusion as a result of taunting of the spinal ligaments pushing in on a disk protrusion
- Neurophysiologic effects of pain inhibition
- Straightens the spinal curve
- Mobilizes the facet joints (nonspecific)
- Stretches spinal muscles

BOX 4.9	Indications for Spinal Traction

- Spinal nerve root impingement (deep tendon reflexes, numbness, weakness, and positive straight leg raise [SLR] test)
- Peripheralization of leg pain with lumbar backward bending
- Positive crossed SLR test (45 degrees)
- Lower extremity pain that centralizes with lumbar traction

BOX 4.10	Contraindications and Precautions of Spinal Traction

- Movement is contraindicated
- Acute strains/inflammation
- Hypermobility/instability
- Rheumatoid arthritis
- Respiratory problems
- Compromised structural integrity
  - Malignant disease
  - Tumor
  - Osteoporosis
  - Infection
- Current pregnancy
- Uncontrolled hypertension
- Aortic aneurysm
- Severe hemorrhoids
- Cardiovascular disease
- Abdominal hernia
- Hiatal hernia

BOX 4.11	Lumbar Traction

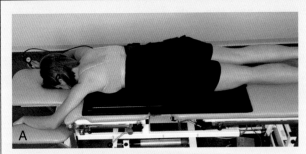
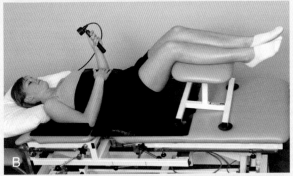

FIG. 4.18 A, Prone lumbar traction set up with portable hydraulic lumbar traction device. B, Supine lumbar traction set up with portable hydraulic lumbar traction device.

Compared with the other impairment-based classifications, the subgroup of patients who receive traction has not been studied extensively. A systematic review found a lack of quality studies and studies that were somewhat inconclusive regarding the effectiveness of lumbar traction.[155] Historically, lumbar traction tends to be used in conditions that do not respond well to other manual therapy or exercise-based approaches. This group of patients may also proceed to surgical interventions, most commonly lumbar discectomy/laminectomy. There is conflicting evidence for the efficacy of lumbar traction for patients with LBP.[58] There is moderate evidence that clinicians should not use intermittent or static lumbar traction for reducing symptoms in patients with acute or subacute, nonradicular LBP or in patients with CLBP.[58] There is preliminary evidence that a subgroup of patients with signs of nerve root compression along with peripheralization of symptoms or a positive crossed SLR will benefit from intermittent lumbar traction in the prone position.[58]

Fritz et al.[154] reported data to support favorable outcomes in a subgroup of patients with lumbar radiculopathy (leg pain with signs of nerve root compression) who had peripheralization of symptoms with lumbar extension or had a positive crossed SLR test (45 degrees). Patients with low back and leg pain and signs of nerve root compression (positive SLR or lower extremity neurologic signs) were randomly assigned to one of two treatment groups: lumbar extension exercise protocol for 6 weeks or lumbar traction for 2 weeks combined with the lumbar extension exercise protocol.[154] At the 2-week follow-up examination, the lumbar traction group showed improvements in disability and fear-avoidance beliefs, but no between-group differences were seen at the 6-week follow-up period.[154] However, further analysis of the participant baseline examination results revealed that the subgroup of patients with symptoms that peripheralized with extension or with positive crossed SLR test showed significantly better outcomes at 2 and 6 weeks if they received the lumbar traction.[154]

In a separate randomized trial, 120 patients with LBP and signs of nerve root compression were either treated with extension-oriented exercise treatment approach (EOTA) or provided this same intervention plus lumbar traction for 6 weeks with up to 12 treatment sessions.[156] After 6 weeks and at 12 month follow-up, both groups had similar positive outcomes with reduction of pain and disability.[156] Mechanical traction combined with EOTA did not provide superior outcomes compared with stand alone EOTA and subgrouping criteria (a positive crossed SLR or peripheralization of symptoms) were not found to modify the effect of mechanical traction in this study.[156] Therefore this study did not support the use of mechanical lumbar traction even in the previously identified subgroup.

Positional distraction is an alternative to lumbar traction that can be performed both in the clinic and at the patient's home. Box 4.12 shows a positional distraction demonstration. Advantages of positional distraction are that it can isolate the spinal level to maximally open the effected neuroforamen, it is inexpensive (a bolster can be made at home by tightly rolling a pillow in a sheet), and it is under the control of the patient.[157] Creighton[158] showed with radiographic evidence that positional distraction that combines isolated lumbar flexion, lateral flexion away from the targeted neuroforamen, and rotation toward the affected side focused to a spinal segment via manual therapy techniques can maximally open a targeted neuroforamen. Once the patient is placed in positional distraction, he or she should be monitored to ensure patient comfort. For the intervention to be effective, the patient should report relief of leg pain shortly after placement in the position. The treatment sessions typically last 10 to 20 minutes, and the patient can perform the procedure at home three to six times per day. Positional distraction allows frequent intermittent unloading of the effected nerve root, which is believed to have positive clinical effects. The patient gradually progresses into an exercise program as the intensity of leg symptoms subsides. However, the effectiveness of positional distraction has not been tested in high-quality clinical trials.

Clinicians should also consider using lower-quarter neural mobilization procedures to reduce pain and disability in patients with subacute and CLBP and radiating pain.[58] A subgroup of patients exists with LBP with related lower extremity symptoms but whose symptoms do not improve with flexion- or extension-oriented exercises.[159] George[159] demonstrated positive clinical outcomes from a case series study with the use of neural mobilization procedures combined with exercise and manual therapy for patients with LBP and leg symptoms distal to the buttock, a positive slump test, and the exclusion of

patients with a positive SLR (<45 degrees). Cleland et al.[160] used the same inclusion/exclusion criteria for an RCT of 30 patients with LBP and leg pain who were randomized to receive lumbar spine nonthrust mobilization and exercise or lumbar spine nonthrust mobilization, exercise, and nerve mobilization with a slump stretching neural mobilization exercise. The slump stretching exercise uses a slump test position (Fig. 4.30D) with passive neck flexion movement induced by the therapist or the patient to the point of symptom reproduction and is held for 30 seconds for five repetitions. All patients were treated in physical therapy twice weekly for 3 weeks for a total of six visits. At discharge, patients who received slump stretching demonstrated significantly greater improvements in disability, pain, and centralization of symptoms. The results suggest that slump stretching is beneficial for improving short-term disability, pain, and centralization of symptoms for a subgroup of patients.[160] Future studies should examine whether these benefits are maintained at a longer-term follow-up.

If the patient has a positive SLR (<45 degrees), the slump stretch exercise will likely be too aggressive. Less aggressive lower extremity nerve mobilization exercises may still be indicated, such as use of modified straight leg exercise with active or passive knee extension movements applied to the point of a tension sensation in the leg. This could be progressed to holding the end-range knee extension position while adding active or passive dorsiflexion of the ankle (Fig. 4.21A). Nerve mobilization would not be used as a standalone treatment but rather incorporated into an impairment-based approach that combines mobilization/manipulation and therapeutic exercise. Basson et al.[161] completed a systematic review of neural mobilization and concluded that neural mobilization shows positive neurophysiologic effects of reduced intraneural edema, and a high level of evidence was identified for use of slump sit and straight leg raise neural mobilization interventions to improve pain and disability in a subgroup of patients with chronic LBP and associated leg pain.

Postsurgical Lumbar Rehabilitation

Success rates after surgery for a lumbar disk herniation have been reported to range from 62% to 84% depending on what measures are used to determine success.[162,163] Long-term follow-up studies have demonstrated that 70% to 75% of patients who had a lumbar discectomy/laminectomy surgery will continue to experience LBP, with 13% to 23% experiencing severe, constant/heavy LBP.[164,165] Up to 45% of the patients will continue to experience sciatica.[164] Return-to-work rates at 12 months after lumbar surgery have been reported as 70% after a discectomy and 45% after lumbar fusion surgery. Reoperation rates have been reported to range from 7% to 14% after a lumbar disk herniation surgery.[163–165]

A systematic review of the literature regarding postoperative lumbar intervertebral disk surgery management concluded that strong evidence exists for intensive exercise programs to enhance functional status and faster return to work and that no evidence exists that these programs increase the reoperation rates.[166] No studies investigated whether active

Box 4.12 Positional Distraction

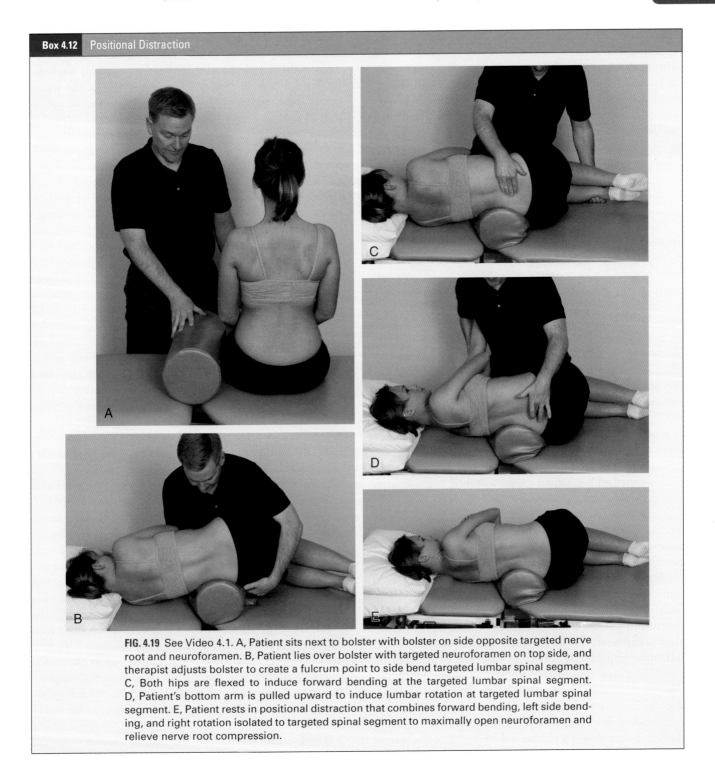

FIG. 4.19 See Video 4.1. A, Patient sits next to bolster with bolster on side opposite targeted nerve root and neuroforamen. B, Patient lies over bolster with targeted neuroforamen on top side, and therapist adjusts bolster to create a fulcrum point to side bend targeted lumbar spinal segment. C, Both hips are flexed to induce forward bending at the targeted lumbar spinal segment. D, Patient's bottom arm is pulled upward to induce lumbar rotation at targeted lumbar spinal segment. E, Patient rests in positional distraction that combines forward bending, left side bending, and right rotation isolated to targeted spinal segment to maximally open neuroforamen and relieve nerve root compression.

rehabilitation programs should start immediately after surgery or start 4 to 6 weeks later.[166] In a separate systematic review of postoperative physical therapy programs that started 4 to 6 weeks after surgery, the results of several studies were pooled to draw the following conclusions: patients who participated in exercise programs reported slightly less short-term pain and disability than those who received no treatment, and patients who participated in high-intensity programs reported slightly less short-term pain and disability than those in low-intensity

programs.[167] None of the included studies reported that active programs increased the rate of repeated surgery, nor did the evidence suggest that patients should restrict their activities after lumbar disk surgery.[167]

Scrimshaw and Maher[168] investigated the effects of neural mobilization after lumbar dissection, fusion, or laminectomy. The results of a 12-month follow-up demonstrated that neural mobilization did not provide additional benefits to traditional postoperative care. However, the patients in this study exhibited a SLR test ROM that was within normal limits, suggesting that perhaps performing neural mobilizations on patients with a normal SLR may not be beneficial in decreasing pain and disability.[160] However, if the SLR test demonstrates a limitation on the symptomatic leg after a lumbar surgery, sound clinical reasoning would dictate that neural mobilization exercises that repeatedly move the lower extremity to the point of reproduction of leg tension without significant reproduction of acute symptoms would be a useful adjunct to management of the patients after lumbar surgery, but further research is needed to study the effects of this intervention for this subgroup of patients.

Yilmaz et al.[169] demonstrated that an 8-week program of dynamic LSEs improved pain relief, function, and strength of the trunk muscles in patients who have undergone microdiscectomy compared with a control group. Kulig et al.[170] demonstrated greater reduction in disability and greater improvement in distance walked in patients who had undergone a single-level microdiscectomy who received an intensive 12-week back extensor and endurance training with mat and upright therapeutic exercises compared with a control group that only received an education program. The exercise program started 4 to 6 weeks after surgery, but no long-term follow-up for these patients was reported beyond the 12-week treatment period. Likewise, Dolan et al.[171] demonstrated improved clinical and disability outcomes in patients who participated in a 4-week exercise program that began 6 weeks after lumbar microdiscectomy designed to improve strength and endurance of the back and abdominal muscles compared with a control group, and these improvements were maintained at 12 months after surgery.

The clinical assumption after lumbar disk surgery is that functional instability with motor coordination impairments of the core muscles results from the surgery and that the patient needs to be progressed into a spinal movement control and conditioning program with emphasis on retraining the motor control of the deep abdominal and multifidus muscles. A thorough examination should be conducted of the surrounding structures, including thoracic spine, pelvis, and hips, to determine impairments that could hinder a full recovery; if identified, these impairments should be addressed in the plan of care. The patient should be cautioned on sitting for longer than 15 to 20 minutes at a time for the first 6 to 12 weeks after lumbar disk surgery to avoid unnecessary loading of the intervertebral disk structures. The patient needs to be guided through progression of a lumbar stabilization/movement control exercise program (Boxes 4.4–4.6 for phases I to III of a lumbar stabilization program). A walking program is also advisable in most circumstances.

Sacroiliac Joint-Related Pain (Pelvic Girdle Pain)
ICF Classification: Low Back Pain With Movement Coordination Impairments

ICF Classification: Low Back Pain With Mobility Deficits
The estimated prevalence of SIJ-related pain in patients with nonspecific CLBP is approximately 13% to 30%.[172] SIJ dysfunctions tend to occur more commonly in women for the following reasons: smaller joint surfaces in the SIJ in women, flatter and smoother joint surfaces, and SIJ mechanical disadvantage in women because the axis of the hip is farther from the line of gravity, which places more torque on the SIJ from a longer lever arm.[173] In addition, hormonal changes, childbirth strains, and intercourse strains can also contribute to development of SIJ-related pain dysfunctions in women. The SIJ is a likely source of symptoms in females during and after pregnancy because of the hypermobility and sensitivity of tissues that results from the release of the hormone relaxin. Approximately 20% of women will experience pelvic girdle pain while they are pregnant.[174,175] Risk factors for developing pelvic girdle pain during pregnancy include a history of previous LBP and previous trauma to the pelvis.[174] Pelvic girdle pain is commonly associated with sensitivity of the sacroiliac and symphysis pubis joints and surrounding ligaments and impaired motor function of the lumbopelvic/hip muscles.

SIJ-related pain can be diagnosed by pain provocation tests and pain palpation tests, such as the long dorsal ligament test and palpation of the symphysis pubis.[174] Laslett et al.[176] used a standard of three of five positive SIJ provocation tests to make the diagnosis of a painful SIJ; this diagnosis was tested against the gold standard of a double SIJ anesthetic and cortisone injection. The five tests were anterior superior iliac spine (ASIS) distraction, thigh thrust, Gaenslen's test, ASIS compression, and sacral thrust. When the results of a cluster of three of five of these provocation tests were combined with ruling out the diagnosis of a SIJ-related pain with centralization or peripheralization of symptoms with repeated movement testing, there was a moderate shift in probability of ruling in and ruling out an SIJ dysfunction. With this clinical reasoning, the combination of three or more positive provocation SIJ test results and no centralization or peripheralization is up to 20 times more likely in patients with positive diagnostic SIJ injection results than in patients with negative injection results. The SIJ provocation tests used in this study were found in a previous study by Laslett and Williams[177] to have good to excellent reliability. These studies support the clinical reasoning concept that the SIJ can be source of nociception that can contribute to a patient's perception of lumbopelvic pain, and a cluster of clinical provocation tests can be used to make this diagnosis.

However, SIJ movement dysfunction is not well supported with contemporary research evidence, and patient education that includes description of SIJ displacements or instabilities can create fear and anxiety in patients that will contribute to pain perception and can be detrimental to recovery.[178]

Much clinical speculation exists that a hypermobile SIJ can displace and can be detected clinically as hypomobility and altered positioning of the ilium and sacrum. Unfortunately, studies that have assessed the reliability of palpation examination procedures designed to detect pelvic position and mobility have shown poor reliability.[179] In clinical situations, therapists rarely use passive joint mobility examinations in isolation.

Rather, they combine the results of the single assessment with those of other examination procedures. Cibulka and Koldehoff[180] showed excellent interrater reliability in assessing the SIJ (kappa = 0.88) by using a cluster of four examination procedures and requiring that three of the four results be positive to diagnose a sacroiliac dysfunction. Cibulka and colleagues[13,180] used tests for position, mobility, and provocation of SIJ impairments. However, Potter and Rothstein[179] showed poor reliability when studying each of those same four examination procedures in isolation. Cibulka's study seems to more closely emulate how therapists actually assess patients in the clinic. Likewise, Arab et al.[181] reported substantial to excellent intra- and interexaminer reliability of clusters of motion palpation and provocation tests with kappa scores ranging from 0.44 to 1.00 and 0.52 to 0.92. This confirms that clusters of motion palpation combined with provocation tests have adequate reliability for use in clinical assessment of the SIJ.

Lee[182] describes the function of the pelvis as the transference of loads from the trunk to the lower extremities and from the lower extremities to the trunk. The active SLR (ASLR) test (Fig. 4.33) has been shown to be an effective functional screen and provides a means to differentiate SIJ symptoms that occur from lack of motor control of the pelvis either from the anterior (TrA) or posterior (multifidus) musculature.[174,183] In patients with pelvic girdle pain, there seems to be less efficient use of the abdominal and pelvic floor muscles noted with the ASLR test resulting in a decreased ability to lift the straight leg and generate force.[184–186] There is also a perception of increased effort and changes in breathing with increased intraabdominal pressure noted with lifting the leg on the symptomatic side.[184–186] Enhancement of pelvis control with manual compression of the iliac (i.e., ASLR test) tends to reverse these differences and provides confirmation that training the TrA to enhance functional motor control of the pelvis and SIJs is indicated.[43,186]

For clinical management purposes, it is helpful to classify sacroiliac conditions into three categories: arthralgia, movement coordination impairments, and mobility deficits. The signs and symptoms of SIJ-related pain or arthralgia tend to include pain and sensitivity well localized over the SIJ, ipsilateral muscle guarding of the thoracolumbar erector spinae, and positive pain provocation test results. The treatment could include support with an SIJ belt, relative rest to avoid activities that strain the involved structures, and manual therapy and exercise to treat any surrounding dysfunctions of the lumbar spine and hip. The manual therapy in the lumbopelvic region will facilitate a neurophysiologic response including pain modulation through central nervous system activation of endogenous descending inhibition and influence muscle activity in a therapeutic manner.[178]

Movement coordination impairments can also be a component of SIJ-related pain and might be related to repetitive minor trauma, childbirth strains, hypermobility or a history of trauma which may sensitize the joints and connective tissues of the pelvis. The signs and symptoms may include a dull ache on assuming a fixed posture with occasional referred pain to the posterior thigh, periodic episodes of sharper or more acute pain associated with displacement of the SIJ, hypermobility with passive mobility assessments, and positive pain provocation test results.[157] These patients often present with a positive active straight leg test indicative of poor ability to stabilize the lumbopelvic region. Treatment may include use of a pelvic compression belt (Fig. 4.20A and B) to be worn 24 hours per day for up to 6 to 12 weeks and treatment of surrounding joint dysfunctions and muscle imbalances with use of exercise and manual therapy.[187] The pelvic compression belt can be weaned as the patient gains proper control of the local lumbopelvic muscles and becomes less symptomatic. An exercise program that focuses on specific motor control exercises that target the multifidus and TrA muscles has been shown to attain positive outcomes in patients with pelvic girdle pain after pregnancy.[187]

In a systematic review of the use of pelvic compression belts, Arumugam et al.[188] determined that there is moderate evidence to support the role of external pelvic compression in decreasing laxity of the SIJ, changing lumbopelvic kinematics, altering selective recruitment of stabilizing musculature, and reducing pain. There is limited evidence for the effects of external pelvic compression on decreasing sacral mobility and affecting strength of muscles surrounding the SIJ.[188] Patient response to the use of a pelvic compression belt must be monitored closely because not all patients with pelvic girdle pain respond the same. For instance, Beales et al.[185] found that application of pelvic compression with the ASLR test with patients with chronic pelvic girdle pain resulted in seven patients displaying decreased EMG activity of the trunk muscles and the other five patients demonstrating increased EMG activity. Clinically, a portion of patients respond favorably to the use of a pelvic compression belt, and it serves as a helpful adjunct to the management of the condition. There are, however, patients who respond with excessive muscle reaction, tension, and guarding with intensification of symptoms. This can usually be determined during the clinical session, and it is useful to have the patient use the belt while performing functional activities, such as walking on the treadmill to monitor the patient's response. If symptoms intensify, the patient is not a good candidate for the use of the pelvic compression belt, and this may be a sign of excessive force closure.[189]

O'Sullivan and Beales[189] describe two types of "peripherally mediated pelvic girdle pain disorders": reduced force closure and excessive force closure. Reduced force closure is characterized by sensitized painful SIJ and surrounding connective tissues with signs of hypermobility and poor motor control of the lumbopelvic and hip muscles. The maladaptive motor control leads to impaired load transfer through the pelvis acting as a mechanism for ongoing strain and pain at the SIJ. Hormonal influences may be a contributing factor to this condition. These patients have positive ASLR test results with poor motor control patterns of force closure of the pelvis involving poor control of the local lumbopelvic muscles (pelvic floor, TrA,

BOX 4.13 | Pelvic Compression Belts

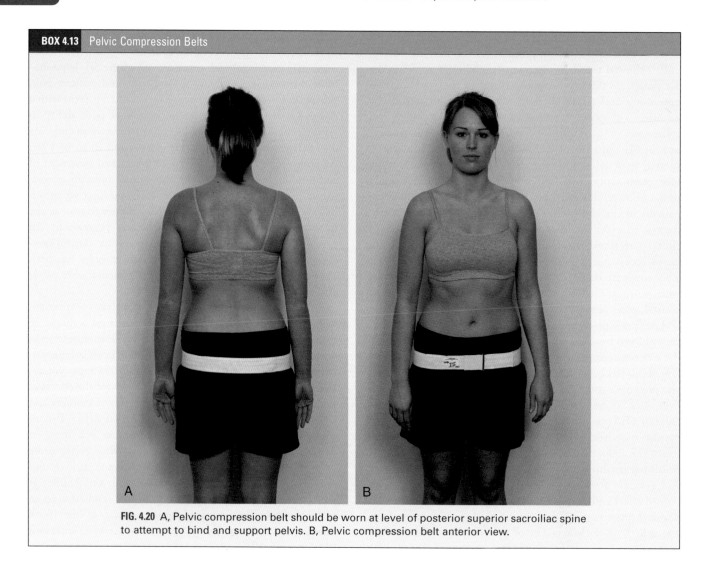

FIG. 4.20 A, Pelvic compression belt should be worn at level of posterior superior sacroiliac spine to attempt to bind and support pelvis. B, Pelvic compression belt anterior view.

multifidus, iliopsoas, and gluteal muscles) and excessive activation of the more global spinal muscles.[190] Pain is seen with weight-bearing postures (such as sitting, standing, and walking) and loaded activities that induce rotation pelvic strain coupled with spine- and hip-loading activities.[189] The pain may be relieved with an SIJ belt, training optimal dynamic postural alignment of the spine and pelvis, and retraining of the local lumbopelvic muscles with inhibition of the thoracopelvic muscles. These disorders may gain temporary relief with manual therapy techniques, but for long-term improvements, a comprehensive motor control exercise program is necessary.[187,189]

Excessive force closure is associated with excessive, abnormal, and sustained loading of sensitized pelvic structures by excessive activation of the local and global lumbopelvic muscle systems. This patient group has positive SIJ provocation test results and localized pain of the SIJ and surrounding ligamentous and myofascial tissues.[189] These patients do not have positive ASLR test results (no feeling of heaviness), and pelvic compression belts and manual pelvic compression tend to make the symptoms worse.[189,191,192] The patients commonly

hold habitual erect lordotic lumbopelvic postures associated with high levels of cocontraction across various muscles, such as the abdominal wall, pelvic floor, piriformis, and local spinal muscles.[189] These patients often have had extensive physical therapy and are preoccupied with concern with "pelvic alignment" and beliefs of being "unstable" or "displaced."[189] Often these patients have been engaged in intensive stabilization exercise programs and are commonly anxious and under high levels of stress.[189] Management of this disorder focuses on reducing force closure across the pelvic structures with targeted relaxation strategies, breathing control, muscle inhibitory techniques, enhancement of passive/relaxed spinal postures, pacing strategies, hydrotherapy, cessation of stabilization exercise training, and focus on cardiovascular exercise, such as the elliptical trainer.[189]

With management of SIJ and pelvic pain conditions, manual therapy and exercise interventions should address the surrounding impairments, such as hip stiffness, tightness of the hip flexors or iliotibial bands, or thoracolumbar hypomobility. Most patients ultimately need to be progressed into a lumbopelvic movement control exercise program.[174]

Assessment and treatment of pelvic floor muscle function may also facilitate a positive clinical outcome. Ultrasound imaging has been used to demonstrate that women with LBP and pelvic girdle pain tend to have lower pelvic floor muscle function than women without LBP and others may develop increased activity of the pelvic floor muscles that may need to be treated with intravaginal manual therapy techniques.[193,194]

Theoretically, a sacroiliac displacement is thought to be caused by a hypermobile joint overriding an articular prominence or by severe trauma to the joint.[157] This is purely speculative and must not be provided to the patient as a viable explanation for their SIJ-related pain condition because of the potential for increased fear of movement and intensification of pain perception that may result.[178] A better patient explanation is that in response to SIJ-related pain, the lumbopelvic muscles have reacted by tensing and guarding resulted in lumbopelvic mobility deficits. Signs and symptoms may include a lowered iliac crest (on sitting and standing), restricted passive motion, and positive provocation test results. If the lower iliac crest is the symptomatic SIJ with provocation testing and limited mobility assessment, in theory, the symptomatic SIJ is considered to be displaced in posterior rotation. If the higher iliac crest side is the symptomatic and restricted side, in theory, this SIJ is considered to be displaced in anterior rotation. Treatment should include SIJ mobilization/manipulation in the direction opposite the suspected displacement followed by treatment as outlined by lumbopelvic movement coordination impairments once the motion is restored. Patient explanation for the effects of the manual therapy techniques should include promotion of muscle relaxation and inhibition of pain that should assist in allowing further movement and exercise, which will further inhibit pain and restore normal motor control.

The lumbopelvic movement control exercise program must be progressed with caution to avoid straining the sensitive pelvic structures by forcing hip motions into directions that provoke symptoms. For instance, if anterior rotation motions of the pelvis provoke a patient's symptoms, the prone hip extension exercise should not be prescribed until the patient can perform this exercise pain free and with good control. Instead, hip flexion stabilization exercises (such as supine hook lying marching with stabilization) should be used early in the program, and the multifidus muscles can be trained with static stabilization postures that are challenged in the standing position, such as shoulder extension theraband exercises (Fig. 4.14F).

Chronic Low Back Pain
ICF Classification: Chronic Low Back Pain With Related Generalized Pain and/or Acute or Subacute Low Back Pain With Related Cognitive or Affective Tendencies

CLBP is commonly described as LBP or low back–related lower extremity pain with symptom duration of more than 3 months.[58] CLBP may include generalized pain not consistent with other impairment-based classification criteria and may be associated with the presence of depression, fear-avoidance beliefs, and pain catastrophizing behaviors.[58] In the absence of depression, anxiety, excessive fear-avoidance beliefs, and pain catastrophizing behaviors, an impairment-based approach can be used that may include use of mobilization/manipulation, soft tissue mobilization, and mobility and motor control exercises. The longer a patient has LBP, the more deconditioned the patient seems to become and the more secondary impairments seem to develop, including movement impairments and muscle imbalances (Box 4.14).

Cecchi et al.[195] randomly assigned 210 patients with chronic, nonspecific LBP to receive back school that included group exercise and ergonomic education; physiotherapy that included exercise, passive nonthrust mobilization, and soft-tissue treatment; or spinal thrust manipulation for four to six 20-minute sessions once a week. Good improvements in pain and disability were reported for all three interventions, but the spinal thrust manipulation group demonstrated higher functional improvement and better short-term and long-term (12 months) pain relief than the back school or physiotherapy treatment groups. A trial of mobilization/manipulation should be incorporated with overall management of the spinal disorder to address the impairments found in the patient examination. In CLBP conditions, RCTs support the application of mobilization/manipulation directed to enhance thoracic and hip mobility as the patient is progressed into a lumbar motor control and conditioning program.[196,197]

A systematic review and metaanalysis that included 51 clinical trials for treating CLBP[198] concluded that there is moderate-quality evidence that thrust manipulation may produce small-moderate reduction in pain intensity and reduction of disability compared with other active comparators, such as exercise. The effect seems to increase over time at 3 and 6-month follow-up. There is moderate-quality evidence that nonthrust mobilizations are likely to have minimal effect compared with other active comparators in terms of reducing pain intensity or disability.[198] The research is heterogeneous, and questions remain about optimal treatment duration and dosage and the characteristics of patients

---

BOX 4.14 Factors That Compound Complex Chronic Back Pain

- Psychosocial components of chronic pain
  - Elevated fear-avoidance beliefs
  - Depression
  - Anxiety disorders
  - Sleep impairments
- Underlying pathology
  - Rheumatoid arthritis
  - Osteoarthritis
  - Ankylosing spondylitis
  - Fibromyalgia
  - Central sensitization
- Movement impairments
- Muscle imbalances
- Multiple joint impairments
- Deconditioning

who may benefit the most. The review also concluded that both mobilization/manipulation appear to be safe and multimodal programs may be a promising option, such as combining mobilization/manipulation with exercise.[198]

In another systematic review and metaanalysis that included 47 RCTs with 9211 participants of the benefits and harms of spinal manipulative therapy (SMT; thrust and nonthrust mobilization/manipulation) for treatment of CLBP,[199] concluded that SMT produces similar effects to other guideline recommended therapies for CLBP, such as exercise and medication for treatment of CLBP and results in clinically better effects for short-term improvement in function compared with nonrecommended therapies (no treatment, waiting list, light soft tissue massage, etc.), sham therapy, or when added as an adjuvant therapy. About half of the studies examined adverse and serious adverse events and most of the observed adverse events were musculoskeletal related, transient in nature, and of mild to moderate severity. The authors suggest that clinicians should inform their patients of the potential risks of mild side effects associated with SMT.[199]

Goldby et al.[200] conducted an RCT for patients with CLBP and compared manual physical therapy, stabilization exercise, and education. The long-term and short-term follow-up results for measures of pain and disability showed improvements in all three treatment groups, but the greatest improvement was noted in the spinal stabilization exercise group. In patients with CLBP and higher initial pain rating scores (>50), the patients in the manual physical therapy group had better outcomes than the education-only group, which shows that mobilization/manipulation can assist in pain reduction with patients with CLBP and high pain scores.[200] This study supported the concept that an active program of spinal stabilization (motor control) exercises is an effective approach for most patients with CLBP, but manual therapy techniques can be used to reduce pain and assist in transitioning patients into an active exercise program.

Cook et al.[201] performed a retrospective observational study that assessed the results of a RCT for individuals ($n = 63$) with CLBP where the intervention group received four sessions of nonthrust lumbar mobilizations over 2 weeks and found that those that experienced a 33% or higher pain reduction by 2 weeks had a 6.98 times higher odds of 50% improvement on the Global Rating of Change score and 4.74 times higher odds of 50% improvement on the ODI score at 6 months. Therefore the therapist should be able to determine in the first 2 weeks of treatment the potential success of a trial of manual therapy for patients with CLBP. If the patient does not respond favorably, the focus should be shifted to other interventions, such as motor control exercise and cognitive-behavioral therapy.

Multidimensional screening through intake forms (see Ch. 2) and a detail personal interview at the initial visit can assist in identification of high levels of stress, anxiety, depressed mood, and fear-avoidance beliefs in addition to levels of sleep disturbance.[202] The therapist must create a therapeutic alliance with the patient to determine which of these factors can be modified and which may need intervention from other professionals. The physical examination will identify movement pattern alterations and pain responses to movements and postures. Manual therapy examination and treatment can assist with identification and treatment of muscle guarding and tissue sensitivity. Once a multidimensional profile is established, the therapist must educate the patient on pain mechanisms and work to alleviate fear of movement.[202] Graded exposure can also be used to correct altered movement patterns that are likely increasing the tissue sensitivity, and education on lifestyle changes can assist with management of anxiety and sleep.

As a movement control exercise program is instructed and progressed, muscle imbalances should also be addressed through mobility and stretching exercises (Box 4.15) (Fig. 4.21), strengthening exercise, and use of myofascial techniques to target myofascial tightness or weakness noted in the examination of both the trunk and the lower extremities. Janda[203] describes the pathogenesis of spinal syndromes as originating from imbalances in muscle function between the phasic and postural muscles. Based on clinical and electromyographic observations, the postural muscles have a tendency to develop tightness, hypertonia, and shortening when in dysfunction. The following muscles are included as predominantly postural muscles: triceps, rectus femoris, thigh adductors, hamstrings, iliopsoas, tensor fasciae latae, some trunk erectors, quadratus lumborum, sternal portion of the pectoralis major, upper part of the trapezius, levator scapulae, and upper extremity flexors.[203]

The muscles with a predominantly phasic function show a tendency for hypotonia, inhibition, and weakening; are less readily activated in most movement patterns; and atrophy more easily and to a greater extent when in dysfunction. Janda[203] states that imbalance between these two muscle systems creates imbalances across joints and leads to pain and degeneration. Motor performance is evaluated with assessment of the sequence of activation of certain movement patterns. For instance, with prone hip extension, the opposite side multifidus should fire first and strongest in comparison with the ipsilateral multifidus and erector spinae. If the erector spinae fires first and strongest, tightness and guarding of the erector spinae (postural) and weakness of the multifidus (phasic) tends to occur.

Standardized intake forms, such as the Four-Item Patient Health Questionnaire (PHQ-4) (see Table 7.4), FABQ (see Fig. 2.5), the Central Sensitization Inventory (see Fig. 2.7), and the STarT Back Screening Tool (see Fig. 2.4) should be used to screen for signs of depression, anxiety disorders, fear avoidance beliefs, central sensitization, and pain catastrophizing behaviors. When these conditions are noted, they need to be addressed as part of the physical therapy program. There is evidence that patients with idiopathic CLBP and fibromyalgia may develop augmented central pain processing (central sensitization), which is demonstrated by higher reports of pain with lower levels of tactile pressure and more widespread areas of brain activation noted with functional MRI scans in response to pressure pain stimuli compared with healthy

BOX 4.15 Lower Extremity Stretching Exercises and Myofascial Techniques

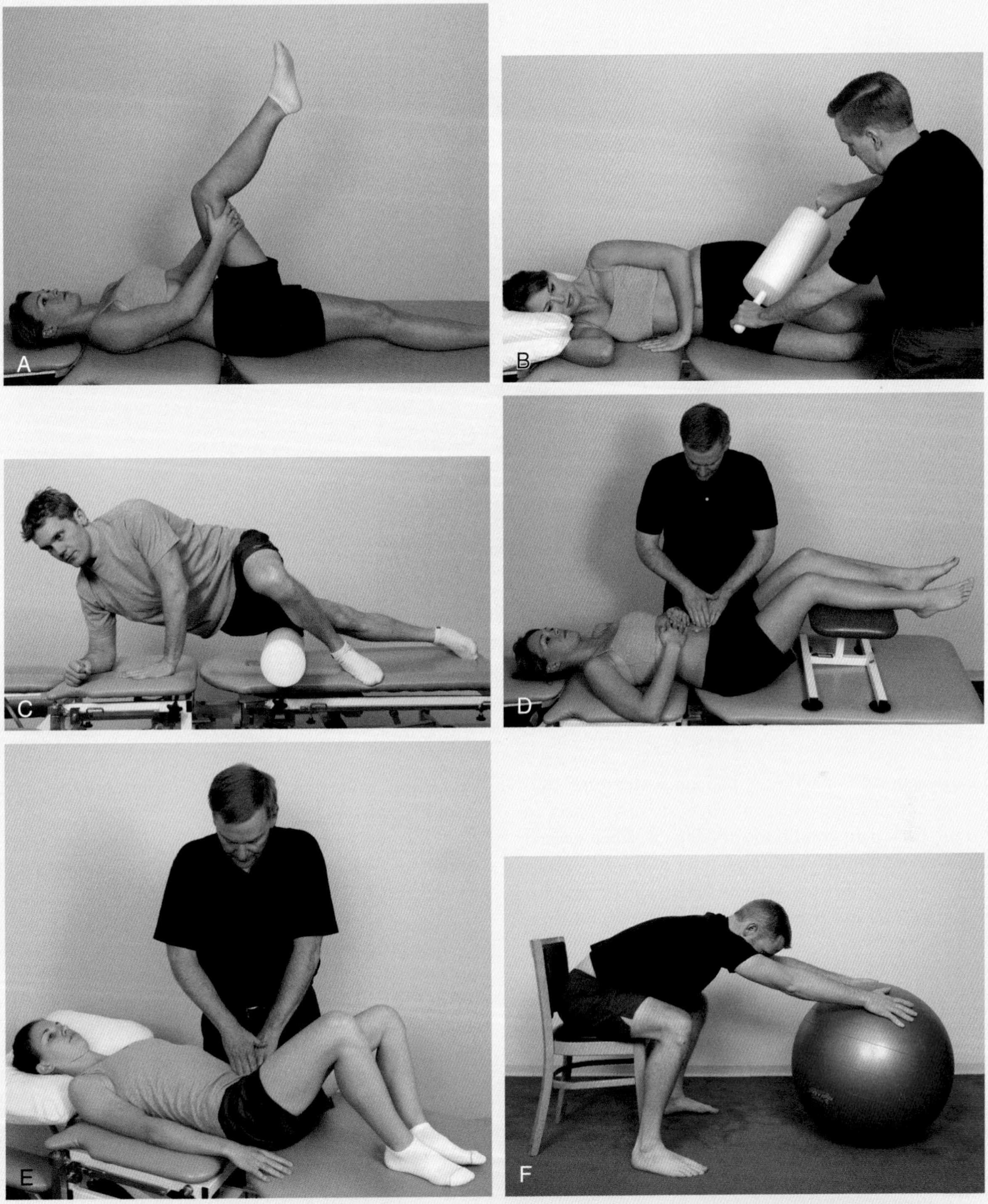

FIG. 4.21 A, Hamstring stretch if sustained for 30 seconds; sciatic nerve glide exercise if performed to the point of tension and repeated without use of sustained end range stretch. This could be progressed to include repeated ankle dorsiflexion. B, Myofascial foam rolling technique to loosen lateral quadriceps muscle and iliotibial band. C, Self-myofascial foam rolling technique to loosen iliotibial band. D, Psoas release. Slowly sink into lower abdomen and sustain pressure on psoas until tension subsides in tight guarded muscle. E, Bent knee fall out hip motions can be combined with the psoas release technique to release and stretch the psoas muscle. F, Physioball trunk flexion stretch. This is a useful stretch for patients who do not tolerate the quadruped position because of knee or wrist conditions.

Continued

BOX 4.15 Lower Extremity Stretching Exercises and Myofascial Techniques—cont'd

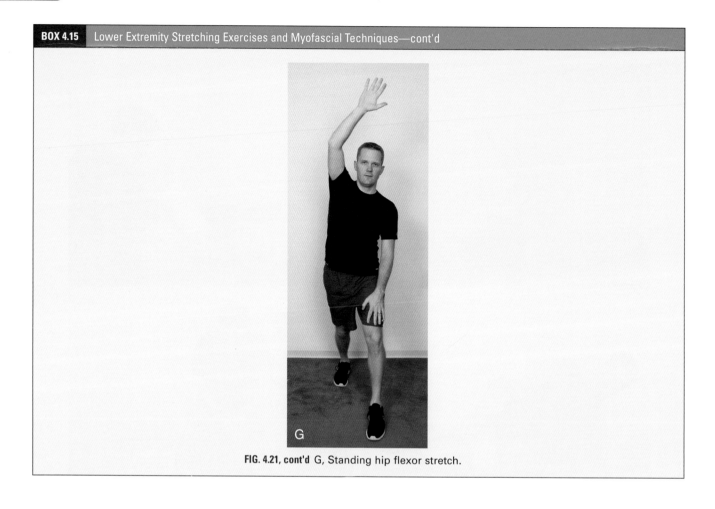

FIG. 4.21, cont'd G, Standing hip flexor stretch.

control participants.[204] In addition, patients with greater psychosocial issues and fear avoidance beliefs are more likely to have chronic back pain conditions develop.[205] When central sensitization is combined with a high level of fear-avoidance beliefs or psychologic distress (such as anxiety or depression), a psychologically informed pain management physical therapy approach needs to be used (Box 4.16) combined with pain neuroscience education (see Ch. 3).

To adopt a physical therapy pain management approach, a clinician needs to accept the concept that persistent LBP can be compatible with a low level of disability and a low level of use of health care.[206] The fear-avoidance model (FAM) for pain-related disability is a psychologic model for chronic musculoskeletal pain that has been suggested to help guide clinical decision making. The FAM could be incorporated into the pain management plan when it is identified that a person with back pain believes strongly that the pain is an indication of injury and that certain activities could make the pain (and thus the injury) worse, this belief could lead to fear of pain, avoidance of those activities, and eventually generalized disability.[206] The FAM of musculoskeletal pain proposes that the primary affective and cognitive components influencing pain perception are anxiety and pain-related fear, including fear of movement and reinjury.[207] Interventions based on this approach involve encouraging patients to confront and overcome their fears and unhelpful beliefs by performing the previously avoided activities.[207–209]

Although several psychologic constructs have potential to influence a patient's response to pain, pain-related fear has received much attention in the physical therapy literature. In addition to identification of fear of movement noted in the patient interview and examination, the FABQ is a helpful tool to measure fear of physical activity and fear of work. High FABQ scores about work with patients with acute LBP can be used to predict which patients are likely to develop more chronic disability and longer-term absences from work at a 4-week follow-up examination, after controlling for initial levels of pain intensity, physical impairment, disability, and the type of therapy received.[210] Likewise, in a cohort of patients with LBP that was not work related, FABQ work scale scores of greater than 20 indicated an increased risk of reporting no improvement in 6-month ODI scores.[211]

Patient education based on a fear-avoidance model encourages confrontation of the feared activities and consists of educating the patient that pain is a common condition rather than a serious disease that needs careful protection.[212] FABQ physical activity subscale scores that exceed 15/24 are considered high.[1] George, Bialosky, and Fritz[213] describe a case report with a progressively graded monitored specific exercise and education approach for successful treatment of a patient with LBP

Basic Cognitive-Behavioral Methods Used in Pain Management

1. Cognitive-behavioral analysis
   - Observe when and where problem behaviors occur and their consequences for the patient.
   - Identify beliefs and expectations associated with problem behaviors (e.g., catastrophizing).
   - Develop a formulation of relationships between these domains.
2. Creation of cognitive-behavioral change plan (with patient's involvement)
   - Identify specific (behavioral) goals that the patient wants to achieve (goal setting).
   - Break down goals into specific subgoals (e.g., walking time) that can be upgraded in steps (e.g., "pacing up" by preset activity or time quotas).
   - Develop a plan for dealing with likely obstacles (e.g., at home and at work).
   - Reinforce activities performed according to the plan.
3. Implementation of plan
   - Explain to and discuss with the patient the formulation for problem behaviors and experiences (including pain) and obtain the patient's agreement.
   - Ensure that the patient attempts activities previously avoided because of pain or fear of pain or reinjury, not just at the clinic but also at home and at work, using pacing quotas.
   - Help the patient deal with obstacles to progress and setbacks.
   - Provide skills training as needed (e.g., identify and challenge unhelpful thoughts and beliefs).
   - Monitor and reinforce (with charts or diaries) the performance of planned tasks.
   - Terminate treatment when goals are achieved and provide a plan for dealing with relapses.

(Modified from Nicholas MK, George SZ. Psychologically informed interventions for low back pain: an update for physical therapists. *Phys Ther.* 2011;91:765-776.)

BOX 4.17 Patient Advice and Education for Effective Treatment of Low Back Pain

Patient education and counseling strategies for patients with low back pain (LBP) should emphasize the following:

1. Promotion of the understanding of the structural strength inherent in the human spine
2. Neuroscience that explains pain perception
3. Favorable prognosis of LBP
4. The use of active pain coping strategies that decrease fear and catastrophizing
5. Early resumption of normal or vocational activities, even when still experiencing pain
6. The importance of improvement in activity levels, not just pain relief

Clinicians should not use patient education and counseling strategies that either directly or indirectly increase the perceived threat or fear associated with LBP, such as education and counseling strategies that do the following:

1. Promote extended bed rest
2. Provide in-depth, pathoanatomic explanations for the specific cause of the patient's LBP

(Modified from Delitto A, George SZ, Van Dillen L, et al. Low back pain. *J Orthop Sports Phys Ther.* 2012;42(4):A1-A57.)

and high FABQ scores. Pain levels were monitored throughout the treatment sessions but did not influence the treatment sessions exercise quota. At a 6-month follow-up examination, the patient had partial return of fear-avoidance beliefs but only minimal increase in perception of disability.[213]

Educational programs tailored to reducing the fear of movement with LBP have been shown to have positive effects on fear-avoidance beliefs and on self-report of disability in patients with high levels of fear.[214] In a randomized trial of patients with CLBP, Moseley et al.[215] provided one group with an explanation about the neurophysiologic processes involved in pain perception and another group with an explanation that was more anatomically oriented (i.e., "back school"). The patients who received an explanation of the neurophysiology of pain demonstrated better improvements in attitudes about pain, pain catastrophizing, and leg raising and forward bending.[215] Similarly, Siemonsma et al.[216] showed statistically significant and clinically relevant improvements in patient-relevant physical activities for patients with CLBP at 18 weeks after an education program focused on illness perceptions concerning CLBP. These findings provide support for including such education in

therapeutic interventions, but to achieve meaningful functional gains (such as return to work or resumption of household chores), the education must be combined with other interventions, such as therapeutic exercise.[206] Pengel et al.[217] found that a combination of advice (about pain) and graded exercise is more effective than either alone or a placebo treatment in patients with subacute LBP. The clinician should address the patient's specific concerns and misconceptions about pain and the potential for reinjury (Box 4.17), and this education should be coupled with an active approach, such as graded activity and exposure that incorporates performing the feared activity.[206]

Through the use of specific behavioral goals (quotas) and systematic reinforcement for effort or achievement, a graded-exercise approach can be used in which pain is not used to determine exercise or activity levels.[206] Dosage follows a quota system, in which a patient's baseline exercise or activity level is first determined by having the patient perform a task until pain limits the patient's ability to perform the task. This level of exercise or activity provides the initial therapeutic quota. Subsequent sessions are based on this quota, and if the patient meets the quota, reinforcement (e.g., verbal praise) is provided. The quota is gradually increased across sessions in a process called "pacing up." If the patient does not meet the quota, the therapist does not offer reinforcement and instead discusses the importance of continuing activity with the patient and encourages the patient to meet the quota at the next session.[206]

Graded exposure is a behavioral approach that strives to increase the performance of fearful activities through a combination of education and activity implementation.[207] Patients receive education that decreases the fear and threat associated with LBP and also receive positive reinforcement for performing fearful activities and utilizing beneficial coping strategies.[207]

Graded exposure involves introduction of a highly feared activity into the rehabilitation program, first at a low level that elicits minimal fear.[206,207] The activities that a patient avoids determine the focus of treatment. Dosage based on graded exposure follows a hierarchical exposure approach. First, patients are asked to identify activities that they are highly fearful of performing because of LBP.[206] Next, the level of the activity is increased slightly to increase the level of fear, it is performed until fear ratings decline, and then exposure is increased again.[207] A key aspect of graded exposure is that the exposure also must occur outside the clinical setting.[206] An example of graded exposure is a patient who is afraid of bending forward. First, the forward bending motion could be incorporated into a supine exercise program. Once the patient is less afraid of this motion in supine, forward bending in quadruped could be added, followed by forwarding bending in sitting and eventually forward bending from a standing position. This could next be incorporated into a forward bending activity, such as lifting a box in the clinic, and later transitioned to a home or work environment. At each phase, the patient is given positive reinforcement for performing the activity and through repetition; the patient's fears lessen, at which point the next level of the motion is introduced. Similar concepts can be used in work conditioning programs where the focus is to enhance patient performance and tolerance to work-related activities with a goal of returning the patient to work. Loisel et al.[218] showed that incorporation of a workplace context into the treatment plan is associated with better return-to-work outcomes than purely clinic-based interventions.

Macedo et al.[219] completed an RCT that compared motor control exercises designed to improve control and coordination of trunk muscles with graded activity under the principles of cognitive-behavioral therapy for treatment of patients with chronic nonspecific LBP. Patients in both groups received 14 sessions of individualized, supervised exercise therapy. Results showed that there were no significant differences between treatment groups at any of the time points (2, 6, and 12 months after intervention) for any of the outcomes studied. The results of this study suggest that motor control exercises and graded activity have similar effects for patients with chronic nonspecific LBP.[219] Future research needs to address if there are subgroups of patients with CLBP who would benefit from each type of exercise-based approach.

Further research is also needed to determine whether subgroups of patients with CLBP would respond best to mobilization/manipulation, exercise, education, or a combination of the three approaches. The use of an impairment-based approach that includes examination of both the movement-related impairments and psychosocial impairments will guide the clinical decisions on the best treatment approach for CLBP. If psychosocial factors are low, the therapist can focus on treatment of mobility and motor control impairments. If psychosocial factors are high, a psychologically informed pain management approach should be incorporated into the physical therapy program with emphasis on an active therapeutic exercise approach that combines motor control exercise, graded exposure,

and education on the neurophysiology of pain. In addition, moderate- to high-intensity exercise should be included in the treatment approach for patients with CLBP without generalized pain, and progressive, low-intensity fitness and endurance activities should be incorporated into the pain management and health promotion strategies for patients with CLBP with generalized pain.[58]

There are educational principles that would be helpful to incorporate with all patients dealing with longer-term pain conditions, such as instruction in wellness principles related to nutrition, stress management, and sleep. Edwards et al. found that sleeping less than 6 hours per night or more than 9 hours per night was associated with increased frequency and intensity of chronic pain the following day.[220]

Population-based longitudinal studies demonstrate that sleep impairments reliably predict new incidents and exacerbations of chronic pain, and sleep impairments are a stronger, more reliable predictor of pain than pain is of sleep impairments.[221] Healthy sleep facilitates immune functions, and impaired sleep quality or quantity can result in low-grade inflammatory responses with increased levels of interleukin 6, prostaglandin E2, and nitric oxide.[222,223]

Anxiety, stress, and depression are commonly associated with both chronic pain and insomnia. Insomnia in adults is defined as more than 30 minutes of sleep latency and/or minutes awake after sleep onset for more than 3 days per week for more than 3 months.[222] If a patient indicates that they get less than the recommended 7 to 8 hours of sleep per night or require medication to sleep at night, a sleep questionnaire, such as the Jenkins Sleep Questionnaire, should be administered to further quantify the nature and degree of sleep impairment (see Box 2.5). If patients are not getting adequate quantity and quality of sleep, sleep hygiene and cognitive-behavioral therapy strategies should be used (Box 4.18). Sleep hygiene education has been shown to improve sleep quality and reduce pain and fatigue in people with chronic pain and fibromyalgia.[224–226]

Cognitive-behavioral therapy is a psychosocial intervention that aims to change unhelpful thoughts, beliefs, and attitudes to improve coping skills, self-regulation, and healthy behavior.[222] It is widely used to treat chronic pain and depression.[222] Cognitive-behavioral therapy is recommended over sedative drugs or hypnotics to improve sleep quality because the changes are more sustainable, there is lower risk of side effects, and it is effective for both management of pain and sleep.[222,227]

People with insomnia have difficulty getting to sleep and are awake frequently during the night resulting in a low ratio of sleep per time in bed, that is, poor sleep efficiency.[222] Bed time restrictions can address poor sleep efficiency that include getting into bed at a later time, when actually sleepy, and sticking to the same getting up time to reduce the amount of time spent in bed and to increase sleep drive at bedtime.[222] If sleep efficiency increases to 85% or more, the upward titration is initiated by adding 15 minutes to time in bed to eventually work toward a target of 7 to 8 quality hours of sleep per night.[222]

BOX 4.18	Strategies to Enhance Sleep Quality (Sleep Hygiene Education)

1. Complete vigorous exercise at least 3 hours before bedtime
2. Moderate to vigorous exercise during the day can improve sleep quality at night
3. Refrain from drinking alcohol or smoking at least 3 to 4 hours before bedtime
4. Avoid eating a large meal or spicy food 2 to 3 hours before going to bed
5. Limit daytime naps to 30 minutes or less and avoid evening naps
6. No caffeine for at least 6 hours before bedtime
7. Set a regular bedtime routine, be calm, and prepare for sleep
8. Use your bed for only sleeping and sexual activity
9. Create a cool, dark, quiet, comfortable sleep environment and remove distractions
10. No bright, blue light devises for at least 30 minutes before bedtime
11. Body alignment—find what is comfortable and use pillows to position
12. Tune out negative thoughts and encourage positive thoughts about sleep
13. Wake up to natural light when possible

(Modified from Teyhen DS, Boland DM, Silvernail JL, Rhon D. Sleep: the impact of sleep on pain, healing and wellness. CSM 2019, February 2019; and Siengsukon CF, Al-dughmi M, Stevens S. Sleep health promotion: practical information for physical therapists. *Phys Ther.* 2017;97:826-836.)

Cognitive-behavioral therapy also involves changing negative thoughts about sleep to decatastrophize the consequences of sleep loss.[222] This approach should target the patient's individualized negative thoughts and feelings regarding sleep in a more positive manner. Hall et al.[228] determined in a systematic review that cognitive-behavioral interventions led by physical therapists with proper training and resources can be an effective treatment for CLBP.

SELECTED SPECIAL TESTS FOR LUMBOPELVIC EXAMINATION

▶ Lumbar Extension/Side Bending/Rotation Combined Motion

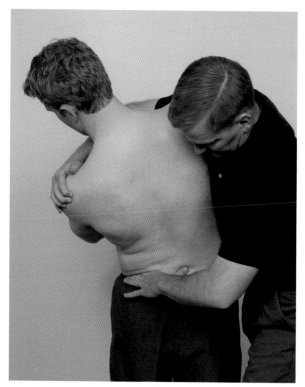

FIG. 4.22 See Video 4.2. Lumbar extension/side bending/rotation combined motion.

PURPOSE	The purpose of this motion test is to assess the amount of motion and pain provocation with the combined motion of backward bending, side bending, and rotation.
PATIENT POSITION	The patient is standing.
THERAPIST POSITION	The therapist stands at the side opposite to the direction of side bending and rotation.
HAND PLACEMENT	The right hand is positioned with the arm across the patient's chest, holding the patient's left shoulder.
	The left hand is positioned with the radial aspect of the second digit at the lower lumbar spine to create a fulcrum point for the motion.
PROCEDURE	The therapist guides the patient into lumbar extension, left side bending, and left rotation with the right arm as the left hand creates a fulcrum point for the motion.
NOTES	In theory, pain provocation at the low back could result from loading the lumbar facet joints on the side of the combined motions, and leg pain could be provoked with loading and closing the lumbar neuroforamen. Haswell[51] reported a kappa value of 0.29 (0.06–0.52) for intertester reliability in pain provocation with this combined motion test in 35 patients with LBP. Laslet et al.[176] reported sensitivity of 100%, specificity of 22%, +LR of 1.3 and −LR of 0.00, which means that this test provides a valid method to screen for lumbar facet joint pain.

▶ Lumbar Side-Glide (Lateral Shift Correction)

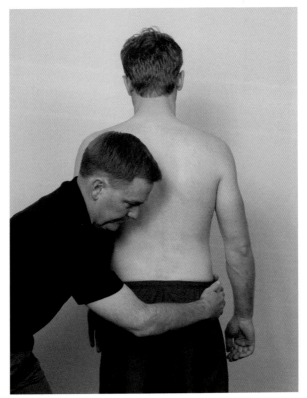

FIG. 4.23 See Video 4.3. Lumbar side-glide (lateral shift correction).

PURPOSE	The purpose of this motion test is to assess the effects of a manual lateral shift correction on the intensity and location of low back and leg pain.
PATIENT POSITION	The patient is standing.
THERAPIST POSITION	The therapist places the left shoulder at the lateral aspect of the thorax on the side of the lateral shift and overlaps the hands at the lateral aspect of the pelvis on the opposite side of the shoulders.
PROCEDURE	The therapist guides the patient into a lateral shift correction with a force couple of laterally directed forces of the therapist's left shoulder toward the right and hands pulling the pelvis toward the left. The patient is monitored for the effect on symptoms, and the procedure is repeated up to 10 times until determination of whether the correction has no effect, peripherizes symptoms, or centralizes symptoms.
NOTES	If the lateral shift correction centralizes symptoms, the correction is repeated as part of the treatment program with other repeated movements that have a centralization effect on the patient's symptoms. If symptoms peripheralize into the lower extremity with this maneuver, further assessment is needed to determine whether other repeated movements, manipulation, exercise, or traction are required to affect the symptoms in a more positive way. Although a lateral shift posture is commonly associated with the presence of a herniated disk, other impairments (such as spinal facet joint, pelvic, and myofascial system dysfunctions) can cause a patient to assume this posture. A thorough analysis of the patient's history and examination of the lumbopelvic structures is needed to develop a treatment plan of care to address the impairments that contribute to a lateral shift posture.

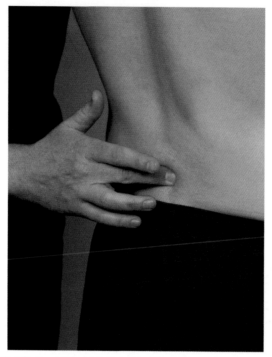

FIG. 4.24 See Video 4.4. Palpation for a lower lumbar step.

PATIENT POSITION	The patient stands with good posture and arms relaxed at the sides.
THERAPIST POSITION	The therapist stands to the side and slightly behind the patient.
PROCEDURE	The pad of the long finger is used to palpate the spinous process of each lumbar vertebra. The fingers of the other hand are spread across the patient's upper chest to provide gentle counter support to the patient's chest.
NOTES	Note the presence of a step between adjacent vertebrae. A palpable step is suspected to be a sign of lumbar instability and can be accompanied by a band of paraspinal muscle guarding across the lumbar vertebrae. A positive finding should be followed up with further instability and mobility testing for detection of other signs of instability.

Collaer et al.[229] reported interrater reliability that was assessed by pair-wise comparison of the findings of three therapists palpating the spinous processes on 30 subjects with LBP. Validity was evaluated by comparing the findings of one therapist to a reference standard of plain film radiographs in 44 patients for detection of spondylolisthesis.[229] The pair-wise kappa values were poor to fair at 0.179, 0.394, and 0.314. Validity testing revealed a sensitivity of 0.60 (95% CI, 14.7–94.7) and a specificity of 0.87 (95% CI, 72.6–95.7%).[229] The +LR was 4.68 (95% CI, 1.57–13.88) and the −LR was 0.458 (95% CI, 0.155–1.35).[229] Both LRs produced only a small change in pre- to posttest probabilities. Based on these results, static spinous process palpation by itself is not a definitive method for the detection of spondylolisthesis, and this test result must be correlated with other signs and symptoms of instability before making a diagnosis.

▶ Lumbar Posterior Shear Test

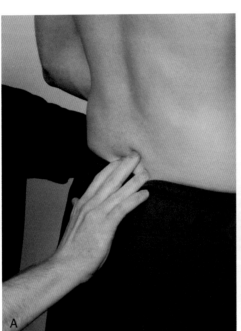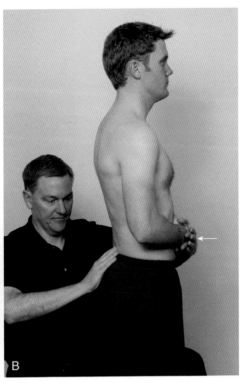

FIG. 4.25 See Video 4.5. A, Finger placement for lumbar posterior shear test. B, Hand placement for lumbar posterior shear test.

PURPOSE	The test is used to assess for instability of lumbar segments L1–L2 through L5–S1.
PATIENT POSITION	The patient stands with hands folded across the abdomen.
THERAPIST POSITION	The therapist kneels to the side and slightly behind the patient.
HAND PLACEMENT	Left hand: The left hand is placed on the patient's hands.
	Right hand: The pad of the long finger is used to palpate the specified spinous process; the index and fourth fingers are used to block the transverse processes of the inferior vertebra; and the heel (thenar/hypothenar eminences) of the hand is used to block the sacrum.
PROCEDURE	The pad of the long finger on the right hand is used to palpate the spinous process of L5. The heel of the right hand blocks the sacrum. The left hand is used to give an anterior to posterior force through the patient's hands and forearms. The pad of the long finger on the right hand is used to palpate for posterior translation of the specified lumbar segment. The procedure is repeated with palpation of the spinous processes of L4, L3, L2, and L1. The amount of posterior translation at each segment is compared, and positive test results include provocation of familiar symptoms or detection of excessive anterior to posterior mobility.
NOTES	Patient relaxation (of abdominal muscles) is vital for proper performance of this technique. Excessive posterior translation at a segment may indicate instability at that segment. This technique should be used in conjunction with other tests to confirm the signs and symptoms of lumbar instability. Reliability testing for this procedure has been reported at a kappa value of 0.35 with 74% agreement when 69 patients with LBP were examined by three pairs of examiners.[91] Fritz, Piva, and Childs[102] tested 49 patients with LBP and found intertester reliability of 64% agreement and a kappa value of 0.27 (0.14, 0.41) with sensitivity 0.57 (0.37,0.75), specificity 0.48 (0.26, 0.7), +LR 1.1 (0.7, 1.8), and −LR 0.9 (0.5, 1.5).

▶ Prone Instability Test

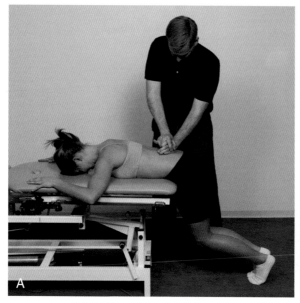
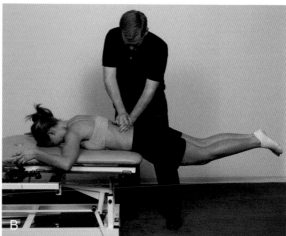

FIG. 4.26 See Video 4.6. A, Prone instability test start position. B, Prone instability test position.

PURPOSE	The test is used to assess for instability of lumbar segments L1–L2 through L5–S1.
PATIENT POSITION	The patient lies prone with the body on the examining table, the legs over the edge of the table, and the feet resting on the floor.
THERAPIST POSITION	The therapist stands at the side of the patient's lumbar spine.
HAND PLACEMENT	Left hand: The ulnar aspect of the hypothenar eminence (just distal to the pisiform) is placed at the targeted spinous process with the wrist extended and the forearm perpendicular to the angle of the contour of the lumbar spine.
	Right hand: The second and third digits are interlaced across the radial aspect of the left hand to support the position of the left hand.
PROCEDURE	The examiner applies a posteroanterior pressure to each targeted lumbar vertebra. If provocation of pain is reported, the patient lifts the feet off the floor and the pressure is reapplied at the symptomatic vertebrae. Test results are positive if the pain is present in the first position but is not reproduced to the same severity when pressure is reapplied to the symptomatic vertebra with the second position (i.e., feet lifted off the floor).
NOTES	This technique should be used in conjunction with other tests to confirm the signs and symptoms of lumbar instability. This test is reliable with a kappa value of 0.87 and 91% agreement when 69 patients with LBP were examined by three pairs of examiners.[91] Alyazedi[83] also reported good interexaminer reliability with kappa of 0.71 with 90% agreement. This test also was included in the CPR developed by Hicks for patients with favorable responses to spinal stabilization exercise programs.[51] Therefore positive test results were correlated with patients with favorable responses, and negative test results were correlated with patients without favorable responses to spinal stabilization exercise programs.[51] This test was one of four variables identified and reported in Table 4.8 in the CPR for lumbar spinal stabilization exercise program success and failure. Fritz, Piva, and Childs[102] tested 49 patients with LBP and found intertester reliability of 85% agreement and a kappa value of 0.69 (0.59, 0.79) for the prone instability test with sensitivity 0.61 (0.41,0.78), specificity 0.57 (0.34, 0.77), +LR 1.4 (0.8, 2.5), and −LR 0.9 (0.7, 1.2).

▶ Prone Lumbar Extension Test

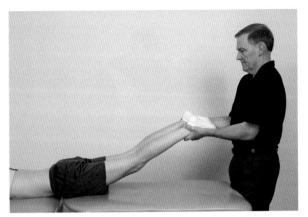

FIG. 4.27 See Video 4.7. Prone lumbar extension test.

PURPOSE	This test is used to determine lumbar instability and is positive if LBP is provoked with the test.
PATIENT POSITION	Patient lies in the prone position.
THERAPIST POSITION	The therapist stands at the foot of the treatment table.
HAND PLACEMENT	The therapist firmly grasps a foot with each hand.
PROCEDURE	The therapist lifts both legs concurrently off the table to a height of 30 cm from the table while maintaining the knees extended and the gently pulling the legs. The test is positive when passively lifting the legs provokes characteristic pain in the lumbar region that is relieved when the legs are lowered back to the table.
NOTES	Kasai et al.[103] compared the results of this test with flexion/extension radiographic evidence of lumbar instability and found sensitivity of 0.84 and specificity of 0.90 with a +LR of 8.84 (4.51, 17.33) and –LR of 0.2 (0.1, 0.4). Alquarni et al.[230] rated the Kasai et al. study as a high-quality study with a 18/26 quality assessment of diagnostic accuracy studies (QUADAS) score. Rabin et al.[231] reported interrater agreement of kappa = 0.76; (95% CI, 0.46–1.00) in using the prone lumbar extension test in a separate study with 26 patients with LBP. Alyazedi[83] reported kappa = 0.46 with 73% agreement.

▶ Femoral Nerve Tension Test (Ely's Test)

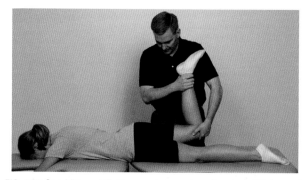

FIG. 4.28 See Video 4.8. Femoral nerve tension test (Ely's test).

PURPOSE	The test is used to assess for irritation of the femoral nerve.
PATIENT POSITION	The patient is prone.
THERAPIST POSITION	The therapist stands at the edge of the table.
HAND PLACEMENT	Cranial hand: The cranial hand supports the lower leg of the test lower extremity.
	Caudal hand: The caudal hand supports the thigh of the test lower extremity.
PROCEDURE	The therapist passively flexes the test leg knee to 90 degrees and then lifts the hip into full extension. Positive test results are found with provocation of anterior thigh pain with the stretch position.
NOTES	This test position can be considered both a muscle length test for the rectus femoris muscle and a nerve tension test for the femoral nerve. The results of this test should be correlated with other neurologic examination procedures to diagnose involvement of the femoral nerve.

▶ Iliotibial Band Length Tests

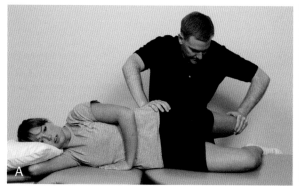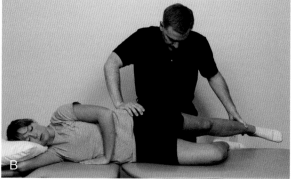

FIG. 4.29 See Videos 4.9 and 4.10. A, Ober test position. B, Modified Ober test position.

▶ Iliotibial Band Length Tests—cont'd

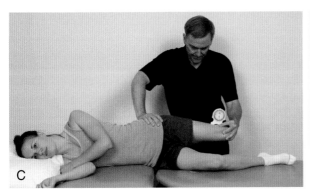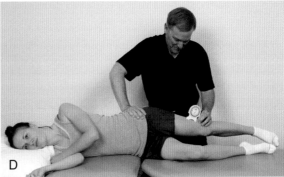

FIG. 4.29, cont'd C, Ober test measured with an inclinometer. D, Modified Ober test measured with an inclinometer.

PURPOSE	This test assesses the length of the iliotibial band.
PATIENT POSITION	The patient is in a side-lying position with the test leg on top and the body positioned near the back edge of the table.
THERAPIST POSITION	The therapist stands along the side of the table behind the patient.
HAND PLACEMENT	Cranial hand: This hand is placed on the lateral aspect of the iliac crest.
	Caudal hand: This hand supports the test leg at the knee.
PROCEDURE	**Modified Ober test:** With the test leg fully extended, the therapist lifts the top leg into a fully abducted position in 10 degrees of extension; with this leg-to-trunk alignment maintained, the test leg is lowered toward the floor. The pelvis must be stabilized throughout the procedure. Hip adduction of 10 degrees is considered normal iliotibial band length.
	Ober test: With the knee flexed to 90 degrees, the therapist lifts the top leg into a fully abducted position with the hip in 10 degrees of extension. With this leg-to-trunk alignment maintained, the test leg is lowered toward the floor. The pelvis must be stabilized throughout the procedure. Hip adduction of 10 degrees is considered normal iliotibial band length.
NOTES	The therapist can use the anterior aspect of his hip and pelvis to support the foot of the test leg during the Ober test. Use of an inclinometer to measure the degree of hip adduction improves the reliability of this test (Fig. 4.29C and D). Reese and Bandy[232] reported intraexaminer reliability for the Ober test as a kappa value of 0.90 and for the modified Ober test as a kappa value of 0.91. Piva et al.[233] used an inclinometer positioned just distal to the lateral knee joint to quantify the Ober test and reported ICC value of 0.97 with 95% CI, 0.93–0.98 and standard error of measurement (SEM) of 2.1 degrees for interexaminer reliability in assessment of 30 patients with patellofemoral pain syndrome.

The Slump Test[234]

PURPOSE	This test is used to determine irritability and extensibility of the central spinal canal and dural tissues.
PATIENT POSITION	The patient sits back on the edge of the treatment table with the posterior knee crease at the edge of the side or foot of the table.
THERAPIST POSITION	The therapist stands at the side of the patient.
HAND PLACEMENT	Left hand: The left hand is positioned across the upper back, neck, and head.
	Right hand: The right hand holds one of the patient's feet.
PROCEDURE	1. The patient begins in an erect sitting position and is asked about any symptoms.

2. The patient is asked to slump the back through the full range of thoracic and lumbar flexion and at the same time prevent the head and neck from flexing. Once this position is achieved, gentle overpressure is applied to the upper thoracic area to stretch the thoracic and lumbar spines into full flexion (Fig. 4.30A)

3. As thoracic/lumbar flexion is maintained, the patient is asked to fully flex the neck, bringing the chin to the sternum. The therapist applies gentle overpressure to the fully flexed spine (Fig. 4.30B).

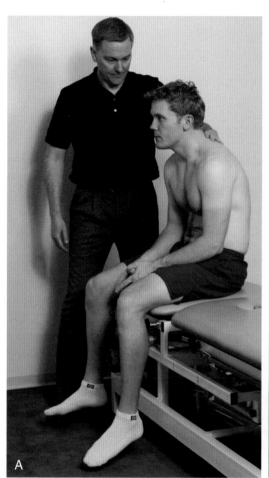
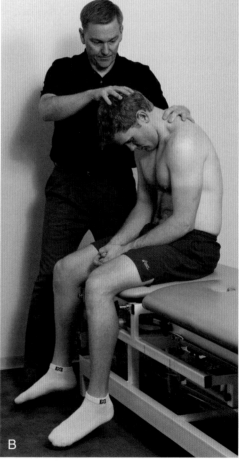

FIG. 4.30 See Video 4.11. A and B, Slump test.

The Slump Test—cont'd

4. As overpressure is maintained to the fully flexed spine, the patient is asked to extend one knee. The range and pain response are noted (Fig. 4.30C).

5. With this position maintained, active ankle dorsiflexion is added to the knee extension and the pain response is noted (Fig. 4.30D).

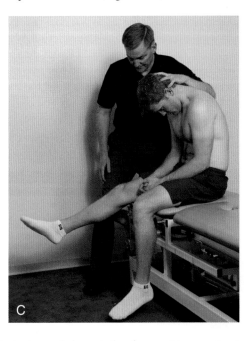

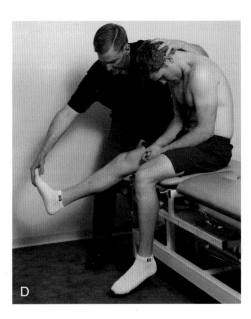

6. With the leg and thoracic/lumbar positions maintained with therapist overpressure, the patient is asked to extend the neck into a neutral position. The patient is asked to report any change in symptoms and is asked to fully extend the knee (if the patient was unable to fully extend the knee when the entire spine was held in flexion). The range of knee extension and pain response are noted in this new position (Fig. 4.30E).

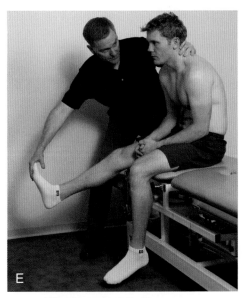

FIG. 4.30, cont'd C–E, Slump test.

NOTES This test should be performed on patients with cervical, thoracic, or lumbar symptoms. Positive test results are seen when lower extremity symptoms are reproduced and knee extension is limited in the slump sit position and when symptoms are alleviated and knee ROM is improved with a return of the neck to a neutral position. Treatment includes treatment of joint and soft tissue restrictions throughout the spine and use of the slump sit position to perform active and passive ROM and sustained stretch (if less irritable) exercises to improve nerve and dural tissue mobility.

The Slump Test—cont'd

Majlesi et al.[235] found sensitivity of the slump test to be 0.84 and specificity to be 0.83 in testing 75 patients with positive MRI finding for a lumbar HNP and 37 control patients with no imaging signs of HNP.

Walsh and Hall[236] tested 45 participants with unilateral leg pain with the straight leg test and slump tests, and when symptoms were reproduced, the ankle was dorsiflexed. Reproduction of presenting symptoms, which were intensified by ankle dorsiflexion, was interpreted as a positive test. There was substantial agreement between SLR and slump test interpretation (kappa = 0.69) with good correlation in ROM between the two tests (r = 0.64) on the symptomatic side.[236] In participants who had positive results, ROM for both tests was significantly reduced compared with ROM on the contralateral side and ROM in participants who had negative results.[236] The study supports the concept that both the slump test and the SLR test primarily test lumbosacral neural tissue mechanosensitivity.

▶ Straight Leg Raise

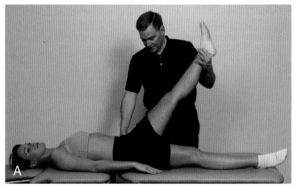

FIG. 4.31 See Video 4.12. A, Straight leg raise (SLR) test position.

PURPOSE	This test is used to determine whether the cause of leg symptoms is a lumbar herniated disk compressing a lumbar nerve root in the lower lumbar spine and is considered a test of lumbosacral neural tissue mechanosensitivity.
PATIENT POSITION	The patient lies supine on a treatment table.
THERAPIST POSITION	The therapist stands on the side to be tested.
HAND PLACEMENT	Cranial hand: This hand palpates the patient's pelvis to monitor pelvic motion during the test or supports the test leg at the posterior knee.
	Caudal hand: This hand supports the foot and ankle of the leg to be tested.

Straight Leg Raise—cont'd

PROCEDURE

The patient's hip is slowly flexed as the knee is maintained in full extension. The patient is asked to respond to the movement, and the degree of hip flexion that is attained when symptoms are reported is recorded with inquiries about the location and nature of the symptoms. For differentiation of a muscle length restriction of the hamstring from neural irritation, three cycles of a 10-second isometric hamstring contraction are applied, followed by attempts to further flex the hip. If greater than 15-degree hip flexion is attained with this maneuver, a muscle tightness component likely exists to the initial finding. Further neural tension sensitizing maneuvers can be applied with either adding hip adduction to the SLR movement or adding ankle dorsiflexion before raising the leg (Fig. 4.31B). In addition, passive neck flexion can be added to increase dural tension during the SLR test (Fig. 4.31C).

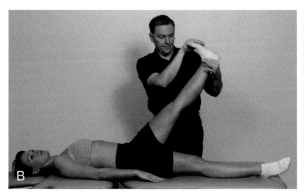 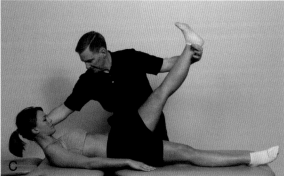

FIG. 4.31, cont'd B, SLR with ankle dorsiflexion. C, SLR with neck flexion.

NOTES

If symptoms are reported with less ROM during the retest with the addition of the sensitizing maneuvers, a neural irritation is likely contributing to the report of the leg symptoms. A positive SLR for reproduction of lower leg pain at 30 degrees of hip flexion or less has been more strongly correlated with herniated disk of the lower lumbar spine.[237] The contralateral leg should also be tested, and if the SLR of the contralateral leg causes symptoms on the involved leg (positive cross SLR), a herniated disk as the cause of the leg pain (i.e., nerve root irritation) is suspected.[237] Deville et al.[238] pooled the results of 11 studies on the SLR test for detection of a lumbar disk herniation at surgery and calculated pooled sensitivity of 0.91 (0.82, 0.94), specificity of 0.26 (0.16, 0.38), +LR of 1.2, and −LR of 3.5. The pooled sensitivity for the cross straight leg test was 0.29 (0.24, 0.34), the pooled specificity was 0.88 (0.86, 0.90), the predictive value of a positive test was 0.92, and the negative predictive value was 0.22.[238]

Majlesi et al.[235] found sensitivity of the SLR test to be 0.52 and specificity to be 0.89 in testing 75 patients with positive MRI finding for a lumbar HNP and 37 control patients with no imaging signs of HNP. Vroomen et al.[239] found the SLR test to be a useful screen for nerve root compression and reported sensitivity of 0.97, specificity of 0.57, +LR of 2.23, and −LR of 0.05.

▶ Modified Straight Leg Raise Test

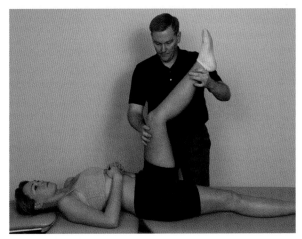

FIG. 4.32 See Video 4.13. Modified straight leg raise test.

PURPOSE	This test is used to test the length of the hamstring muscles.
PATIENT POSITION	The patient is positioned supine with the opposite leg extended.
THERAPIST POSITION	The therapist stands at the edge of the table.
HAND PLACEMENT	Cranial hand: The cranial hand supports the test leg at the anterior distal femur.
	Caudal hand: The caudal hand supports the test leg at the posterior aspect of the ankle.
PROCEDURE	The therapist first flexes the test leg hip to 90 degrees with the knee fully flexed and then slowly extends the patient's knee to end ROM. A neutral lumbopelvic spine position should be maintained.
NOTES	Normal hamstring length is considered a –10 degree angle of the knee extension with the hip in 90 degrees of flexion. Reliability is enhanced if a goniometer is used to measure the knee angle with the test position. This test position can be used as a sustained stretch position for the patient or a hold/relax stretch can be applied to attempt to lengthen the hamstring muscles. In the presence of sciatic nerve root irritation, provocation of leg pain may occur with this test position. Bandy et al.[149] reported ICC levels of 0.97 for intratester reliability in testing hamstring length on 20 participants with this method.

▶ Active Straight Leg Raise Test

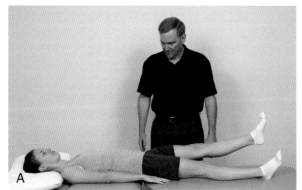
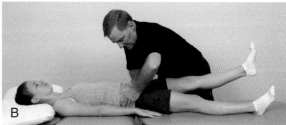
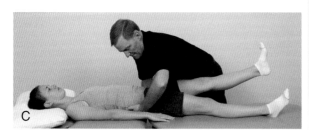
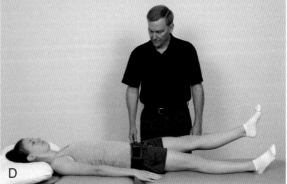

FIG. 4.33 See Video 4.14. A, Active straight leg raise (ASLR). B, ASLR with anterior pelvic compression. C, ASLR with posterior pelvic compression. D, ASLR test with pelvic compression belt.

PURPOSE	This test assesses the ability of the lumbopelvic region to accept the load applied from the lower extremities. When the test results are positive, the assumption is that a lack of motor control exists for dynamic stabilization of the pelvis.
PATIENT POSITION	The patient is positioned supine with the legs straight on a treatment table.
THERAPIST POSITION	The therapist stands at the side of the patient.
PROCEDURE	The therapist asks the patient to slowly and actively raise a straight leg off the treatment table 20 cm (8 inches), pause, and then slowly lower the leg to the table (Fig. 4.33A). The movement is repeated on each side. The therapist observes the patient's ability to stabilize at the lumbopelvic region during the active leg raising and lowering and asks the patient to rate the level of difficulty in raising the leg and pain provocation with the ASLR. If the patient admits to difficulty in raising the leg or symptoms are provoked with the ASLR, the ASLR is repeated with the therapist providing compression of the anterior pelvis at the level of the pubic symphysis to simulate action of the anterior pelvic floor muscles and the TrA (Fig. 4.33B). If symptoms are relieved or the ease of leg raising is improved with pelvic compression, the test results are positive. The ASLR is repeated with compressive forces applied at the posterior pelvis at the level of the posterior superior sacroiliac spine (PSIS) to simulate action of the sacral multifidus (Fig. 4.33C). If symptoms are relieved or ease of leg raising is improved with posterior compression, the test results are positive. The test motion can also be repeated after application of a pelvic compression belt. If there is less pain and greater ease of raising the leg after application of a pelvic compression belt (Fig. 4.33D), the test is also positive.

Active Straight Leg Raise Test—cont'd

NOTES   Positive test results with anterior pelvic compression are an indication of a lack of neuromuscular control provided by the anterior pelvic floor and TrA muscles. Positive test results with posterior pelvic compression are an indication of a lack of neuromuscular control provided by the lumbopelvic multifidus muscles.

Mens et al.[183] reported that test-retest reliability of the ASLR test in identification of women with posterior pelvic pain with pregnancy had a Pearson's correlation coefficient of 0.87. The sensitivity of the test was 0.87, and the specificity was 0.94.[183]

In the Mens et al.[183] original description of the ASLR test, the postpartum patient was asked to score the perceived effort to perform the test on a six-point (0–5) scale: not difficult at all, minimally difficult, somewhat difficult, fairly difficult, very difficult, or unable to perform; and the confirmatory anterior and posterior pelvic compression maneuvers were not used. The ASLR test was considered positive by Mens et al.[183] if a patient graded the perceived effort to perform the test to be a 1 (minimally difficult) or greater for either leg. Rabin et al.[231] reported intertester reliability scores for 25 patients with LBP as kappa = 0.53 (95% CI, 0.20–0.84) and performed the test with the Mens et al.[183] original description.

Roussel et al.[240] reported interexaminer reliability of kappa = 0.70 when the ASLR was used to assess 36 patients with chronic nonspecific LBP. They calculated the Cronbach coefficient for internal consistency of the Trendelenberg (Fig. 4.37A) and ASLR tests to be greater than 0.73, suggesting that these tests assess the same dimension of dynamic neuromuscular control.

Supine Hook-Lying Lumbopelvic Control Test

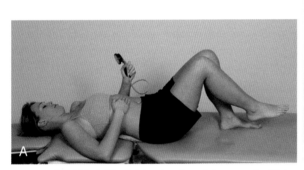
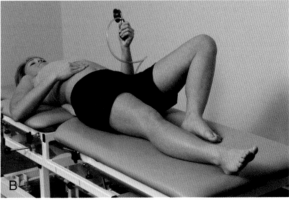

FIG. 4.34 A, Hook-lying lumbopelvic control with lower extremity marching motion. B, Hook-lying lumbopelvic control with lower extremity bent knee fall out motion and opposite hip in neutral.

PURPOSE   This test assesses the ability of the TrA to control lumbopelvic motion while imparting lower extremity motions to challenge the system.

PATIENT POSITION   The patient is in the supine hook-lying position with a pressure bag positioned at the lumbosacral region (bottom edge at S2).

THERAPIST POSITION   The therapist stands beside the patient to provide instructions and to palpate the TrA just medial to the ASIS for tactile feedback.

Supine Hook-Lying Lumbopelvic Control Test—cont'd

PROCEDURE   The pressure feedback bag is inflated to 40 mm Hg, and the patient is instructed to contract and hold the TrA muscle by performing the "drawing in" abdominal maneuver.[241] The pressure gauge either increases 2 to 3 mm Hg with the contraction or stays the same. The patient should practice 10-second isometric holds in this position. For further testing of the ability to stabilize the lumbopelvic spine, leg motions can be induced as the patient attempts to maintain the pressure gauge reading steady throughout the movement. The leg movements that can be used (in order of difficulty) include a heel slide, a 3-inch march (Fig. 4.34A), a bent-knee fall out (hip abduction with external rotation; Fig. 4.34B and D), and an SLR (8–10 inches; Fig. 4.34C).

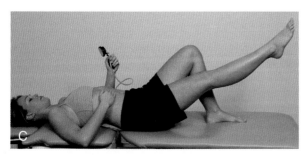 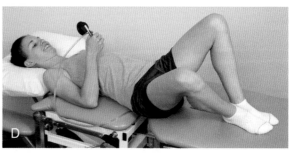

FIG. 4.34, cont'd C, Hook-lying lumbopelvic control with lower extremity straight leg raise motion. D, Hook-lying lumbopelvic control with lower extremity bent knee fall out motion.

NOTES   If the patient is unable to stabilize the lumbopelvic spine with leg movements, the home program should focus on isolated sustained (10-second) isometric holds of the TrA. Once the patient can master this maneuver, a gradual progression of leg movements can be superimposed on the stable neutral lumbopelvic position as the TrA contraction is maintained (see Boxes 4.4–4.6 for further progression of lumbopelvic stabilization exercises).

Prone Transversus Abdominis Test

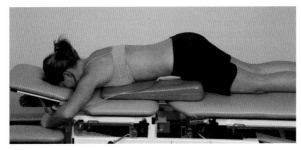

FIG. 4.35 Biofeedback pressure bag is positioned under lower abdomen for prone transversus abdominis test.

PURPOSE	The purpose of this test is to assess the ability to isolate TrA muscle control in the absence of overdominance of the global abdominal muscles.
PATIENT POSITION	The patient lies prone with the arms at the side, and the pressure biofeedback unit is placed under the abdomen with the navel in the center of the bag and the distal edge of the bag in line with the right and left ASIS. If the patient does not tolerate the prone position well, a firm foam wedge can be positioned under the pelvis.
THERAPIST POSITION	The therapist stands at the side of the patient with hands at the sides of the patient's lower trunk to facilitate the drawing in maneuver.
PROCEDURE	The pressure pad is inflated to 70 mm Hg. The patient is instructed to breathe in and out and then, without breathing in, slowly draw in the abdomen to lift the abdomen off the bag, keeping the spine position steady. Once the contraction has been achieved, the patient should return to relaxed normal breathing. A successful performance of the test reduces the pressure by 6 to 10 mm Hg, which indicates that the patient can perform an isolated TrA contraction. Normal strength is achieved when the patient can sustain up to 10 repetitions of 10-second holds of an isolated drawing in maneuver.[241]
NOTES	The therapist must ensure that the patient is not just tilting the pelvis or flexing the spine to attain the change in pressure. The drawing in maneuver is the foundation of successful lumbopelvic motor control training, and the pressure biofeedback device can be used to facilitate progression of a stabilization and motor control exercise program.

▶ Prone Hip Extension Neuromuscular Control Test

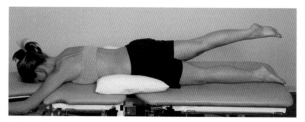

FIG. 4.36 See Video 4.15. Prone hip extension neuromuscular control test.

PURPOSE	This test is used to assess the strength, control, and firing pattern of the lumbopelvic stabilizers and hip extensor muscles during active hip extension.
PATIENT POSITION	The patient is prone with a pillow positioned under the pelvis for maintenance of a neutral spine position.
THERAPIST POSITION	The therapist stands at the side of the table to observe and palpate muscle firing action with the test.
PROCEDURE	The patient is instructed to lift a straight leg 8 to 10 inches off the table. The therapist observes for the patient's ability to maintain a neutral spine position during this test and for the muscle firing pattern, which should progress as ipsilateral gluteus maximus/hamstrings, contralateral multifidus, ipsilateral multifidus, contralateral erector spinae, and ipsilateral erector spinae.[203] Pain provocation is also noted and may occur with poor ability to stabilize the lumbopelvic spine during this test.
NOTES	When a patient has a poor ability to stabilize the lumbopelvic region with this maneuver, a pattern of overdominance of the global erector spinae muscles and delayed or poor firing of the deep local muscles (multifidus and TrA) is common. With delayed firing and weakness of the gluteus maximus, reduction in the degree of hip extension and compensation with an anterior pelvic tilt of the pelvis, hyperlordosis, and increased pressure on the lumbar segments of the spine are often found.[242] With training of the local muscles, the patient can often begin to perform this test with better control and less pain. The abdominal drawing in maneuver can be used to limit excessive anterior pelvic tilt and reduce the overactivity of the erector spinae muscle, which enhances the control of prone hip extension.[243]

Murphy et al.[244] determined interrater reliability for 42 patients with chronic lower back pain for assessment of lumbar   deviation during active prone hip extension into one of three patterns: (1) rotation of the lumbar spine such that the spinous processes appear to move toward the side of hip extension; (2) lateral shift of the lumbar spine toward the side of hip extension; or (3) extension of the lumbar spine. Two clinicians simultaneously observed and independently assessed the left and right prone hip extension test, and the kappa scores were reported as 0.72 for the left leg and 0.76 for the right leg.[244] |

⏵ Trendelenburg Test

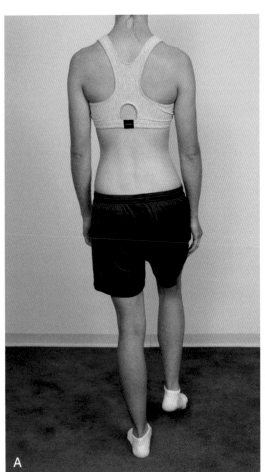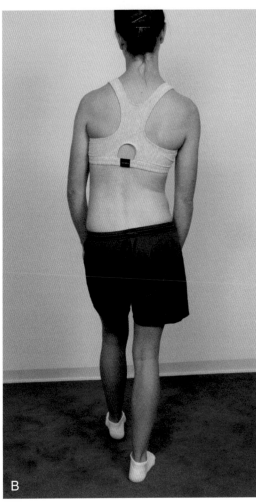

FIG. 4.37 See Video 4.16. A, Negative Trendelenburg sign. B, Positive Trendelenburg sign.

PURPOSE	This test is used to determine neuromuscular control of the hip, pelvis, and trunk with emphasis on gluteus medius strength, function, and control to stabilize the pelvis during single leg stance.
PATIENT POSITION	Patient is in a standing position.
THERAPIST POSITION	Therapist stands behind the patient.
HAND PLACEMENT	No palpation required.
PROCEDURE	The patient is asked to balance on one leg by flexing the contralateral hip to 30 degrees. The position is maintained for 30 seconds and then repeated for the other side. From the posterior view, the therapist observes the angle formed by a line that connects the iliac crest and a line vertical to the testing surface.
NOTES	The test is negative if the pelvis on the nonstance side can be elevated and maintained for 30 seconds. The test is positive if one of the following criteria are met: (1) the patient is unable to hold the elevated pelvic position for 30 seconds; , (2) no elevation is noted on the nonstance side; and/or (3) the stance hip adducts allowing the pelvis on the nonstance side to drop downward below the level of the stance side pelvis. The patient is allowed to touch the table with one finger to correct for potential balance problems.

Trendelenburg Test—cont'd

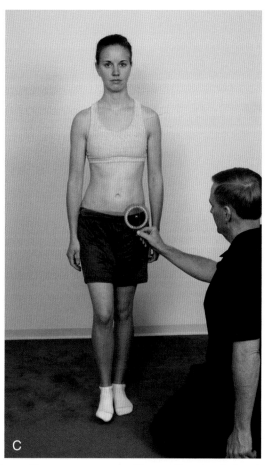

FIG. 4.37, cont'd C, Pelvic position measurement with a goniometer during the Trendelenburg test.

A goniometer may be used to quantify the amount of pelvic movement (Fig. 4.37C). The axis of the goniometer is placed on the ASIS, the stationary arm along an imaginary line between the two ASIS landmarks, and the moving arm along the anterior midline of the femur.[245] Youdas[246] measured intratester reliability in 90 healthy participants and reported intratester reliability for measurement of the hip adduction angle is 0.58 and SEM is 2 degrees. The minimal detectable change (MDC) is 4 degrees.[246]

Bird et al.[247] tested the validity of the Trendelenburg sign for detection of gluteus medius tendon tears in 24 women with lateral hip pain and reported sensitivity of 0.72 and a specificity of 0.76 with the intraexaminer kappa of 0.676 (95% CI, 0.270–1.08) for 12 of the patients who were retested 2 months later. Roussel et al.[240] reported an interexaminer reliability of kappa = 0.83 for the left side and 0.75 for the right side after assessing 36 patients with chronic nonspecific LBP. The Cronbach coefficient for internal consistency of the Trendelenburg and ASLR tests was greater than 0.73.[240] These data provide evidence favoring the test-retest reliability and internal consistency of the Trendelenburg and ASLR (Fig. 4.33A) tests in patients with chronic nonspecific LBP, suggesting that these tests assess similar dimensions.[240]

Hip Abductor Neuromuscular Control Test

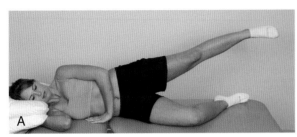
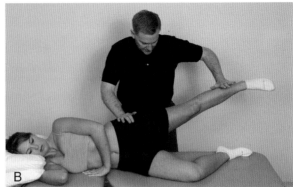

FIG. 4.38 A, Active hip abduction neuromuscular control test. B, Resisted hip abduction with isolation of gluteus medius muscle strength.

PURPOSE	The purpose of this test is to assess muscle firing pattern, strength, and control of hip abductors and lumbopelvic stabilizers.
PATIENT POSITION	The patient lies in a side-lying position with the bottom hip and knee flexed at 30 degrees and the top leg extended and aligned with the plane of the trunk.
THERAPIST POSITION	The therapist stands at the edge of the table behind the patient.
PROCEDURE	The patient is instructed to actively lift the top leg approximately 24 inches off the table while keeping the leg in line with the trunk (Fig. 4.38A). The therapist observes the quality of the movement. A leg that flexes at the hip joint as it abducts is a sign of weakness of the gluteus medius and overdominance or compensation with the tensor fasciae latae. The patient may also have an inability to stabilize the pelvis in this position, which could be an indication of poor control of local trunk stabilizers. A gluteus medius muscle isometric (brake) strength test should also be performed with positioning of the hip at 35 degrees of abduction, 10 degrees of extension, and 10 degrees of external rotation and application of a brake test into adduction (Fig. 4.38B). The patient should be able to hold this position with a moderate level of force to show normal strength of the gluteus medius.
NOTES	Normal gluteus medius strength and control is required for lumbopelvic dynamic stability and proper lower extremity function. Overactivation of the tensor fasciae latae muscle to compensate for weakness of the gluteus medius often results in tightness of the iliotibial band, which can contribute to lumbopelvic, hip, and knee impairments. Bird et al.[247] compared the results of resisted hip abduction for weakness or pain provocation with MRI findings of a complete or partial gluteus medius tendon tear in 24 patients with lateral hip pain and found a sensitivity of 0.72 and specificity of 0.46. Rabin[231] reported poor interexaminer reliability for the active hip abduction test with kappa of −0.09 (−0.035, 0.27) with testing on 25 patients with LBP in which the examiners assessed the quality and control of the movement.

▶ Gillet Marching Test

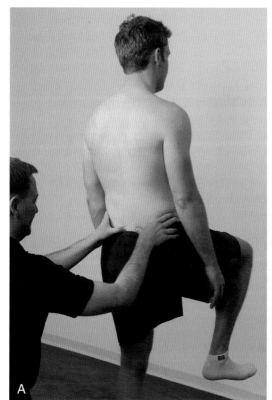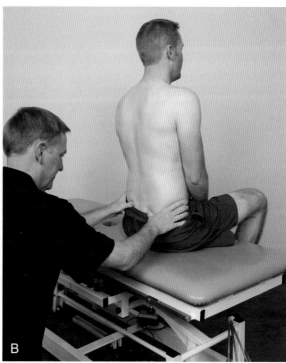

FIG. 4.39 See Video 4.17. A, Gillet marching test. B, Gillet marching test in sitting.

PURPOSE	This test is used to assess for mobility deficits of the lumbopelvic region and SIJ.
PATIENT POSITION	The patient stands or sits on a firm level treatment table and faces away from the therapist.
THERAPIST POSITION	The therapist kneels or sits on a low stool behind the patient with eyes level with the patient's PSIS.
PROCEDURE	The therapist uses the thumb to palpate the PSIS on the side to be tested; the other thumb is on the spinous process of S1. The patient is instructed to fully flex one hip as if marching. The therapist should observe for the ipsilateral PSIS to move caudally as the hip is flexed. An alternative technique is palpation of both PSISs with the thumbs for comparison of relative movement of one PSIS with the other PSIS.
NOTES	Test results are considered positive for sacroiliac/lumbopelvic mobility deficits if the PSIS does not move caudally with hip flexion. The therapist should observe for a Trendelenburg sign while the patient is standing on one leg. The test can be performed in the seated position when the patient has balance or strength deficits that limit the ability to balance on one leg. Although the test is described as a SIJ mobility assessment, false-positive findings could be produced with L5–S1/lower lumbar mobility deficits. Therefore L5–S1 PIVM should be assessed before a SIJ dysfunction is diagnosed. When compared with a reference standard of anesthetic blocks of the SIJ in patients with LBP, the Gillet test has shown a sensitivity of 0.43, a specificity of 0.68, a −LR of 0.84, and a +LR of 1.3.[248] Flynn et al.[50] found a kappa value of 0.59 for intertester reliability in the examination of 71 patients with LBP. When this test is positive, manipulation techniques, such as the lumbopelvic lift manipulation that move lower lumbar and pelvic joints can often be used to restore mobility and inhibit pain. This test can serve as an excellent pre- and posttest for the lumbopelvic lift manipulation. (Fig. 4.69)

Distraction Provocation (Anterior Superior Iliac Spine Gap) Sacroiliac Joint Test

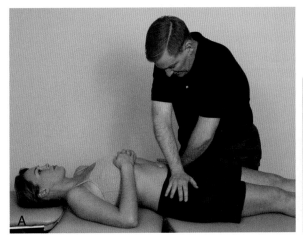
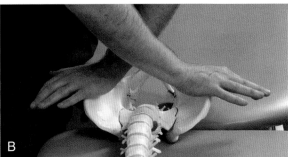

FIG. 4.40 See Video 4.18. A, Anterior superior iliac spine (ASIS) gap test. B, ASIS gap test hand placement.

PURPOSE	This test assesses the level of reactivity of the SIJ and provokes SIJ pain (arthralgia).
PATIENT POSITION	The patient is supine with the head on a pillow.
THERAPIST POSITION	The therapist stands next to the patient.
PROCEDURE	The therapist crosses arms and contacts the medial aspect of each ASIS with the soft spot of each palm. A gentle force is applied to gap the ASIS pushing in a posterior lateral direction, and the force is gradually increased over approximately 10 seconds. The patient should report any pain provoked by the test. If no discomfort is reported, an impulse is given at the end of the application of the force. Again, the patient is instructed to report any pain provoked by the test.
NOTES	The test results are positive if the test provokes pain at the SIJ or symphysis pubis. The test results are not considered positive if pain is provoked at the ASIS as a result of therapist hand placement. This technique can be performed over the patient's clothing. Laslett and Williams[177] reported a kappa value of 0.69 for interexaminer reliability for assessment of 51 patients with LBP with and without radiation into the lower extremities.

Anterior Superior Iliac Spine Compression Provocation Sacroiliac Joint Test

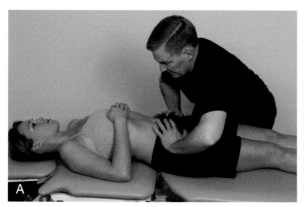 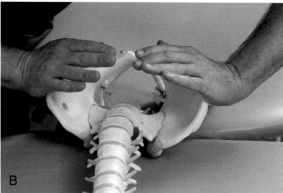

FIG. 4.41 See Video 4.19. A, Anterior superior iliac spine (ASIS) compression test. B, ASIS compression test hand placement.

PURPOSE	This test is used to assess the level of reactivity of the SIJ and provoke SIJ-related pain (arthralgia).
PATIENT POSITION	The patient is supine with the head on a pillow.
THERAPIST POSITION	The therapist stands next to the patient with a diagonal stance and leans over to place the chest directly over the patient's pelvis.
PROCEDURE	The therapist contacts the lateral aspect of each ASIS with the soft spot of each palm. A gentle force is applied to compress the ASIS toward midline, and the force is gradually increased over approximately 10 seconds. The patient should report any pain provoked by the test. If no discomfort is reported, an impulse is given at the end of the application of the force. Again, the patient is instructed to report any pain provoked by the test.
NOTES	The test results are positive if the test provokes pain at the SIJ or symphysis pubis. The test results are not considered positive if pain is provoked at the ASIS as a result of therapist hand placement. This technique can be performed over the patient's clothing. Russell et al.[249] reported a sensitivity of 0.70, a specificity of 0.90, a +LR of 7.0, and a −LR of 0.33 for identification of patients with ankylosing spondylitis (AS) with reference standard of radiographically confirmed AS. Laslett and Williams[177] reported kappa value of 0.73 for interexaminer reliability for assessment of 51 patients with LBP with and without radiation into the lower extremities.

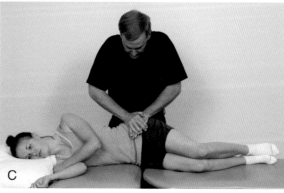

FIG. 4.41, cont'd See Video 4.20.C, ASIS compression test in the side-lying position.

ALTERNATIVE TECHNIQUE	The ASIS compression provocation SIJ test can also be performed in a side-lying position with both hands used on the lateral aspect of the top ASIS to apply a compressive force through the pelvis (Fig. 4.41C).

Sacroiliac Joint Posterior Gapping Test and Thigh Thrust Provocation Test

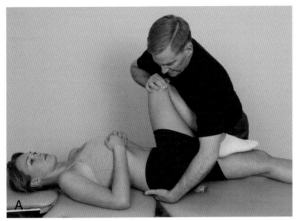 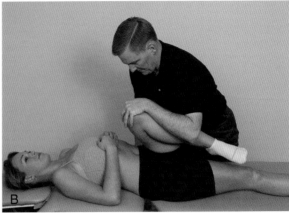

FIG. 4.42 See Video 4.21. A, Palpation of opposite side sacroiliac joint (SIJ) gapping with knee to opposite chest movement. B, Palpation of same side SIJ gapping with knee to opposite chest movement.

PURPOSE	This test evaluates the mobility of the SIJ to gap and to provoke SIJ-related pain (arthralgia).
PATIENT POSITION	The patient is supine with the head on a pillow.
THERAPIST POSITION	The therapist stands next to the patient.
HAND PLACEMENT	Caudal hand: The pads of the index and long fingers are used to palpate the medial aspect of the PSIS.
	Cranial hand: This hand is used to grasp the patient's knee on the side to be tested.
PROCEDURE	The therapist stands on the patient's left side and flexes the patient's right hip and knee to approximately 90 degrees. The patient's hip is adducted so that the right side of the pelvis comes off of the table. The pads of the index and long fingers are used to palpate the medial edge of the patient's right PSIS. The patient's pelvis is rolled back onto the left hand, and the patient's right hip is flexed and adducted toward the left shoulder (Fig. 4.42A). The therapist palpates for the right PSIS to move laterally and the SIJ to gap. The amount of gapping and pain provocation are noted.
	The procedure is repeated to assess the left SIJ. The amount of movement/pain provocation is noted and compared with the right side (Fig. 4.42B).

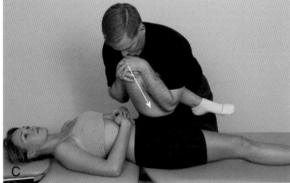

FIG. 4.42, cont'd See Video 4.22. C, Thigh thrust overpressure for SIJ pain provocation test.

The thigh thrust test uses similar hand placement and patient position, but instead of palpation of SIJ mobility, posteriorly directed force through the femur at varying angles of abduction/adduction are used to attempt to reproduce posterior buttock pain (Fig. 4.42C).

Sacroiliac Joint Posterior Gapping Test and Thigh Thrust Provocation Test—cont'd

NOTES	The test results are considered positive if the joint does not gap or if the patient's symptoms are reproduced at the SIJ. The motion should be graded as normal, hypomobile (decreased movement), or hypermobile (increased movement). Dreyfuss et al.[248] reported a sensitivity of 0.36, a specificity of 0.50, a +LR of 0.7, and a −LR of 1.28 for the thigh thrust test with an intraarticular injection anesthetic block of the SIJ used as a reference standard. Laslett and Williams[177] reported kappa of 0.88 for interexaminer reliability for assessment of 51 patients with LBP with and without radiation into the lower extremities. This test has also been called the *posterior pelvic pain provocation (P4)* test.[187]

▶ Gaenslen's Provocation Sacroiliac Joint Test

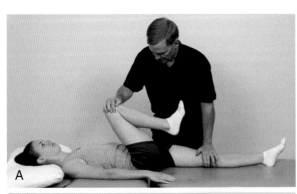
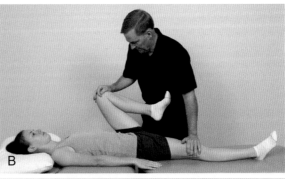
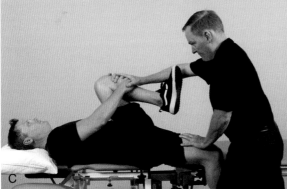
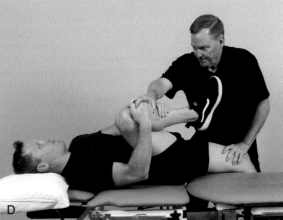

FIG. 4.43 See Video 4.23. Gaenslen's provocation sacroiliac joint test.

PURPOSE	Gaenslen's provocation SIJ test is used to assess the level of reactivity of the SIJ and to provoke SIJ-related pain.
PATIENT POSITION	The patient is supine with the head on a pillow and both legs extended.
THERAPIST POSITION	The therapist stands with a diagonal stance next to the patient.
PROCEDURE	The therapist fully flexes the patient's hip and brings the patient's knee toward the chest while the opposite hip remains in extension. Overpressure is applied to both legs at the end range of hip flexion and hip extension. If the patient has good hip flexibility, the extended hip lower extremity can be positioned over the side of the table to apply greater strain to the hip and pelvis (Fig. 4.43C and D). Symptoms could be produced on either side. The test is repeated by flexing the opposite hip.

Gaenslen's Provocation Sacroiliac Joint Test—cont'd

NOTES   The test results are positive if the test provokes pain at the SIJ region. For assurance that the opposite hip remains in full extension, the leg can be extended over the edge of the table. Laslett and Williams[177] reported kappa of 0.72 for interexaminer reliability for assessment of 51 patients with LBP with and without radiation into the lower extremities. Dreyfuss et al.[248] reported interexaminer agreement of 82% and kappa of 0.61 with reported a sensitivity of 0.71, a specificity of 0.26, a +LR of 1.0, and a −LR of 1.12 for Gaenslen's test with the reference standard of intraarticular injection anesthetic block of the SIJ.

▶ Sacral Thrust Provocation Sacroiliac Joint Test

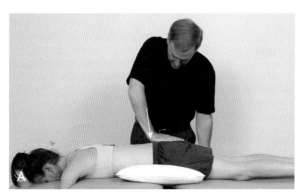
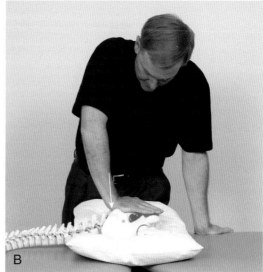

FIG. 4.44 See Video 4.24. A, Sacral thrust provocation sacroiliac test hand placement. B, Sacral thrust provocation sacroiliac test hand placement on a spine model.

PURPOSE   This test assesses the level of reactivity of the SIJ and provokes SIJ-related pain.

PATIENT POSITION   The patient is prone with pillow supporting the pelvis.

THERAPIST POSITION   The therapist stands with a diagonal stance next to the patient.

PROCEDURE   The therapist contacts the posterior base and mid portion of the sacrum and gradually increases a posteroanterior force over approximately 10 seconds. The patient is instructed to report pain provocation. If no discomfort is reported, an impulse is given at the end of the application of the force and pain provocation is assessed.

NOTES   The test results are positive if the test provokes pain at the SIJs. This technique can be performed over the patient's clothing. An alternative method is use of a second hand to reinforce the primary contact and assist in force application. Laslett and Williams[177] reported an interrater reliability of kappa value of 0.56 with testing of 51 patients with LBP with and without leg pain.

▶ Flexion, Abduction, and External Rotation (Patrick or FABER) Test

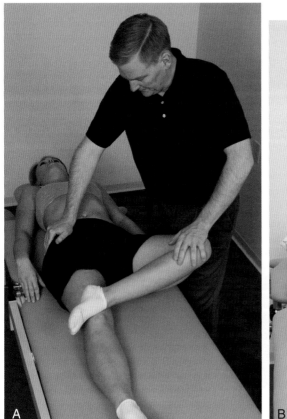 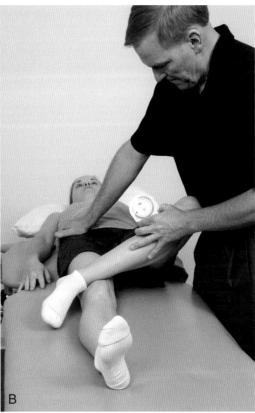

FIG. 4.45 See Video 4.25. A, Flexion, abduction, and external rotation (FABER) test. B, FABER test measured with an inclinometer.

PURPOSE	This test is both a provocation test for the SIJ-related and hip joint pain and a general mobility screen of the hip joint.
PATIENT POSITION	The patient is supine with one leg extended and the test leg crossed over the extended leg just above the knee. The test leg hip is flexed, abducted, and externally rotated (flexion, abduction, and external rotation [FABER] position).
HAND PLACEMENT	Cranial hand: This hand is used to stabilize the opposite side of pelvis at the ASIS.
	Caudal hand: This hand is placed on the medial aspect of the knee joint of the test leg.
PROCEDURE	The therapist applies gentle overpressure of the hip into flexion, abduction, and external rotation by pressing the test leg knee down toward the table and applying a stabilizing force at the opposite ASIS.
NOTES	Positive test results are reached with reproduction of buttock or groin pain, which could be an indication of irritation of either the SIJ or hip joint. The test leg tibia should attain a horizontal position to be considered at full ROM. More importantly, significant difference in mobility between sides should be noted and can be further quantified by use of an inclinometer placed at the medial aspect of the tibia just distal to the knee (Fig. 4.45B).[250] Interexaminer reliability has been reported as a kappa value of 0.62 by Dreyfuss et al[248] and a kappa value of 0.60 by Flynn et al.[50]

Flexion, Abduction, and External Rotation (Patrick or FABER) Test—cont'd

Sutlive et al.[250] reported ICC interexaminer reliability values of 0.90 (0.78–0.96), SEM of 2.6 degrees, MDC of 7.2 degrees with use of an inclinometer to quantify the Patrick test with testing of 72 patients with hip pain. Sutlive et al.[250] also reported that FABER test of less than 60 degrees of hip external rotation correlated with radiographic evidence of hip osteoarthritis with sensitivity of 0.57 (0.34–0.77), specificity of 0.71 (0.56–0.82), +LR of 1.9 (1.1–3.4), and −LR of 0.61 (0.36–1.00), which indicates that a positive FABER test is not a good indicator of hip osteoarthritis. Cliborne[246] reported ICC values of 0.87 with 95% CI range of 0.78 to 0.94 for pain reproduction and ICC of 0.96 with 95% CI range of 0.92 to 0.98 with SEM of 2.9 degrees for ROM measurements on 35 participants with lower extremity symptoms.

Martin[251] assessed the intertester reliability of the FABER test in people seeking care for intraarticular, nonarthritic hip joint pain. The examiners demonstrated 84% agreement and a kappa value of 0.63 (95% CI, 0.43–0.83) indicating substantial reliability. In a separate study, Martin[252] assessed the diagnostic accuracy of the FABER test. Using pain relief with a diagnostic injection as the comparison, the sensitivity and specificity of the FABER test was reported to be 0.60 (95% CI, 0.41–0.77) and 0.18 (95% CI, 0.07–0.39), respectively. The +LR was 0.73 (95% CI, 0.50–1.1) and the −LR was 2.2 (95% CI, 0.8–6).[252]

In their study to detect intraarticular hip pathology, including osteoarthritis, Maslowski[253] also assessed the diagnostic accuracy of the FABER test. Using pain relief with a diagnostic injection as the comparison, the sensitivity and specificity of the FABER test was reported to be 0.82 (95% CI, 0.34–0.82) and 0.25 (95% CI, 0.09–0.48), respectively.[253] The positive predictive value was 0.46 (95% CI, 0.28–0.65) and the negative predictive value was 0.64 (95% CI, 0.27–0.91).[253]

⊙ Flexion, Adduction, Internal Rotation (FADIR) Impingement Test

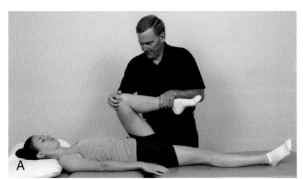 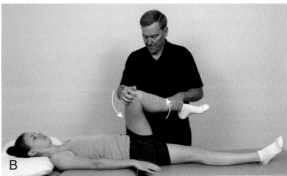

FIG. 4.46 See Video 4.26. A, Flexion, adduction, internal rotation (FADIR) test start position. B, FADIR with passively moving the hip into internal rotation with adduction.

PURPOSE	This test is used to assess for painful impingement between the femoral neck and acetabulum in the anterosuperior region and to assess for specific pathology of the acetabular labrum.
PATIENT POSITION	Patient is in the supine position.
HAND PLACEMENT	Therapist supports the lower extremity to be tested at the knee and ankle.
PROCEDURE	The hip and knee are flexed to 90 degrees. Maintaining the hip at 90 degrees of flexion, the hip is then internally rotated and adducted as far as possible (Fig. 4.46B). The patient is asked what effect the motion has on symptoms. The test is considered positive if the patient reports a production of, or increase in, the anterior groin, posterior buttock, or lateral hip pain consistent with the patient's presenting pain complaint. If the test is negative, the test is repeated with the hip placed in full flexion.
NOTES	Martin[251] assessed the intertester reliability of the flexion, adduction, and internal rotation (FADIR) test in patients seeking care for intraarticular, nonarthritic hip joint pain and reported a kappa value of 0.58 (95% CI, 0.29–0.87), indicating moderate reliability, which may be explained in part by the high proportion of positive findings in the study participants.

Two studies report the FADIR test characteristics specific to pain provocation. In both studies, the participants were patients who reported pain consistent with intraarticular, nonarthritic hip joint pain. Martin[251] compared the results of the FADIR to diagnostic injection and reported the sensitivity and specificity of the FADIR test to be 0.78 (95% CI, 0.59–0.89) and 0.10 (95% CI, 0.03–0.29), respectively. The +LR was 0.86 (95% CI, 0.67–1.1) and the −LR was 2.3 (95% CI, 0.52–10.4).

In their study to detect intraarticular hip pathology (including osteoarthritis), Maslowski[253] assessed the diagnostic accuracy of a test that is similar to the FADIR test, called the internal rotation with overpressure (IROP). Using pain relief with a diagnostic injection as the comparison, the sensitivity and specificity of the IROP test was reported to be 0.91 (95% CI, 0.68–0.99) and 0.18 (95% CI, 0.05–0.40), respectively. The positive predictive value was 0.88 (95% CI, 0.67–0.98), and the negative predictive value was 0.17(95% CI, 0.04–0.40).[253]

▶ **Hip Scour Test**

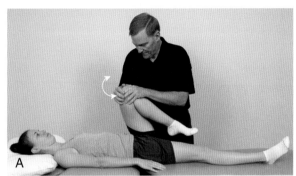 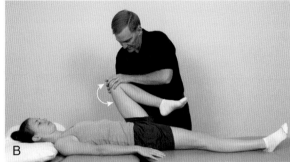

FIG. 4.47 See Video 4.27. A, Hip scour test start position: flexion and adduction of the hip. B, Hip is moved into an arc of motion from adduction to abduction with long axis compression.

PURPOSE

This test is used to detect tissue irritability of the hip joint and surrounding tissues.

PATIENT POSITION

Patient is in the supine position with both legs extended.

HAND PLACEMENT

The therapist supports the patient's leg at the knee and the foot as the hip is moved into the test position. The compressive axial load is applied with both hands positioned at the anterior aspect of the knee.

PROCEDURE

The hip is flexed and adducted until resistance to the movement is detected. The therapist then maintains hip flexion into resistance and moves the hip into an arc of abduction, which is repeated through two full arcs of motion. If the no pain is reported, the examiner repeats the test while applying long-axis compression through the femur.

NOTES

ROM is not assessed with this test. The test is positive if the patient reports reproduction of the primary symptoms in the hip, groin, thigh, or buttock. Cliborne et al.[231] reported interexaminer ICC values of 0.87 (0.76–0.93) for pain reproduction when tested on 35 patients with lower extremity symptoms. Sutlive[250] reported sensitivity of 0.62 (0.39–0.81), specificity of 0.75 (0.60–0.85), +LR of 2.4 (1.4–4.3), and −LR of 0.51 (0.29–0.89) for detection of radiographic evidence of osteoarthritis of the hip and kappa values of 0.52 (0.08–0.96) and 86.7% agreement for reproduction of hip symptoms when tested on 72 patients. Five variables formed a CPR developed for detection of hip osteoarthritis, including: (1) self-reported squatting as an aggravating factor, (2) scour test with adduction causing groin or lateral pain, (3) active hip flexion causing lateral pain, (4) active hip extension causing hip pain, and (5) passive hip internal rotation 25 degrees or less.[250] If at least four of five variables were present, the +LR was 24.3 (95% CI, 4.4–142.1), increasing the probability of hip osteoarthritis to 91%.[250]

▶ Thomas Test

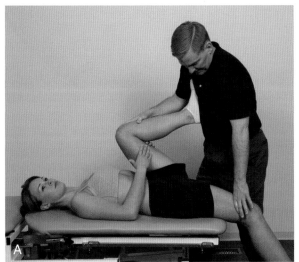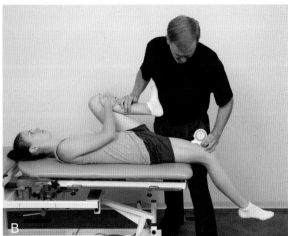

FIG. 4.48 See Video 4.28. A, Thomas test end position. B, Thomas test position measured with an inclinometer.

PURPOSE	The Thomas test is used to assess the length of the hip flexor muscles.
PATIENT POSITION	The patient is supine at the foot of the table.
THERAPIST POSITION	The therapist stands at the foot of the table.
HAND PLACEMENT	The hands and chest are used to control both of the patient's legs during the procedure.
PROCEDURE	The patient starts sitting at the edge of the foot of the treatment table. The therapist supports the patient and guides the patient into a supine position with both knees and hips fully flexed. The therapist holds one leg in full flexion and guides the test leg down into hip extension. The thigh should come parallel with the table to attain full normal hip flexor muscle length. The therapist then uses his leg to flex the test leg knee to 90 degrees. If the hip flexes when knee flexion is added, the rectus femoris muscle is tight. An inclinometer or goniometer can be used to further quantify the positive test result (Fig. 4.48B).
NOTES	Hip abduction in the test position is an indication of iliotibial band tightness. The test position can be used to provide a hold/relax stretch technique or a sustained stretch for the hip flexors. Wang et al.[254] reported ICC of 0.97 for Thomas test intraexaminer reliability on 10 participants. Clapis et al.[255] reported high interexaminer reliability for both the inclinometer and goniometric measurements for hip extension using the Thomas test on 42 healthy participants with ICC = 0.89–0.92. They also reported high correlation between the results of the use of the goniometer and inclinometer with ICC = 0.86–0.92 indicating that the two measurement devices could be used interchangeably for this test.

Hip Passive Rotation Range of Motion Test (Supine)

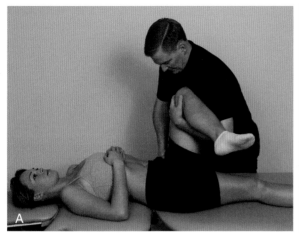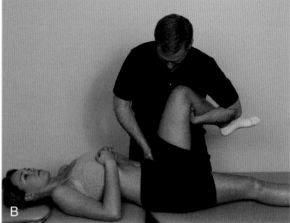

FIG. 4.49 See Video 4.29. A, Hip external rotation passive range of motion (ROM) test. B, Hip internal rotation passive ROM test.

PURPOSE	The test assesses passive ROM of the hip joint.
PATIENT POSITION	The patient is supine with the opposite leg extended and the test leg supported by the therapist.
THERAPIST POSITION	The therapist stands with a diagonal stance at the edge of table.
HAND PLACEMENT	Cranial hand: The thumb and fingers are placed at the ASIS to monitor and prevent pelvic motion. Caudal hand: The forearm is placed under the patient's lower leg, and the hand is under the knee to support the knee and hip at 90 degrees of flexion.
PROCEDURE	The therapist palpates and stabilizes the pelvis with the cranial hand and uses the caudal arm to induce hip rotation. Overpressure can be given at end ROM to assess tissue end feel and to assess for pain provocation.
NOTES	A goniometer can be used to measure the amount of passive rotation attained with this test. The advantage of this test position is that the therapist can limit pelvic motion that may tend to compensate for limited hip motion and the therapist can get a sense of hip joint end feel.

Hip Passive Rotation Range of Motion Test (Prone)

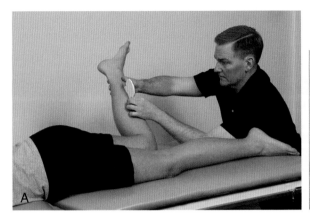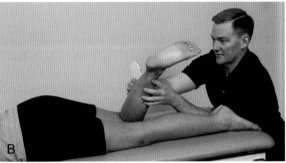

FIG. 4.50 See Video 4.30. A, Use of inclinometer to measure prone hip internal rotation. B, Use of inclinometer to measure prone hip external rotation.

PURPOSE	The purpose of this test is to measure hip rotation ROM in the prone position.
PATIENT POSITION	The patient is prone with the test leg (right) knee flexed at 90 degrees and hip in neutral abduction and the opposite leg knee extended and hip abducted to 30 degrees.
THERAPIST POSITION	The therapist kneels at the foot of the treatment table.
HAND PLACEMENT	Inclinometer hand: This hand holds the gravity inclinometer at the distal one-third of the tibia on the lateral side of the tibia to measure external rotation and is placed on the medial aspect of the tibia to measure internal rotation.
	Other hand: The other hand is placed on the tibia on the opposite side of the inclinometer to guide hip motion.
PROCEDURE	The therapist guides the tibia medially to test hip external rotation and laterally to test hip internal rotation. The angle measured on the inclinometer is read at the end ROM and is recorded in degrees.
NOTES	The pelvis should remain flat on the table during the hip motion. The pelvis rising from the table is an indication that the end range of hip motion has been attained. Hip internal rotation of 35 degrees or greater was one of the components of the CPR for manipulation success for treatment of acute LBP, and Flynn et al.[50] used this method of measurement in developing the CPR. Bullock-Saxton and Bullock[256] reported a kappa value of 0.99 for external rotation and a kappa value of 0.98 for internal rotation for intertester reliability with use of an inclinometer to measure these hip motions.

Sutlive et al.[250] reported kappa values of 0.51 (0.19–0.83) for detection of capsular and noncapsular hip end feels and interexaminer ICC values of 0.88 (0.74–0.94), SEM of 1.8 degrees, and MDC of 5.0 degrees for measurement of ROM when tested on 72 patients with hip pain. Sutlive et al.[250] also reported that passive internal rotation less than 25 degrees was a moderately good indicator of hip joint osteoarthritis with a sensitivity of 0.76 (0.52–0.91), specificity of 0.61 (0.46–0.74), +LR of 1.9 (1.3–3.0), and −LR of 0.39 (0.18–0.86).

Five variables formed a CPR developed for detection of hip osteoarthritis, including: (1) self-reported squatting as an aggravating factor, (2) scour test with adduction causing groin or lateral pain, (3) active hip flexion causing lateral pain, (4) active hip extension causing hip pain, and (5) passive hip internal rotation less than or equal to 25 degrees.[250] If at least four of five variables were present, the +LR was equal to 24.3 (95% CI, 4.4–142.1), increasing the probability of hip osteoarthritis to 91%.[250]

In patients with hip osteoarthritis, Pua[257] reported ICCs of 0.93 (95% CI, 0.83–0.97; SEM, 3.4 degrees) and 0.96 (95% CI, 0.91–0.99; SEM, 3.1 degrees) for internal and external rotation. Ellison[258] reported ICCs for hip internal and external rotation ranging from 0.96 to 0.99 in healthy individuals and 0.95 to 0.97 in people with LBP.

▶ Patella Pubic Percussion Test

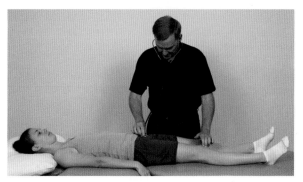

FIG. 4.51 See Video 4.31. Patella pubic percussion test.

PURPOSE	This test is designed to detect the presence of a hip or femur fracture to determine whether further imaging is necessary to confirm the diagnosis.
PATIENT POSITION	Patient is in the supine position with both legs extended on the treatment table.
THERAPIST POSITION	The therapist stands at the side of the patient and positions a stethoscope on the anterior aspect of the patient's pubic symphysis.
PROCEDURE	The therapist firmly taps (percusses) the patella of one knee while auscultating the pubic symphysis. The procedure is repeated with tapping each patella.
NOTES	A positive test is a diminished percussion note on the symptomatic side. A negative test is no difference between the two sides. A tuning fork can be used in place of the percussion. Tiru et al.[259] tested 290 patients with suspected occult hip fractures and used radiographs, bone scintigraphy, MRI, and CT scan as reference standards to make the diagnosis and reported sensitivity of 0.96 (0.87, 0.99), specificity of 0.86 (0.49, 0.98), +LR of 6.73, and −LR of 0.14, which demonstrates that this test is a good screening tool for hip fractures.

ACCESSORY MOTION TESTING AND MANIPULATION OF THE HIP JOINT

 Hip Long Axis Distraction Test and Manipulation

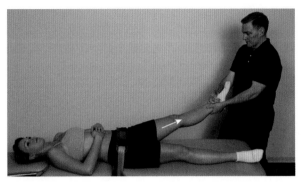

FIG. 4.52 See Video 4.32. Hip long axis distraction test and manipulation.

PURPOSE	This test is used to test the capsular mobility of the hip joint and to mobilize a joint capsule with mobility deficits.
PATIENT POSITION	The patient is supine with the pelvis stabilized by a belt or second examiner.
THERAPIST POSITION	The therapist stands with a diagonal stance at the foot of the table.
HAND PLACEMENT	Both hands are wrapped around the distal tibia just proximal to the ankle joint.
PROCEDURE	The therapist positions the patient's test leg hip in a loose packed position of 30 degrees abduction and 30 degrees flexion. The therapist slowly applies a force to the hip by pulling the leg toward the body in the plane of the test leg. The amount of joint play at one joint is compared with the other hip joint.
NOTES	If muscle holding is seen at the hip joint, the pelvis tends to move as soon as distraction forces are applied to the leg, and the patient may have difficulty relaxing the leg. In osteoarthritic hip joints, this procedure often alleviates the patient's hip area pain. When limitations in hip joint mobility are noted, this procedure can be turned into a joint manipulation by sustaining end-range forces or applying a thrust impulse at the end of the available ROM.

▶ Inferior Glide Accessory Hip Motion Test and Manipulation

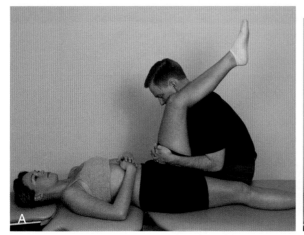
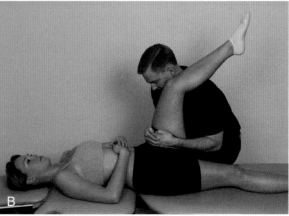
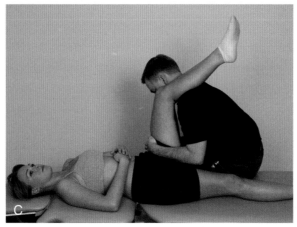

FIG. 4.53 See Video 4.33. A, Inferior glide accessory hip motion test and manipulation. B, Inferior lateral glide accessory hip motion test. C, Inferior medial glide accessory hip motion test.

PURPOSE	This test is used to evaluate the capsular mobility of the hip joint and to mobilize a joint capsule with mobility deficits.
PATIENT POSITION	The patient is supine with the test leg resting on the therapist's shoulder.
THERAPIST POSITION	The therapist sits on the edge of the table with the patient's test leg resting on a shoulder.
HAND PLACEMENT	The therapist overlaps their hands at the anterior aspect of the proximal thigh with the fifth digits of both hands at the crease formed by the flexed hip position.
PROCEDURE	An inferiorly directed force is applied through the femur to produce an inferior glide. The therapist shifts the hands laterally and the body and forearms medially to produce an inferior medial glide. The therapist shifts the hands medially and the forearms and body laterally to produce an inferior lateral glide. The amount of joint play at one joint is compared with the other hip joint.
NOTES	If muscle holding or capsular tightness is present at the hip joint, the pelvis tends to move as soon as gliding forces are applied to the leg, and the patient may have difficulty relaxing the leg. In osteoarthritic hip joints, this procedure often alleviates the patient's hip area pain. When limitations in hip joint mobility are noted, this procedure can be turned into a joint manipulation by sustaining end range forces or applying a thrust impulse at the end of the available ROM.

PASSIVE INTERVERTEBRAL MOTION TECHNIQUES

▶ **Lumbar Forward-Bending Passive Intervertebral Motion Test: Side-Lying With Single Leg Flexion**

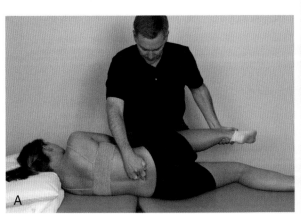
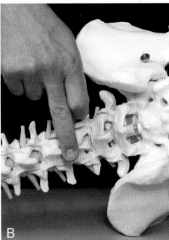

FIG. 4.54 See Video 4.34. A, Lumbar forward-bending passive intervertebral motion (PIVM) test. B, Finger placement for lumbar forward-bending PIVM test.

PURPOSE	This test is used to evaluate the passive forward-bending motion of lumbar segments L5–S1 through T12–L1.
PATIENT POSITION	The patient is in a side-lying position facing the therapist.
THERAPIST POSITION	The therapist stands next to the patient with feet parallel to the table, hips and knees flexed approximately 30 degrees, and weight on the forefeet.
HAND PLACEMENT	Caudal hand: The caudal hand supports the patient's top leg just proximal to the ankle.
	Cranial hand: The pad of the long finger (third digit) is used to palpate the interspinous space of the lumbar segment.
PROCEDURE	The patient's bottom leg is positioned in approximately 30 degrees of hip and knee flexion. The patient's top leg is positioned in approximately 90 degrees of hip and knee flexion. The tibial tuberosity of the patient's top leg should rest on the therapist's anterior hip. The caudal hand is used to support the top leg just proximal to the ankle. With the anterior hip, slight counterpressure is applied through the patient's upper leg to prevent the patient's pelvis from rotating. The therapist induces lumbar forward bending by shifting the body weight toward the patient's head while flexing the patient's hip. The hip is flexed with small amplitude motions, and the pad of the long finger on the cranial hand is used to palpate the interspinous space of the targeted lumbar segment. The therapist palpates for the interspinous space to gap during lumbar forward bending as the inferior vertebra's spinous process of the spinal segment moves inferiorly in relationship to the superior vertebra's spinous process. The amount of passive forward-bending motion available at each lumbar segment is noted and compared.
NOTES	The assessment of PIVM begins at L5–S1 and proceeds cranially. As the assessment proceeds cranially, the amount of hip flexion is increased, but how far the hip is returned toward extension with each successive segment is reduced. This technique can be performed with the patient's top hip adducted (because of the height of the therapist), but the patient's pelvis/trunk should not be allowed to rotate. In patients with wide hips and a narrow waist, a towel roll can be placed under the patient's waist to prevent lateral flexion in the lumbar spine.

Lumbar Forward-Bending Passive Intervertebral Motion Test: Side-Lying With Bilateral Leg Flexion

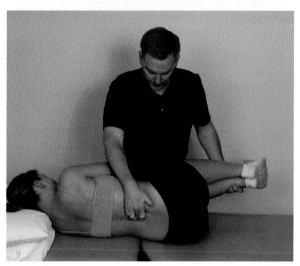

FIG. 4.55 See Video 4.35. Lumbar forward-bending passive intervertebral motion test: side-lying with bilateral leg flexion.

PURPOSE	This test is used to evaluate the passive forward-bending motion of lumbar segments L5–S1 through T12–L1.
PATIENT POSITION	The patient is in a side-lying position facing the therapist and near the edge of the table with hips and knees flexed.
THERAPIST POSITION	The therapist stands in front of the patient with feet parallel to the table and weight on the balls of the feet.
HAND PLACEMENT	Caudal hand: This hand supports the patient's lower leg just proximal to the ankle.
	Cranial hand: The pad of the long finger is used to palpate the interspinous space of the lumbar segment.
PROCEDURE	The patient's legs are positioned together in approximately 90 degrees of hip and knee flexion. The tibial tuberosity of the patient's lower leg should rest on the therapist's anterior hip. The caudal hand is used to support the lower leg just proximal to the ankle. With the therapist's anterior hip, slight counterpressure is applied through the patient's lower leg. The therapist induces lumbar forward bending by shifting body weight toward the patient's head while flexing the patient's hips. The top leg continues to rest on top of the lower leg throughout the procedure. The hip is flexed with small amplitude motions, and the pad of the long finger of the cranial hand is used to palpate the interspinous space of the targeted lumbar segment. The therapist palpates for the interspinous space to gap during lumbar forward bending as the inferior vertebra's spinous process of the spinal segment moves inferiorly in relationship to the superior vertebra's spinous process. The amount of passive forward-bending motion available at each lumbar segment is noted and compared.
NOTES	Assessment of PIVM begins at L5–S1 and proceeds cranially. As the assessment proceeds cranially, the amount of hip flexion is increased, but how far the hip is returned toward extension with each successive segment is reduced. In patients with wide hips and a narrow waist, a towel roll can be placed under the patient's waist to prevent lateral flexion in the lumbar spine.

▶ Modification for Lumbar Backward-Bending Passive Intervertebral Motion Test

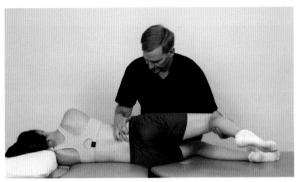

FIG. 4.56 See Video 4.36. Lumbar backward-bending passive intervertebral motion test.

PROCEDURE MODIFICATION

The same therapist palpation and patient positioning can be modified to assess PIVM lumbar backward bending by moving the patient's hips toward extension from the 90-degree hip flexion start position. The therapist's caudal arm and hand support the patient's top leg as the patient's hip is moved into extension to induce passive segmental backward bending. The palpation begins at L5–S1 and proceeds cranially as the legs are moved further toward extension.

NOTES

Abbott et al.[104] reported on the validity of the use of lumbar forward and backward bending PPIVM testing and lumbar posteroanterior PAIVM testing for use in detection of LSI using lumbar flexion/extension radiographs as the reference standard on 138 patients with LBP. Flexion PPIVM tests were highly specific for the diagnosis of translation LSI (specificity 0.99; CI, 0.97–1.00) but showed very poor sensitivity (0.05; CI, 0.01–0.22). LR statistics for flexion PPIVM tests were not statistically significant. Extension PPIVM tests performed better than flexion PPIVM tests, with slightly higher sensitivity (0.16; CI, 0.06–0.38) resulting in a +LR of 7.1 (95% CI, 1.7–29.2) for translation LSI. This research indicates that PIVM test procedures have moderate validity for detecting segmental motion abnormality.[104] Alqarni et al.[260] rated the Abbott et al. study[104] as a moderately high-quality study with a QUADAS score of 19/26.

Lumbar Side Bending (Lateral Flexion) Passive Intervertebral Motion Test in Prone Position

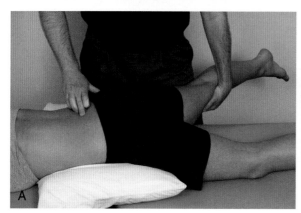

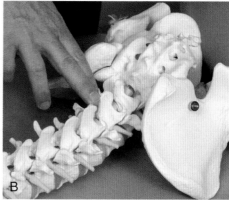

FIG. 4.57 See Video 4.37. A, Lumbar side bending passive intervertebral motion (PIVM), prone lying with hip abduction. B, Hand placement for lumbar side bending PIVM.

PURPOSE	This test evaluates the passive side bending (lateral flexion) motion in the lumbar segments L5–S1 through T12–L1.
PATIENT POSITION	The patient is prone with a pillow under the abdomen and pelvis.
THERAPIST POSITION	The therapist stands next to the patient.
HAND PLACEMENT	Caudal hand: The caudal hand supports the patient's right leg at the knee while avoiding compression of the patient's patella.
	Cranial hand: The pad of the long finger is used to palpate the lateral aspect of the interspinous space of the lumbar segment.
PROCEDURE	The therapist stands on the patient's right side and induces lumbar side bending to the right by abducting the patient's right hip with the caudal hand. The hip is abducted, and the pad of the long finger on the cranial hand is used to palpate the right lateral aspect of the interspinous space of the specified lumbar segment. The therapist palpates for the interspinous space to close down into the palpating finger by palpating the lateral edge of the inferior spinous process in relation to the lateral edge of the superior spinous process. The amount of passive side bending motion available at each segment is noted and compared. Lumbar side bending to the left is induced with the therapist standing on the patient's left side and repeating the procedure abducting the left hip. The amount of passive side bending motion available at each segment and in each direction is noted and compared.

Lumbar Side Bending (Lateral Flexion) Passive Intervertebral Motion Test in Prone Position—cont'd

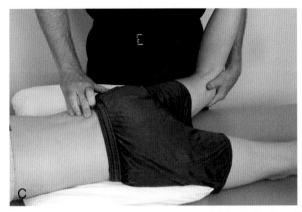

FIG. 4.57, cont'd C, Lumbar side bending PIVM, prone lying with hip abduction with the knee flexed.

PROCEDURE MODIFICATION	This technique can also be performed with the patient's knee slightly flexed (Fig. 4.57C). However, the therapist should avoid excessive knee flexion with tightness of the rectus femoris muscle.
NOTES	Assessment of PIVM begins at L5–S1 and proceeds cranially. As the assessment proceeds cranially, the amount of hip abduction is increased, but the range through which the hip is adducted with each successive segment is decreased. With support of the patient's leg, hip extension and compression of the patella should be avoided.

Prone Lumbar Side Bending Passive Intervertebral Motion Test With a Mobilization Table

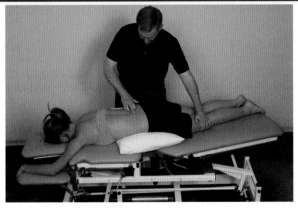

FIG. 4.58 See Video 4.38. Use of mobilization table to assess prone side bending.

PROCEDURE MODIFICATION	This technique can be modified with use of a mobilization table. The cranial palpating hand remains the same, but the spinal side-bending motion is induced by moving the lower half of the table laterally, with the patient's legs resting on the table.

Lumbar Side Bending (Lateral Flexion) Passive Intervertebral Motion Test: Side-Lying With Rocking the Pelvis

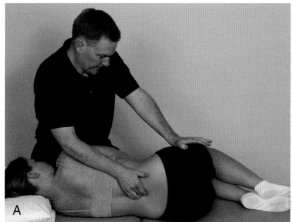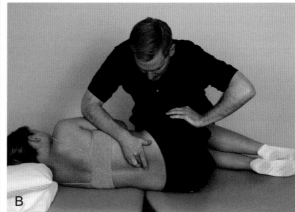

FIG. 4.59 See Video 4.39. A, Lumbar side bending left passive intervertebral motion (PIVM), side-lying with rocking the pelvis. B, Lumbar side bending right PIVM, side-lying with rocking the pelvis.

PURPOSE   This test is used to evaluate the passive side bending segmental motion in the lumbar segments L5–S1 through T12–L1.

PATIENT POSITION   The patient is in a side-lying position facing the therapist with the hips and knees flexed to 90 degrees.

THERAPIST POSITION   The therapist stands with a diagonal stance in front of the patient and facing the patient's pelvis.

HAND PLACEMENT   Caudal hand: The palm of the hand is placed on the patient's greater trochanter.

Cranial hand: The pad of the long finger is used to palpate the lateral aspect of the interspinous space of the lumbar segment.

PROCEDURE   With the patient in a left side-lying position, both legs are positioned in 90 degrees of hip and knee flexion. The superior aspect of the greater trochanter is contacted with the heel of the caudal hand. Lumbar side bending to the left is induced with the caudal hand pushing the patient's greater trochanter caudally (Fig. 4.59A). The pad of the long finger on the cranial hand is used to palpate the left lateral aspect of the interspinous space of the specified lumbar segment. The therapist palpates for the interspinous space to close down into the palpating finger on the concavity formed with the side-bend motion. The amount of passive side-bending motion available at each segment is noted and compared.

Lumbar side bending to the right is induced with the caudal hand pushing the patient's greater trochanter cranially (Fig. 4.59B). The pad of the long finger on the cranial hand is used to palpate the right lateral aspect of the interspinous space of the specified lumbar segment. The therapist palpates for the interspinous process to close down into the palpating finger. The amount of passive side-bending motion available at each segment for both directions is noted and compared.

NOTES   Assessment of PIVM begins at L5–S1 and proceeds cranially. The forearm should be positioned parallel to the direction of the force applied through the greater trochanter. The procedure can be performed with the patient in a right side-lying position, with caudal movement of the pelvis inducing right side bending and cranial movement of the pelvis inducing left side bending. Assessment of lumbar side bending with this technique (e.g., rocking the pelvis) is useful for patients with hip pathology (the hip needs to be protected).

Lumbar Rotation Passive Intervertebral Motion Test: Prone Lying With Rolling the Legs

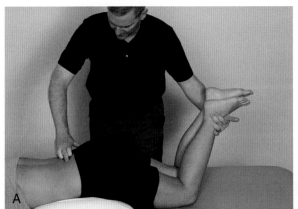
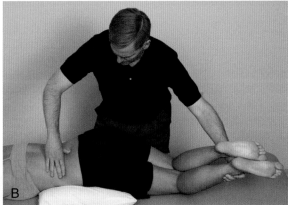
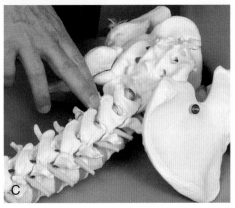

FIG. 4.60 See Video 4.40. A, Lumbar right rotation passive intervertebral motion (PIVM), prone lying with rolling the legs. B, Lumbar left rotation PIVM, prone lying with rolling the legs. C, Finger placement for palpation for lumbar rotation PIVM.

PURPOSE	This test evaluates the passive rotation of lumbar segments L5–S1 through T12–L1.
PATIENT POSITION	The patient is prone with a pillow under the abdomen and pelvis.
THERAPIST POSITION	The therapist stands next to the patient.
HAND PLACEMENT	Caudal hand: The caudal hand supports both of the patient's legs at the ankles.
	Cranial hand: The pad of the long finger is used to palpate the lateral aspect of the interspinous space of the lumbar segment.
PROCEDURE	Both of the patient's knees are flexed to approximately 45 to 60 degrees, and the legs are supported at the ankles with the caudal hand and forearm. Right rotation of the lumbar spine is induced with rolling the legs toward the patient's right side (Fig. 4.60A). The pad of the long finger on the cranial hand is used to palpate the right lateral aspect of the interspinous space of the specified segment. The therapist palpates for the spinous process of the lower member of the segment to rotate or press into the palpating finger in relation to the superior member of the segment's spinous process. The amount of right rotation available at each segment is noted and compared. Left rotation is induced with rolling the legs toward the patient's left side (Fig. 4.60B). The pad of the thumb can be used to palpate the left lateral aspect of the interspinous space of the specified segment. The therapist palpates for the spinous process of the lower member of the segment to rotate or press into the palpating finger (Fig. 4.60C). The amount of left rotation available at each segment is noted and compared. The amount of rotation available in each direction is compared.

Lumbar Rotation Passive Intervertebral Motion Test: Prone Lying With Rolling the Legs—cont'd

NOTES	Assessment of PIVM begins at L5–S1 and proceeds cranially. As the assessment progresses cranially, the amount of rotation of the legs is increased, but the amount of rotation back toward the midline with each successive segment is decreased. This technique follows the rule of the leg, which states that the direction of the movement of the legs is the same as the direction of the rotation of the lumbar spine (i.e., rolling the legs to the right induces right rotation of the lumbar spine). The direction of rotation is based on the direction of rotation of the vertebral body of the superior member of the spinal segment in relation to the inferior member of the segment.

Lumbar Rotation Passive Intervertebral Motion Test: Prone Lying With Raising the Pelvis

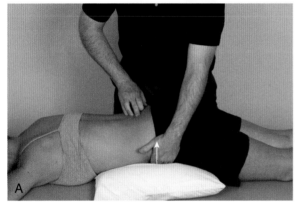 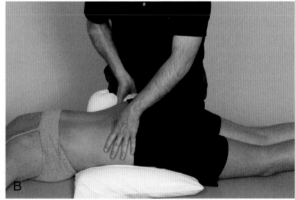

FIG. 4.61 See Video 4.41. A, Lumbar right rotation, prone lying with raising the pelvis. B, Lumbar left rotation, prone lying with raising the pelvis.

PURPOSE	This test is used to evaluate the passive rotation of lumbar segments L5–S1 through T12–L1.
PATIENT POSITION	The patient is prone with a pillow under the abdomen and pelvis.
THERAPIST POSITION	The therapist stands next to the patient.
HAND PLACEMENT	Caudal hand: The fingers grasp the patient's pelvis under the ASIS.
	Cranial hand: The pad of the long finger palpates the lateral aspect of the interspinous space.

Lumbar Rotation Passive Intervertebral Motion Test: Prone Lying With Raising the Pelvis—cont'd

PROCEDURE   With the therapist standing on the patient's right side, the fingers of the caudal hand are used to grasp the patient's pelvis under the left ASIS. Right lumbar rotation is induced with gentle lifting of the pelvis in a rotary manner. The pad of the long finger on the cranial hand palpates the right lateral aspect of the interspinous space of the specified lumbar segment. The therapist palpates for the spinous process of the lower member of the segment to rotate or press into the palpating finger. The amount of passive rotation available at each segment is noted and compared. Left lumbar rotation is induced with grasping the patient's pelvis under the right ASIS (with the fingers of the caudal hand) and gently lifting the pelvis in a rotary manner. The pad of the long finger or thumb on the cranial hand is used to palpate the left lateral aspect of the interspinous space of the specified lumbar segment. The therapist palpates for the spinous process of the lower member of the segment to rotate or press into the palpating finger. The amount of passive rotation available at each segment is noted and compared. The amount of rotation available in each direction is compared.

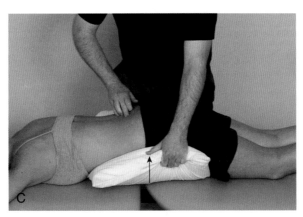

FIG. 4.61, cont'd C, Lumbar right rotation, prone lying raising the pelvis with assistance of a pillow.

NOTES   Assessment begins at L5–S1 and proceeds cranially. The amount of lifting of the pelvis is increased with assessment of each successive cranial segment. This technique can be performed with the therapist standing on the same side of the patient to assess both right and left rotation (as described), or the therapist can switch sides to assess the rotation available in each direction. When this technique is performed, the therapist should be aware that just placing the hand under the patient's pelvis can induce enough movement to rotate L5–S1. To prevent this occurrence, the therapist should push the hand into the pillow/table to allow the patient's pelvis to remain in a neutral position. This technique can also be performed with the pillow used to lift the pelvis (Fig. 4.61C). Assessment of lumbar rotation with this technique (e.g., lifting the pelvis) is useful for patients with hip pathology (the hip needs to be protected).

Lumbar Rotation Passive Accessory Intervertebral Motion Test: Spring Testing Through the Transverse Processes

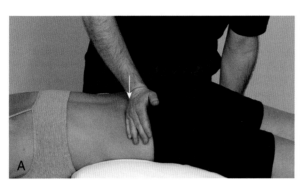

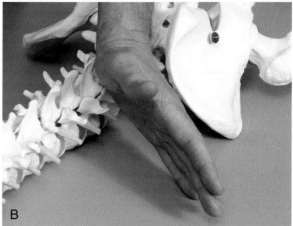

FIG. 4.62 See Video 4.42. A, Lumbar rotation, spring testing through left L3 transverse process. B, Hand placement for lumbar rotation, spring testing through the left L3 transverse process.

PURPOSE	This test evaluates the passive rotation of lumbar segments L5–S1 through L2–L3 and assesses the level of reactivity of lumbar segments L5–S1 through L2–L3 (pain provocation test).
PATIENT POSITION	The patient is prone with a pillow under the abdomen and pelvis.
THERAPIST POSITION	The therapist stands next to the patient.
HAND PLACEMENT	Caudal hand: This hand supports the therapist's body weight on the edge of the treatment table.
	Cranial hand: The proximal ulnar aspect of the fifth metacarpal contacts the transverse process (Fig. 4.62A and B).
PROCEDURE	With the therapist standing on the patient's right side, the ulnar aspect of the fifth metacarpal on the caudal hand locates the iliac crest on the patient's left side. The ulnar aspect of the fifth metacarpal locates the 12th rib on the patient's left side. The hands make a V shape (Fig. 4.62C).

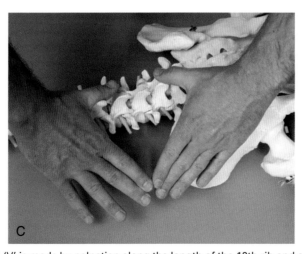

FIG. 4.62, cont'd C, A 'V' is made by palpation along the length of the 12th rib and along the iliac crest angle to identify L2–L4 transverse processes.

Lumbar Rotation Passive Accessory Intervertebral Motion Test: Spring Testing Through the Transverse Processes—cont'd

The transverse process of L3 is located at the point of the V. The ulnar aspect of the fifth metacarpal of the cranial hand is used to "sink into" the middle of the V at the location of the L3 transverse process (see Fig. 4.62A and B). The therapist should take up the slack and spring (i.e., midrange thrust) the transverse process of L3. The amount of passive right rotation available at the segment is noted (spring testing the transverse process of L3 assesses the mobility of the L3–L4 segment). Pain provocation is also noted. The procedure is repeated with the transverse processes of L2 (located just inferior to the 12th rib, segment L2–L3) and L4 (located just superior to the iliac crest, segment L4–L5). L5–S1 is tested with placement of the middle crease of the cranial hand on the patient's right PSIS with the thenar eminence on the sacral sulcus (Fig. 4.62D). The therapist takes up the slack and springs the L5–S1 segment by giving a posteroanterior force. The amount of passive right rotation available at the segment is noted. Pain provocation is also noted. The procedure is repeated with assessment of the opposite side spinal segments (Fig. 4.62E). The amount of rotation available and the level of reactivity in each direction at each segment are compared.

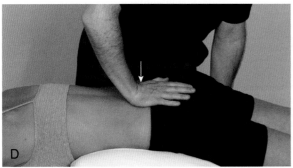 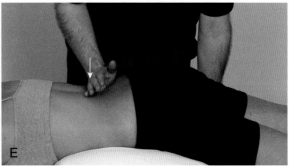

FIG. 4.62, cont'd D, Lumbar rotation, spring testing through the right posterior superior sacroiliac spine and sacral sulcus to target right L5S1 motion. E, Lumbar rotation, spring testing through the right L2 transverse process.

NOTES   The therapist is recommended to spring with the cranial hand to remain specific and consistent with this technique. Spring testing of segments L2–L3 through L4–L5 on the left induces right rotation, and spring testing segment L5–S1 (through the PSIS and sacral base) on the left induces left rotation. The forearm of the arm that gives the impulse should be near to parallel to the direction of the force applied. Assessment of rotation tests the ability of the facet joint on the ipsilateral side to gap (i.e., right rotation tests the ability of the right facet joint to gap). Pain provocation with spring testing the L5–S1 segment could indicate tissue sensitivity at that segment or the SIJ.

▶ Central Posteroanterior Passive Accessory Intervertebral Motion Test

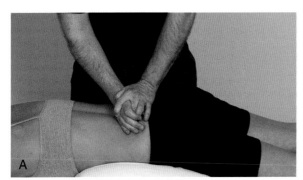
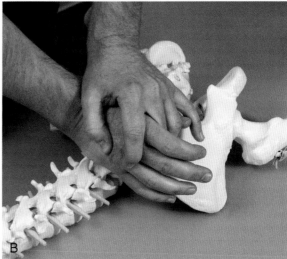

FIG. 4.63 See Video 4.43. A, Central posteroanterior passive accessory intervertebral motion (PAIVM) test, two-handed technique. B, Hand positioning for central posteroanterior PAIVM test.

PURPOSE	This test is used for PAIVM or pain provocation of the lumbar spinal segments. For intervention, the appropriate grade of mobilization (I–IV) to treat pain or hypomobility is used.
PATIENT POSITION	The patient lies prone over a pillow with the arms by the body or hanging off the edge of the table. A pillow can be placed under the lower legs for comfort.
THERAPIST POSITION	The therapist stands at the side of patient.
HAND PLACEMENT	Right hand: The right hand is placed on the patient's back so that the ulnar border of the hand just distal to the pisiform is in contact with the spinous process of the vertebrae to be mobilized. The shoulders are directly over the patient. The right wrist is fully extended with the forearm midway between supination and pronation.
	Left hand: The right hand is reinforced with the left hand so that the second and third digits of the left hand envelop the second metacarpal phalangeal joint of the right hand. The elbows are allowed to slightly flex.
PROCEDURE	The therapist applies a posteroanterior force on each spinous process examined and performs a total of three slow repetitions. First pressures should be applied gently; amplitude and depth of the movement are increased if no pain response occurs. The therapist assesses the quality of movement through the range and the end feel and compares it with the levels above and below.
NOTES	A midrange of passive movement thrust (spring test) could also be used with this technique to assess tissue resistance and pain provocation.
	A positive response is movement that reproduces the comparable sign (pain or resistance or muscle guarding). This PAIVM test can be modified as a nonthrust mobilization treatment technique for graded oscillations I to IV.

Central Posteroanterior Passive Accessory Intervertebral Motion Test—cont'd

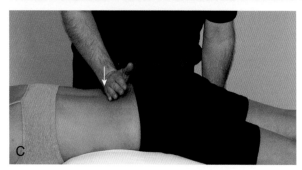

FIG. 4.63, cont'd C, Central posteroanterior PAIVM test, one-handed technique commonly used for spring testing.

PROCEDURE MODIFICATION This technique could also be done as a one-handed technique with the cranial hand contacting the spinous process just distal to the pisiform, the elbow flexed, and the forearm perpendicular with the angle of the contour of the surface of the spine (Fig. 4.63C). The caudal hand rests at the edge of the table to support the therapist's upper body weight with leaning over the patient.

NOTES The two-handed posteroanterior PAIVM test was used in development of CPRs for both stabilization and manipulation and has been included as one of the primary findings in clinical decision making for identification of patients who respond to stabilization if hypermobility is noted and to manipulation if hypomobility is noted with this PAIVM procedure.[50,51] Fritz et al.[102] reported intertester reliability ($n = 49$ patients with LBP) for findings of hypomobility of 77% agreement with a kappa value of 0.38 (0.22, 0.54), for findings of hypermobility of 77% agreement with a kappa value of 0.48 (0.35, 0.61), and for findings of pain provocation of 85% agreement with a kappa value of 0.57 (0.43, 0.71). The finding of lack of hypomobility with central posteroanterior PAIVM testing combined with lumbar flexion of more than 53 degrees showed a +LR of 12.8 for correlation with radiographic evidence of lumbar instability.[102] Alqarni et al.[260] rated the Fritz et al.[102] study as a very high - quality study with a QUADAS score of 25/26.

Abbott et al.[104] reported on the validity of the use of lumbar forward and backward bending PIVM testing and posteroanterior PAIVM testing for use in detection of LSI, using lumbar flexion/extension radiographs as the reference standard on 138 patients with LBP. PAIVMs were specific for the diagnosis of translation LSI (specificity 0.89, CI, 0.83–0.93), but showed poor sensitivity (0.29, CI, 0.14–0.50). A positive test results in a +LR of 2.52 (95% CI, 1.15–5.53). This research indicates that PIVM test procedures have moderate validity for detecting segmental motion abnormality.[104] Alqarni et al.[260] rated the study by Abbott et al. as a moderately high - quality study with a QUADAS score of 19/26.

MANIPULATION TECHNIQUES FOR LUMBAR SPINE, PELVIS, AND HIPS

▶ Lumbopelvic Manipulation in Supine

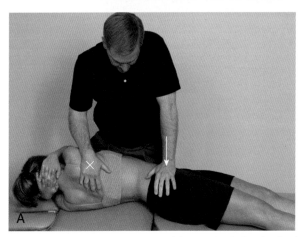

FIG. 4.64 See Video 4.44. A, Lumbopelvic manipulation in Supine.

PURPOSE	This technique restores lumbopelvic mobility and reduces lumbopelvic pain.
PATIENT POSITION	The patient is supine on the treatment table.
THERAPIST POSITION	The therapist stands on the side opposite the side to be manipulated.
PROCEDURE	The pelvis is translated toward the therapist's side of the table (Fig. 4.64B). The therapist maximally side bends the patient's lower extremities and trunk to the right (Fig. 4.64C). Without losing the right side bending, the therapist lifts and left rotates the trunk so that the patient rests on her left shoulder (Fig. 4.64D).

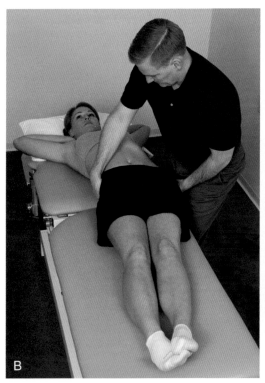

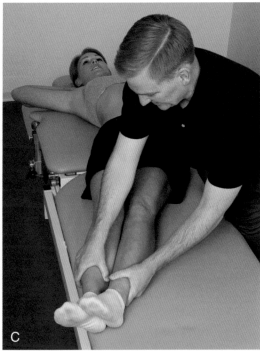

FIG. 4.64, cont'd B, Therapist translates pelvis toward therapist side of table. C, Maximally side bend patient's lower extremities and trunk to the right.

Lumbopelvic (Sacroiliac Region) Manipulation—cont'd

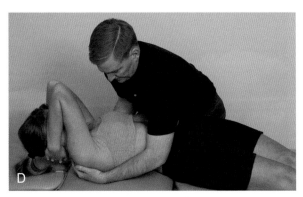

FIG. 4.64, cont'd D, Lift and rotation of patient's upper body.

The patient's right ASIS and ilium is contacted in a broad comfortable manner with the therapist's left hand. The top shoulder and scapula are grasped with the therapist's right hand, and the trunk is rotated to the left with the right side bending maintained. Once the right ASIS starts to elevate, a counter anterior-to-posterior force is applied through the ASIS to further take up the tissue slack, and once a firm barrier to motion is reached, a high-velocity, low-amplitude thrust is performed through the pelvis in an anterior-to-posterior direction.

PROCEDURE MODIFICATION An alternative method is use of the cranial forearm and hand across the scapula, thoracic, and lumbar spine to maintain the locked spinal position (Fig. 4.64E).

PROCEDURE MODIFICATION An alternative method to assist in maintaining lumbar side bending is to hook the patient's ipsilateral heel over the opposite edge of the treatment table (Fig. 4.65F).

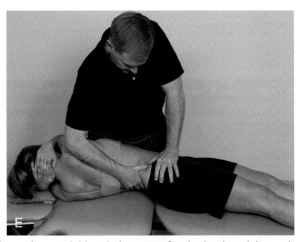

FIG. 4.64, cont'd E, Alternative cranial hand placement for the lumbopelvic manipulation technique.

NOTES Flynn et al.[50] used this technique to develop the CPR for manipulation for treatment of acute LBP. This CPR was validated by Childs et al.[48] who also used this technique with a different sample of patients and clinicians. This technique could be used to treat hypomobility impairments of the lower lumbar spine, lumbosacral junction, and SIJ on the targeted side.

Lumbar Rotation Manipulation in Side-Lying

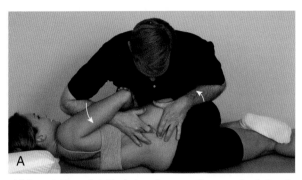

FIG. 4.65 See Videos 4.45 and 4.46. A, Lumbar rotation manipulation in side-lying.

PURPOSE	This technique manipulates a specific lumbar segment (L1–L2 through L5–S1) into rotation.
PATIENT POSITION	The patient is positioned side-lying facing the therapist with the bottom leg in approximately 30 degrees of hip and knee flexion.
THERAPIST POSITION	The therapist stands in front of the patient with feet parallel with the table, weight on the balls of the feet, and hips and knees slightly flexed in an athletic stance position. The patient's top knee is positioned in the "hip hollow" at the anterior hip shelf of the therapist created by slight flexing of the hips and knees, and the therapist presses the front of the hip into the patient's knee to support the top leg.
HAND PLACEMENT	Caudal hand: The technique begins with grasping of the patient's top leg just proximal to the ankle to induce hip flexion and lumbar forward bending. Cranial hand: The pad of the long finger contacts the interspinous space of the targeted spinal segment to assess forward bending to begin the technique setup.
PROCEDURE	The single-leg forward-bending PIVM technique is used to forward bend the lumbar spine up to the segment to be manipulated, and then the hip and spine are slightly extended to maintain the spinal segment inferior to the targeted segment in a forward bent position and to maintain the targeted segment in neutral. Once this point is reached, the top leg is "hooked" onto the bottom leg (i.e., the foot of the top leg rests behind the knee of the bottom leg) (Fig. 4.65B).

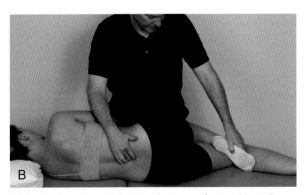

FIG. 4.65, cont'd B, Hook top leg on bottom leg once forward-bending position has been reached for lumbar rotation technique.

Lumbar Rotation Manipulation in Side-Lying—cont'd

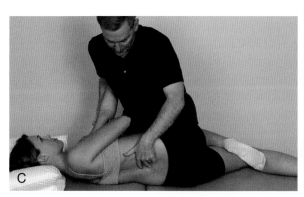
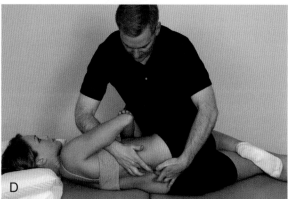

FIG. 4.65, cont'd C, Rotation of spine to include segment above the level to be manipulated. D, Hand and arm positioning to set up lumbar rotation technique.

The position of the hands are now switched so that the pad of the third digit of the caudal hand now palpates the interspinous space of the targeted segment and the second digit palpates one segment above. The spine is rotated to include the segment superior to the segment to be manipulated, but the segment to be manipulated is maintained in neutral. This is accomplished by pulling the patient's bottom arm (from proximal to the elbow) in a forward and upward rotary motion with the cranial hand (Fig. 4.65C). Next, fold the patient's arms loosely across the patient's chest (Fig. 4.65D).

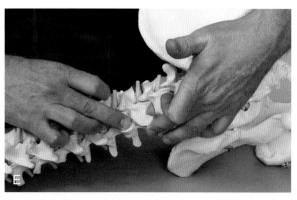

FIG. 4.65, cont'd E, Finger placement for lumbar rotation manipulation.

The cranial hand slides underneath the patient's top arm, and the pad of the long finger contacts the top right lateral side of the spinous process of the cranial member of the segment (Fig. 4.65E). The pad of the long finger of the caudal hand is used to contact the left lateral (bottom) side of the spinous process of the caudal member of the segment (Fig. 4.65E).

The cranial leg is used to step into the edge of the table toward the patient so that the caudal leg leaves the ground and the knee on the patient's upper leg slides down the thigh of the therapist's caudal leg (Fig. 4.65F). Equal and opposite forces through the forearms (with contact with the patient's right anterior shoulder and chest and the right posterior hip and pelvis) are used to take up the slack and induce right rotation of the specified segment. The manipulation is coordinated with the patient's breathing, with progressive oscillation into more rotation each time.

Lumbar Rotation Manipulation in Side-Lying—cont'd

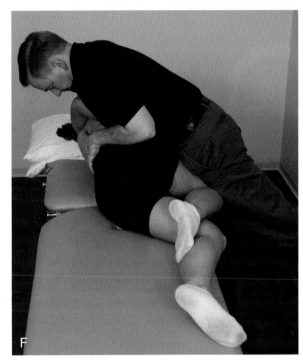

FIG. 4.65, cont'd F, Lumbar rotation manipulation caudal view to illustrate therapist body position.

The manipulation is repeated through approximately three breathing cycles. Once an end-range barrier is established, a short-amplitude, high-velocity thrust may be imparted. After completion of the manipulation, the spine is derotated to a neutral position and PIVM of the specified segment can be retested. For manipulation of a lumbar segment into left rotation, the procedure is repeated with the patient in the right side-lying position.

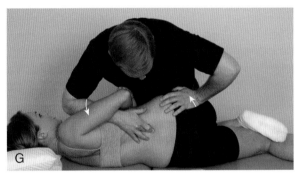

FIG. 4.65, cont'd See Video 4.47. G, An alternative caudal hand/arm position for the lumbar rotation manipulation technique, to target L5S1.

PROCEDURE MODIFICATION   An alternative caudal hand/arm position can assist in creation of greater leverage and can further lock the spine for production of an effective thrust manipulation, especially at the L5–S1 segment (Fig. 4.65G).

NOTES   Impairment-based indications for use of the right rotation manipulation technique are decreased right rotation PIVM or PAIVM testing and limited AROM of the lumbar spine. Indications for use of the left rotation manipulation technique are decreased left rotation PIVM or PAIVM testing and limited AROM of the lumbar spine. This technique is best performed as a progressive oscillation and is best combined with deep breathing for mechanical effects. Acute disk involvement, spondylolysis, or spondylolisthesis are considered precautions for performance of this technique.

Lumbar Rotation Manipulation in Side-Lying—cont'd

Further adjustments can be made in the technique to enhance the success of high-velocity thrust manipulation. The technique set up is the same for the thrust, but emphasis is placed on use of the therapist forearms as the points of contact. Once the spinal segment is isolated with locking out the segments above and below as previously described, log-rolling the patient toward the therapist is helpful to create a 45-degree angle of the patient's pelvis in relation to the table and allow better use of gravity. The therapist's caudal forearm and body weight rotate the pelvis and lumbar spine toward the floor, and a counterforce is applied through the thorax with the cranial forearm.

If the patient has difficulty relaxing during a direct manipulation, use of an isometric manipulation technique can be effective. Once the segment is isolated and the spine is locked superior and inferior to the targeted segment as previously described, the patient is instructed to actively press the pelvis back into the therapist's forearm. After this force output (about 50% of maximum) is resisted for 10 seconds, the patient is asked to relax as the therapist takes up the tissue slack to apply a greater stretch and hold for 10 seconds. At this new barrier point, the isometric rotation is repeated and immediately followed by further stretching. After this sequence is repeated three to four times, the therapist applies further end range oscillations, or a sustained stretch, or a thrust manipulation.

After application of the manipulation, the patient is gently repositioned in a neutral side-lying position, and muscle tone and passive lumbar mobility are reassessed to determine the effectiveness of the manipulation. If objective or subjective improvements are noted, the patient is progressed to active lumbar ROM exercises, spinal stabilization exercises, or functional activities, such as walking on a treadmill. In general, it is advisable to have the patient functionally use the new mobility gained with the manipulation after the procedure. The follow-up activities also allow the therapist further opportunity to assess the effectiveness of the manual therapy interventions.

▶ Modification: Lumbar Rotation Manipulation Initiated Caudally

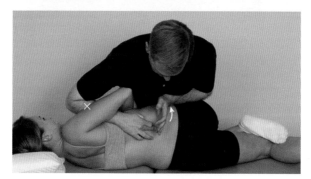

FIG. 4.66 See Video 4.48. Modification: Lumbar rotation manipulation initiated caudally.

PROCEDURE MODIFICATION

The setup and hand placement are the same as in the side-lying lumbar rotation manipulation, but instead of equal and opposite forces used with both arms, the cranial arm stabilizes as the caudal forearm provides the manipulative force. This variation should be used when spinal segments cranial to the targeted segment are either highly reactive or unstable.

▶ Modification: Lumbar Rotation Manipulation Initiated Cranially

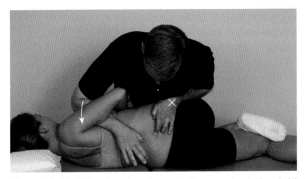

FIG. 4.67 See Video 4.49. Modification: Lumbar rotation manipulation initiated cranially.

PROCEDURE MODIFICATION   The setup and hand placement are the same as in the side-lying lumbar rotation manipulation, but instead of equal and opposite forces used with both arms, the caudal arm stabilizes the pelvis and lower spinal segments as the cranial forearm provides the manipulative force (Fig. 4.67). This variation should be used when spinal segments caudal to the targeted segment are either highly reactive or unstable.

▶ Modification: Lumbar Rotation Manipulation With Lateral Flexion

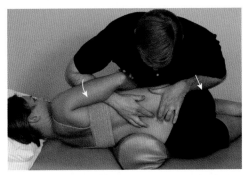

FIG. 4.68 See Video 4.50. Modification: Lumbar rotation manipulation with lateral flexion.

PROCEDURE MODIFICATION   The setup and hand placement are the same as in the side-lying lumbar rotation manipulation, but the patient starts the procedure by lying over a bolster to induce lateral flexion to the opposite direction of the rotation (Fig. 4.68). The caudal forearm can also rock the lateral (top) aspect of the pelvis inferiorly and downward to induce further lateral flexion. Lateral flexion could be used as either the primary or secondary lever with the technique. If lateral flexion is used as the primary lever, the manipulative force is with the caudal arm. If lateral flexion is used as the secondary lever to assist in taking up tissue slack, the manipulative force is with equal and opposite forces from both arms or either the caudal or cranial forces are emphasized. Care must be taken to maintain the lumbar spine in neutral or slight backward bending at the targeted segment when lateral flexion is used as a primary or secondary lever.

▶ Lumbosacral Lift Manipulation

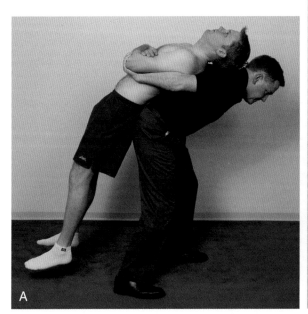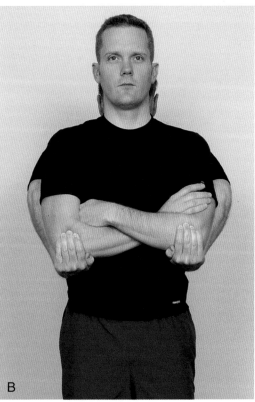

FIG. 4.69 See Video 4.51. A, A Lumbosacral lift manipulation. B, Patient arm position and therapist hand placement.

PURPOSE	This technique is used to manipulate the lumbosacral junction (L5–S1) with a distractive force.
PATIENT POSITION	The patient stands with the arms folded firmly across the chest (Fig. 4.69B).
THERAPIST POSITION	The therapist stands with a diagonal stance with the back to the patient.
HAND PLACEMENT	Each hand is cupped across the inferior aspect of the patient's elbows.
PROCEDURE	The therapist leans forward, hinging at the hips, with the lumbar spine stabilized in a neutral position, to backward bend the patient to the lumbosacral junction and lift the patient's feet off the floor. The therapist's buttock should contact the patient's lumbosacral junction. The therapist can apply the thrust by rising up on the toes and dropping the heels abruptly to the ground or by jumping off the ground and landing with the legs and trunk held rigidly. In this way, the ground reaction forces cause the manipulative thrust.
NOTES	If the patient is taller than the therapist, the patient may need to spread the legs to assure the correct alignment of the therapist's buttock to the patient's lumbosacral junction. If the patient is much shorter than the therapist, the therapist needs to flex a greater degree at the hips and knees to create the proper patient-to-therapist alignment. Joint distraction at the lumbosacral junction occurs with the initial lift position and may be all the force that is needed for an effective technique. The therapist is advised to first lift the patient without applying the thrust and to reassess the patient's tolerance to the positioning before resetting the technique and applying the thrust. In addition to restoring mobility at the lumbosacral junction, this technique can be used to correct sacroiliac dysfunctions.

Lumbar Spine Side Bending (Lateral Flexion) Manipulation: Prone Abducting the Leg With a Thumb or Finger Block

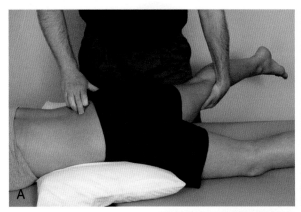
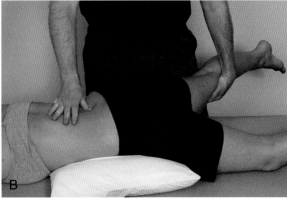
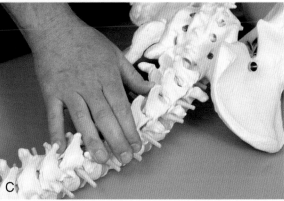

FIG. 4.70 See Video 4.52. A, Lumbar spine lateral flexion manipulation, prone abducting the leg with finger block. B, Lumbar spine lateral flexion manipulation, prone abducting the leg with thumb block. C, Thumb placement to create fulcrum for lumbar spine lateral flexion manipulation, prone abducting the leg with thumb block.

PURPOSE	This technique is used to manipulate a specific lumbar segment (L1–L2 through L5–S1) into side bending.
PATIENT POSITION	The patient is prone with a pillow under the abdomen and pelvis.
THERAPIST POSITION	The therapist stands next to the patient.
HAND PLACEMENT	Caudal hand: The caudal hand supports the patient's right leg at the knee but avoids patella compression.
	Cranial hand: The pad of the thumb or long finger is used to block the lateral aspect of the spinous process of the cranial member of the segment.
PROCEDURE	The therapist stands on the patient's right side and uses the pad of the thumb or long finger of the cranial hand to block the right lateral aspect of the spinous process of the cranial member of the specified segment. Lumbar side bending to the right is induced by abducting the patient's right hip with the caudal hand and keeping the leg even with the top of the table to avoid excessive hip extension/lumbar lordosis (Fig. 4.70). The therapist takes up the slack and oscillates. On completion of the manipulation, lumbar side bending is retested.
	The spinal segment is manipulated into side bending to the left with the therapist standing on the patient's left side and repeating the procedure abducting the left hip.

Lumbar Spine Side Bending (Lateral Flexion) Manipulation: Prone Abducting the Leg With a Thumb or Finger Block—cont'd

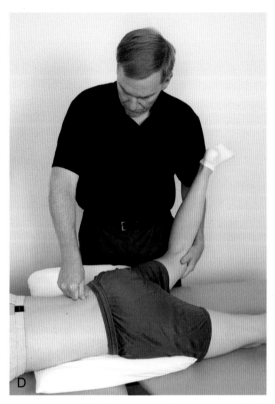

FIG. 4.70, cont'd D, Lumbar spine lateral flexion manipulation, prone abducting the leg with finger block with the knee flexed.

PROCEDURE MODIFICATION This technique can also be performed with the patient's knee slightly flexed (Fig. 4.50D).

NOTES Impairment-based indications for use of the right side bending manipulation technique are decreased lumbar AROM and right side bending PIVM testing of a specific lumbar segment (L1–L2 through L5–S1). Indications for use of the left side bending manipulation technique are decreased lumbar AROM and left side bending of a specific lumbar segment (L1–L2 through L5–S1). With proper handling of the patient's leg, excessive hip extension and compression of the patella are avoided. However, excessive knee flexion with tightness of the rectus femoris muscle should be avoided. This technique is most commonly used as a grade III (nonthrust) mobilization for mechanical effects. Hip pathologic conditions are a precaution with this technique.

Lumbar Spine Side Bending (Lateral Flexion) Manipulation With a Mobilization Table and a Thumb Block

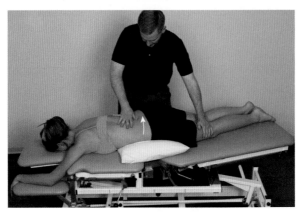

FIG. 4.71 See Video 4.53. Lumbar spine side bending (lateral flexion) manipulation with a mobilization table and a thumb block.

PROCEDURE MODIFICATION   The prone lumbar spine side bending manipulation is even more effective with use of a mobilization table. The cranial hand function remains the same; but instead of abduction of the hip to induce lateral flexion, the lateral flexion function of the table is used to swing both legs and the lumbar spine into a lateral flexion passive motion (Fig. 4.71).

Side Bending Myofascial Stretch

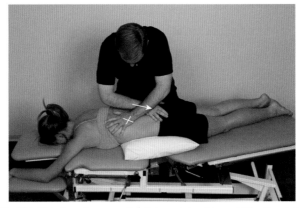

FIG. 4.72 Side bending myofascial stretch with mobilization table.

PROCEDURE   A side bending myofascial stretch can also be applied with the use of the mobilization table with placement of the hands on the upper and lower lumbar spine as the stretch is applied (Fig. 4.72). The stretch should be sustained for at least 30 seconds and repeated three to four times.

Lumbar Spine Side Bending Manipulation: Side-Lying Raising and Lowering the Legs

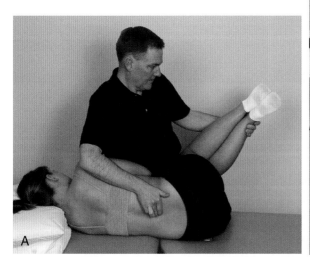
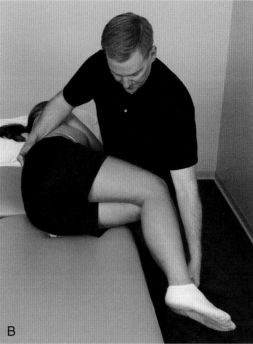

FIG. 4.73 See Videos 4.54 and 4.55. A, Lumbar spine side bending manipulation, side-lying raising the legs. B, Lumbar spine side bending manipulation lowering the legs.

PURPOSE	This manipulation is used to move a specific lumbar segment (L1–L2 through L5–S1) into side bending.
PATIENT POSITION	The patient is positioned side-lying facing the therapist with the hips and knees flexed to 90 degrees.
THERAPIST POSITION	The therapist stands with a diagonal stance in front of the patient facing the patient's thighs with the caudal leg forward, flexed, and supporting the patient's bottom thigh.
HAND PLACEMENT	Caudal hand: This hand holds the patient's bottom leg just proximal to the ankle.
	Cranial hand: The pad of the long finger is used to block the lateral aspect of the spinous process of the cranial member of the segment.
PROCEDURE	With the patient in a left side-lying position, both legs are positioned in 90 degrees of hip and knee flexion. For manipulation of the segment into right side bending, the pad of the long finger on the cranial hand is used to block the right lateral aspect of the spinous process of the cranial member of the segment (Fig. 4.75D). The patient's legs are lifted until side bending is induced at the targeted segment (Fig. 4.73A). The therapist takes up the slack and oscillates through the leg. On completion of the manipulation, side bending to the right is retested. For the leg lowering variation of the technique, the pad of the long finger of the cranial hand is used to block the left lateral aspect of the spinous process of the cranial member of the segment (Fig. 4.75B). The legs are lowered until side bending is induced at the targeted segment. The therapist takes up the slack and oscillates through the leg. On completion of the manipulation, side bending is retested to the left.

Lumbar Spine Side Bending Manipulation: Side-Lying Raising and Lowering the Legs—cont'd

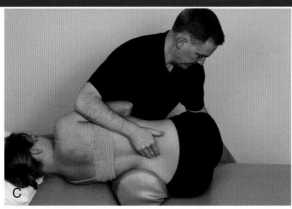

FIG. 4.73, cont'd C, Further stretch can be induced with lowering the legs manipulation technique by having the patient lie over a bolster.

PROCEDURE MODIFICATION　　The leg-lowering manipulation technique can be further facilitated by placing the patient over the top of the bolster, with the apex of the bolster positioned to induce lateral flexion at the targeted segment (Fig. 4.73C).

NOTES　　Impairment-based indications for use of the right side bending manipulation technique are decreased lumbar AROM and PIVM right side bending of a specific lumbar segment (L1–L2 through L5–S1). Indications for use of the left side bending manipulation technique are decreased lumbar AROM and PIVM left side bending of a specific lumbar segment (L1–L2 through L5–S1).

Isometric Lumbar Manipulation With the Side Bending Leg Lowering Technique

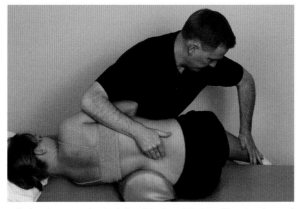

FIG. 4.74 Isometric lumbar manipulation with the side bending leg lowering technique.

PROCEDURE MODIFICATION　　An isometric manipulation can be used with the side bending leg lowering manipulation by applying resistance in the leg-raising direction followed by further stretching into the leg-lowering direction (Fig. 4.74). The isometric contraction is held for 10 seconds and followed by a 10-second stretch. This sequence is repeated for three to four bouts.

▶ Lumbar Spine Side Bending Manipulation: Side-Lying Rocking the Pelvis

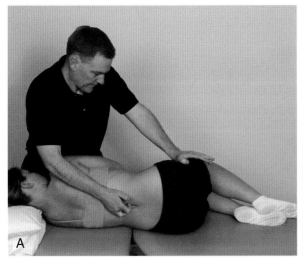
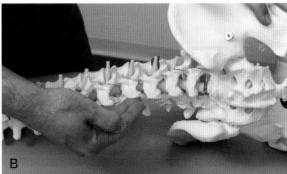

FIG. 4.75 See Video 4.56. A, Lumbar spine side bending manipulation, side-lying rocking the pelvis. B, Finger placement for blocking the spinous process for lumbar

PURPOSE	The purpose of this technique is to manipulate a specific lumbar segment (L1–L2 through L5–S1) into side bending.
PATIENT POSITION	The patient is in a side-lying position facing the therapist.
THERAPIST POSITION	The therapist stands next to the patient.
HAND PLACEMENT	Caudal hand: The palm of the hand is placed on the patient's greater trochanter.
	Cranial hand: The pad of the long finger is used to block the lateral aspect of the spinous process of the cranial member of the segment.
PROCEDURE	With the patient in a left side-lying position, both legs are positioned in 90 degrees of hip and knee flexion. The pad of the long finger of the cranial hand is used to block the left lateral aspect of the spinous process of the cranial member of the segment (Fig. 4.75B). The superior aspect of the greater trochanter is contacted with the heel of the caudal hand, with the elbow straight and the arm in line with the direction of the force. Lumbar side bending is induced to the left with the caudal hand pushing the patient's greater trochanter caudally (Fig. 4.75A). The therapist takes up the slack and oscillates. On completion of the manipulation, side bending to the left is retested.

Lumbar Spine Side Bending Manipulation: Side-Lying Rocking the Pelvis—cont'd

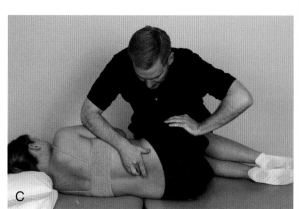

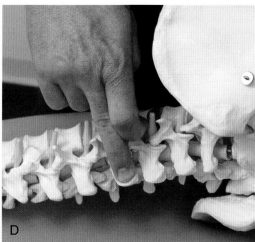

FIG. 4.75, cont'd spine left side bending. C, Lumbar spine side bending manipulation, side-lying rocking the pelvis. D, Finger placement for blocking the spinous process for lumbar right side bending

For manipulation of the segment into right side bending, the pad of the long finger on the cranial hand is used to block the right lateral aspect of the spinous process of the cranial member of the segment (Fig. 4.75D). The caudal hand pushes the patient's greater trochanter cranially, with the forearm lined up in frontal plane parallel to the direction of the force (Fig. 4.75C). The therapist takes up the slack and oscillates. On completion of the manipulation, side bending to the right is retested.

NOTES   Because of the small lever arm, use of grade I and II oscillations is most appropriate for this technique. The forearm should be positioned parallel to the direction of the force applied through the greater trochanter. The procedure can be performed with the patient in a right side-lying position, with caudal movement of the pelvis inducing right side bending and cranial movement of the pelvis inducing left side bending. Mobilization of lumbar side bending with this technique (e.g., rocking the pelvis) is useful for patients with hip pathologic conditions (the hip joint is not stressed).

▶ Lumbar Rotation Manipulation: Oscillation Through the Transverse Process

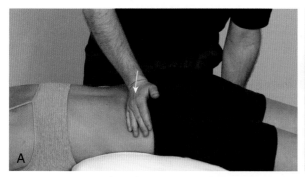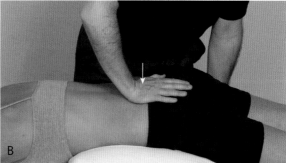

FIG. 4.76 See Video 4.57. Lumbar rotation manipulation. A, Oscillation through the left L3 transverse process. B, L5–S1 posteroanterior mobilization.

PURPOSE	This technique manipulates a specific lumbar segment (L1–L2 through L5–S1) into rotation.
PATIENT POSITION	The patient is prone with a pillow under the abdomen and pelvis.
THERAPIST POSITION	The therapist stands next to the patient.
HAND PLACEMENT	Caudal hand: The caudal hand is used to support the therapist's body weight on the edge of the treatment table.
	Cranial hand: The ulnar proximal aspect of the fifth metacarpal is used to contact and apply force through the transverse process.
PROCEDURE	With the therapist standing on the patient's right side, the ulnar aspect of the fifth metacarpal on the caudal hand is used to locate the iliac crest on the patient's left side. The ulnar aspect of the fifth metacarpal locates the 12th rib on the patient's left side. The two hands make a V shape on the patient's back. The transverse process of L3 is located at the point of the V (4.62C). The ulnar proximal aspect of the fifth metacarpal of the cranial hand is used to "sink into" the middle of the V at the location of the L3 transverse process. For mobilization into right rotation, the therapist takes up the slack and oscillates the left transverse process of L3. On completion of the mobilization, right rotation is retested. The procedure can be repeated with the transverse processes of L2 (located just inferior to the 12th rib, segment L2–L3) and L4 (located just superior to the iliac crest, segment L4–L5). The therapist manipulates L5–S1 by placing the middle crease of the cranial hand on the patient's right PSIS with the thenar eminence on the sacral sulcus. The therapist takes up the slack and oscillates the L5–S1 segment by giving a posteroanterior force (Fig. 4.76B).
	For manipulation of the lumbar segments into left rotation, the procedure is repeated by oscillating through the right transverse processes of L2–L4 and through the left PSIS/sacral sulcus.
NOTES	This technique is commonly used to induce grade I and II oscillations for the purpose of pain inhibition. Therefore a painful reactive facet joint or surrounding soft tissues are indications for this technique.

▶ Prone Lumbar Isometric Manipulation

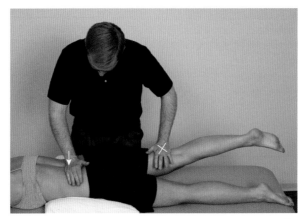

FIG. 4.77 See Video 4.58. Lumbar isometric manipulation combined with direct mobilization of targeted segment with posteroanterior pressure through the transverse process.

PURPOSE	The purpose of this technique is to mobilize a lumbar segment (L1–L2 though L5–S1) with a painful facet joint entrapment.
PATIENT POSITION	The patient is prone with a pillow under the abdomen and pelvis.
THERAPIST POSITION	The therapist stands next to the patient.
HAND PLACEMENT	Caudal hand: The caudal hand is placed across the posterior aspect of the patient's upper leg.
	Cranial hand: The ulnar proximal aspect of the fifth metacarpal is used to contact the transverse process of the superior member of the targeted segment.
PROCEDURE	After the reactive or stiff facet joint is identified with a posteroanterior force at the transverse process with the cranial hand, the posteroanterior force is held with the cranial hand at the targeted transverse process and the patient is asked to extend the opposite hip. Isometric resistance is applied to the hip extension for a 10-second hold. After the patient rests the leg back on the table, posteroanterior oscillations are applied to the targeted segment for 10 seconds and then the isometric hip extension is repeated. This sequence is repeated three to four times until improved mobility and reduced joint reactivity is noted with the posteroanterior force at the transverse process.
NOTES	Opposite hip extension is used to facilitate an isometric contraction of the multifidus muscle on the side of the targeted facet joint. The patient may have difficulty actively extending the hip for the first one or two isometric contractions. Commonly, the patient is able to generate greater force with each subsequent contraction. The segment can be further isolated by side bending the lumbar spine to the targeted segment.

Posterior Ilial Rotation Sacroiliac Joint Manipulation

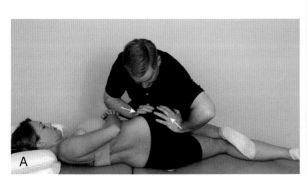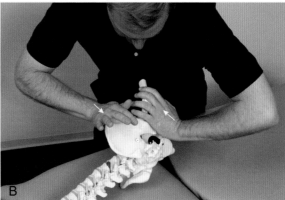

FIG. 4.78 See Video 4.59. A, Posterior ilial rotation sacroiliac joint (SIJ) manipulation. B, Posterior rotation SIJ manipulation hand placement.

PURPOSE	This technique is used to manipulate an anterior ilial rotation displacement SIJ dysfunction and to restore posterior rotation of the ilium. This technique can also be used as an SIJ-related pain provocation test.
PATIENT POSITION	The patient is positioned side-lying facing the therapist.
THERAPIST POSITION	The therapist stands with a diagonal athletic stance in front of the patient.
HAND PLACEMENT	Caudal hand: The palm is used to contact the patient's ischial tuberosity.
	Cranial hand: The palm is used to contact the patient's ASIS.
PROCEDURE	The patient's bottom leg is flexed to approximately 30 degrees of hip and knee flexion. The top hip is flexed to approximately 90 degrees, and the foot of the top leg is hooked at the knee of the bottom leg. The spine is rotated to include the L5–S1 segment with pulling the patient's bottom arm (from proximal to the elbow) in a forward and upward rotary motion with the cranial hand. The patient's arms are loosely folded across the chest. The palm of the cranial hand is used to contact the patient's top ASIS, and the palm of the caudal hand is used to contact the patient's top ischial tuberosity. A force couple is created with pushing the ASIS posteriorly and pushing the ischial tuberosity anteriorly. The force is gradually increased over 10 to 30 seconds. End-range oscillations or a thrust can be used.

Posterior Ilial Rotation Sacroiliac Joint Manipulation—cont'd

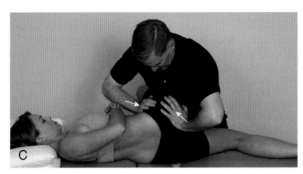

FIG. 4.78, cont'd See Video 4.60. C, Posterior rotation SIJ manipulation with leg positioned for an isometric manipulation.

PROCEDURE MODIFICATION   For further mechanical advantage and for an isometric manipulation, the therapist should follow the procedure as described previously; but before application of the force couple, the therapist can step inside the patient's top leg and alternate a direct manipulation, using the force couple, with an isometric manipulation by using isometric hip extension of the top leg (patient instructed to push the thigh into the front hip of the therapist; Fig. 4.78C). The therapist takes up the slack and holds for 10 seconds and then instructs the patient to isometrically extend the hip for 10 seconds. The force couple of the direct manipulation is maintained as the isometric manipulation is performed. The procedure is repeated for a total of three to four repetitions. Once the slack is fully taken up, a small-amplitude, high-velocity thrust manipulation can also be used.

NOTES   Patients who tend to loose mobility or "redisplace" into anterior rotation of the SIJ between treatment sessions can turn this technique into a self-isometric manipulation: In supine position, the ipsilateral hip is flexed and both hands are used to hold the thigh in a flexed position. The hip is isometrically extended into the hands and held for 10 seconds; repeat three to four times.

▶ Anterior Ilial Rotation Sacroiliac Joint Manipulation

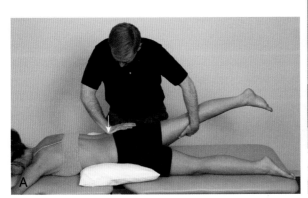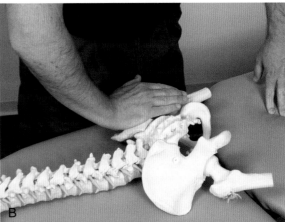

FIG. 4.79 See Video 4.61. A, Anterior ilial rotation sacroiliac joint (SIJ) manipulation. B, Anterior rotation SIJ manipulation hand

PURPOSE	The purpose is to manipulate a posterior ilial rotation displacement SIJ dysfunction and restore anterior rotation of the ilium. This technique can also be used as an SIJ-related pain provocation test.
PATIENT POSITION	The patient is prone with a pillow under the pelvis.
THERAPIST POSITION	The therapist stands with a diagonal athletic stance next to the patient.
HAND PLACEMENT	Caudal hand: The caudal hand grasps the anterior thigh just proximal to the knee.
	Cranial hand: The hypothenar eminence is used to contact the PSIS, with the fingers pointing toward the patient's thigh (to keep the hands off the lumbar spine) (Fig. 4.79B).
PROCEDURE	The hypothenar eminence of the cranial hand is used to contact the PSIS, and the caudal hand is used to extend the hip just enough to take up the slack in the hip. The cranial hand forces the PSIS toward the table and approximately 10 to 20 degrees laterally. An isometric manipulation can be added by following the procedure as described previously; but before the application of the direct manipulation force, the patient is instructed to isometrically flex the hip into the therapist's hand and hold for 10 seconds. After the isometric hip flexion hold, the therapist further extends the patient's hip and progressively oscillates with the caudal hand to take up the slack and repeats three to four times. At the end range of the available motion, a thrust can be applied with the cranial hand directed to the pelvis.

Anterior Ilial Rotation Sacroiliac Joint Manipulation—cont'd

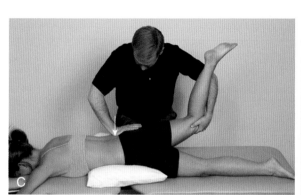
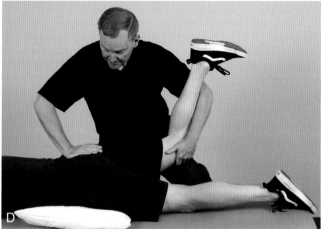

FIG. 4.79, cont'd placement. C, Anterior ilial rotation SIJ manipulation with knee flexed. D, Anterior ilial rotation SIJ manipulation with patient's flexed knee on table to assist in holding patient's leg.

PROCEDURE MODIFICATION   The patient's knee can be flexed during the performance of this technique (Fig. 4.79C). It may also be helpful for the therapist to position their caudal flexed knee under the patient's thigh to assist in holding the patient's hip in extension during this procedure (Fig. 4.79D).

NOTES   This technique can be turned into a self-isometric manipulation: in the prone position with a pillow under the pelvis, the unaffected leg is placed off the lateral edge of the bed with the foot on the floor. The hip is isometrically flexed on the affected side by pushing the knee into the bed and holding for 10 seconds. The procedure is repeated three to four times. Patients who tend to loose lumbopelvic mobility between therapy sessions are instructed to perform this self-manipulation as part of a home program.

▶ Sacral Mobilization and Myofascial Stretch

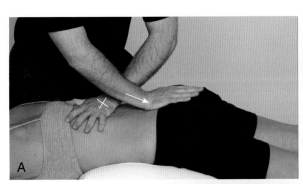
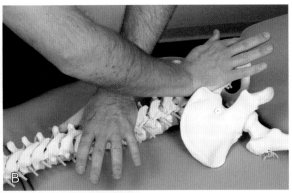
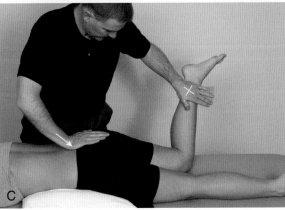

FIG. 4.80 See Videos 4.62 and 4.63. A, Myofascial stretch and sacral mobilization. B, Myofascial stretch and sacral mobilization hand placement. C, Isometric manipulation of sacrum with hip lateral rotators.

PURPOSE	This manipulation inhibits muscle tone at the lumbosacral junction and, in theory, corrects suspected sacral torsional displacements.
PATIENT POSITION	The patient is in a prone position with a pillow supporting the pelvis.
THERAPIST POSITION	The therapist stands with a diagonal athletic stance against the edge of treatment table.
HAND PLACEMENT	Cranial hand: The heel of the hand is placed at the base of the patient's sacrum.
	Caudal hand: The palm of hand is placed across the upper lumbar spine and erector spinae muscles.
PROCEDURE	The cranial hand gradually sinks into the myofascial tissues over the base of the sacrum and applies a caudally directed anterior force as the tissue tone relaxes. The caudal hand applies a gradual counterforce directed anteriorly and superiorly. The forces start gentle and gradually are increased as the muscle tone relaxes. For further mobilization of the sacrum, the caudal hand can move the hip into medial rotation and isometrically resist lateral rotation as the cranial hand sustains pressure at the base of the sacrum (Fig. 4.80C). In theory, the isometric contraction of the lateral rotators of the hip pulls one side of the base of the sacrum anteriorly to mobilize the SIJ and inhibit muscle tone in the region. The isometric force should be sustained for 10 seconds and repeated three to four times with a 10-second rest between contractions. The sacral force is sustained throughout and between the isometric contractions.

Lumbosacral Manual Traction With a Mobilization Table

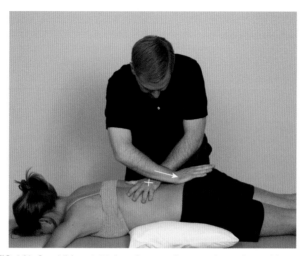

FIG. 4.81 See Video 4.64. Lumbosacral manual traction with a mobilization table.

PROCEDURE   The direct sacral mobilization technique can be modified to apply traction at the lower lumbar spine with use of a mobilization table. The table can be released to allow the lower section to separate as the manual traction force is sustained at the sacrum and counterforce is applied at the upper lumbar spine.

Coccyx Direct Internal Manipulation

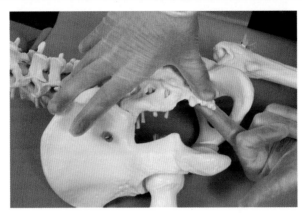

FIG. 4.82 Coccyx direct internal manipulation hand placement.

PURPOSE	This manipulation is used to mobilize the coccyx to restore coccyx mobility, correct a coccygeal displacement, and to inhibit pelvic floor muscle tone.
PATIENT POSITION	The patient is prone over two or three pillows with the hips abducted and internally rotated.
THERAPIST POSITION	The therapist stands at the side of the patient.
HAND PLACEMENT	Caudal hand: With a latex glove with lubricating gel worn on the long finger, the finger is eased through the anus into the rectum, with the volar pad of the finger facing dorsally to palpate the anterior surface of the coccyx.
	Cranial hand: The thumb is placed on the external dorsal surface of the coccyx.
PROCEDURE	Once the proper finger placement is obtained, a distraction force is applied along the long axis of the coccyx. If a lateral flexed or rotation deviation is noted, correction can be attempted during application of the distraction force. The distraction force is sustained for 30 seconds for three to four repetitions.
NOTES	The primary finding for indication of coccyx manipulation is coccyx pain with sitting, pain with contraction of the gluteus maximus muscle, and pain provocation with direct pressure at the coccyx. Pelvic floor muscle dysfunctions can contribute to coccyx pain and should be addressed as part of the treatment plan of care. Stress reduction strategies, such as use of a coccyx pillow with a square cut out of the posterior edge of the cushion, should be used on a consistent basis to unload the coccyx when seated.

▶ Coccyx Isometric Manipulation (Lateral Flexion)

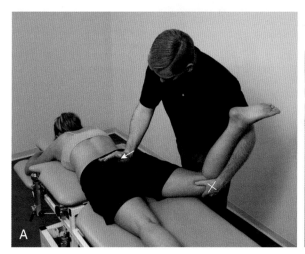 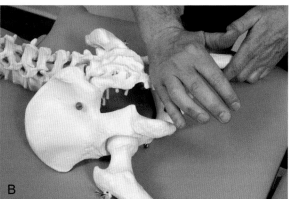

FIG. 4.83 See Video 4.65. A, Coccyx isometric manipulation (lateral flexion). B, Coccyx isometric manipulation hand placement.

PURPOSE	This technique is used to manipulate the sacrococcygeal joint into a lateral flexion direction to restore sacrococcygeal joint mobility.
PATIENT POSITION	The patient is in a prone position lying over a pillow with the knee flexed on the side to be manipulated.
THERAPIST POSITION	The therapist stands at the side of the patient.
HAND PLACEMENT	Cranial hand: The hypothenar eminence is placed at the lateral edge of the base of the coccyx just distal to the sacrococcygeal joint on the side of the therapist. Caudal hand: The caudal hand cups the medial and anterior aspect of the patient's knee on the leg closest to the therapist.
PROCEDURE	A medially directed force is applied at the sacrococcygeal joint with the cranial hand as the caudal hand abducts the patient's hip. Once full hip abduction is obtained, hip adduction is resisted isometrically and held for 10 seconds. The patient rests for 10 seconds and then repeats the isometric hold after the tissue slack is taken up with further hip abduction and direct force. The procedure is repeated three to four times, and the direct force is maintained with the cranial hand throughout the hold/relax sequence with the hip.
NOTES	In theory, gliding the sacrococcygeal joint toward the midline from the right to the left moves the coccyx into right lateral flexion because the proximal coccyx is a convex joint surface moving a concave distal sacrum. Pelvic floor muscle dysfunctions can contribute to coccyx pain and should be addressed as part of the treatment plan of care. Stress reduction strategies, such as regular use of a coccyx pillow with a square cut out of the posterior edge of the cushion, should be used on a consistent basis to unload the coccyx when seated.

Coccyx Isometric Manipulation (Rotation)

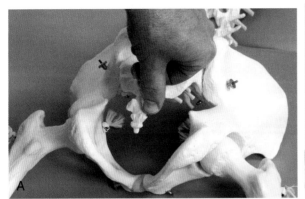
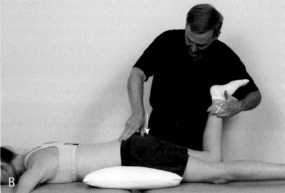
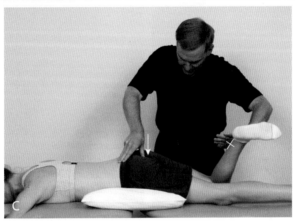

FIG. 4.84 See Video 4.66.   A, Thumb placement for coccyx isometric rotation manipulation. B, Coccyx isometric rotation manipulation with resisted hip external rotation. C, Coccyx isometric rotation manipulation with resisted hip internal rotation.

PURPOSE	This technique is used to manipulate the sacrococcygeal joint into a rotation direction to restore sacrococcygeal mobility.
PATIENT POSITION	The patient is in a prone position lying over a pillow with the knee flexed on the side to be manipulated.
THERAPIST POSITION	The therapist stands at the side of the patient.
HAND PLACEMENT	Cranial hand: The pad of the thumb is placed at the posterior base of one side the coccyx just distal to the sacrococcygeal joint on the side of the therapist.
	Caudal hand: The caudal hand holds the patient's leg just proximal to the ankle on the leg closest to the therapist.
PROCEDURE	A unilateral posteroanterior directed force is applied at the sacrococcygeal joint with the cranial hand as the caudal hand internally rotates the patient's hip. Once full hip internal rotation is obtained, hip external rotation is resisted isometrically and held for 10 seconds (Fig. 4.84B). The patient rests for 10 seconds and then repeats the isometric hold after the tissue slack is taken up with further hip internal rotation and direct unilateral posteroanterior force. The procedure is repeated three to four times, and the direct force is maintained with the cranial hand throughout the hold/relax sequence with the hip. This technique can also be performed by moving the hip into external rotation and resisting hip internal rotation (Fig. 4.84C). The decision on which direction of hip rotation to resist is based on assessment of the movement barrier and finding a firm barrier to the hip motion as posteroanterior pressure is maintained at the coccyx.

Coccyx Isometric Manipulation (Rotation)—cont'd

NOTES   In theory, providing a unilateral posteroanterior force at the sacrococcygeal joint will rotate the coccyx to the opposite direction of the side the force is applied. The isometric force of the hip rotators and gluteal muscles will facilitate this mobilization. Pelvic floor muscle dysfunctions can contribute to coccyx pain and should be addressed as part of the treatment plan of care.

▶ Hip Abduction/Adduction Isometric Manipulation

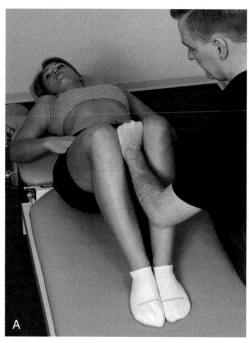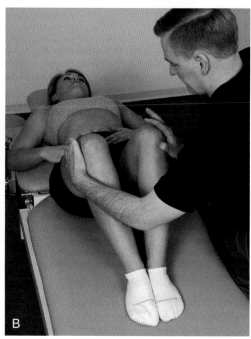

FIG. 4.85 See Video 4.67. A, Hip adduction isometric manipulation. B, Hip abduction isometric manipulation.

PURPOSE   General isometric manipulation of the pelvis is used to relax muscle tone, balance alignment of the pelvis and to inhibit pain.

PATIENT POSITION   The patient is supine in the hook-lying position.

THERAPIST POSITION   The therapist stands at the edge of the table.

PROCEDURE   For the hip adduction isometric technique, the therapist places a closed fist between the patient's knees and asks the patient to squeeze the fist between the knees. The isometric contraction is held for 10 seconds and repeated three to four times, with a 10-second rest between contractions.

For the hip abduction isometric technique, the therapist places the hands along the lateral aspect of both of the patient's knees and asks the patient to pull the knees apart. The contraction is held for 10 seconds and repeated three to four times, with a 10-second rest between contractions.

NOTES   A useful method is to finish a manual therapy session with these isometric techniques to relax muscle tone of the pelvic region before the therapy session is completed. Theoretically, the symphysis pubis and SIJs are both mobilized with these isometric techniques. Alternating between the abduction and adduction isometric techniques is often helpful. These isometric techniques can be done as a self-mobilization technique with use of a belt to resist hip abduction and use of a small soft ball to resist hip adduction.

▶ Hip Joint Manipulation With a Mobilization Belt

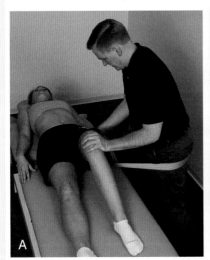
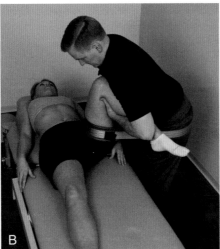
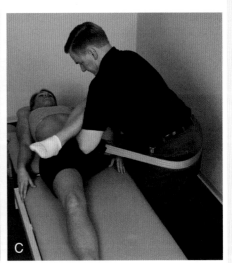

FIG. 4.86 See Videos 4.68, 4.69, and 4.70. A, Hip joint manipulation with a mobilization belt. B, Lateral distraction hip joint manipulation with belt combined with passive hip internal rotation. C, Lateral distraction hip joint manipulation with belt combined with passive hip external rotation.

PURPOSE	The purpose of this manipulation is to stretch the hip joint capsule and restore full hip mobility.
PATIENT POSITION	The patient is supine, lying close to the edge of the table on the side of the hip to be manipulated.
THERAPIST POSITION	The therapist stands, in a diagonal stance with the caudal foot back, at the edge of the table on the side of the hip to be manipulated.
PROCEDURE	The mobilization belt is positioned at the proximal thigh near the crease formed by flexing the patient's hip to 30 degrees of flexion and looped around the therapist's buttock. The therapist stabilizes the patient's pelvis and distal femur while leaning in an inferior and posterior direction in line with the 120-degree angle at the neck of the patient's femur. Mobilization with movement: The distraction technique can be modified by flexing the hip to 90 degrees. The therapist uses the chest to stabilize the distal femur, the cranial hand to stabilize the pelvis, and the caudal hand/arm to rotate the hip either into internal or external rotation. The distraction is sustained as the hip is stretched repeatedly into the end range of hip internal or external rotation motion (Fig. 4.86B and C).
NOTES	The therapist should follow the hip mobilization techniques with AROM exercises, such as the bent knee fall out exercise (Fig. 4.11G), to have the patient move into the new ROM obtained with the manipulation procedure. Many patients with LBP have limitations in hip capsular mobility and can benefit from this technique.

▶ Hip Joint Anterior Glide Manipulation

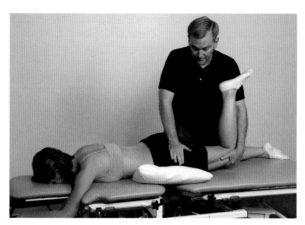

FIG. 4.87 See Video 4.71. Hip joint anterior glide manipulation with hip in extension.

PURPOSE	This manipulation is used to stretch the anterior hip joint capsule to improve hip extension ROM.
PATIENT POSITION	The patient is prone lying over a pillow.
THERAPIST POSITION	The therapist stands on the side of the table opposite the hip to be manipulated.
PROCEDURE	The therapist lifts and holds the patient's hip in extension with the caudal hand and applies an anterior lateral force parallel to the angle of the acetabulum at the posterior aspect of the proximal femur near the greater trochanter.
NOTES	Typically, a progressive oscillation or a grade III mobilization force is used with this technique to attempt to improve hip extension. If the leg is too heavy for the therapist to hold, the femur could be supported in an extended position with a pillow or towel roll. Patients with CLBP conditions, such as spinal stenosis, commonly have limited hip extension and may benefit from use of an anterior glide manipulation to attempt to improve hip mobility.

Hip Joint Anterior Glide Manipulation—cont'd

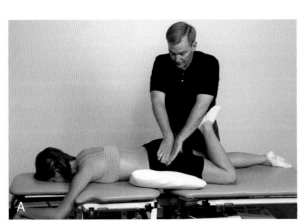
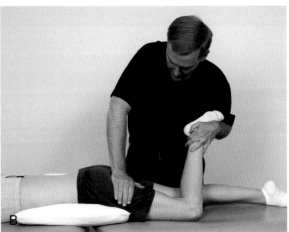

FIG. 4.88 See Video 4.72. A, Alternate technique for hip joint anterior glide manipulation with hip positioned in external rotation. B, The hip anterior glide manipulation can also be performed with one hand holding the leg in external rotation and the other hand applying the anterior hip-gliding mobilization.

PROCEDURE MODIFICATION The anterior glide manipulation can be performed with the targeted hip placed in an end-range external rotation position with the patient's tibia resting on the opposite leg in a frog leg position (Fig. 4.88A). This position allows the therapist to use the web space of both hands to apply an anterior lateral force at the posterior aspect of the proximal femur. Fig. 4.88B illustrates another variation where the leg is supported in external rotation with the caudal hand and the cranial hand applies the anterior glide manipulation. Theoretically, this manipulation technique should assist in restoring both hip extension and external rotation.

CASE STUDIES AND PROBLEM SOLVING

The following case studies are provided as a way for physical therapy students to practice clinical reasoning with an impairment-based evidence-based approach. Basic objective and subjective information is provided, and students are asked to develop a physical therapy diagnosis, problem list, and treatment plan. Students should also consider the following questions:

1. What additional historical/subjective information would you like to have?
2. What additional diagnostic tests should be ordered, if any?
3. What additional tests and measures would be helpful in making the diagnosis?
4. What impairment-based classification does the patient most likely fit? What other impairment-based classifications did you consider?
5. What are the primary impairments that should be addressed?
6. What treatment techniques that you learned in this textbook will you use to address these impairments?
7. How do you plan to progress and modify the interventions as the patient progresses?

Mr. Acute Back

History

A 30-year-old factory worker bent over to put down his dog's dish and strained his lower back 2 weeks before the initial evaluation. The pain is focused in the right lumbosacral junction and radiates into the right buttock and posterior thigh (Fig. 4.89). Pain is made worse with sitting, bending forward, twisting, and walking and is relieved with lying supine in a 90/90 position. The patient is a heavy smoker and has had LBP episodes in the past but never this intense or prolonged. An MRI scan 2 years previous showed a degenerative disk at L5–S1. FABQ work subscale score is l6.

Tests and Measures

1. Structural examination reveals a ½ inch leg length discrepancy, with the left leg shorter, and the patient is shifted to the left in standing, avoiding full weight on the right lower extremity
2. Active motion testing: 50% forward bending with provocation of pain, 25% left side bending, 50% right side bending, 25% right rotation, 50% left rotation, and 15% backward bending with provocation of pain
3. Neurologic testing results are negative
4. Palpation: Guarded/tight/tender right L5–S1 area

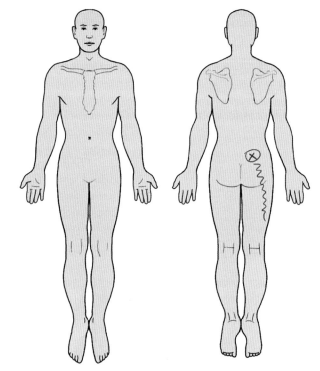

FIG. 4.89 Body chart for Mr. Acute Back.

5. PIVM: Significant restriction L5–S1 forward bending and left and right rotation
6. PAIVM (spring) test: Positive pain provocation right L5–S1 facet and limited mobility with posteroanterior testing at L5-S1
7. Strength: 4/5 multifidus, abdominal, and hip muscles
8. Muscle length: Moderately tight right psoas and both hamstrings
9. Hip AROM: 65 degrees external rotation, 38 degrees internal rotation bilaterally

Evaluation

Diagnosis
Problem list
Goals
Treatment plan/intervention

Mr. Chronic Back

History

A 55-year-old man with a 14-month history of LBP and sciatica received 2 months of physical therapy with good relief of sciatica but still has LBP. The patient works as a machine operator and has to stand on concrete all day and wants to work 6 more years before he retires. LBP is constant and focused centrally across the lower lumbar region (Fig. 4.90). Pain is worse with prolonged sitting, standing, or bending. The patient was injured at work by falling on a wet spot left by a leaky air conditioner. The patient works on light duty with a 25-pound lifting restriction. Pain is worse (7/10) at the end of the day.

Tests and Measures

1. Structural examination: Good symmetry, but step noted at L3–L4 with increased lumbar lordosis and rotund abdomen
2. AROM: All planes 75% with limited lower lumbar motion and fulcrum at L3–L4
3. PIVM: Limited L5–S1 and L4–L5 in all motions; hypermobile L3–L4 all motions with positive pain provocation spring testing results L3–L4
4. Prone instability test: Negative
5. Palpation: Myofascial tightness with minimal tenderness lumbar paraspinals
6. Muscle length: Moderately tight bilateral hamstrings and iliopsoas
7. Muscle strength: Abdominals and multifidus 3/5
8. Endurance: Poor

Evaluation

Diagnosis
Problem list
Goals
Treatment plan/intervention

Ms. Lucy Goosey

History

A 25-year-old woman who works at a department store as a cashier has right upper lumbar pain and left upper thoracic area pain that is provoked with prolonged standing and work activities (Fig. 4.91). The patient admits to being fairly sedentary when not at work. The patient describes pain as achiness that intensifies with sustained postures and is relieved with lying down.

Tests and Measures

1. Posture: Moderate forward head posture with protracted scapulae and flat lumbar spine
2. Cervical AROM: At 75% in all planes with stiffness noted in upper thoracic spine and pain reported with end-range left rotation
3. Lumbar AROM: Nearly 100% in all planes with poor muscle control (aberrant motion) noted with forward bending and stiffness noted in lower thoracic spine
4. SLR: 95 degrees bilaterally
5. Prone instability test: Positive

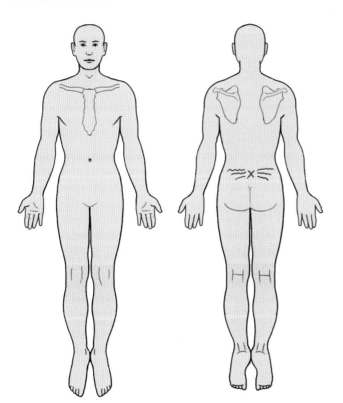

FIG. 4.90 Body chart for Mr. Chronic Back.

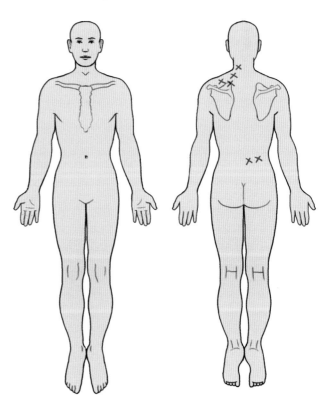

FIG. 4.91 Body chart for Ms. Lucy Goosey.

6. PIVM: Hypermobile in mid-cervical segments; moderately restricted upper thoracic right rotation and forward bending; hypermobile upper lumbar; moderately restricted T9–T10 and T10–T11 right rotation
7. Palpation: Mildly tender and moderately guarded left upper thoracic tissues and right lower thoracic; moderately tender left lower cervical facet joint tissues and right upper lumbar tissues
8. Strength: Poor positive scapular stabilizers, lumbar, and cervical multifidus
9. Other observations: Systemic hypermobility noted in fingers, elbows, and knees

Evaluation

Diagnosis
Problem list
Goals
Treatment plan/intervention

REFERENCES

1. Burton A, Tollotson K, Main C, et al. Psychosocial predictors of outcome in acute and subchronic low back trouble. *Spine*. 1995; 20:722-728.
2. Balague F, Mannion AF, Pellise F, et al. Non-specific low back pain. *Lancet*. 2012;379:482-491.
3. Truchon M. Determinants of chronic disability related to low back pain: towards an integrated biopsychosocial model. *Disabil Rehabil*. 2001;23:758-767.
4. Dieleman JL, Baral R, Birger M, et al. U.S. spending on personal health care and public health 1996–2013. *JAMA*. 2016;316:2627-2646.
5. Hoy D, March L, Brooks P, et al. The global burden of low back pain: estimates from the global burden of disease study. *Ann Rheum Dis*. 2014;73(6):968-974.
6. Froud R, Patterson S, Eldridge S, et al. A systematicreview and meta-synthesis of the impact of low back pain on people's lives. *BMC Musculoskelet Disord*. 2014;15:50.
7. Dagenais S, Caro J, Haldeman S. A systematic review of low back pain cost of illness studies in the United States and internationally. *Spine J*. 2008;8(1):8-20.
8. Stanton TR, Latimer J, Maher CG, et al. Definitions of recurrence of an episode of low back pain: a systematic review. *Spine (Phila Pa 1976)*. 2009;34(9):E316-E322.
9. Lambeek LC, van Tulder MW, Swinkels IC, et al. The trend in total cost of back pain in The Netherlands in the period 2002 to2007. *Spine (Phila Pa 1976)*. 2011;36(13):1050-1058.
10. Stubbs B, Koyanagi A, Thompson T, et al. The epidemiology of back pain and its relationship with depression, psychosis, anxiety, sleep disturbances, and stress sensitivity: Data from 43 low- and middle-income countries. *Gen Hosp Psychiatry*. 2016;43:63-70.
11. Fenuele J, Birkmeyer N, Abdu W, et al. The impact of spinal problems on the health status of patients: have we underestimated the effect? *Spine*. 2000;25:1509-1514.
12. Deyo R, Gray D, Dreuter W, et al. United States trends in lumbar fusion surgery for degenerative conditions. *Spine*. 2005;30:1441-1445.
13. Weinstein JN. US trends and regional variations in lumbar spine surgery 1992-2003. *Spine*. 2006;31(2):2707-2714.
14. Waddell G, Feder G, McIntosh A. *Low Back Pain Evidence Review*. London: Royal College of General Practitioners; 1999.
15. Iglehart JK. The new era of medical imaging—progress and pitfalls. *N Engl J Med*. 2006;354:2822-2828.
16. Iglehart JK. Health insurers and medical-imaging policy—a work in progress. *N Engl J Med*. 2009;360:1030-1037.
17. Shuford H, Restrepo T, Beaven N, et al. Trends in components of medical spending within workers compensation: results from 37 states combined. *J Occup Environ Med*. 2009;51:232.
18. Graves JM, Fulton-Kehoe D, Jarvik JG, et al. Early imaging for acute low back pain. *Spine*. 2012;37(18):1617-1627.
19. Brinjikji W, Luetmer PH, Comstock B, et al. Systematic literature review of imaging features of spinal degeneration in asymptomatic populations. *AJNR Am J Neuroradiol*. 2015;36:811-816.
20. Weber C, Giannadakis C, Rao V, et al. Is there an association between radiological severity of lumbar spinal stenosis and disability, pain, or surgical outcome? A multicenter observational study. *Spine (Phila Pa 1976)*. 2016;41(2):E78-E83.
21. Magel J, Hansen P, Meier W, et al. Implementation of an alternative pathway for patients seeking care for low back pain: a prospective observational cohort study. *Phys Ther*. 2018;98(12):1000-1009.

22. Fritz JM, Childs JD, Wainner RS, et al. Primary care referral of patients with low back pain to physical therapy. *Spine*. 2012; 37(25):2114-2121.
23. Foster NE, Anema JR, Cherkin D, et al. Low back pain 2: prevention and treatment of low back pain: evidence, challenges, and promising directions. *Lancet*. 2018;391:2368-2383.
24. American Medical Association. *Guides to the Evaluation of Permanent Impairment*, ed 3. Chicago: AMA; 1988.
25. Troke M, Moore AP, Maillardet FJ, et al. A normative database of lumbar spine ranges of motion. *Man Ther*. 2005;10(3):198-206.
26. Wattananon P, Ebaugh D, Biely SA, et al. Kinematic characterization of clinically observed aberrant movement patterns in patients with non-specific low back pain: a cross-sectional study. *BMC Musculoskelet Disord*. 2017;18:455.
27. Norris CM. Spinal stabilization 2: limiting factors to end-range motion in the lumbar spine. *Physiotherapy*. 1995;81(2):64-72.
28. Inufusa A, An HS, Lim T, et al. Anatomic changes of the spinal canal and intervertebral foramen associated with flexion-extension movement. *Spine*. 1996;21(21):2412-2420.
29. Nachemson A. The load on lumbar disks in different positions of the body. *Clin Orthop*. 1966;45:107-122.
30. Paris SV. Anatomy as related to function and pain. *Orthop Clin North Am*. 1983;14(3):475-489.
31. Pearcy MJ, Tibrewal SB. Axial rotation and lateral bending in the normal lumbar spine measured by three-dimensional radiography. *Spine*. 1984;9:582-587.
32. Panjabi MM, Oxland TR, Yamamoto I, et al. Mechanical behavior of the lumbar and lumbosacral spine as shown by three-dimensional load-displacement curves. *J Bone Joint Surg (Am)*. 1994;76:413-424.
33. Plamondon A, Gagnon M, Maurais G. Application of a stereoradiographic method for the study of intervertebral motion. *Spine*. 1988;13:1027-1032.
34. Lund T, Nydegger T, Schlenzka D, et al. Three-dimensional motion patterns during active bending in patients with chronic low back pain. *Spine*. 2002;27(17):1865-1874.
35. Legaspi O, Edmond S. Does the evidence support the existence of lumbar spine coupled motion? A critical review of the literature. *J Orthop Sports Phys Ther*. 2007;27(4):169-178.
36. Bergmark A. Stability of the lumbar spine: a study in mechanical engineering. *Acta Orthop Scand Suppl*. 1989;230(60):2-54.
37. Taylor JR, O'Sullivan P. Lumbar segmental instability: pathology, diagnosis, and conservative management. In: Twomey LT, Taylor JR, editors. *Physical Therapy of the Low Back*. London: Churchill Livingstone; 2000.
38. Macintosh JE, Bogduk N. The biomechanics of the lumbar multifidus. *Clin Biomech*. 1986;1:205-213.
39. Str[u]resson B, Selvik G, Uden A. Movements of the sacroiliac joints: a roentgen stereophotogrammetric analysis. *Spine*. 1989;14(2): 162-165.
40. Neumann DA. *Kinesiology of the Musculoskeletal System*. St. Louis: Mosby; 2000.
41. Adams MA, Bogduk N, Burton K, et al. *The biomechanics of Back Pain*, ed 2. Edinburgh: Churchill Livingstone; 2006.
42. Vleeming A, Snijders CJ, Stoeckart R, et al. The role of the sacroiliac joints in coupling between spine, pelvis, legs and arms. In: Vleeming A, et al., editors. *Movement, Stability and Low Back Pain*. Edinburgh: Churchill Livingstone; 1997.

43. Richardson CA, Snijders CJ, Hides JA, et al. The relation between the transversus abdominis muscles, sacroiliac joint mechanics, and low back pain. *Spine*. 2002;27(4):399-405.

44. Koes BW, van Tulder MW, Oselo R, et al. Clinical guidelines for the management of low back pain in primary care: an international comparison. *Spine*. 2001;26(22):2504-2514.

45. Koes BW, van Tulder M, Lin CWC, et al. An updated overview of clinical guidelines for the management of non-specific low back pain in primary care. *Eur Spine J*. 2010;19:2075-2094.

46. Airaksinen O, Brox JI, Cedrashi C, et al. On behalf of the COST B13 working group on guidelines for chronic low back pain: European guidelines for the management of chronic nonspecific low back pain. *Eur Spine J*. 2006;15:192-300.

47. Brennan GP, Fritz JM, Hunter SJ, et al. Identifying subgroups of patients with acute/subacute "nonspecific" low back pain: results of a randomized clinical trial. *Spine*. 2006;31(6):623-631.

48. Childs J, Fritz J, Flynn T, et al. A clinical prediction rule to identify patients with low back pain most likely to respond to spinal manipulation: a validation study. *Ann Intern Med*. 2004;141(12): 922-928.

49. Delitto A, Erhard RE, Bowling RW. A treatment-based classification approach to low back syndrome: identifying and staging patients for conservative treatment. *Phys Ther*. 1995;75(6):470-485.

50. Flynn T, Fritz J, Whitman J, et al. A clinical prediction rule for classifying patients with low back pain who demonstrate short-term improvement with spinal manipulation. *Spine*. 2002;27: 2835-2843.

51. Hicks GE, Fritz JM, Delitto A, et al. Preliminary development of a clinical prediction rule for determining which patients with low back pain will respond to a stabilization exercise program. *Arch Phys Med Rehabil*. 2005;86:1753-1762.

52. Fritz JM, Delitto A, Vignovic M, et al. Interrater reliability of judgments of the centralization phenomenon and status change during movement testing in patients with low back pain. *Arch Phys Med Rehabil*. 2000;81:57-61.

53. McKenzie R. *The Lumbar Spine: Mechanical Diagnosis and Therapy*. Waikanae, New Zealand: Spinal Publication; 1981.

54. Werneke M, Hart DL. Centralization phenomenon as a prognostic factor for chronic low back pain and disability. *Spine*. 2001; 26:758-765.

55. Werneke M, Hart DL. Categorizing patients with occupational low back pain by use of the Quebec Task Force classification system versus pain pattern classification procedures: discriminant and predictive validity. *Phys Ther*. 2004;84:243-254.

56. Long A, Donelson R. Does it matter which exercise? A randomized trial of exercise for low back pain. *Spine*. 2004;29:2593-2602.

57. Waddell G. Clinical assessment of lumbar impairment. *Clin Orthop Related Res*. 1987;221:110-120.

58. Delitto A, George SZ, Van Dillen L, et al. Low back pain. *J Orthop Sports Phys Ther*. 2012;42(4):A1-A57.

59. Fritz JM, Delitto A, Erhard RE. Comparison of a classification-based approach to physical therapy and therapy based on clinical practice guidelines for patients with acute low back pain: a randomized clinical trial. *Spine*. 2003;28:1363-1372.

60. Bigos S, Bowyer O, Braen G, et al. *Acute Low Back Problems in Adults*. Rockville, MD: Agency for Health Care Policy and Research, Public Health Service; 1994.

61. Cho R, Juffman LH. Nonpharmacologic therapies for acute and chronic low back pain: a review of the evidence for an American Pain Society/American College of Physicians Clinical Practice Guideline. *Ann Intern Med*. 2007;147:492-504.

62. Chou F, Qaseem A, Snow V, et al. Diagnosis and treatment of low back pain: a joint clinical practice guideline from the American College of Physicians and American Pain Society. *Ann Intern Med*. 2007;147:478-491.

63. Kuczynski JJ, Schwieterman B, Columber K, et al. Effectiveness of physical therapist administered spinal manipulation treatment of low back pain: a systematic review of the literature. *Int J Sports Phys Ther*. 2012;7(6):647-662.

64. Department of Defense/Veterans' Affairs (DoD/VA). *Low Back Pain Guidelines*. Falls Church, VA: DoD/VA; 1999.

65. ACC and National Health Committee. *New Zealand Acute Low Back Pain Guide*. Wellington, NZ: ACC and National Health Committee; 1997.

66. Coulter ID, Crawford C, Hurwitz EL, et al. Manipulation and mobilization for treating chronic low back pain: a systematic review and meta-analysis. *Spine J*. 2018;18:866-879.

67. Whitman JM, Flynn TW, Childs JD, et al. A comparison between two physical therapy treatment programs for patients with lumbar spinal stenosis. *Spine*. 2006;31(22):2541-2549.

68. Cleland J, Fritz JM, Whitman JM, et al. The use of a lumbar spine manipulation technique by physical therapists in patients who satisfy a clinical prediction rule: a case series. *J Orthop Sports Phys Ther*. 2006;36(4):209-214.

69. Mohseni-Bandpei MA, Critchley J, Staunton T, et al. A prospective randomised controlled trial of spinal manipulation and ultrasound in the treatment of chronic low back pain. *Physiotherapy*. 2006;92(1):34-42.

70. von Heymann WJ, Schloemer P, Timm J, et al. Spinal high-velocity low amplitude manipulation in acute nonspecific low back pain: a double-blinded randomized controlled trial in comparison with diclofenac and placebo. *Spine*. 2013;38:540-548.

71. Cleland JA, Fritz JM, Kulig K, et al. Comparison of the effectiveness of three manual physical therapy techniques in a subgroup of patients with low back pain who satisfy a clinical prediction rule: a randomized clinical trial. *Spine*. 2009;34(25):2720-2729.

72. Cook C., Learman K., Showalter C, et al. Early use of thrust manipulation versus non-thrust manipulation: a randomized clinical trial. *Man Ther*. 2013;13:191-190.

73. Fritz JM, Whitman JM, Flynn TW, et al. Factors related to the inability of individuals with low back pain to improve with a spinal manipulation. *Phys Ther*. 2004;84:173-190.

74. Fritz JM, Whitman JM, Childs JD. Lumbar spine segmental mobility assessment: an examination of validity for determining intervention strategies in patients with low back pain. *Arch Phys Med Rehabil*. 2005;86:1745-1752.

75. Hancock MJ, Maher CG, Latimer J, et al. Independent evaluation of a clinical prediction rule for spinal manipulative therapy: a randomised controlled trial. *Eur Spine J*. 2008;17:936-943.

76. Roenz D, Broccolo J, Brust S, et al. The Impact of pragmatic vs. prescriptive study designs on the outcomes of low back and neck pain when using mobilization or manipulation techniques: a systematic review and meta-analysis. *J Man Manip Ther*. 2018;26(3):123-135.

77. Panjabi MM. The stabilizing system of spine: part II: neutral zone and instability hypothesis. *J Spinal Disord*. 1992;5:390-397.

78. Panjabi MM, Lydon C, Vasavada A, et al. On the understanding of clinical instability. *Spine*. 1994;23:2642-2650.

79. Oxland TR, Panjabi MM. The onset and progression of spinal injury: a demonstration of neutral zone sensitivity. *J Biomechanics*. 1992;25:1165-1172.

80. Beazell JR, Mullins M, Grindstaff TL. Lumbar instability: an evolving and challenging concept. *J Man Manip Ther*. 2010;18(1):9-14.

81. Knutsson F. The instability associated with disk degeneration in the lumbar spine. *Acta Radiol.* 1944;25(5):593-609.

82. Paris S. Physical signs of instability. *Spine (Phila Pa 1976).* 1985;10:277-279.

83. Alyazedi FM, Lohman EB, Swen W, et al. The inter-rater reliability of clinical tests that best predict the subclassification of lumbar segmental instability: structural, functional and combined instability. *J Man Manip Ther.* 2015;23(4):197-204.

84. Panjabi MM. The stabilizing system of the spine: part I: function, dysfunction, adaptation, and enhancement. *J Spinal Disord.* 1992;5:383-389.

85. Hohl M. Normal motions in the upper portion of the cervical spine. *J Bone Joint Surg.* 1978;46(8):1777-1779.

86. Panjabi MM, Krag MH, Chung TQ. Effects of disc injury on mechanical behavior of the human spine. *Spine.* 1984;9:707-713.

87. White AA, III, Johnson RM, Panjabi MM, et al. Biomechanical analysis of clinical instability in the cervical spine. *Clin Orthop Related Res.* 1975;109:85-96.

88. Frymoyer JW, Selby DK. Segmental instability: rationale for treatment. *Spine.* 1985;10:280-286.

89. Ogon M, Bender BR, Hooper DM, et al. A dynamic approach to spinal instability, part I: sensitization of intersegmental motion profiles to motion direction and load condition by instability. *Spine.* 1997;22:2841-2858.

90. Paris SV. *Introduction to Spinal Evaluation and Manipulation.* Atlanta: Institute Press; 1986.

91. Hicks GE, Fritz JM, Delitto A, et al. Interrater reliability of clinical examination measures for identification of lumbar segmental instability. *Arch Phys Med Rehabil.* 2003;84:1858-1864.

92. Biely SA, Silfies SP, Smith SS, et al. Clinical observation of standing trunk movements: what do the aberrant movement patterns tell us? *J Orthop Sport Phys.* 2014;44(4):262-272.

93. Fritz JM, Erhard RE, Hagen BF. Segmental instability of the lumbar spine. *Phys Ther.* 1998;78:889-896.

94. Shippel AH, Robinson GK. Radiological and magnetic resonance imaging of cervical spine instability: a case report. *J Manipulative Physiol Ther.* 1987;10:317-322.

95. Twomey LT. A rationale for the treatment of back pain and joint pain by manual therapy. *Phys Ther.* 1992;72:885-892.

96. Olson KA, Joder D. Cervical spine clinical instability: a resident's case report. *J Orthop Sports Phys Ther.* 2001;31(4):194-206.

97. Gonnella C, Paris SV, Kutner M. Reliability in evaluating passive intervertebral motion. *Phys Ther.* 1982;62:436-444.

98. Richardson CA, Jull GA. Muscle control-pain control: what exercises would you prescribe? *Man Ther.* 1995;1:2-10.

99. Tippets RH, Apfelbaum RI. Anterior fusion with the caspar instrumentation system. *Neurosurgery.* 1988;22:1008-1013.

100. Jull G, Bogduk N, Marsland A. The accuracy of manual diagnosis for cervical zygapophysial joint pain syndromes. *Med J Aust.* 1988;148:233-236.

101. Pope MH, Frymoyer JW, Krag MH. Diagnosing instability. *Clin Orthop Related Res.* 1992;279:60-67.

102. Fritz JM, Piva SR, Childs JD. Accuracy of the clinical examination to predict radiographic instability of lumbar spine. *Eur Spine J.* 2005;14:743-750.

103. Kasai Y, Morishita K, Kawakita E, et al. A new evaluation method for lumbar spinal instability: passive lumbar extension test. *Phys Ther.* 2006;86:1661-1667.

104. Abbott JH, McCane B, Herbison P, et al. Lumbar segmental instability: a criterion-related validity study of manual therapy assessment. *BMC Musculoskelet Disord.* 2005;6(56):1-10.

105. Teyhan DS, Flynn FW, Childs JD, et al. Arthrokinematics in a subgroup of patients likely to benefit from lumbar stabilization exercise program. *Phys Ther.* 2007;87(3):313-325.

106. Herkowitz HN, Rothman RH. Subacute instability of the cervical spine. *Spine.* 1984;9:348-357.

107. Rabin A, Shashua A, Pizem K, et al. A clinical prediction rule to identify patients with low back pain who are likely to experience short-term success following lumbar stabilization exercises—a randomized controlled validation study. *J Orthop Sports Phys Ther.* 2014;44(1):6-18.

108. Hodges PW, Richardson CA. Inefficient muscular stabilization of the lumbar spine associated with low back pain: a motor control evaluation of transversus abdominis. *Spine.* 1996;21:2640-2650.

109. Moseley GL, Hodges PW, Gandevia SC. Deep and superficial fibers of the lumbar multifidus muscle are differentially active during voluntary arm movements. *Spine.* 2002;27(2):E29-E36.

110. Kjaer P, Bendix T, Sorensen JS, et al. Are MRI-defined fat infiltrations in the mulfidus muscles associated with low back pain? *BMC Med.* 2007;5:1-10.

111. Hides JA, Jull GA, Richardson CA. Long-term effects of specific stabilizing exercises for first-episode low back pain. *Spine.* 2001;26(11):E243-E248.

112. Hodges PW, Richardson CA. Contraction of the abdominal muscles associated with movement of the lower limb. *Phys Ther.* 1997;77:132-142.

113. Hides J, Wilson S, Stanton W, et al. An MRI investigation into the function of the transversus abdominis muscle during "drawing-in" of the abdominal wall. *Spine.* 2006;31(6):E175-E178.

114. Hides JA, Gilmore C, Stanton W, et al. Multifidus size and symmetry among chronic LBP and healthy asymptomatic subjects. *Man Ther.* 2008;13:43-49.

115. Wallwork TL, Warren RS, Freke M, et al. The effect of chronic low back pain on size and contraction of the lumbar multifidus muscle. *Man Ther.* 2009;14:496-500.

116. O'Sullivan PB, Twomey LT, Allison GT. Evaluation of specific stabilizing exercise in the treatment of chronic low back pain with radiographic diagnosis of spondylolysis or spondylolisthesis. *Spine.* 1997;22(24):2959-2967.

117. Urquhart DM, Hodges PW, Allen TJ, et al. Abdominal muscle recruitment during a range of voluntary exercises. *Man Ther.* 2005;10:144-153.

118. Koppenhaver SL, Hebert JJ, Fritz JM, et al. Reliability of rehabilitative ultrasound imaging of transversus abdominis and lumbar multifidus muscles. *Arch Phys Med Rehabil.* 2009;90:87-94.

119. Teyhen DS, Bluemle LN, Dolbeer JA, et al. Changes in lateral abdominal muscle thickness during the abdominal drawing-in maneuver in those with lumbopelvic pain. *J Orthop Sports Phys Ther.* 2009;39:791-798.

120. Hebert JJ, Koppenhaver SL, Magel JS, et al. The relationship of transversus abdominis and lumbar multifidus activation and prognostic factors for clinical success with a stabilization exercise program: a cross-sectional study. *Arch Phys Med Rehabil.* 2010;91:78-85.

121. Costa LOP, Maher CG, Latimer J, et al. Motor control exercise for chronic low back pain: a randomized placebo-controlled trial. *Phys Ther.* 2009;89:1275-1286.

122. Tsao H, Druitt TR, Schollum TM, et al. Motor training of the lumbar paraspinal muscles induces immediate changes in motor coordination in patients with recurrent low back pain. *J Pain.* 2010;11:1120-1128.

123. Grooms DR, Grindstaff TL, Croy T, et al. Clinimetric analysis of pressure biofeedback and transversus abdominis function in individuals with stabilization classification low back pain. *J Orthop Sports Phys Ther.* 2013;43(3):184-193.

124. Schmidt RA. *Motor Control and Learning*, ed 2. Champaign, IL: Human Kinetics Publishers; 1988.

125. Donelson R, Aprill C, Medcalf R, et al. A prospective study of centralization of lumbar and referred pain: a predictor of symptomatic discs and annular competence. *Spine.* 1997;22(10):1115-1122.

126. Beattie P, Arnot CE, Donley JW, et al. The immediate reduction in low back pain intensity following lumbar joint mobilization and prone press-ups is associated with increased diffusion of water in the L5S1 intervertebral disc. *J Orthop Sports Phys Ther.* 2010;40(5):256-264.

127. Werneke MW, Hart DL, Cutrone G, et al. Association between directional preference and centralization in patients with low back pain. *J Orthop Sports Phys Ther.* 2011;41(1):22-31.

128. Aina A, May S, Clare H. Systematic review: the centralization phenomenon of spinal symptoms: a systematic review. *Man Ther.* 2004;9:134-143.

129. Surkitt LK, Ford JJ, Hahne AJ, et al. Efficacy of directional preference management for low back pain: a systematic review. *Phys Ther.* 2012;92:652-665.

130. Miller ER, Schenk RJ, Karnes JL, et al. A comparison of the McKenzie approach to a specific spine stabilization program for chronic low back pain. *J Man Manipulative Ther.* 2005;13(2):103-112.

131. Paatelma M, Kilpikoski S, Simonen R, et al. Orthopaedic manual therapy, McKenzie method or advice only for low back pain in working adults: a randomized controlled trial with one year follow-up. *J Rehabil Med.* 2008;40:858-863.

132. Peterson T, Larsen K, Dordsteen J, et al. The McKenzie method compared with manipulation when used adjunctive to information and advice in low back patients presenting with centralization or pepherialization; a randomized controlled trial. *Spine.* 2011;36(24):1999-2010.

133. Schenk R, Dionne C, Simon C, et al. Effectiveness of mechanical diagnosis and therapy in patients with back pain who meet a clinical prediction rule for spinal manipulation. *J Man Manipulative Ther.* 2012;20(1):43-49.

134. Browder DA, Childs JD, Cleland JA, et al. Effectiveness of an extension-oriented treatment approach in a subgroup of subjects with low back pain: a randomized clinical trial. *Phys Ther.* 2007;87(12):1608-1618.

135. Riddle DL, Rothstein JM. Intertester reliability of McKenzie's classifications of the syndrome types present in patients with low back pain. *Spine.* 1993;18:1333-1344.

136. Garcia AN, Menezes Costa L, De Souza FS, et al. Reliability of mechanical diagnosis and therapy system in patients with spinal pain: a systematic review. *J Orthop Sports Phys Ther.* 2018;48(12):923-933.

137. Fritz JM, Erhard RE, Delitto A, et al. Preliminary results of the use of a two-stage treadmill test as a clinical diagnostic tool in the differential diagnosis of lumbar spinal stenosis. *J Spinal Disord.* 1997;10(5):410-416.

138. Tomkins-Lane C, Melloh M, Lurie J, et al. ISSLS Prize Winner: Consensus on the clinical diagnosis of lumbar spinal stenosis. Results of an international Delphi study. *Spine (Phila Pa 1976).* 2016;41(15):1239-1246.

139. Fritz JM, Erhard RE, Vignovic M. A nonsurgical treatment approach for patients with lumbar spinal stenosis. *Phys Ther.* 1997;77(9):962-972.

140. Lurie JD, Tosteson TD, Tosteson A, et al. Long-term outcomes of lumbar spinal stenosis. Eight-year results of the spine patient outcomes research trial (SPORT). *Spine (Phila Pa 1976).* 2015;40(2):63-76.

141. Delitto A, Piva SR, Moore CG, et al. Surgery versus nonsurgical treatment of lumbar spinal stenosis: a randomized Trial. *Ann Intern Med.* 2015;162:465-473.

142. Deyo RA, Mirza SK, Martin BI, et al. Trends, major medical complications, and charges associated with surgery for lumbar spinal stenosis in older adults. *JAMA.* 2010;303(13):1259-1265.

143. Park D, An H, Lurie J, et al. Does multilevel lumbar stenosis lead to poorer outcomes? A subanalysis of the Spine Patient Outcomes research. *Spine.* 2010;35(4):439-446.

144. Backstrom KM, Whitman JM, Flynn TW. Lumbar spinal stenosis—diagnosis and management of the aging spine. *Man Ther.* 2011;16:308-317.

145. Burgstaller JM, Schuffler PJ, Buhmann JM, et al. Is there an association between pain and magnetic resonance imaging parameters in patients with lumbar spinal stenosis? *Spine (Phila Pa 1976).* 2016;41(17):E1053-E1062.

146. Murphy DR, Hurwitz EL, Gregory AA, et al. A non-surgical approach to the management of lumbar spinal stenosis: a prospective observational cohort study. *BMC Musculoskelet Disord.* 2006;7:16.

147. Pua YH, Cai CC, Lim KC. Treadmill walking with body weight support is no more effective than cycling when added to an exercise program for lumbar spinal stenosis: a randomised controlled trial. *Aust J Physiother.* 2007;53:83-89.

148. Nicola W, Mok NW, Brauer SG, et al. Changes in lumbar movement in people with low back pain are related to compromised balance. *Spine.* 2010;36(1):E45-E52.

149. Gatti R, Faccendini S, Tettamanti A, et al. Efficacy of trunk balance exercises for individuals with chronic low back pain: a randomized clinical trial. *J Orthop Sports Phys Ther.* 2011;41(8):542-552.

150. Saal JA, Saal JS. Nonoperative treatment of herniated lumbar intervertebral disc with radiculopathy an outcome study. *Spine.* 1989;14(4):431-436.

151. Weber H. Lumbar disc herniation: a controlled prospective study with ten years of observation. *Spine.* 1983;8:131-140.

152. Thomas KC, Fisher CG, Boyd M, et al. Outcome evaluation of surgical and nonsurgical management of lumbar disc protrusion causing radiculopathy. *Spine.* 2007;12(13):1414-1422.

153. Saunders HD, Saunders R. *Evaluation*, Treatment, and Prevention of Musculoskeletal Disorders, vol. 1. Chaska, MN: Saunders; 1993.

154. Fritz JM, Lindsay W, Matheson JW, et al. Is there a subgroup of patients with low back pain likely to benefit from mechanical traction? Results of a randomized clinical trial and subgrouping analysis. *Spine.* 2007;32(26):E793-E800.

155. Van der Heijden GJMG, Beurskens AJHM, Koes BW, et al. The efficacy of traction for back and neck pain: a systematic, blinded review of randomized clinical trial methods. *Phys Ther.* 1995;75(2):93-104.

156. Thackeray A, Fritz J, Childs J, et al. The effectiveness of mechanical traction among subgroups of patients with low back pain and leg pain: a randomized trial. *J Orthop Sports Phys Ther.* 2016;46(3):144-154.

157. Paris SV. Physical therapy approach to facet, disc, and sacroiliac syndrome of the lumbar spine. In: White AH, editor. *Conservative Care of Low Back Pain.* Baltimore: Williams and Wilkins; 1990.

158. Creighton DS. Positional distraction: a radiological confirmation. *J Man Manipulative Ther.* 1993;1(3):83-86.

159. George SZ. Characteristics of patients with lower extremity symptoms treated with slump stretching: a case series. *J Orthop Sports Phys Ther.* 2002;32:391-398.

160. Cleland JA, Childs JD, Palmer JA, et al. Slump stretching in the management of non-radicular low back pain: a pilot clinical trial. *Man Ther.* 2006;11:279-286.

161. Basson A, Olivier B, Ellis R, et al. The effectiveness of neural mobilization for neuromusculoskeletal conditions: a systematic review and meta-analysis. *J Orthop Sports Phys Ther.* 2017; 47(9):593-615.

162. Korres DS, Loupassis G, Stamos K. Results of lumbar discectomy: a study using 15 different evaluation methods. *Eur Spine J.* 1992;1:20-24.

163. Loupasis GA, Stamos K, Katonis PG, et al. Seven- to 20-year outcome of lumbar discectomy. *Spine.* 1999;24:2313-2317.

164. Dvorak J, Valach L, Fuhrimann P, et al. The outcome of surgery for lumbar disc herniation. II. A 4–17 years' follow-up with emphasis on psychosocial aspects. *Spine.* 1988;13:1423-1427.

165. Yorimitsu E, Chiba K, Toyama Y, et al. Long-term outcomes of standard discectomy for lumbar disc herniation: a follow-up study of more than 10 years. *Spine.* 2001;26:652-657.

166. Ostelo RWJG, deVet CW, Waddell G, et al. *Rehabilitation after Lumbar Disc Surgery.* Oxford: The Cochrane Library; 2002.

167. Ostelo RWJG, Costa LOP, Maher CG, et al. *Rehabilitation after Lumbar Disc Surgery.* Available at http://summaries. cochrane.org/CD003007/rehabilitation-after-lumbar-disc-surgery. Accessed December 8, 2013.

168. Scrimshaw SV, Maher CG. Randomized controlled trial of neural mobilization after spinal surgery. *Spine (Phila Pa 1976).* 2001;26:2647-2652.

169. Yilmaz F, Yilmaz A, Merdol F, et al. Efficacy of dynamic lumbar stabilization exercise in lumbar microdiscectomy. *J Rehabil Med.* 2003;35:163-167.

170. Kulig K, Beneck GJ, Selkowitz DM, et al. An intensive, progressive exercise program reduces disability and improves performance in patients after single-level lumbar microdiscectomy. *Phys Ther.* 2009;89:1145-1157.

171. Dolan P, Greenfield K, Nelson RJ, et al. Can exercise therapy improve the outcome of microdiscecomy? *Spine.* 2000;25(12): 1523-1532.

172. Schwarzer A, Aprill C, Bogduk N. The sacroiliac joint in chronic low back pain. *Spine.* 1995;20:31-37.

173. Hayne CR. Manual transport of loads by women. *Physiotherapy.* 1981;67(8):226-231.

174. Vleeming A, Albert HB, Ostgaard HC, et al. European guidelines for the diagnosis and treatment of pelvic girdle pain. *Eur Spine J.* 2008;17(6):794-819.

175. Albert HB, Modskesen M, Westergaard JG. Incidence of four syndromes of pregnancy-related pelvic joint pain. *Spine.* 2002; 27(24):2831-2834.

176. Laslett M, Young SB, Aprill CN, et al. Diagnosing painful sacroiliac joints: a validity study of a McKenzie evaluation and sacroiliac provocation tests. *Aust J Physiother.* 2003;49:89-97.

177. Laslett M, Williams M. The reliability of selected pain provocation tests for sacroiliac joint pathology. *Spine.* 1994; 19:1243-1249.

178. Palsson TS, Gibson W, Darlow B, et al. Changing the narrative in diagnosis and management of pain in the sacroiliac joint area. *Phys Ther.* 2019;99(11):1511-1519.

179. Potter NA, Rothstein JM. Intertester reliability for selected tests of the sacroiliac joint. *Phys Ther.* 1985;65:1671-1975.

180. Cibulka M, Koldehoff R. Clinical usefulness of a cluster of sacroiliac joint tests in patients with and without low back pain. *J Orthop Sports Phys Ther.* 1999;29(2):83-92.

181. Arab AM, Abdollahi I, Joghataei MT, et al. Inter- and intra-examiner reliability of single and composites of selected motion palpation and pain provocation tests for sacroiliac joint. *Man Ther.* 2009;14:213-221.

182. Lee D. *The Pelvic Girdle: an Approach to the Examination and Treatment of the Lumbopelvic-Hip Region.* Edinburgh: Churchill Livingstone; 2004.

183. Mens JMA, Vleeming A, Snijders CJ, et al. Reliability and validity of the active straight leg raise test in posterior pelvic pain since pregnancy. *Spine.* 2001;26(10):1167-1171.

184. de Groot M, Pool-Goudzwaard AL, Spoor CW, et al. The active straight leg raising test (ASLR) in pregnant women: differences in muscle activity and force between patients and healthy subjects. *Man Ther.* 2008;13:68-74.

185. Beales DJ, O'Sullivan PB, Briffa NK. Motor control patterns during an active straight leg raise in chronic pelvic girdle pain subjects. *Spine.* 2009;34(9):861-870.

186. O'Sullivan PB, Beales DJ, Beetham JA, et al. Altered motor control strategies in subjects with sacroiliac joint pain during the active straight-leg-raise test. *Spine.* 2002;27(1):E1-E8.

187. Stuge B, Lacrum E, Kirkesola G, et al. The efficacy of a treatment program focusing on specific stabilizing exercises for pelvic girdle pain after pregnancy: a randomized controlled trial. *Spine.* 2004;29(4):351-359.

188. Arumugam A, Milosavljevic S, Woodley S, et al. Effects of external pelvic compression on form closure, force closure, and neuromotor control of the lumbopelvic spine: a systematic review. *Man Ther.* 2012;17:275-284.

189. O'Sullivan PB, Beales DJ. Diagnosis and classification of pelvic girdle pain disorders: part I: a mechanism based approach within a biopsychosocial framework. *Man Ther.* 2007;12:86-97.

190. O'Sullivan P. Classification of lumbopelvic pain disorders: why is it essential for management. *Man Ther.* 2006;11:169-170.

191. Mens JM, Damen L, Snijders CJ, et al. The mechanical effect of a pelvic belt in patients with pregnancy-related pelvic pain. *Clin Biomech.* 2006;21(2):122-127.

192. Ostgaard HC, Zetherstrom G, Roos-Hansen E, et al. Reduction of back and posterior pelvic pain in pregnancy. *Spine.* 1994;19(8):894-900.

193. Arab AM, Behbahani RB, Lorestani L, et al. Assessment of pelvic floor muscle function in women with and without low back pain using transabdominal ultrasound. *Man Ther.* 2010;15(3): 235-239.

194. Stuge B, Saetre K, Braekken IH. The association between pelvic floor muscle function and pelvic girdle pain–a matched case control 3D ultrasound study. *Man Ther.* 2012;17:150-156.

195. Cecchi F, Molino-Lova R, Chiti M, et al. Spinal manipulation compared with back school and with individually delivered physiotherapy for the treatment of chronic low back pain: a randomized trial with one-year follow-up. *Clin Rehabil.* 2010;24:26-36.

196. Zafereo J, Wang-Price S, Roddey T, et al. Regional manual therapy and motor control exercises for chronic low back pain: a randomized clinical trial. *J Man Manip Ther.* 2018;26(4):193-202.

197. de Oliveira RF, Liebano RE, Costa Lda C, et al. Immediate effects of region-specific and non–region-specific spinal manipulative

therapy in patients with chronic low back pain: a randomized controlled trial. *Phys Ther.* 2013;93:748-756.

198. Coulter ID, Crawford C, Hurwitz E, et al. Manipulation and mobilization for treating chronic low back pain: a systematic review and meta-analysis. *Spine J.* 2018;18(7):1109-1302.

199. Rubinstein SM, de Zoete AM, van Middelkoop M, et al. Benefits and harms of spinal manipulative therapy for treatment of chronic low back pain: systematic review and meta-analysis of randomized controlled trials. *BMJ.* 2019;364:l689.

200. Goldby LJ, Moore AP, Doust J, et al. A randomized controlled trial investigating the efficiency of musculoskeletal physiotherapy on chronic low back disorder. *Spine.* 2006;31(10):1083-1093.

201. Cook C, Petersen S, Donaldson M, et al. Does early change predict long-term (6 months) improvements in subjects who receive manual therapy for low back pain? *Physiotherapy Theory Pract.* 2017;33(9):716–724.

202. O'Sullivan P, Caneiro JP, O'Keefe M, et al. Unraveling the complexity of low back pain. JOSPT. *Orthop Sports Phys Ther.* 2016;46(11):932-937.

203. Janda V. *Postural and Phasic Muscles in the Pathogenesis of Low Back Pain.* Dublin: Proceedings of the XIth Congress ISRD; 1968.

204. Giesecke T, Gracely R, Grant M, et al. Evidence of augmented central pain processing in idiopathic chronic low back pain. *Arthritis Rheum.* 2004;50(2):613-623.

205. Clare HA, Adams R, Maher CG. A systematic review of efficacy of McKenzie therapy for spinal pain. *Aust J Physiother.* 2004;50:209-216.

206. Nicholas MK, George SZ. Psychologically informed interventions for low back pain: an update for physical therapists. *Phys Ther.* 2011;91:765-776.

207. George SZ, Zeppieri G. Physical Therapy utilization of graded exposure for patients with low back pain. *Orthop Sport Phys Ther.* 2009;39(7):496-505.

208. Vlaeyen JW, de Jong J, Geilen M, et al. Graded exposure in vivo in the treatment of pain-related fear: a replicated single-case experimental design in four patients with chronic low back pain. *Behav Res Ther.* 2001;39:151-166.

209. Vlaeyen JW, de Jong J, Geilen M, et al. The treatment of fear of movement/(re)injury in chronic low back pain: further evidence on the effectiveness of exposure in vivo. *Clin J Pain.* 2002;18:251-261.

210. Fritz JM, George SZ, Delitto A. The role of fear-avoidance beliefs in acute low back pain: relationships with current and future disability and work status. *Pain.* 2001;94:7-15.

211. George SZ, Fritz JM, Childs JD. Investigation of elevated fear-avoidance beliefs for patients with low back pain: a secondary analysis involving patients enrolled in physical therapy clinical trials. *J Orthop Sports Phys Ther.* 2008;38(2):50-58.

212. Waddell G, Newton M, Handerson I, et al. A fear-avoidance beliefs questionnaire (FABQ) and the role of fear-avoidance beliefs in chronic low back pain and disability. *Pain.* 1993;52:157-168.

213. George SZ, Bialosky JE, Fritz JM. Physical therapist management of a patient with acute low back pain and elevated fear-avoidance beliefs. *Phys Ther.* 2004;84(6):538-549.

214. Burton AK, Waddell G, Tillotson KM, et al. Information and advice to patients with back pain can have a positive effect: a randomized controlled trial of a novel educational booklet in primary care. *Spine (Phila Pa 1976).* 1999;24:2484-2491.

215. Moseley GL, Nicholas MK, Hodges PW. A randomized controlled trial of intensive neurophysiology education in chronic low back pain. *Clin J Pain.* 2004;20:324-330.

216. Siemonsma PC, Stuive I, Roorda LD, et al. Cognitive treatment of illness perceptions in patients with chronic low back pain: a randomized controlled trial. *Phys Ther.* 2013;93:435-448.

217. Pengel LH, Refshauge KM, Maher CG, et al. Physiotherapist-directed exercise, advice, or both for subacute low back pain: a randomized trial. *Ann Intern Med.* 2007;146:787-796.

218. Loisel P, Lemaire J, Poitras S, et al. Cost-benefit and cost-effectiveness analysis of a disability prevention model for back pain management: a six year follow up study. *Occup Environ Med.* 2002;59:807-815.

219. Macedo LG, Latimer J, Maher CG, et al. Effect of motor control exercises versus graded activity in patients with chronic nonspecific low back pain: a randomized controlled trial. *Phys Ther.* 2012;92:363-377.

220. Edwards RR, Almeida DM, Klick B, et al. Duration of sleep contributes to next-day pain report in the general population. *Pain.* 2000;137:202-207.

221. Finan PH, Goodin BR, Smith MT. The association of sleep and pain: an update and a path forward. *J Pain.* 2013;14:1539-1552.

222. Nijs J, Mairesse O, Neu D, et al. Sleep disturbances in chronic pain: neurobiology, assessment, and treatment in physical therapist practice. *Phys Ther.* 2018;98:325-335.

223. Haack M, Sanchez E, Mullington JM. Elevated inflammatory markers in response to prolonged sleep restriction are associated with increased pain experience in healthy volunteers. *Sleep.* 2007;30:1145-1152.

224. Cho S, Kim GS, Lee JH. Psychometric evaluation of the sleep hygiene index: a sample of patients with chronic pain. *Health Qual Life Outcomes.* 2013;11:213.

225. Orlandi AC, Ventura C, Gallinaro AL, et al. Improvement in pain, fatigue, and subjective sleep quality through sleep hygiene tips in patients with fibromyalgia [Article in English, Portuguese]. *Rev Bras Reumatol.* 2012;52:666-678.

226. Siengsukon CF, Al-dughmi M, Stevens S. Sleep health promotion: practical information for physical therapists. *Phys Ther.* 2017;97:826-836.

227. Tang NK, Goodchild CE, Salkovskis PM. Hybrid cognitive-behaviour therapy for individuals with insomnia and chronic pain: a pilot randomised controlled trial. *Behav Res Ther.* 2012;50:814-821.

228. Hall A, Richmond H, Copsey B, et al. Physiotherapist-delivered cognitive-behavioural interventions are effective for low back pain, but can they be replicated in clinical practice? A systematic review. *Disabil Rehabil.* 2018;40:1-9.

229. Collaer JW, McKeough DM, Boissonnault WG. Lumbar isthmic spondylolisthesis detection with palpation interrater reliability and concurrent criterion-related validity. *J Man Manip Ther.* 2006;14(1):22-29.

230. Alquarni AM, Schneiders AG, Hendrick PA. Clinical tests to diagnose lumbar segmental instability: a systematic review. *J Orthop Sports Phys Ther.* 2011;41(3):130-140.

231. Rabin L, Shashua A, Pizem K, et al. The interrater reliability of physical examination tests that may predict the outcome or suggest the need for lumbar stabilization exercises. *J Orthop Sports Phys Ther.* 2013;43(2):83-90.

232. Reese N, Bandy W. Use of an inclinometer to measure flexibility of the iliotibial band using the Ober test and the Modified Ober test: difference in magnitude and reliability of measurements. *J Orthop Sports Phys Ther.* 2003;33:326-330.

233. Piva SR, Fitzgerald K, Irrgang JJ, et al. Reliability of measures of impairments associated with patellofemoral pain. Syndrome. *BMC Musculoskelet Disord.* 2006;7:33.

234. Maitland G, Hengeveld E, Banks K, et al. *Maitland's Vertebral Manipulation*, ed 7. Edinburgh: Elsevier Butterworth Heinemann; 2005.

235. Majlesi J, Togay H, Ünalan H, et al. The sensitivity and specificity of the slump and the straight leg raising tests in patients with lumbar disc herniation. *J Clin Rheumatol*. 2008;14(2):87-91.

236. Walsh J, Hall T. Agreement and correlation between the straight leg raise and slump tests in subjects with leg pain. *J Manipulative Physiol Ther*. 2009;32:184-192.

237. Urban LM. The straight leg raise test: a review. *J Orthop Sports Phys Ther*. 1981;2(3):117-133.

238. Deville W, van der Windt D, Dzaferagic A, et al. The test of Laseque: systematic review of the accuracy in diagnosing herniated discs. *Spine*. 2000;25:1140-1147.

239. Vroomen P, de Krom M, Wilmink J, et al. Diagnostic value of history and physical examination in patients suspected of lumbosacral nerve root compression. *J Neurol Neurosurg Psychiatry*. 2002;72(5):630-634.

240. Roussel NA, Nijs J, Truijen S, et al. Low back pain: clinimetric properties of the Trendelenburg test, active straight leg raise test, and breathing pattern during active straight leg raising. *J Manipulative Physiol Ther*. 2007;30:270-278.

241. Richardson C, Jull G, Hodges P, et al. *Therapeutic Exercise for Spinal Segmental Stabilization in Low Back Pain: Scientific Basis and Clinical Approach*. Edinburgh: Churchill Livingstone; 1999.

242. Janda V. *Rational Therapeutic Approach of Chronic Back Pain Syndromes*. Turku, Finland: Proceedings of the Symposium; 1985.

243. Oh JS, Cynn HS, Won JH, et al. Effects of performing an abdominal drawing-in maneuver during prone hip extension exercises on hip and back extensor muscle activity and amount of anterior pelvic tilt. *J Orthop Sports Phys Ther*. 2007;37(6):320-324.

244. Murphy DR, Byfield D, McCarthy P, et al. Interexaminer reliability of the hip extension test for suspected impaired motor control of the lumbar spine. *J Manipulative Physiol Ther*. 2006;29:374-377.

245. Youdas JW, Mraz ST, Norstad BJ, et al. Determining meaningful changes in pelvic-on-femoral position during the Trendelenburg test. *J Sport Rehabil*. 2007;16:326-335.

246. Cliborne AV, Wainner RS, Rhon DI, et al. Clinical hip tests and a functional squat test in patients with knee osteoarthritis: reliability, prevalence of positive test findings, and short-term response to hip mobilization. *J Orthop Sports Phys Ther*. 2004;34:676-685.

247. Bird PA, Oakley SP, Shnier R, et al. Prospective evaluation of magnetic resonance imaging and physical examination findings in patients with greater trochanteric pain syndrome. *Arthritis Rheum*. 2001;44(9):2138-2145.

248. Dreyfuss P, Michaelson M, Pauza M, et al. The value of medical history and physical examination in diagnosing sacroiliac joint pain. *Spine*. 1996;21:2594-2602.

249. Russell A, Maksymowych W, LeClercq S. Clinical examination of the sacroiliac joints: a prospective study. *Arthritis Rheum*. 1981;24:1575-1577.

250. Sutlive TG, Lopez HP, Schnitker DE, et al. Development of a clinical prediction rule for diagnosing hip osteoarthritis in individuals with unilateral hip pain. *J Orthop Sports Phys Ther*. 2008;38(9):542-550.

251. Martin RL, Sekiya JK. The interrater reliability of 4 clinical tests used to assess individuals with musculoskeletal hip pain. *J Orthop Sports Phys Ther*. 2008;38:71-77.

252. Martin RL, Irrgang JJ, Sekiya JK. The diagnostic accuracy of a clinical examination in determining intra-articular hip pain for potential hip arthroscopy candidates. *Arthroscopy*. 2008;24:1013-1018.

253. Maslowski E, Sullivan W, Forster Harwood J, et al. The diagnostic validity of hip provocation maneuvers to detect intra-articular hip pathology. *PM R*. 2010;2:174-181.

254. Wang SS, Whitney SL, Burdett RG, et al. Lower extremity muscular flexibility in long distance runners. *J Orthop Sports Phys Ther*. 1993;17:102-107.

255. Clapis PA, Davis SM, Davis RO. Reliability of inclinometer and goniometric measurements of hip extension flexibility using the modified Thomas test. *Physiother Theory Pract*. 2008;24(2):135-141.

256. Bullock-Saxton J, Bullock M. Repeatability of muscle length measures around the hip. *Physiother Can*. 1994;46:105-109.

257. Pua YH, Wrigley TV, Cowan SM, et al. Intrarater test-retest reliability of hip range of motion and hip muscle strength measurements in persons with hip osteoarthritis. *Arch Phys Med Rehabil*. 2008;89(6):1146-1154.

258. Ellison JB, Rose SJ, Sahrmann SA. Patterns of hip rotation range of motion: a comparison between healthy subjects and patients with low back pain. *Phys Ther*. 1990;70:537-541.

259. Tiru M, Goh S, Low B. Use of percussion as a screening tool in the diagnosis of occult hip fractures. *Singapore Med J*. 2002;43:467-469.

260. Alqarni AM, Scheiders AG, Hendrick PA. Clinical tests to diagnose lumbar segmental instability: a systematic review. *J Orthop Sports Phys Ther*. 2011;41(3):130-140.

CHAPTER 5

Examination and Treatment of Thoracic Spine Disorders

OVERVIEW

This chapter covers the kinematics of the thoracic spine and rib cage, describes common thoracic spine disorders, and provides a detailed description of special tests, manual examination, mobilization/manipulation, and exercise procedures for the thoracic spine and rib cage. Video clips of the majority of the examination and manual therapy procedures are also included.

OBJECTIVES

1. Describe the significance and impact of thoracic spine disorders.
2. Describe thoracic spine and rib cage biomechanics.
3. Utilize clinical reasoning to cClassify thoracic spine disorders based on signs and symptoms.
4. Determine the most effective and pPerform manual therapy and therapeutic exercise interventions for thoracic spine and rib cage disorders.
5. Demonstrate and interpret thoracic spine examination procedures.
6. Demonstrate mobilization/manipulation techniques of the thoracic spine and rib cage.
7. Instruct exercises for thoracic spine disorders.
8. Incorporate psychologically informed education and management principles for treatment of patients with thoracic spine and rib cage disorders.

▶ To view videos pertaining to this chapter, please visit the eBook.

SIGNIFICANCE OF THORACIC SPINE DISORDERS

Although the full impact of thoracic spine disorders is not fully appreciated because little research has been completed on these disorders compared with cervical and lumbar disorders, a systematic literature review found that the 1-year prevalence of thoracic spinal pain ranged between 3% and 55% with most occupational groups having medium of about 30% 1-year prevalence.[1] A study of a Norwegian population, found a 1-year prevalence of thoracic spinal pain of 13% compared with 43% and 44% for low back and neck pain respectively.[2] In another study investigating a working population in France, an incidence of thoracic spine pain was reported of 5.2 per 100 male workers and 10.0 per 100 female workers.[3] The researchers also found a coexistence of neck and/or low back pain in 41% of male and 36% of female workers with thoracic spinal pain.[3]

THORACIC SPINE AND RIB CAGE KINEMATICS: FUNCTIONAL ANATOMY AND MECHANICS

The thorax consists of the thoracic spine, the rib cage, and the sternum. The thorax is a fairly rigid structure whose function is to provide a stable base for muscles to control the craniocervical region and shoulder girdle, to protect internal organs, and to create a mechanical bellows for breathing.[4] The structure consists of 12 thoracic vertebrae and 12 corresponding ribs on each side. A natural thoracic kyphosis is created by a bony slope of 3.8 degrees from posterior to anterior at each vertebral body, which creates a 45-degree kyphotic angle for the entire thoracic spine.[5]

Anatomically and functionally, the thoracic spine is commonly divided into the upper thoracic (T1–T4), the middle thoracic (T5–T9), and the lower thoracic (T10–T12), with

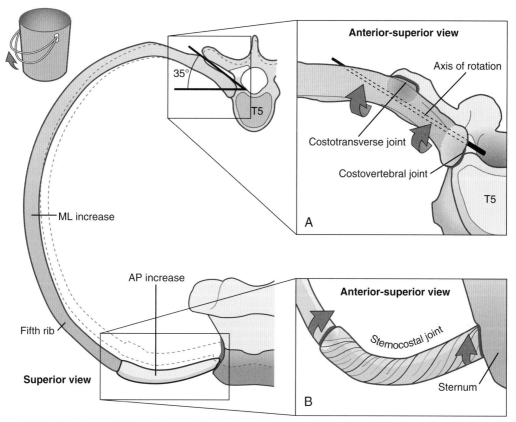

FIG. 5.1 Top view of fifth rib shows "bucket-handle" mechanism of elevation of the ribs during inspiration. The *ghosted* outline of the rib indicates its position before inspiration. Elevation of the rib increases both anteroposterior (*AP*) and mediolateral (*ML*) diameters of thorax. Rib connects to vertebral column via costotransverse and costovertebral joints (A) and to sternum via the sternocostal joint (B). During elevation, neck of the rib moves about an axis of rotation that courses between each costotransverse and costovertebral joint. Elevating rib creates torsion in the cartilage associated with sternocostal joint. (From Neumann DA. *Kinesiology of the Musculoskeletal System*, ed 3. St Louis: Elsevier; 2017.)

the upper thoracic functioning as a transition zone from the cervical spine to the thoracic spine and the lower thoracic functioning as a transition zone from thoracic spine to lumbar spine.[5] The mid-thoracic region is the most rigid because of the rib articulations, with the T11 and T12 vertebrae being more mobile because of the lack of complete anterior rib attachment with the "floating ribs" at T11 and T12.[5] The upper thoracic region moves with the cervical spine and with similar mechanics to the cervical spine.

The facet joints of the thoracic vertebrae are generally in the frontal plane with a mild slope that varies between 0 and 30 degrees from the vertical.[4] The spinous processes of the thoracic vertebrae tend to angle downward and extend to the level of the caudal vertebrae's transverse processes. In identification of the vertebral level through palpation, the transverse processes can be found lateral to the most prominent aspect of the spinous process of the vertebra one level above.[6] This trend is consistent throughout the upper and middle thoracic spine but is less consistent at lower thoracic levels (especially T11 and T12).[6]

The costotransverse and costovertebral joints allow movement of the ribs in relation to the spine and function during

ventilation. The costovertebral joints connect the heads of each of the 12 ribs to the corresponding sides of the bodies of the thoracic vertebrae. The costotransverse joints connect the articular tubercles of the ribs 1 to 10 to the transverse processes of the corresponding thoracic vertebrae. Ribs 11 and 12 usually lack costotransverse joints.[4] The sternocostal joints provide a functional link of the ribs from the sternum to the thoracic spine (Fig. 5.1).

The costovertebral joints connect the head of the rib with a pair of costal facets at adjacent vertebral bodies and the adjacent margin of the intervertebral disk. The articular surfaces of the costovertebral joints are slightly ovoid and are held together by capsular and radiate ligaments.[4] Costotransverse joints connect the articular tubercle of a rib to the costal facet on the transverse process of a corresponding thoracic vertebra. An articular capsule surrounds this synovial joint, and the costotransverse ligament firmly anchors the neck of the rib to the entire length of a corresponding transverse process.[4]

Approximately 30 to 40 degrees of forward bending and 15 to 20 degrees of backward bending are available throughout the thoracic region.[4] A two-dimensional (2D) photographic analysis study measured mean range of motion of 11.5 degrees

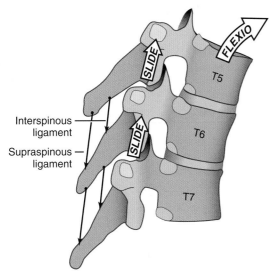

FIG. 5.2 Kinematics at thoracic region. Kinematics of thoracolumbar flexion are shown through 85-degree arc: sum of 35 degrees of thoracic flexion and 50 degrees of lumbar flexion. (From Neumann DA. *Kinesiology of the Musculoskeletal System*, ed 3. St Louis: Elsevier; 2017.)

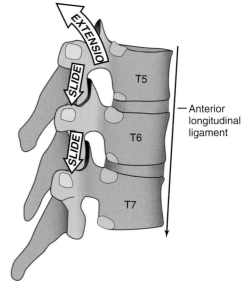

FIG. 5.3 Kinematics at thoracic region. Kinematics of thoracolumbar extension are shown through arc of 35 to 40 degrees: 20 to 25 degrees of thoracic extension and 15 degrees of lumbar extension. (From Neumann DA. *Kinesiology of the Musculoskeletal System*, ed 3. St Louis: Elsevier; 2017.)

forward bending and 8.7 degrees backward bending in the standing position in 40 young, asymptomatic adults.[7] In an unloaded position (prone or quadruped), the mean thoracic backward bending increases to approximately 14.5 degrees with approximately 60% of the motion occurring in the upper six thoracic segments and remaining 40% of the motion in the lower half of the thorax.[7] The kinematics of forward bending occur with a superior and slightly anterior sliding (i.e., upglide) of the inferior facet surfaces of the superior member of the vertebral segment moving on the superior facet surfaces of the lower member of the vertebral segment (Fig. 5.2). Backward bending occurs with just the opposite movements: inferior and slightly posterior sliding (i.e., downglide) of the inferior facet surfaces of the superior member of the vertebral segment moving on the superior facet surfaces of the lower member of the vertebral segment (Fig. 5.3).

Approximately 25 to 35 degrees of axial rotation occurs to each side throughout the thoracic region.[4] Rotation occurs in the mid-thoracic spine as the frontal plane–aligned inferior articular facets of the superior member of the spinal segment slide a short distance in relation to the superior facets of the inferior member of the vertebral segment.[4] The amount of axial rotation tends to decrease from the upper to lower thoracic spine because the greater vertically oriented facet joints tend to block the horizontal plane movement (Fig. 5.4).[4]

Approximately 25 to 30 degrees of lateral flexion occur to each side in the thoracic region.[4] The motion is limited by the ribs and remains fairly constant from one segment to another throughout the thorax. Lateral flexion occurs as the inferior facet surface of the superior member of the spinal segment slides superiorly (i.e., upglides) on the opposite direction of the lateral flexion and inferiorly (i.e., downglides) on the same

side of the lateral flexion. The ribs drop slightly on the same side of the lateral flexion and rise slightly on the opposite side (Fig. 5.5). Coupling patterns for lateral flexion and rotation are inconsistent in the middle and lower thoracic spine and seem to vary from individual to individual and from one study to another.[4,8]

The thorax changes shape during ventilation with movement at five articulations: the manubriosternal, sternocostal, interchondral, costotransverse, and costovertebral joints. During inspiration, the shaft of the ribs elevates in a path perpendicular to the axis of the rotation that courses between the costotransverse and costovertebral joints. The downward-sloped shaft of the ribs rotates upward and outward, increasing the intrathoracic volume in both anteroposterior and mediolateral diameters.[4] During expiration, the muscles of inspiration relax to allow the ribs and sternum to return to their preinspiration positions. The lowering of the body of the ribs combined with the inferior and posterior movements of the sternum decreases the anteroposterior and mediolateral diameters of the thorax.[4]

The muscles of the thorax are organized into three layers: superficial, intermediate, and deep.[4] The superficial layer includes primarily shoulder girdle muscles including the trapezius, latissimus dorsi, rhomboids, levator scapula, and serratus anterior. Bilateral activation of the muscles of the superficial layer assists in extension of the thorax, and unilateral activation of these muscles laterally flexes and rotates the region. For example, the right middle trapezius assists with right lateral flexion and left axial rotation of the upper thoracic region.[4] The intermediate layer of muscles includes the serratus posterior superior and serratus posterior inferior. They are relatively

Thoracolumbar axial rotation

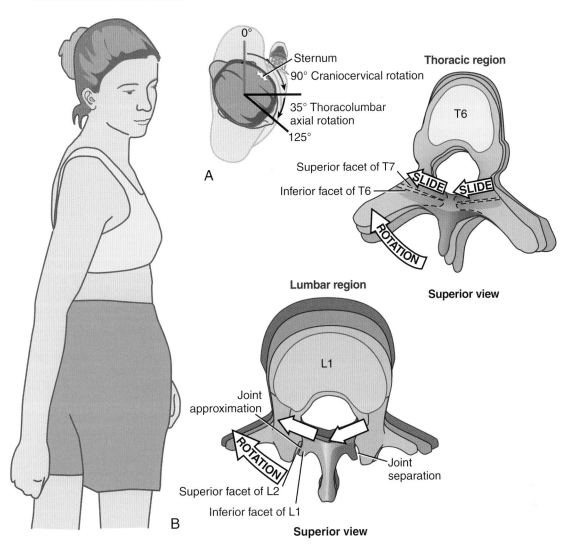

FIG. 5.4 Kinematics of thoracolumbar axial rotation are depicted as the subject rotates her face 125 degrees to the right. The thoracolumbar axial rotation is shown through a 35-degree arc: the sum of 30 degrees of thoracic rotation and 5 degrees of lumbar rotation. A, Kinematics at the thoracic region. B, Kinematics at the lumbar region. (From Neumann DA. *Kinesiology of the Musculoskeletal System*, ed 3. St Louis: Elsevier; 2017.)

thin muscles that offer little contribution to trunk movements and are more likely involved in ventilation.[4]

The deep layer of back muscles in the thoracic region includes the erector spinae group, transversospinal group, and short segmental group (Fig. 5.6). The erector spinae muscle group consists of the spinalis, longissimus, and the iliocostalis muscles. The bulk of the erector spinae muscles have a common attachment on a broad and thick common tendon, located in the region of the sacrum (Fig. 5.7). The erector spinae design is more suited to produce gross trunk movements across regions of the spine rather than controlling intervertebral motions. Bilateral contraction produces backward bending of the trunk. Unilateral contraction

of the iliocostalis produces lateral flexion and unilateral contraction of the upper portions of the longissimus, and iliocostalis muscles assist with ipsilateral axial rotation.[4] Located deep to the erector spinae muscles is the transversospinal muscle group: the semispinalis, multifidus, and rotatores (Figs. 5.8 and 5.9). The transversospinalis muscles tend to originate at the transverse processes and angle superiorly and medially to attach at spinous processes (Fig. 5.10). These muscles are well situated to provide fine segmental control of spinal motions. When contracting bilaterally, the transversospinal muscles produce backward bending, and when contracting unilaterally, they produce contralateral axial rotation.[4]

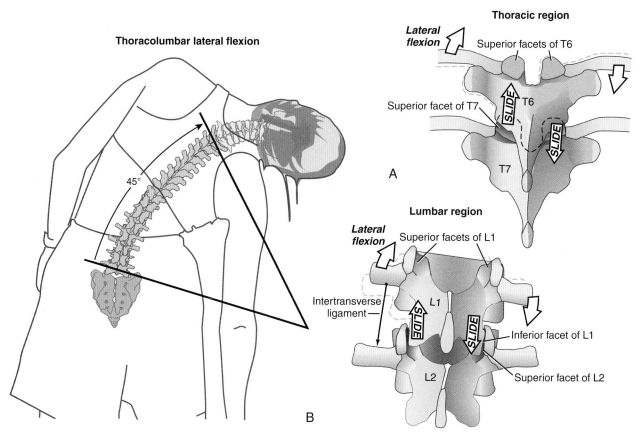

FIG. 5.5 Kinematics of thoracolumbar lateral flexion are shown through approximate 45-degree arc: sum of 25 degrees of thoracic lateral flexion. A, Kinematics at thoracic region. B, Kinematics at lumbar region. Note slight contralateral coupling pattern between axial rotation and lateral flexion in lumbar region. Elongated and taut tissue is indicated by the *thin black arrow*. (From Neumann DA. *Kinesiology of the Musculoskeletal System*, ed 3. St Louis: Elsevier; 2017.)

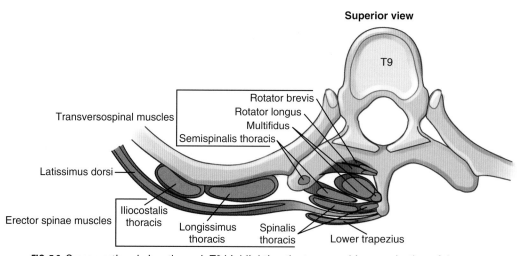

FIG. 5.6 Cross-sectional view through T9 highlighting the topographic organization of the erector spinae and the transversospinal group of muscles. The short segmental group is not shown. (From Neumann DA. *Kinesiology of the Musculoskeletal System*, ed 3. St Louis: Elsevier; 2017.)

Posterior view

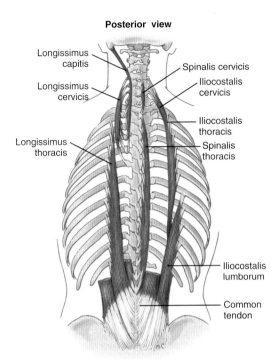

FIG. 5.7 Muscles of erector spinae. For clarity, the left iliocostalis, left spinalis, and the right longissimus muscles are cut just superior to the common tendon. (Modified from Luttgens K, Hamilton N. *Kinesiology: Scientific Basis of Human Motion,* ed 9. Madison, WI: Brown and Benchmark; 1997; Neumann DA. *Kinesiology of the Musculoskeletal System,* ed 3. St Louis: Elsevier; 2017.)

Posterior view

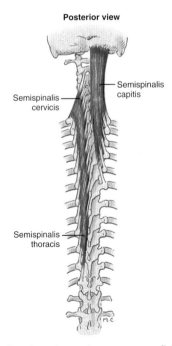

FIG. 5.8 A posterior view shows the more superficial semispinalis muscles within the transversospinal group. For clarity, only the left semispinalis cervicis, left semispinalis thoracis, and right semispinalis capitis are included. (Modified from Luttgens K, Hamilton N. *Kinesiology: Scientific Basis of Human Motion,* ed 9. Madison, WI: Brown and Benchmark; 1997; Neumann DA. *Kinesiology of the Musculoskeletal System,* ed 3. St Louis: Elsevier; 2017.)

Posterior view

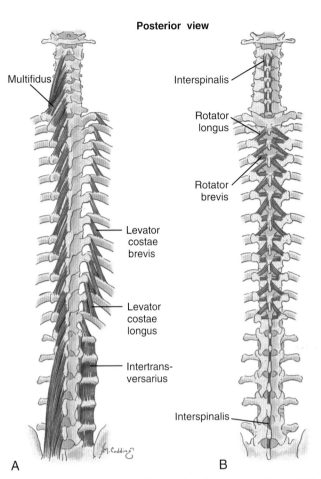

A   B

FIG. 5.9 A posterior view shows the deeper muscles within transversospinal (multifidi on entire left side of A; rotatores bilaterally in B). The muscles within the short segmental group (intertransversarius and interspinalis) are depicted in A and B, respectively. Note that the intertransversarius muscles are shown for the right side of the lumbar region only. (Modified from Luttgens K, Hamilton N. *Kinesiology: Scientific Basis of Human Motion,* ed 9. Madison, WI: Brown and Benchmark; 1997; Neumann DA. *Kinesiology of the Musculoskeletal System,* ed 3. St Louis: Elsevier; 2017.)

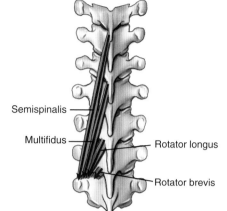

MUSCLE GROUP	RELATIVE LENGTH AND DEPTH	AVERAGE NUMBER OF CROSSED INTERVERTEBRAL JUNCTIONS
Semispinalis	Long; superficial	6 to 8
Multifidi	Intermediate	2 to 4
Rotatores	Short; deep	1 to 2

FIG. 5.10 Simplified depiction of the spatial orientation of muscles within the left transversospinal muscle group. Additional information is listed in tabular form. (Note that the muscles illustrated normally exist bilaterally, throughout the entire cranial-caudal aspect of the vertebral column; their unilateral location is the figure is simplified for the sake of clarity.) (From Neumann DA. *Kinesiology of the Musculoskeletal System*, ed 3. St Louis: Elsevier; 2017.)

TABLE 5.1	Classification of Causes of Acute Thoracic Pain

Painful Conditions of Thoracic Spine

Serious conditions	Infection, fracture, neoplastic disorders, inflammatory disorders, and disk protrusion
Mechanical conditions	Discogenic pain; zygapophyseal joint pain; rib dysfunctions: costotransverse and costovertebral joint pain, muscle imbalances and myofascial pain, and postural deviations

Conditions Referring Pain to Thoracic Spine

Somatic conditions	Disorders of cervical facet joints, muscles, and intervertebral disks
Visceral conditions	Myocardial ischemia, dissecting thoracic aortic aneurysm, peptic ulcer; acute cholecystitis; pancreatitis; renal colic; and acute pyelonephritis

(Modified from National Health and Medical Research Council. Acute thoracic spinal pain. In: *Australian Acute Musculoskeletal Pain Guidelines: Evidence-Based Management of Acute Musculoskeletal Pain.* Brisbane: Australian Academic Press; 2003.)

TABLE 5.2	Alerting Features (Red Flags) of Serious Conditions Associated With Acute Thoracic Spinal Pain

FEATURE OR RISK FACTOR	CONDITION
Minor trauma (if >50 years of age, history of osteoporosis, and corticosteroid use)	Fracture
Major trauma in younger population	Fracture
Fever Night sweats Risk factors of infection (e.g., underlying disease process, penetrating wound, and tuberculosis)	Infection
History of malignant disease Age >50 years No improvement with treatment Unexplained weight loss Pain at multiple sites Pain at rest Night pain	Tumor
Chest pain or heaviness No effect on pain with movement/change in posture Abdominal pain Shortness of breath; cough	Other serious conditions

(Modified from National Health and Medical Research Council. Acute thoracic spinal pain. In: *Australian Acute Musculoskeletal Pain Guidelines: Evidence-Based Management of Acute Musculoskeletal Pain.* Brisbane: Australian Academic Press; 2003.)

DIAGNOSIS, CLASSIFICATION, AND MANAGEMENT OF DISORDERS

Thoracic spine pain conditions are commonly caused by mechanical musculoskeletal impairments of the joints and soft tissues. An impairment-based classification system has not been fully developed and validated; and in general, little research is found on the effectiveness of commonly used interventions for thoracic spine pain.[9] Likewise, a World Health Organization (WHO)'s International Classification of Functioning, Disability, and Health (ICF) classification relative to the thoracic spine has not been published in the literature. The potential causes of thoracic spine pain include referral from other structures, such as the cervical spine; visceral issues; fractures from osteoporosis or malignancy; spinal infections; and mechanical musculoskeletal impairments. Table 5.1 outlines a classification for potential causes of acute and subacute musculoskeletal thoracic pain.

A number of serious medical conditions can be the source of acute thoracic pain. Table 5.2 provides an outline of the conditions that must be screened before initiation of treatment of the thoracic spine and additional details regarding red flag screening can be found in Chapter 2. Appropriate referrals for further medical diagnostic testing should be made if these features or risk factors are identified in patients with acute thoracic spinal pain. After screening for red flags associated with these serious conditions, an impairment-based approach is used to address impairments noted in the examination (Table 5.3).

TABLE 5.3	Impairment-Based Classification for Thoracic Spine Pain Disorders	
CLASSIFICATION	**EXAMINATION FINDINGS**	**PROPOSED INTERVENTIONS**
Thoracic mobility deficits	• Thoracic spine mobility deficits with AROM • Mobility deficits with PIVM testing of the thoracic spine and ribs • No upper extremity radicular symptoms • Muscle imbalances • Postural deviations	• Mobility exercises • Thoracic spine and rib mobilization/manipulation • Self-mobilization techniques • Postural exercises
Thoracic mobility deficits with upper extremity referred pain	• Thoracic spine mobility deficits with AROM • Mobility deficits with PIVM testing of the upper thoracic spine and ribs • Upper extremity symptoms • Positive ULND test results • Muscle imbalances • Postural deviations	• Mobility exercises • Thoracic and rib mobilization/manipulation • ULND mobilization/exercise • Self-mobilization techniques • Postural exercises
Thoracic mobility deficits with neck pain	• Thoracic spine mobility deficits with cervical AROM • Mobility deficits with PIVM testing of the thoracic spine and ribs • No symptoms distal to shoulder • Neck pain with associated cervical spine impairments • Muscle imbalances • Postural deviations	• Thoracic and rib mobilization/manipulation • Mobility exercises • Self-mobilization techniques • Postural exercises • Treatment of cervical impairments
Thoracic mobility deficits with shoulder impairments	• Thoracic spine mobility deficits with shoulder AROM • Mobility deficits with PIVM testing in upper thoracic spine and ribs • Shoulder impingement/rotator cuff signs • Muscle imbalances • Postural deviations	• Mobility exercises • Thoracic and rib mobilization/manipulation • Self-mobilization techniques. • Postural exercises • Rotator cuff exercises
Thoracic mobility deficits with low back pain	• Thoracic spine mobility deficits with thoracolumbar AROM Mobility deficits with PIVM testing • Lumbar impairments • Muscle imbalances • Postural deviations	• Mobility exercises • Thoracic and rib mobilization/manipulation • Lumbar rehabilitation program • Self-mobilization techniques • Postural exercises
Thoracic clinical instability	• History of trauma or thoracic surgery • Provocation of symptoms with sustained weight-bearing posture • Relief of symptoms with nonweight-bearing postures • Hypermobility with loose end feel with PIVM testing • Poor strength (2/5) of thoracic multifidus, erector spinae, and parascapular muscles • Shaking/poorly controlled (aberrant) motion with thoracic AROM (i.e., movement coordination impairments)	• Postural education • Thoracic stabilization exercise program • Parascapular muscle strengthening exercises • Thoracic ring mobilization with movement • Mobilization/manipulation above and below hypermobilities • Ergonomic correction

AROM, Active range of motion; *PIVM,* passive intervertebral motion; *ULND,* upper limb neurodynamic.

The cervical spine must be screened as a possible source of referral pain to the thoracic spine. Experimental studies in healthy volunteers and in patients have shown that pain from structures in the cervical spine can be referred into the upper thoracic spinal region. Referred pain into the upper thoracic spine region can arise from the lower cervical facet joints,[10–12] the cervical muscles,[13] or the cervical intervertebral disks.[14] Cervical screening examination testing should include active range of motion (AROM) testing, Spurling test, cervical distraction test, palpation, and passive intervertebral motion (PIVM) testing.[15] If upper extremity symptoms are reported, upper limb neurodynamic (ULND) testing should also be carried out.[15] Chapter 6 provides a detailed description of these cervical spine examination procedures.

Osteoporosis

Osteoporosis is a condition associated with loss of bone density that is most common in women after menopause and that can result in vertebral fractures and excessive thoracic kyphotic deformity. Osteoporosis leads to nearly 9 million fragility fractures annually worldwide.[16] Fragility fractures are fractures that result from mechanical forces that would not ordinarily result in fracture, known as low-level trauma.[17] The WHO has quantified this as forces equivalent to a fall from a standing height or less.[18] Reduced bone density is a major risk factor for fragility fracture. Other factors that may affect the risk of fragility fracture include the use of oral or systemic glucocorticoids, age, female sex, previous fractures, and a family history of osteoporosis.[18]

The prevalence rate of vertebral fractures associated with osteoporosis dramatically increases in women aged 65 years and older[19] with a 6.5% prevalence rate in those 50 to 59 years of age and a 77.8% prevalence rate in those older than 90 years of age.[20] The most common sites of vertebral fractures are at the T7, T8, T11, and L1 vertebrae.[20] A triggering event for an osteoporotic fracture is often not present. In a hospital-based case series of 30 patients with acute thoracolumbar vertebral compression fractures (VCFs), 46% of cases were classified as spontaneous, 36% were associated with a trivial strain, and 18% were associated with moderate or severe injury.[21] The severity of vertebral deformity has been correlated with more severe back pain and disability. Women with deformities of more than four standard deviations (SDs) below the mean had a 1.9 times higher risk of moderate to severe back pain and a 2.6 times higher risk of disability involving the back.[22]

An estimated 30% of postmenopausal white women in the United States have osteoporosis, and one in four has at least one vertebral deformity; however, two-thirds of vertebral fractures remain undiagnosed.[23] In a group of 3000 American White women aged 65 to 70 years, two-thirds reported back pain during the previous 12 months.[24] At least one vertebral deformity was found in 60% of these women, and 24% had deformities three SDs or more below the mean.[24] After a clinically diagnosed vertebral fracture, survival rate decreases gradually from the rate expected without fracture.[23] Women with severe vertebral deformities have a consistently higher risk of back pain and height loss.[23] The clinical impact of a single vertebral fracture may be minimal, but the effects of multiple fractures are cumulative and often result in acute and chronic back pain, limitation of physical activity, and progressive kyphosis and height loss. Depression and low self-esteem accompany the loss of functional abilities and the inability to take part in recreational activities. Pain and fear of additional fractures cause decreased physical activity, which in turn exacerbates osteoporosis and increases the risk of fracture.[23]

Risk factors for developing osteoporosis include age 50 years and older; female gender; Caucasian or Asian race; menopause (especially early or surgically induced); family history of osteoporosis or fragility fractures; northern European ancestry; long periods of inactivity or immobilization; depression; use of alcohol (more than three drinks/day), tobacco, or caffeine (more than four cups/day); amenorrhea (abnormal absence of menses); and a thin body build.[25] Individuals with these risk factors should have a bone density test to detect osteoporosis before a fracture occurs. Central bone densitometry (DXA) measures bone density at the hip and spine where bone loss most rapidly occurs and provides a T score based on the number of SDs from the mean bone density of a healthy 30-year-old adult.[26] A T score of −1.0 or greater is considered normal; −1.0 to −2.5 is considered osteopenia with early evidence of low bone mass; and −2.5 or less is diagnosed as osteoporosis.[26] Therefore the lower the T score, the lower the bone density, and people with a T score of −2.5 and lower should consider taking osteoporosis medication.[26]

Roman et al.[27] evaluated clinical findings of 1400 patients seen in an adult spine surgery clinic over a 4-year period and determined that the cluster of five findings listed in Box 5.1 are useful to screen for osteoporotic VCFs. A finding of two of five positive tests or fewer demonstrated high sensitivity of 0.95 (95% confidence interval [CI], 0.83–0.99) and low negative likelihood ratio (−LR) of 0.16 (95% CI, 0.04–0.51), providing moderate value to rule out osteoporotic VCF. Four of five yielded a positive likelihood ratio (+LR) of 9.6 (95% CI, 3.7–14.9), providing moderate value in ruling in the diagnosis of osteoporotic VCF.[27]

BOX 5.1	Diagnostic Cluster to Screen for Osteoporotic Vertebral Compression Fracture

1. Age >52 years
2. No presence of leg pain
3. Body mass index <22 kg/m²
4. Does not exercise regularly
5. Female gender

A finding of two of five positive tests or fewer demonstrated high sensitivity of 0.95 (95% CI, 0.83–0.99) and low −LR of 0.16 (95% CI, 0.04–0.51) providing moderate value to rule out osteoporotic VCF. Four of five yielded a +LR of 9.6 (95% CI, 3.7–14.9) providing moderate value in ruling in the diagnosis of osteoporotic VCF.

CI, Confidence interval; *LR,* likelihood ratio; *VCF,* vertebral compression fracture. (Modified from Roman M, Brown C, Richardson W, et al. The development of a clinical decision making algorithm for detection of osteoporotic vertebral compression fracture and wedge deformity. *J Man Manipulative The.* 2010;18:45-50.)

Osteoporosis is considered a contraindication to thrust manipulation techniques to the thoracic spine and rib cage, especially techniques performed in the prone or supine position. Manual therapy techniques performed to the thoracic spine in the prone position for all patients should be performed with a pillow placed under the thorax as a precaution to cushion the ribs during posteroanterior (PA) force application. Gentle nonthrust manual therapy techniques performed to the thorax with the patient in the side-lying position are generally safe for patients with osteoporosis and can be effective in restoring mobility and inhibiting muscle tone and pain in the region. In addition, the sitting thoracic techniques can be performed safely because these techniques involve more lifting distraction forces rather than compressive loading of the vertebra and ribs. Therefore osteoporosis is a precaution for the nonthrust techniques performed in side-lying and sitting positions, but osteoporosis is a contraindication for thrust manipulation techniques performed in prone and supine positions.

The physical therapy intervention that can be of greatest assistance for patients with osteoporosis is a program of guided progression of weight-bearing and resistive exercises.[28–30] Posture, strength, balance, endurance, and bone density can also improve with an exercise program guided by a physical therapist.[28,30] Results can ultimately prevent falls and fractures, which limits the potential for pain and disability associated with osteoporosis.

Thoracic Mobility Deficits

The thoracic spine is by design a fairly rigid structure. With postural stresses and in response to stresses, strains, and injury, regions of the thoracic spine tend to further stiffen and be a source of mechanical pain and mobility deficit symptoms. Even in young, healthy adults, thoracic mobility deficits are more likely to be found in people who sit more than 7 hours per day and participate in less than 150 minutes per week of moderate physical exercise.[31] No systematic reviews of treatment for thoracic spinal pain are found, and little published research exists on the effectiveness of the most commonly used treatments for thoracic spine pain.[8] Only one randomized controlled trial (RCT) on the effectiveness of manual physical therapy treatment of the thoracic spine pain could be identified.[32] Schiller[32] compared the use of spinal manipulation with nonfunctional ultrasound placebo in an RCT of 30 patients with mechanical thoracic spinal pain. The group who received manipulation showed significantly better reductions in numeric pain ratings and improvements in lateral flexion at the end of a 2-week to 3-week treatment period.[32] These changes were maintained 1 month later, but results were no longer better than in the placebo group.[32] Oswestry Disability Index scores and McGill Pain Questionnaire results were the same for both groups throughout the study.[32] Because of the small sample size, it is difficult to draw conclusions from this study. However, at least short-term pain relief and improvement in mobility can be provided with the use of thoracic spine manipulation.

Once regions of thoracic mobility deficits are noted with AROM and PIVM testing, further differentiation can be attempted to isolate facet joint versus costotransverse/costovertebral joint hypomobility. Most commonly, both the rib and the thoracic spine PIVM test results show mobility deficits at the affected spinal segments. Overlying muscle holding is also commonly associated with this condition, as are postural deviations, such as excessive thoracic kyphosis. Muscle imbalances, such as weakness of the parascapular muscles (lower trapezius/middle trapezius) and tightness of the pectoral muscles, are commonly found with an increased thoracic kyphosis and forward head posture.

Pain associated with rib dysfunction is commonly provoked with deep breathing and with spring testing the rib as the thoracic vertebra is stabilized (Fig. 5.28). The location of the pain associated with a rib dysfunction is often slightly lateral to the thoracic vertebrae, and symptoms may be referred laterally along the length of the rib angle.

The manual physical therapy approach starts with manipulation to improve thoracic mobility and is followed up with instruction in mobility, self-mobilization, and postural exercises. Once thoracic segmental restrictions are improved, rib techniques can be used to further restore mobility to the region. Case report evidence has shown that nonthrust mobilization to the thoracic spine can decrease tenderness to palpation of the thoracic erector spinae musculature and the associated intercostals spaces of the ribs at the level of the mobilization, increase thoracic side bending AROM, and improve chest expansion that had been limited by pain before the treatment.[33]

Box 5.2 (Fig 5.11) illustrates self-mobilization and mobility exercises, and Box 5.3 (Fig. 5.12) illustrates postural exercises that address common muscle imbalances found with thoracic hypomobility. Thoracic spine PIVM testing for rib and thoracic segmental restrictions and joint mobilization/manipulation techniques for the ribs and thoracic spine are presented in detail later in this chapter.

Upper Thoracic Mobility Deficits With Upper Extremity Referred Pain

Upper thoracic mobility deficits with upper extremity referred pain is commonly called T4 syndrome. T4 syndrome is a classification of thoracic spine disorders that involve upper extremity paresthesia and pain with or without symptoms into the neck or head.[34] This condition is associated with upper thoracic mobility deficits, most commonly peak stiffness at T3–T4 or T4–T5 spinal segments and a positive ULND 1 test.[35] After manipulation (thrust or nonthrust) of the restricted segment, the upper extremity symptoms subside and an immediate improvement in the ULND 1 test is noted, with improved mobility and reduced upper extremity symptoms.[35] The addition of postural and thoracic mobility exercises can further facilitate recovery (Boxes 5.2 and 5.3).

The mechanism for the immediate effect of thoracic manipulation on upper extremity symptoms is not completely understood. Speculation exists that upper thoracic manipulation may influence the autonomic nervous system in a therapeutic manner based on the anatomic location of the sympathetic nerve fibers that leave the spinal nerve from levels T1–L2 to join the sympathetic chain via the white rami communicantes. These then travel within the sympathetic chain from up to six segments before synapsing on four to 20 postganglionic neurons.[35] The postganglionic neurons exit via the gray rami communicantes to join a peripheral nerve that is distributed to target tissues.[36] One preganglionic neuron synapses with numerous postganglionic neurons in the sympathetic chain; therefore it interacts with somatic nerve fibers that supply a variety of target tissues.[29] The head and neck are supplied by levels T1–T4, and the upper trunk and upper limb by T1–T9.[37] Speculation is that dysfunction of the sympathetic nervous system from T4 could result in referred pain in the head, neck, upper thoracic, and upper limb.

Although there is a very little of research evidence to guide the diagnosis and treatment of the T4 syndrome, there is evidence to support the positive neurophysiologic effects of manipulation of the T4 region on the upper extremity and sympathetic nervous system. Both thoracic thrust manipulation and nonthrust mobilization directed between segments T4 and T7 with a supine technique have demonstrated improvement in ULND and slump sit test mobility in asymptomatic subjects with impaired neurodynamic mobility.[38] The effect was enhanced in subjects with a positive expectation of the intervention.[38] In addition, a grade III posterior to anterior rotatory mobilization technique applied to the T4 vertebrae at a frequency of 0.5 Hz produced a side-specific sympathoexcitatory increase in skin conductance in the hand of normal subjects, which was greater than a validated placebo mobilization technique.[39] Evans[36] suggests that the joint itself may not be the causative factor but that sustained or extreme postures may lead to relative ischemia in the tissues of the region. The sympathetic nerves also form a vasoconstriction network on arterioles and capillaries that are stimulated in the presence of ischemia. The manipulation techniques are believed to activate descending inhibitory pain pathways,[40] resulting in a hypoalgesic effect. A close relationship is found between pain reduction and sympathetic excitation,[41,42] which supports the role of spinal manipulation as a treatment option for the T4 syndrome.

The effectiveness of manipulation for T4 syndrome has only been supported by case report evidence;[35,36] more extensive RCTs are needed to support the use of manipulation and exercise for this condition. The authors of a review of the

BOX 5.2   Self-Mobilization and Mobility Exercises for the Thoracic Spine

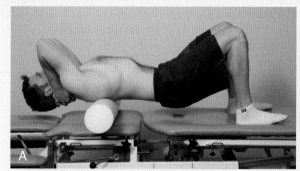

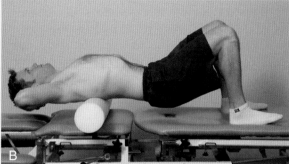

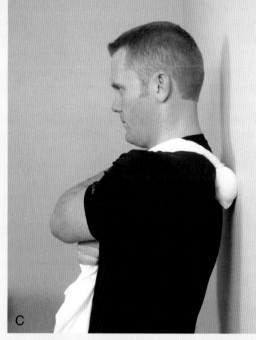

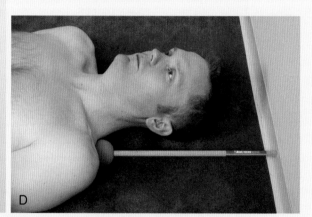

FIG. 5.11 A, Self–soft tissue mobilization of thoracic spine with a foam roll. Patient can bridge and glide across foam roll for 1 to 2 minutes as a self–soft tissue mobilization technique. B, Self–joint mobilization of thoracic spine with foam roll. Once patient identifies a stiff, tender region with initial rolling procedure, sustained pressure can be placed on restricted region, and the patient can extend over the foam roll focused at targeted stiff region of the thorax to attempt to self-mobilize the region. Targeted force can be combined with deep breathing. Sustained stretches of 20 to 30 seconds can be applied to two to three targeted areas of stiffness. This technique works best for segments T3–T4 to T7–T8. C, Tennis ball is held in a pillowcase and used to apply direct pressure to upper thoracic paraspinal tissues against the wall. This allows the patient to self-mobilize the upper thoracic tissues, and the direct pressure can be combined with deep breathing to enhance the mobilization effect. D, A rubber ball on a stick can be used to apply a self-mobilization force to depress the first rib and surrounding tissues. Deep breathing can be used to enhance the mobilization effect.

BOX 5.2   Self-Mobilization and Mobility Exercises for the Thoracic Spine—cont'd

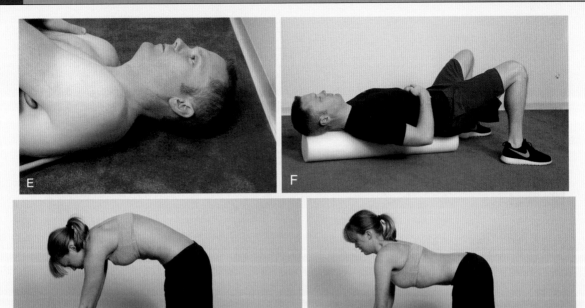

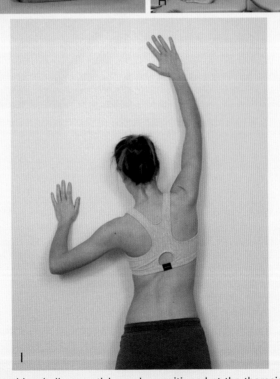

FIG. 5.11, cont'd E, A rubber ball on a stick can be positioned at the thoracic paraspinal area to apply direct pressure to the paraspinal tissues. Deep breathing can be used to enhance the mobilization effect. F, The patient can lie supine over a foam roll that is positioned parallel with the spine. The patient can shift his weight slightly side-to-side to roll the foam roll in a position to apply direct pressure to the paraspinal tissues. Deep breathing can be used to enhance the mobilization effect. G, Cat back exercise: arching thoracolumbar spine into flexion position while in quadruped position can assist in maintaining and enhancing thoracic spine mobility. H, Cat back exercise: sagging thoracolumbar spine into extension position while in quadruped position can assist in maintaining and enhancing thoracic spine mobility. I, Wall dance exercise: patient alternately reaches up and across with each arm in attempt to fully elongate and stretch the lateral thorax. This exercise facilitates side bending of the thorax.

BOX 5.3   Postural Exercises to Address Muscle Imbalances Associated With Thoracic Spine Disorders

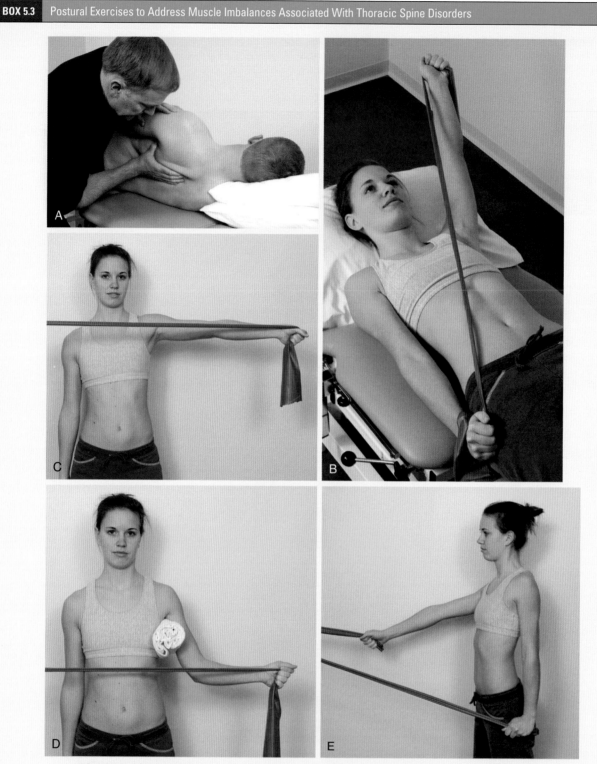

FIG. 5.12 A, Manual resistance can be used to facilitate muscle reeducation and strengthening of the scapular retraction muscles. B, Supine TheraBand Diagonal (D2) shoulder flexion. This exercise targets strengthening the lower trapezius muscle and facilitates reciprocal relaxation of the upper trapezius muscle. C, Standing TheraBand shoulder horizontal abduction. This exercise targets the middle trapezius muscle and posterior rotator cuff muscles. D, Standing TheraBand shoulder external rotation. This exercise targets strengthening of the lateral rotators of the rotator cuff and scapular stabilizer muscles. E, Reciprocal shoulder girdle retraction. Reciprocal motion used with this exercise facilitates thoracic spine rotation motions and at the same time targets strengthening parascapular and thoracic multifidus muscles.

literature on the T4 syndrome concluded that there is no high-quality evidence published about the T4 syndrome; it is a diagnosis of exclusion (advising to rule out thoracic outlet syndrome, carpal tunnel syndrome, lower cervical nerve root lesions, and cardiac issues); and clinicians should be cautious when considering T4 syndrome as a diagnostic classification because of this lack of high-quality evidence.[43]

Thoracic Mobility Deficits With Neck Pain

Thrust manipulation techniques directed to the thoracic spine have also been shown as an effective means to provide relief of neck pain.[44] This is an example of the clinical application of the theory of regional interdependence, which states that impairments in one region of the body can influence the musculoskeletal and neuromuscular function and symptoms in other remote regions of the body.[45,46] Although the regional interdependence theories were initially based on biomechanical and anatomic interrelationships of regions of the body, several authors have expanded on the regional interdependence theory to argue that the primary beneficial effects for use of thoracic manipulation for treatment of neck and shoulder pain conditions can most likely be explained by the regional neurophysiologic effects of the intervention.[47–49]

Cleland[44] developed a clinical prediction rule (CPR) for identification of patients with neck pain who benefit from thoracic spine thrust manipulation to relieve neck pain. The CPR was developed on a group of 78 patients with neck pain who all received thrust manipulation to the upper and middle thoracic spine. The thoracic spine segments that were regarded as having passive mobility deficits from a clinical examination were targeted for manipulation by the physical therapists. Cleland et al.[50] conducted a validation RCT study of the CPR to identify patients with neck pain who benefit from thoracic spine thrust manipulation. Some 140 patients with a primary complaint of neck pain were randomly assigned to receive either five sessions of stretching and strengthening exercises or two sessions of thoracic spine thrust manipulation and cervical range of motion exercises followed by three sessions of stretching and strengthening exercise. The results of the study did not support the validity of the CPR, but the results demonstrated that patients with mechanical neck pain who did not have red flags or contraindications and received thoracic spine thrust manipulation and exercise demonstrated greater improvements in disability at both long- and short-term follow-up periods and in pain at 1-week follow-up compared with patients who received only exercise. A separate study by Cleland[51] demonstrated that thoracic spine thrust manipulation was more effective than thoracic spine nonthrust mobilization in providing short-term follow-up relief of neck pain and reduction in disability. This study also found no differences in frequency, duration, or types of side effects between the thrust and nonthrust techniques.[51]

Gonzalez-Iglesias et al.[52] compared the use of heat plus electrical stimulation alone or combined with thoracic spine thrust manipulation for five treatment sessions over a 3-week duration in a group of 45 patients with mechanical neck pain. The group who received the thrust manipulation (mid-thoracic lift) demonstrated more significant improvements in pain, neck mobility, and disability at the fifth treatment session and at a 4-week follow-up reexamination. Another RCT compared the short-term effects of a supine thoracic thrust manipulation with a prone thrust technique in 60 subjects with chronic nonspecific neck pain targeting the T4 spinal level. Both manipulation techniques improved neck mobility and mechanosensitivity and reduced pain in the short term with no major clinical differences found between the groups.[53] Karas et al.[54] found a similar reduction in neck pain and disability at a 2-week follow-up in patients treated with thoracic manipulation delivered in supine with positioning in both thoracic extension or flexion.[54] In another study by the same researchers, an immediate improvement in neck flexion range of motion and reduction of neck pain with movement was noted following a supine thoracic spine thrust manipulation and to a lesser extent with a seated thoracic distraction manipulation.[55] There is mounting evidence for at least short-term benefits in neck mobility and reduction in pain and disability following thoracic spine manipulation techniques, and there are numerous methods of delivering effective techniques (i.e., sitting, supine, prone, etc.).

A systematic review of the literature confirmed that there is preliminary evidence that thoracic spine thrust manipulation may provide improvements in pain and disability for patients with acute and subacute mechanical neck pain.[56]

In another systematic review to assess and compare the evidence for thoracic spine thrust manipulation and nonthrust mobilization for patients with neck pain, the authors concluded there is no definitive evidence to support the clinical efficacy of the use of thoracic nonthrust mobilization for the treatment of neck pain because of methodologic concerns of the few studies that have been published.[57] In contrast, there is a significant amount of evidence, although of varied quality, that exists to support the use of thoracic thrust manipulation in the treatment of neck pain for short-term improvements in neck pain, range of motion, and disability.[57] Further research is needed to explore the value of thoracic mobilization/manipulation in long-term relief of neck pain.[57]

The majority of these studies used an impairment-based approach clinical reasoning model that includes the use of thoracic spine thrust manipulation directed at mobility deficits of the thoracic spine to demonstrate reduction of pain and disability associated with neck pain. The treatment approach should also include self-mobilization and mobility exercises of the thoracic spine (Box 5.2) and select postural exercises based on the impairments identified (Box 5.3).

Additional interventions to treat the neck are dependent on the cervical spine impairments and symptoms identified by the therapist. A classification system for management of neck pain disorders is outlined in Chapter 6. In an RCT that compared the use of cervical spine thrust manipulation with the use of thoracic spine thrust manipulation techniques followed by neck range of motion exercises (for both groups) for patients with a primary complaint of neck pain, greater improvements were noted for pain and disability at 1 week, 4 weeks, and 6 months for the group that received the cervical spine thrust manipulation techniques.[58] In addition, the patients who received the cervical thrust manipulation also demonstrated fewer transient side effects.[58] This study[58] provides a useful reminder that although thoracic spine thrust manipulation can be a useful adjunct in the treatment of patients with neck pain, the cervical spine impairments must also be addressed with cervical spine manipulation techniques and specific exercises to maximize clinical outcomes.

Another RCT[59] randomly assigned patients with a primary complaint of neck pain to receive either nonthrust cervical mobilization plus neck range of motion exercises or this intervention combined with thoracic spine thrust manipulation for two treatment sessions. At a 1-week follow-up, the individuals with neck pain who received a combination of thoracic spine thrust manipulation and cervical spine nonthrust mobilization demonstrated better overall short-term outcome improvements in pain, disability, and global rating of change.[59] This study further confirms that an impairment-based treatment approach for patients with a primary complaint of neck pain should include manual therapy techniques and exercises directed to the impairments of both the cervical and thoracic spine.

Thoracic Mobility Deficits With Shoulder Impairments

Thoracic spine extension and variable amounts of thoracic rotation and lateral flexion are necessary to fully complete unilateral shoulder flexion and abduction movements.[60,61] Crawford and Jull[62] used an inclinometer to measure thoracic motion on 60 women during bilateral shoulder elevation and reported that bilateral shoulder elevation induces 13 to 15 degrees thoracic extension and that a large thoracic kyphosis is associated with reduced arm elevation in older adults. Edmondston et al.[63] demonstrated that thoracic spine extension normally accompanies bilateral end-range shoulder elevation in young, healthy adult male subjects. The thoracic motion, which was measured with both a photographic and radiographic technique, was on average 10.5 ± 4.4 degrees and 12.8 ± 7.6 degrees. Of the 10.5 degrees of thoracic extension measured with the photographic technique, approximately 30% of the extension motion occurs in the upper thoracic region (six cranial vertebrae) and approximately 70% takes place in the lower thoracic region. Loss of upper and middle thoracic mobility is postulated to lead to increased strain and impingement placed on the rotator cuff, especially at the end range of shoulder motions, which may lead to impingement syndrome, tendonitis, and tears of the rotator cuff. Therefore thoracic mobility should be visually inspected during shoulder AROM testing (Fig. 5.18); if limited mobility is noted with shoulder movements, further examination of the thoracic spine is warranted and should include PIVM testing of the thoracic spinal segments and ribs. If shoulder flexion AROM provokes pain at the end of range, the shoulder girdle should be manually positioned and held into a more retracted position as AROM is retested. If this procedure improves the degree of pain-free AROM, a postural component to the shoulder pain condition is suspected. To improve posture and enhance full shoulder complex flexion/abduction motions, adequate mobility of the thorax is necessary.

Boyles et al.[64] demonstrated reduction in the degree of shoulder pain with resistive shoulder testing and perception of disability with a group of 56 patients with shoulder impingement syndrome at a 48-hour follow-up examination after a one-time treatment session of thrust manipulation to the thoracic spine. Bergman et al.[65] demonstrated improved treatment outcomes in a group of 150 patients with shoulder area symptoms and dysfunctions of the shoulder girdle that received thrust manipulation and nonthrust mobilization techniques to impairments of the cervical and upper thoracic spine and adjacent ribs compared with a control group who received a usual medical management approach. The physical therapists applied techniques based on the location of the spine or rib impairments and the therapist's technique preferences. After completion of treatment (12 weeks), 43% of the intervention group and 21% of the control group reported full recovery. After 52 weeks, approximately the same difference in recovery rate (17 percentage points) was seen between groups.[65] These studies offer support for including spinal manipulation procedures as a useful adjunct to treat shoulder impairments.

In an attempt to determine why thoracic spine thrust manipulation has a positive effect on shoulder rotator cuff tendinopathy conditions, Muth et al.[66] assessed scapular kinematics and electromyography of the shoulder muscles before and after thoracic spine thrust manipulation techniques on patients with evidence of shoulder rotator cuff tendinopathy. Although improvements in shoulder pain with resistive tests were noted immediately after thoracic spine thrust manipulation techniques, minimal changes in scapular kinematics or shoulder muscle activity could be identified. This study further supports the use of thoracic spine thrust manipulation to treat shoulder rotator cuff tendinopathy but was not able to validate a mechanical or physiologic mechanism for why this treatment is effective.

In a systematic review, three RCTs demonstrated that thoracic manual therapy reduced pain and disability at 6, 26, and 52 weeks compared with usual care.[67] Two pre–posttest studies found between 76% and 100% of patients experienced significant pain reduction immediately post-thoracic manual therapy.[67] An additional pre–posttest study and a single-arm trial showed reductions in pain and disability scores 48 hours post-thoracic manual therapy.[67] Thoracic manual therapy accelerated recovery and reduced pain and disability immediately and for up to 52 weeks compared with usual care for nonspecific shoulder pain.[67] Some of the articles included in this review, provided shoulder girdle manual therapy in addition to thoracic manual therapy, which may confuse the interpretation of the results.

Mintken et al.[68] identified five prognostic variables to identify patients with a primary complaint of shoulder pain who will have a favorable response to cervical and thoracic thrust manipulation. If three of the five variables were present, the chance of achieving a successful outcome improved from 61% to 89% with a +LR of 5.3.

A follow-up RCT was unable to validate the CPR,[69] but the results demonstrated superior successful clinical outcomes in Global Rating of Change at 4 weeks and 6 months for the treatment group that used two sessions of thoracic thrust manipulation/cervical nonthrust mobilization plus six sessions of exercise compared with the group that received eight sessions over 4 weeks of cervicothoracic and shoulder exercises alone to treat patients with shoulder pain.[70]

Based on the evidence and clinical reasoning, thoracic spine mobility deficit impairments should be treated with thoracic manipulation (thrust and nonthrust) techniques in patients with shoulder pain. If thoracic and rib mobility deficit impairments are still evident after the thoracic manipulation, rib manipulation techniques should be used. These techniques can be followed up with postural correction training, thoracic self-mobilization and mobility exercises, and exercises to address muscle imbalances across the shoulder girdle complex (Boxes 5.2 and 5.3). In addition, a shoulder rehabilitation program designed to address the specific impairments noted at the shoulder, such as rotator cuff muscle strengthening, should be initiated.

Thoracic Mobility Deficits With Low Back Pain

Although little has been written on this condition in the low back pain literature, thoracic hypomobility is commonly associated with many low back pain conditions. From a biomechanical impairment-based model, the mobility deficits in the thoracic spine place increased mechanical loading on the lumbar spine. The stiffness may be caused by muscle holding of the erector spinae muscles that originate in the middle and lower thoracic spine and connect into the thoracolumbar fascia. Because these global back muscles guard to protect the painful low back condition or to compensate for weak deep local muscles of the lumbar spine, the thoracic spine tends to stiffen. Therefore thoracic manipulation can provide reflexive relaxation of these muscles and also reduce mechanical strain on the lumbar spine once mobility improves.[71] A hypoalgesic effect may also be seen from manipulation of segments superior to the primary pain symptom by applying principles of regional interdependence. Enhanced clinical outcomes have been noted in RCTs with patients with chronic low back pain when manual therapy techniques are added to the treatment program that target the thoracic spine and hips in addition to specific motor control exercises and manual therapy directed to the lumbar spine.[72,73] However, in a recent RCT that compared sham thoracic manipulation with thoracic thrust manipulation and both comparison groups received lumbar exercises and education for three treatment sessions for 90 patients with low back pain (72% chronic), similar positive outcomes were reported.[74]

In a randomized controlled study completed to assess an impairment-based manual physical therapy approach for the treatment of patients with lumbar spinal stenosis, Whitman et al.[75] demonstrated excellent treatment outcomes with the use of mobilization/manipulation of the hip, thoracic, and lumbar spine combined with a flexion-based exercise program and body weight supported treadmill walking. Nearly 60% of the patients in the manual physical therapy treatment group received thrust manipulation techniques, and almost 70% received nonthrust mobilization techniques directed to the thoracic spine.[75] This study provides preliminary evidence of the effectiveness of using thoracic mobilization/manipulation as an adjunct to treatment of chronic lumbar conditions.

Therefore evaluation and treatment of impairments noted in the thoracic spine in patients with lumbar spine conditions is advisable as an adjunct to addressing the primary impairments at the lumbar spine. Further research is needed to further validate this clinical recommendation.

Thoracic Clinical Instability (Movement Coordination Impairments)

Although this condition is thought to be less common than hypomobility disorders of the thoracic spine, clinical instability of the thoracic spine may occur in one or more of the following situations: with systemic hypermobility; with severe postural deviations, such as excessive kyphosis and thoracic scoliosis; after trauma, such as a motor vehicle accident; or after thoracic surgery, such as thoracotomy or thoracic laminectomy. Thoracic laminectomy has been shown on cadavers to increase segmental range of motion by 22% to 30%.[76] Clinical signs and symptoms are similar to instability in other regions of the spine and include achiness with sustained upright postures, relief of pain with recumbent positions, aberrant movements with AROM, and hypermobility noted with PIVM testing. Strength deficits may also be noted with testing the thoracic erector spinae and multifidus and the middle and lower trapezius muscles. Lee[77] describes a mid-thoracic rotation instability syndrome characterized by a "fixation" of the mid-thoracic segment that presents with hypermobility after the fixation is corrected with mobilization/manipulation.

To regain neuromuscular control of the thoracic ring, manual correction of the thoracic ring position can be applied as the patient moves actively. Once a functional movement is found that causes a feeling of tension/restriction at the thorax, manual pressure can be applied at the lateral ribcage with a corrective medial and cranial force. This manual therapy technique is essentially providing a mobilization with movement to correct a thoracic ring "fixation." The therapist will hold this pressure at the thorax as the patient is asked to actively move. Box 5.4 (Fig. 5.13) shows the mobilization of a middle thoracic ring combined with cervicothoracic rotation and trunk forward bending movements. The mobilizing force should be sustained for at least 10 repetitions of the active movement, which should be followed with another five to 10 repetitions of the same active movement without the corrective force to assess a carryover effect from the technique.

Additional treatment for thoracic clinical instability includes postural education and training, thoracic and parascapular muscle strengthening exercises, mobilization/manipulation techniques for segmental restrictions noted above and below the hypermobile spinal region, and ergonomic corrections at home and work to attempt to reduce the strain associated with a kyphotic thoracic spine posture.

Thoracic Outlet Syndrome

When a patient has radiating pain that has been confirmed by a positive neurodynamic tension test (see Ch. 6), the therapist must further examine the patient to determine the sight of the entrapment. Thoracic outlet syndrome (TOS) is a generic

BOX 5.4   Mobilization of a Mid-Thoracic Ring Combined With Cervicothoracic Rotation and Trunk Forward-Bending Movements

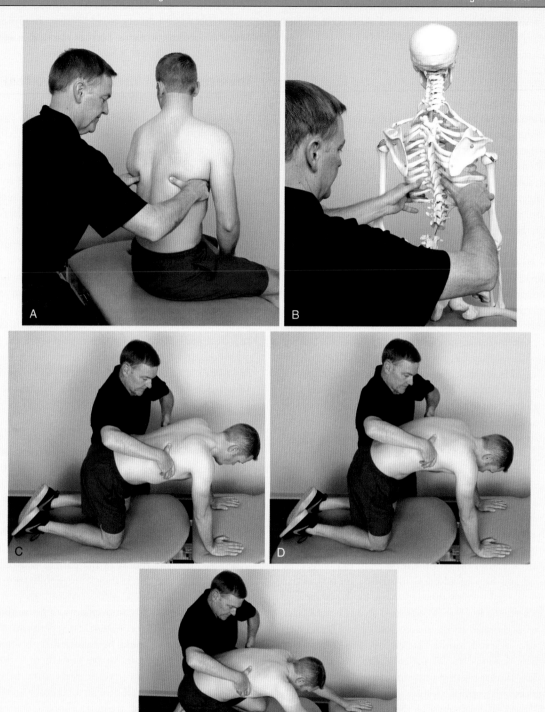

FIG. 5.13 A, Thoracic ring mobilization with movement in sitting: the therapist applies a corrective medial and cranial force and moves with the patient as the patient rotates to the left. The mobilizing force should allow the patient to move further into the range of motion with less pain and is repeated at least 10 repetitions. B, Hand placement on a skeleton for thoracic ring mobilization with movement in sitting. C, Thoracic ring mobilization hand placement in the quadruped position. D, Thoracic ring mobilization in quadruped position with active cat back motion. The mobilizing force should allow the patient to move further into the range of motion with less pain and is repeated at least 10 repetitions. E, Thoracic ring mobilization in quadruped position with active trunk flexion motion. The mobilizing force should allow the patient to move further with less pain and is repeated at least 10 repetitions.

diagnosis for those patients who exhibit symptoms characteristic of entrapment of the brachial plexus and the subclavian-axillary vessels.[78] TOS specifically involves the major portion of the brachial plexus, beginning just distal to the intervertebral foramina and extending laterally to just beyond the coracoid process and the insertion of the pectoralis minor muscle. It also involves the subclavian-axillary vessels as they arch across the first rib from the thorax and follow the brachial plexus.[78] The symptoms most commonly associated with TOS result from the involvement of the ventral rami of C8 and T1 (or the inferior trunk of the brachial plexus) and the ulnar nerve.[78]

The three primary outlet sites where neurovascular entrapment can occur, and the structures compressed that may lead to upper extremity symptoms include the subclavian artery and lower roots of the brachial plexus as they exit from the thoracic cavity and rise superior to the first rib and pass between the anterior and middle scalene muscles. This has been referred to as the cervical outlet or the scalene triangle.[79] The second outlet is where the subclavian artery and vein and lower trunk of the brachial plexus travel beneath the clavicle and superior to the first rib, which is referred to as the costoclavicular space. The final outlet is where the axillary artery and vein and the cords of the brachial plexus pass through the subcoracoid tunnel inferior to the pectoralis minor muscle and coracoid process[78,79] (Fig. 5.14).

TOS may manifest as either a vascular or neurogenic condition. The vascular TOS can be further subdivided into arterial or venous (Table 5.4). Arterial TOS (aTOS) is caused by compression of the subclavian artery, and patients with aTOS complain of arm fatigue and paresthesias with arm movement and exertion.[79,80] Early symptoms may include cold sensitivity of the hand or Raynaud syndrome. Arm blood pressure and radial pulse can be decreased with movement of the arm into an abducted and externally rotated position.[80] Repeated compression

can cause intimal trauma and stenosis of the subclavian artery, and patients may develop poststenotic dilation or aneurysm formation.[80] Patients may present with arterial thrombosis or distal ischemia and gangrene related to emboli lodging in the digital vessels.[80] Angiography can be carried out with the arm in various positions, and visualized compression of the subclavian artery confirms the diagnosis.[80] Venous TOS (vTOS) is caused by subclavian vein compression and will present with venous engorgement, upper extremity edema, pain, cyanosis, fatigability, and a feeling of upper extremity stiffness.[79] Venography performed with the shoulder abducted and externally rotated shows impingement of the subclavian vein at the level of the first rib to confirm the diagnosis.[80] If conservative measures (such as physical therapy) are unsuccessful in treating vascular TOS, surgical decompression of the artery or vein with resection of the first rib or a cervical rib is commonly performed. Additional interventions include thrombolysis, anticoagulation, and endovascular procedures, such as angioplasty plus stent placement.[80]

Neurogenic TOS can be further subdivided into true neurologic TOS (tnTOS) and symptomatic TOS (sTOS) (Table 5.4). tnTOS is caused by traction or compression of the brachial plexus usually as a result of repetitive or significant trauma and result in neurologic weakness or numbness of the upper extremity with upper extremity distribution that corresponds to the compromised portion of the brachial plexus.[79] Pain and paresthesia in the neck, chest, and upper extremity may also accompany tnTOS. sTOS accounts for approximately 90% of the cases of TOS and has the fewest objective findings to base the diagnosis.[78,81] sTOS is characterized by paresthesia and pain most commonly in the ulnar distribution of the hand and forearm that is provoked with repetitive use of the upper extremity and with positioning the arm above shoulder height.[78,81] sTOS typically does not present with objective neurologic compromise of the upper extremity. Double crush

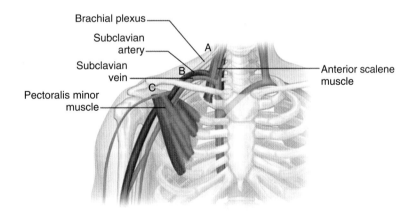

FIG. 5.14 Thoracic outlet anatomy. Three possible sites of compression and structures compressed: *A,* Subclavian artery and lower roots of the brachial plexus may be compressed as they exit from the thoracic cavity and rise up over the first rib and pass between the anterior and middle scalene muscles. *B,* Subclavian artery and vein and/or lower trunk of the brachial plexus beneath the clavicle in the costoclavicular space. *C,* The axillary artery or vein or one of the cords of the brachial plexus in the subcoracoid tunnel. (From Ho V, Reddy G. *Cardiovascular Imaging.* Philadelphia: Saunders; 2011.)

TABLE 5.4	Thoracic Outlet Syndrome Classification and Differential Diagnosis		
CLASSIFICATION	**SYMPTOMS**	**DIFFERENTIAL DIAGNOSIS**	**IMPAIRMENTS**
Vascular thoracic outlet syndrome; arterial TOS (aTOS)	Arm fatigue/paresthesia with use of arm	Decreased blood pressure or pulse with abducted shoulder position	• See sTOS • Loss of pulse with Adson's, hyperabduction maneuvers
Vascular thoracic outlet syndrome; venous TOS (vTOS)	Venous engorgement Upper extremity edema Pain Cyanosis Fatigability Feeling of upper extremity stiffness	Venography performed with shoulder abducted and externally rotated shows impingement of subclavian vein at level of first rib	• See sTOS • Loss of pulse with Adson's, hyperabduction maneuvers
Neurogenic thoracic outlet syndrome; true neurologic TOS (tnTOS)	Pain and paresthesia in the neck, chest, and upper extremity	• Neurologic weakness or numbness of upper extremity with upper extremity distribution that corresponds to compromised portion of brachial plexus • Positive electrodiagnostic test findings for brachial plexus compromise	• See sTOS • Myotomal weakness • Loss of sensation • Loss of DTR
Neurogenic thoracic outlet syndrome; symptomatic (sTOS)	Paresthesia and pain most commonly in the ulnar distribution of hand and forearm that is provoked with repetitive use of upper extremity and with positioning arm above shoulder height	• No objective neurologic compromise of the upper extremity • ULND 1 symptom reproduction in ulnar distribution • Cluster of three out of five positive TOS tests (Adson's, Roos, hyperabduction for pulse, hyperabduction for symptoms, and Tinel sign at the supraclavicular space)	• Forward head posture/protracted scapulas • Upper chest breathing pattern • First rib hypomobility • Upper thoracic hypomobility • Tight/shortened/guarded pectoralis minor, scalene, and levator scapula muscles • Weak/poor neuromuscular control of deep neck flexor, deep neck extensor, and scapular stabilizer muscles

DTR, Deep tendon reflex; *TOS,* thoracic outlet syndrome; *ULND,* upper limb neurodynamic.

syndrome can also occur where nerve entrapment is present at multiple sites throughout the upper extremity, such as the thoracic outlet, the elbow, and the wrist.

TOS is commonly associated with postural deviations that tend to narrow the thoracic outlets such a forward head/protracted scapular positioning and with muscle imbalances, such as tight/shortened pectoralis, levator scapulae, and scalene muscles and weakness of the deep neck flexors, lower trapezius, serratus anterior, and rotator cuff muscles. Scapula mechanics are often poor, and the patient may present with the dropped shoulder condition (scapula depressed, downwardly rotated, or anteriorly tilted).[81] Cervicogenic headaches, along with upper thoracic and cervical pain and muscle tension, commonly accompany TOS, and these impairments need to be addressed as part of the treatment program.[81]

Differential diagnosis of the TOS and the four subtypes of TOS requires screening for other possible causes of the symptoms, including but not limited to cervical radiculopathy and ulnar and median nerve peripheral entrapment neuropathies at the elbow and wrist, with screening procedures, such as Tinel sign at the elbow and wrist and Spurling test. Additional diagnostic tests, such as electromyography/nerve condition studies and cervical magnetic resonance imaging (MRI), further assist in the diagnosis. aTOS and vTOS are often diagnosed with use of magnetic resonance angiography (MRA) and ultrasound Doppler studies, but the specificity and sensitivity of MRA is

questionable. A systematic review by Estilaei and Byl[82] found the current evidence in support of MRA as a valid test for diagnosing aTOS is weak, and studies typically have not used designs with high internal validity.

The ULND 1 test (see Fig. 6.29) can be used to determine the degree of irritability of the neural and surrounding connective tissues of the brachial plexus. Although ULND 1 is designed to bias the median nerve, patients with sTOS commonly report symptoms in an ulnar distribution with this test.[81,83] Ide et al.[84] correlated positive neurogenic TOS provocations tests with the results of a neuroradiograph with contrast in 150 patients with TOS and found that 92 patients (61%) had symptoms provoked with brachial plexus traction maneuvers and concluded that stretching the brachial plexus is an important factor in detecting nerve irritation associated with TOS. The ULND test more effectively elongates the brachial plexus in a controlled manner than the traditional TOS provocation tests. In highly reactive situations, care must be taken to not overstretch the neural tissues, which could create a severe flare-up from the examination.

The traditional TOS provocation tests include Adson's maneuver (Fig. 5.15), the hyperabduction maneuver (Fig. 5.16), and the Roos stress test (elevated arm stress test [EAST; Fig. 5.17]). These tests have been reported as being unreliable and often positive (up to 90%) for radial pulse obliteration in healthy, asymptomatic participants.[79,85–87] Even Wright,[85] who first described the hyperabduction maneuver in 1945, found that 125 of 150 (83%) normal, asymptomatic volunteers had obliteration of the radial pulse when their arm was positioned in full shoulder abduction, which suggests that this test is not diagnostic of a pathologic entity but instead demonstrates a normal physiologic response to fully abducting the arm. Likewise, Rayan[86] assessed the upper extremities of 100 normal, asymptomatic volunteers using the Tinel sign at the supraclavicular and infraclavicular area and Adson's, costoclavicular, and hyperabduction maneuvers for vascular and neurogenic responses. Some 15 (7.5%) extremities had a positive Tinel sign. Vascular responses with elimination of the radial pulse were present in 27 (13.5%) extremities for the Adson's maneuver, 94 (47%) extremities for the costoclavicular maneuver (CCM), and 114 (57%) extremities for the hyperabduction maneuver.[86] The neurogenic, symptomatic response was present in four (2%) extremities for the Adson's maneuver, 20 (10%) extremities for the CCM, and 33 (16.5%) extremities for the hyperabduction maneuver.[86,87] Nord et al.[87] also tested normal subjects and found false positive tests were observed in 20% in the Adson's maneuver, 16% in the CCM, 47% in the Roos test, and 30% in the supraclavicular pressure. Some 56% of the normal subjects had at least one positive TOS diagnostic maneuver.[87] This illustrates the high potential for false positive findings for TOS tests, especially for a positive vascular response.

When using provocation tests that assess for obliteration of the radial pulse for diagnosis of aTOS and vTOS, the therapist should also assess for distal ischemic signs, edema, and cyanosis of the upper extremity; measure the blood pressure in each upper extremity; and auscultate for a bruit in both upper extremities with the arms by the side and in provocation positions.[79,88,89] In cases of tnTOS and sTOS, the provocation tests should be performed not only to obliterate the radial artery pulse but also to recreate the patient's symptoms, and the ULND 1 test should be included in the examination.[81,83] Because of the low specificity of the traditional TOS tests, if these tests are being used for a diagnosis of TOS, a cluster of at least three tests should be positive in a given patient.[79] Gillard[90] reported that using several tests in combination improved specificity so that when five tests were positive, sensitivity and specificity both improved to 0.84 with +LR at 5.25 and −LR at 0.19, which translates to a moderate shift in probability, with five positive TOS tests (Adson's, Roos, hyperabduction for pulse, hyperabduction for symptoms, and Tinel at the supraclavicular space) more accurately ruling in or rule out vascular TOS. However, further research is warranted to develop a more accurate, definitive method to diagnose TOS.

In addition to examination procedures of the irritability and function of the neurovascular bundle, a detailed examination of cervical, thoracic, and shoulder girdle active and passive mobility, muscle length and strength/neuromuscular control testing are important considerations to develop a comprehensive treatment plan. Assessment of first rib position and mobility can also provide useful information on tissue extensibility, muscle tone, and symptom reproduction at the costoclavicular thoracic outlet and surrounding tissues.

Conservative treatment of TOS includes use of manual therapy and self-mobilization techniques to open the cervical and thoracic outlets to decompress the neurovascular bundle (Box 5.2, Fig. 5.11D). Manual treatment of hypomobility of the cervical and upper thoracic spine and rib cage along with techniques to inhibit muscle tone and enhance muscle extensibility of the pectoral, scalene, and upper trap/levator scapula muscles will promote positive outcomes. This should be combined with training the deep neck flexor, deep neck extensor, and scapular stabilizing muscles along with postural education/training.

A therapeutic exercise program designed to restore cervical and thoracic mobility and enhance strength of the cervical and scapular stabilizing muscles was used in a study of 119 patients with sTOS who met the three out of four of the following criteria: a history of aggravation of symptoms with the arm in the elevated position; a history of paresthesia in the C8–T1 dermatome region; tenderness over the brachial plexus supraclavicularly; and a positive Roos maneuver.[91] Eighty-eight percent of the patients reported satisfaction with the treatment and demonstrated improvements of the cervical and thoracic mobility, and 73% were able to return to work and have at least partial resolution of symptoms at a 2-year follow-up after treatment.[91]

Edgelow[83] advocates use of devices (such as the rubber ball on a stick and a foam roll) to enhance self-mobilization of the first rib and thorax and relaxation of the involved muscle groups (Box 5.2, Fig. 5.11D). Training diaphragmatic breathing is another important component of the treatment approach to inhibit habitual overuse of the upper chest breathing muscles (such as the scalenes), and the diaphragmatic breathing should be incorporated and reinforced with the self-mobilization and a home exercise program.[83] Watson advocates use of manual facilitation and taping combined with shoulder girdle strengthening exercises to retrain scapular stabilizer muscles to change the resting and functional position of the scapula for treatment of TOS.[92] Cervical, thoracic, and first rib mobilization techniques, massage, and scalene and pectoral muscle stretches, as well as neural mobilization treatment techniques may also be included in the treatment of TOS.[92] In addition, workplace ergonomics should be addressed as part of the treatment approach because postural strains contribute to development and aggravation of TOS.[92] Further research is warranted to evaluate the effectiveness of manual therapy and therapeutic exercises for treatment of TOS because there is very little high-quality published research available.

Examination of the thoracic spine starts with structural and postural examination followed by AROM testing of the cervical and thoracolumbar spine as described in Chapter 2. Shoulder screening is also an important component of the thoracic examination for determination of the presence of upper extremity signs and symptoms that could be a contributing or perpetuating factor in the thoracic spine disorder. In addition, primary shoulder impairments may have a thoracic spine hypomobility component that needs to be addressed as part of the plan of care.

INSPECTION OF THORACIC MOBILITY WITH SHOULDER ELEVATION ACTIVE RANGE OF MOTION TESTING

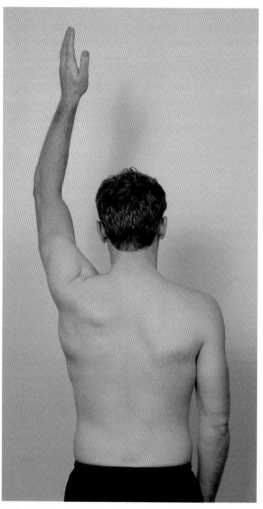

FIG. 5.15 See Video 5.1. Visual inspection for thoracic extension, lateral flexion, and rotation as patient actively forward flexes the shoulder. Compare left with right to judge for limitations and asymmetries in thoracic motion.

Muscle strength of the parascapular muscles should be tested because weakness of these muscles may be a component of thoracic and shoulder postural deviations (Box 5.5) (Fig 5.19).

Other than special tests used to diagnose TOS, few special tests are described specifically for diagnosis of thoracic spine disorders. The primary objective of the manual portion of the thoracic examination is determination of regions of hypomobility, irritability, tenderness, or instability through the thoracic spine and rib cage. This determination is best done with palpation for tissue condition and PIVM testing.

BOX 5.5 Parascapular Manual Muscle Tests

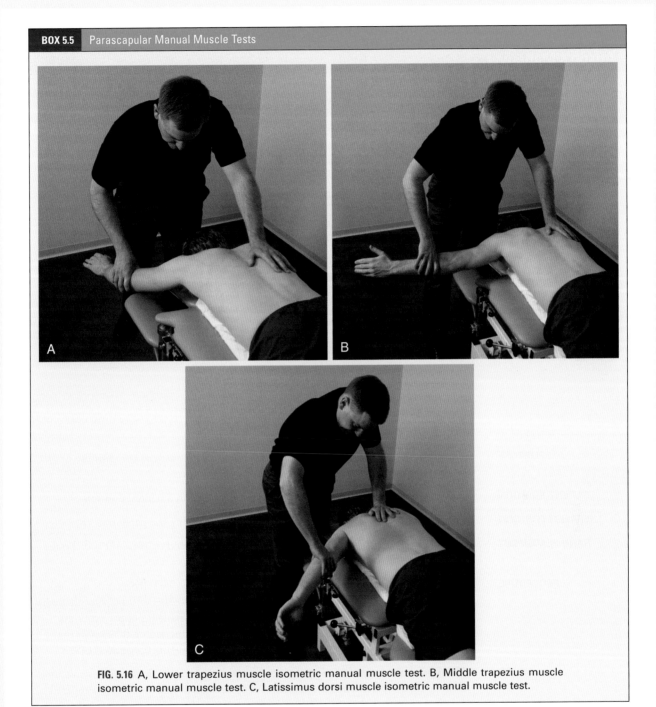

FIG. 5.16 A, Lower trapezius muscle isometric manual muscle test. B, Middle trapezius muscle isometric manual muscle test. C, Latissimus dorsi muscle isometric manual muscle test.

aShould be completed as part of the thoracic spine examination.

SELECTED SPECIAL TESTS FOR THORACIC SPINE EXAMINATION

▶ Adson's Maneuver

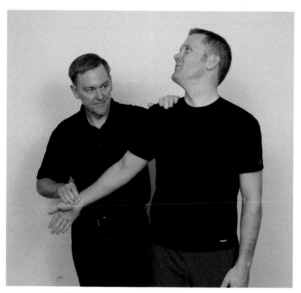

FIG. 5.17 See Video 5.2. Adson's maneuver.

PURPOSE	The purpose of this test is to determine whether there is vascular compromise or peripheral nerve irritation occurring at the thoracic outlet.
PATIENT POSITION	Patient is in the standing position with arms at his side in a neutral position.
THERAPIST POSITION	The therapist stands at the patient's side to be tested facing the patient.
HAND PLACEMENT	The therapist supports the patient's arm with one hand and palpates the radial pulse with the other hand.
PROCEDURE	The patient is asked to take and hold a deep inhalation as he fully extends the neck and rotates the head toward the side being examined. The therapist palpates the radial pulse and asks the patient if the maneuver replicates the patient's upper extremity symptoms. A positive test for vascular compromise is reduction or ablation of the radial pulse. Reproduction of symptoms is associated with a neurogenic sTOS.
NOTES	The Adson's maneuver is designed to implicate the anterior scalene muscle's role in obliterating the pulse when the muscle is fully elongated. In a study that compared the diagnostic accuracy of the Adson's maneuver with Doppler ultrasonography, electrophysiologic investigations, and helical computed tomography angiography to diagnose TOS in 46 patients with suspected TOS, the following results were reported: sensitivity of 0.79, specificity of 0.76, positive predictive value (PPV) of 0.85, and a negative predictive value (NPV) 0.72;[90] therefore +LR can be calculated at 3.29 and −LR at 0.27, which demonstrates only a small shift in posttest probability for use of this test for either ruling in or ruling out the vascular component of TOS with Adson's maneuver. Gillard[90] reported that using several tests in combination improved specificity so that when five tests were positive, sensitivity and specificity both improved to 0.84 with +LR at 5.25 and −LR at 0.19, which translates to a moderate shift in probability that having five positive TOS tests (Adson's, Roos, hyperabduction for pulse, hyperabduction for symptoms, and Tinel at the supraclavicular space) can accurately rule in or rule out TOS.

▶ Hyperabduction Maneuver

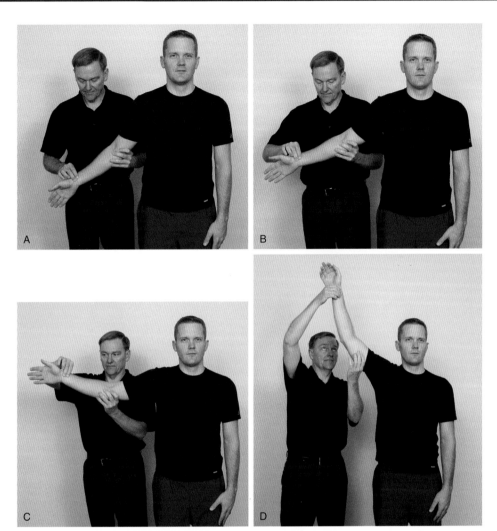

FIG. 5.18 See Video 5.3. A, Hyperabduction maneuver at 30 degrees shoulder abduction. B, Hyperabduction maneuver at 60 degrees shoulder abduction. C, Hyperabduction maneuver at 90 degrees shoulder abduction. D, Hyperabduction maneuver at full shoulder (target 180 degrees) abduction.

PURPOSE	This test is used to determine if there is vascular compromise or brachial plexus nerve irritation occurring at the thoracic outlet.
PATIENT POSITION	Patient is in the standing position with arms at his side in a neutral position with palms facing forward.
THERAPIST POSITION	The therapist stands at the patient's side to be tested facing the patient.
HAND PLACEMENT	The therapist supports the patient's arm with one hand and palpates the radial pulse with the other hand.
PROCEDURE	The test arm is positioned in 30 to 40 degrees elbow flexion and is passively abducted to 30 degrees, 60 degrees, 90 degrees, and 180 degrees with documentation of the angle at which the radial pulse is abolished and the angle at which the patient's symptoms are reproduced. A positive test for vascular TOS is reduction or ablation of the radial pulse. Reproduction of upper extremity paresthesia symptoms could be associated with neurogenic sTOS.

Hyperabduction Maneuver—cont'd

NOTES	The diagnostic accuracy of the hyperabduction maneuver to diagnose TOS in 46 patients with suspected TOS for pulse abolition ($n = 47$) is sensitivity 0.70, specificity 0.53, PPV 72%, and NPV 50%, +LR 1.49 and −LR 0.56; for symptom reproduction ($n = 47$), sensitivity 0.90, specificity 0.29, PPV 69%, and NPV 63%, +LR 0.69 and −LR 0.34;[90] therefore there is very little shift in posttest probability for use of this test for either ruling in or ruling out the vascular component of TOS. Gillard[90] reported that using several tests in combination improved specificity so that when five tests were positive, sensitivity and specificity both improved to 0.84 with +LR at 5.25 and −LR at 0.19, which translates to a moderate shift in probability that having five positive TOS tests (Adson's, Roos, hyperabduction for pulse, hyperabduction for symptoms, and Tinel at the supraclavicular space) can accurately rule in or rule out TOS.

▶ Roos Stress Test (Elevated Arm Stress Test)

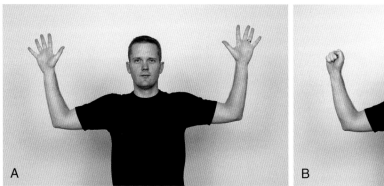 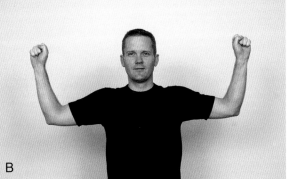

FIG. 5.19 See Video 5.4. A, Roos stress test (elevated arm stress test [EAST]) with hands open. B, Roos stress test (EAST) with fingers flexed.

PURPOSE	The purpose of this test is to determine whether there is vascular compromise or brachial plexus nerve irritation as a result of compression at the thoracic outlet.
PATIENT POSITION	Patient is in the sitting or standing position with head and neck in a neutral position.
THERAPIST POSITION	The therapist stands facing the patient.
HAND PLACEMENT	The therapist does not palpate the patient during this test.
PROCEDURE	The patient positions his arms at 90 degrees shoulder abduction and full external rotation with the elbows flexed at 90 degrees. The patient is then requested to flex and extend the fingers for up to 3 minutes. The test is positive if the patient is unable to maintain the test position for 3 minutes by demonstrating a dropping extremity that could indicate fatigue or arterial compromise. The therapist should also observe the color of the distal extremity comparing left and right and monitor the time of onset of symptoms.
NOTES	The diagnostic accuracy of the Roos stress test to diagnose TOS in 48 patients with suspected TOS is sensitivity 0.84, specificity 0.30; PPV was 68%, and NPV was 50%; +LR can be calculated at 1.2 and −LR at 0.53, which demonstrates a very small shift in probably that the patient has vascular TOS with a positive test or does not have vascular TOS with a negative test.[93] Gillard[90] reported that using several tests in combination improved specificity so that when five tests were positive, sensitivity and specificity both improved to 0.84 with +LR at 5.25 and −LR at 0.19, which translates to a moderate shift in probability that having five positive TOS tests (Adson's, Roos, hyperabduction for pulse, hyperabduction for symptoms, and Tinel at the supraclavicular space) can accurately rule in or rule out TOS.

THORACIC SPINE PASSIVE INTERVERTEBRAL MOTION TESTING

▶ Upper Thoracic Forward-Bending Passive Intervertebral Motion Test

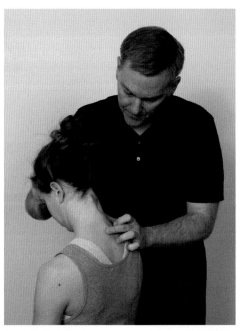

FIG. 5.20 See Video 5.5. Upper thoracic forward bending passive intervertebral motion test.

PURPOSE	This test is used to evaluate the passive forward-bending segmental motion of the thoracic segments C7–T1 through T3–T4.
PATIENT POSITION	The patient sits with the arms supported on two pillows in the lap.
THERAPIST POSITION	The therapist stands to the side and slightly behind the patient.
HAND PLACEMENT	Fig. 5.20 depicts proper hand placement.
	Right hand: The right hand supports the patient's forehead.
	Left hand: The pad of the long finger is used to palpate the interspinous space of the targeted segment.
PROCEDURE	The pad of the long finger on the left hand is used to palpate the interspinous space of the C7–T1 segment. The right hand is used to passively forward bend the patient's head and neck. The therapist palpates for the C7–T1 interspinous space to expand with forward bending by palpating the relative amount of movement of the superior spinous process of the spinal segment in relation to the inferior member of the segment. The amount of passive forward bending available at the segment is noted. The procedure is repeated one segment at a time with palpation of the interspinous spaces of segments T1–T2 through T3–T4. The amount of passive forward bending available at each segment is compared.

Upper Thoracic Forward-Bending Passive Intervertebral Motion Test—cont'd

NOTES   The assessment should begin at C7–T1 and proceed caudally, allowing for easy location of the specified segments with a start at C7, which tends to have a prominent spinous process. The amount of forward bending of the head and neck is increased as the assessment proceeds caudally. However, the head and neck are moved with small oscillations to avoid excessive movement of the patient's neck, which may be painful with large passive movements. Christensen et al.[94] reported an intrarater agreement with a kappa value of 0.60 and an interrater agreement with a kappa value of 0.22 for a sitting upper thoracic PIVM technique performed by a group of chiropractors.

▶ Upper Thoracic Rotation Passive Intervertebral Motion Test

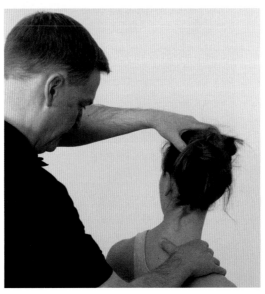

FIG. 5.21 See Video 5.6. Upper thoracic rotation passive intervertebral motion test.

PURPOSE   The purpose of this test is to evaluate the passive rotation of thoracic segments C7–T1 through T3–T4.

PATIENT POSITION   The patient sits on a chair or treatment table with the arms resting on two pillows in the lap.

THERAPIST POSITION   The therapist stands or kneels behind the patient.

HAND PLACEMENT   Fig 5.21 depicts proper hand placement for this test.

Left hand: The left hand gently grasps the top of the patient's head for left rotation. The right hand is on top of the patient's head for right rotation.

Right hand: The pad of the thumb is used to palpate the lateral aspect of the specified segment, and the fingers rest on the patient's shoulder girdle.

Upper Thoracic Rotation Passive Intervertebral Motion Test—cont'd

PROCEDURE

The pad of the thumb on the right hand is used to palpate the right lateral aspect of the interspinous space of the C7–T1 segment. Left rotation is induced with the left hand passively rotating the patient's head to the left. The therapist palpates for the spinous process of the superior member of the segment to press into the palpating thumb in relation to the inferior member of the segments spinous process. The amount of passive rotation available at the segment is noted. The procedure is repeated with palpation of the right lateral aspect of interspinous space for segments T1–T2 through T3–T4. The hand placements are reversed, and the procedure is repeated, with rotation of the patient's head to the right. The amount of passive right rotation available at each segment is noted, and the amount of passive rotation available in each direction is compared.

NOTES

The assessment should begin at C7–T1 and proceed caudally, which allows for easy location of the specified segments with a start at C7. The amount of rotation of the head and neck is increased as the assessment proceeds caudally. However, the therapist should try to move the head and neck as little as possible during the performance of this technique because the patients often have neck pain. During the performance of this technique, the therapist stands directly behind the patient to clearly observe and palpate the motion. If the cervical spine is hypermobile, positioning the cervical spine in a partially forward-bent position can take up tissue slack; then the rotation should occur within the new plane created by the forward-bent position of the neck.

Central Posteroanterior Passive Accessory Intervertebral Motion Test: Backward Bending

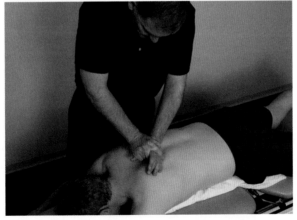

FIG. 5.22 See Video 5.7. Central posteroanterior passive accessory intervertebral motion test: two-handed technique.

PURPOSE

This test is used for passive accessory motion and pain provocation of the thoracic spinal segments. For intervention, one should use the appropriate grade of movement (I to IV) for treatment of pain or hypomobility.

PATIENT POSITION

The patient lies prone with one or two pillows under the thorax and with the arms along the side of the body, hanging off the edge of the table, or supported on the adjustable arms of a mobilization table. Another pillow can be placed under the lower legs for comfort.

Central Posteroanterior Passive Accessory Intervertebral Motion Test: Backward Bending—cont'd

THERAPIST POSITION	The therapist stands at the side of the patient.
HAND PLACEMENT	Left hand: The left hand is placed on the patient's back so that the ulnar border of the hand just distal to the pisiform is in contact with the spinous process of the vertebrae to be tested. The shoulders are directly over the patient. The wrist is fully extended with the forearm midway between supination and pronation.
	Right hand: The left hand is reinforced with the right hand so that the second and third digits of the right hand envelop the second metacarpal phalangeal joint of the left hand. The elbows are allowed to slightly flex.
PROCEDURE	The therapist applies a PA force on each spinous process being examined for a total of three slow repetitions. The first pressures should be applied gently; amplitude and depth of the movement are increased if no pain response occurs. The therapist assesses the quality of movement through the range and the end feel and compares it to the levels above and below.
NOTES	A midrange of movement thrust (spring test) could also be used with this technique for assessment of tissue resistance and pain provocation. A positive response is movement that reproduces the comparable sign (pain or resistance or muscle guarding). The technique assesses for both joint mobility and reactivity. The direction of motion is a direct PA force that produces a relative backward-bending motion of the targeted vertebra in relation to the vertebra below. Christensen et al.[94] reported intrarater reliability with a kappa value of 0.68 and interrater reliability with a kappa value of 0.24 for prone passive accessory intervertebral movement (PAIVM) testing; and for agreement in palpation of tenderness over the facet joint, the intrarater reliability was a kappa value of 0.94 and the interrater reliability was a kappa value of 0.70.
PROCEDURE MODIFICATION	This technique could also be done as a one-handed technique with the cranial hand contacting the spinous process just distal to the pisiform, the elbow flexed, and the forearm perpendicular with the angle of the contour of the surface of the spine (Fig 5.23). The caudal hand rests at the edge of the table to support the therapist's upper body weight as the therapist leans over the patient. Application of force could be done as a gradual PA force or a midrange spring test.

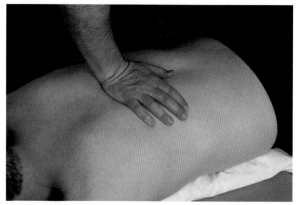

FIG. 5.23 See Video 5.8. Central posteroanterior passive accessory intervertebral motion test: one-handed technique commonly used for spring testing.

Posteroanterior Forward-Bending (Transverse Processes of the Same Vertebra) Passive Accessory Intervertebral Motion Test

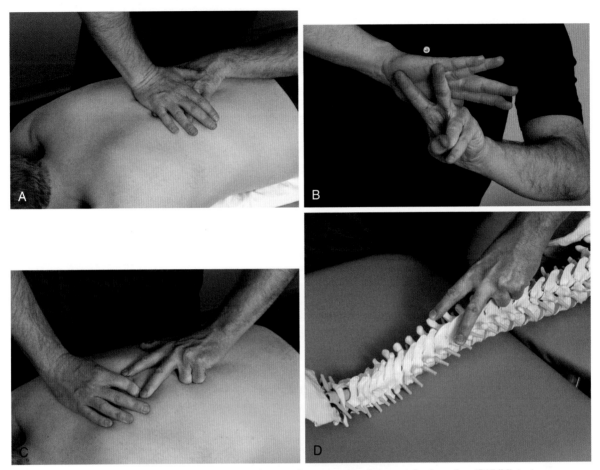

FIG. 5.24 See Video 5.9. A, Posteroanterior passive accessory intervertebral motion (PAIVM) test forward-bending. B, Dummy finger position in relation to manipulative hand for forward bending PAIVM test: posteroanterior transverse processes of same vertebra. C, Use of cranial hand to loosely pinch spinous process to find targeted transverse processes for PAIVM test: posteroanterior transverse processes of same vertebra. D, Finger placement for forward bending PAIVM test: posteroanterior transverse processes of same vertebra.

PURPOSE	This test assesses passive forward-bending motion and the level of reactivity (pain provocation) of thoracic segments T3–T4 through T11–T12.
PATIENT POSITION	The patient lies prone with a pillow under the chest/trunk.
THERAPIST POSITION	The therapist stands next to the patient with a diagonal stance.
HAND PLACEMENT	Caudal hand: The second and third digits are used as "dummy" fingers with the pads of the second and third fingers placed on the transverse processes of the targeted vertebra.
	Cranial hand: The palmar aspect of the fifth metacarpal is placed over the dummy fingers.

Posteroanterior Forward-Bending (Transverse Processes of the Same Vertebra) Passive Accessory Intervertebral Motion Test—cont'd

PROCEDURE

The index finger and thumb of the cranial hand gently pinches the lateral edges of the spinous process of T2. The second and third digits of the caudal hand are placed just lateral to the thumb and index finger of the cranial hand, respectively. This position places the dummy fingers over the transverse processes of T3. The volar aspect of the fifth metacarpal of the cranial hand is placed over the dummy fingers, and the cranial hand takes up the slack (to the joint's midrange) and gives an impulse. The amount of passive forward bending available at the T3–T4 segment and pain provocation are noted. Another variation of this procedure is to gently ease the segment into an end-range position progressively for three or four repetitions to sense the amount of resistance to the passive movement and pain provocation. The procedure is repeated at the transverse processes of T3 through T11 (segments T3–T4 through T11–T12). The amount of passive forward bending available at each segment is compared.

NOTES

This technique can be performed by starting at T3 and proceeding caudally, which allows for easy location of the thoracic vertebrae (by counting down from C7). The forearm of the arm that gives the impulse should be perpendicular to the angle of the contour of the spine being examined. One should note that the transverse processes usually are not palpable, but the dummy fingers should feel a firmness when taking up the soft tissue slack. Also the transverse processes of one thoracic vertebra are located lateral to the spinous process of the superior vertebra.[6] A positive pain provocation test may indicate reactivity of the facet joints and surrounding soft tissues.

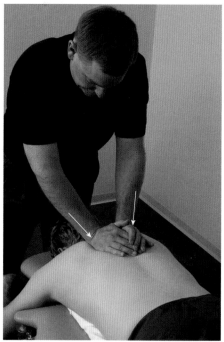

▶ **FIG. 5.25** See Video 5.10. Forward bending passive accessory intervertebral motion test: posteroanterior transverse processes of same vertebra with the two-handed technique.

PROCEDURE MODIFICATION

With the patient lying prone over a pillow, the therapist can stand over the head of the table and position both hypothenar eminences at the transverse processes of the same vertebral (Fig 5.25). As the therapist keeps both elbows straight, a gradual application of PA pressure can be applied to the targeted thoracic vertebra to assess PAIVM at each thoracic spinal segment.

Posteroanterior Rotation (Transverse Processes of Adjacent Vertebrae) Passive Accessory Intervertebral Motion Test

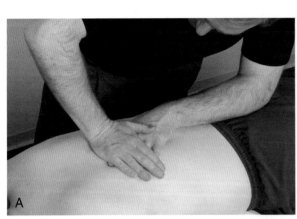

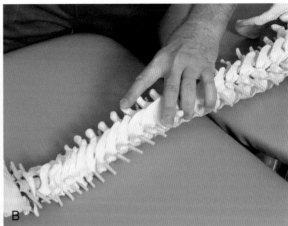

FIG. 5.26 See Video 5.11. A, Passive accessory intervertebral motion (PAIVM) test: posteroanterior transverse processes of adjacent vertebrae for left rotation. B, Finger placement.

PURPOSE	This test is used to assess the passive rotation and level of reactivity of thoracic segments T3–T4 through T11–T12.
PATIENT POSITION	The patient is prone with a pillow under the chest/trunk.
THERAPIST POSITION	The therapist stands with a diagonal stance next to the patient.
HAND PLACEMENT	Caudal hand: The second and third digits are used as dummy fingers, and the pads of the second and third digits are placed on the transverse processes of the specified adjacent vertebrae.
	Cranial hand: The volar aspect of the fifth metacarpal is placed over the dummy fingers.
PROCEDURE	The therapist stands on the patient's right side and places the second digit of the caudal hand approximately a finger's width to the right side of the spinous process of T4, which positions the finger over the right transverse process of T5. The third digit of the caudal hand is placed approximately a finger's width to the left side of the spinous process of T5, which positions the third digit over the left transverse process of T6. The therapist places the volar aspect of the fifth metacarpal of the cranial hand over the pads of the dummy fingers and induces left rotation by using the cranial hand to take up the slack (to the joint's midrange) and give an impulse. Another variation is gradual, repeated moving of the segment into an end-range position to sense the resistance to movement. The amount of passive rotation available at the targeted segment and pain provocation are noted. Right rotation is tested with placement of the cranial dummy finger on the left transverse process of T5 and the caudal dummy finger on the right transverse process of T6. The cranial hand takes up the slack (to the joint's midrange) and gives an impulse. The amount of passive rotation available at the targeted segment and pain provocation are noted. The procedure is repeated at the appropriate transverse processes of T3–T4 through T11–T12, and the amount of passive rotation available in each direction is compared.

Posteroanterior Rotation (Transverse Processes of Adjacent Vertebrae) Passive Accessory Intervertebral Motion Test—cont'd

NOTES   This technique can be performed with starting at T3 and proceeding caudally, which allows for easy location of the thoracic vertebrae (by counting down from C7). The forearm of the arm that gives the impulse should be perpendicular to the angle of the contour of the region of the spine being assessed. This technique follows the rule of the lower finger: "The direction of the rotation of the spinal segment is the same as the side of the lower finger" (e.g., if the lower finger is on the right side, right rotation is being induced). The transverse processes usually are not palpable, but the dummy fingers should feel firmness when taking up the soft tissue slack; and the transverse processes of one thoracic vertebra are located lateral to the spinous process of the superior vertebra. Both mobility and pain provocation are tested with this assessment.

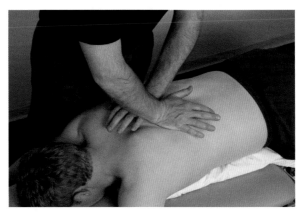

FIG. 5.27 See Video 5.12. Alternative two-handed technique posteroanterior rotation passive accessory intervertebral motion test.

PROCEDURE MODIFICATION   With the patient in a prone-lying position over a pillow, the therapist contacts the adjacent transverse processes of the targeted spinal segment with the hypothenar eminences of each hand. PA force can be applied equally and gradually with both hands (Fig 5.27) or a midrange spring can be applied to assess the PAIVM for thoracic rotation of the targeted segment. It is advisable for students to master the "dummy finger" method before attempting this alternative two-handed technique, because the two-handed technique requires more advanced palpation skills to perform safely and effectively.

RIB PASSIVE ACCESSORY MOTION TESTS AND MANIPULATION TECHNIQUES

▶ Rib Posteroanterior Accessory Motion Test

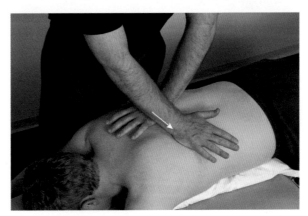

FIG. 5.28 See Video 5.13. Rib posteroanterior accessory motion test.

PURPOSE	This test assesses the mobility and level of reactivity of the costotransverse and costovertebral joints of the targeted rib. If hypomobility is noted, the forces can be modified to convert this technique to a manipulation.
PATIENT POSITION	The patient is prone with a pillow under the chest/trunk.
THERAPIST POSITION	The therapist stands with a diagonal stance next to the patient on the opposite side of the targeted rib.
HAND PLACEMENT	Caudal hand: Hypothenar eminence is placed on the opposite transverse process of the corresponding vertebra.
	Cranial hand: The arm crosses over the top of the caudal hand to place the hypothenar eminence at the posterior rib angle of the targeted rib.
PROCEDURE	As the therapist sustains a firm stabilizing pressure on the transverse process with the caudal hand, the cranial hand applies a PA force to the rib. Either a midrange thrust (i.e., spring) force or a gradually intensified PA force can be used. The amount of passive rib mobility available at the targeted segment and pain provocation are noted. The procedure is repeated from the third to the 12th rib, and left versus right is compared.
NOTES	If pain is provoked with this procedure but not with PA PAIVM tests of the thoracic vertebra, the more irritable joints at the involved segment are likely the rib joints (costotransverse and costovertebral). If pain is provoked with both the thoracic vertebra PAIVM and the rib accessory motion tests, the irritable joints could be either rib or vertebral facet joints or both. This technique can be converted to a mobilization/manipulation technique by varying the depth and frequency of the oscillations.

▶ Rib Forward Rotation Passive Motion Test and Manipulation

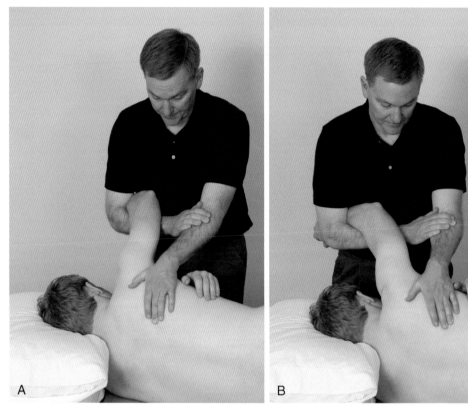

FIG. 5.29 See Video 5.14. A, Rib forward rotation passive mobility assessment for middle ribs. B, Rib forward rotation passive mobility assessment for lower ribs.

PURPOSE	This test is used to assess the mobility of the ribs and surrounding soft tissues. If hypomobility is noted, the forces can be modified to convert this technique to a manipulation.
PATIENT POSITION	The patient is in a side-lying position facing the therapist with the side to be tested on top.
THERAPIST POSITION	The therapist stands with a diagonal stance facing the patient.
HAND PLACEMENT	Caudal hand: The pads of the second and third digits contact the posterior angle of the targeted rib.
	Cranial hand: The therapist hooks the patient's top arm with the forearm and holds the forearm of the caudal arm.
PROCEDURE	As the targeted rib is contacted, the therapist shifts weight posteriorly to move the patient's top arm/shoulder girdle complex forward and pulls the targeted rib forward to assess the ability of the rib to rotate forward.
NOTES	This technique can easily be converted to a rib mobilization technique with holding and pulling the targeted stiff rib into an anterior rotation direction. As lower ribs are targeted, the therapist should progressively flex the patient's top arm and shift his body cranially to maintain the therapist's body in the direction of the manipulative force.

▶ Rib Bucket-Handle Passive Motion Test and Manipulation

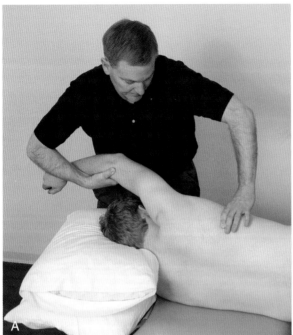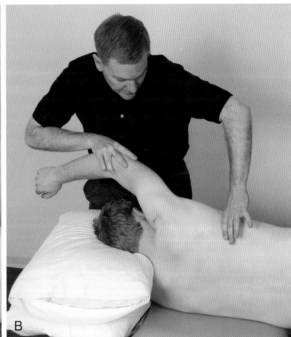

FIG. 5.30 See Video 5.15. A, Rib bucket-handle passive motion assessment. B, Rib bucket-handle technique converted to isometric manipulation of the targeted rib.

PURPOSE	This test is used to assess the mobility of the ribs and surrounding soft tissues in a bucket-handle motion direction. If hypomobility is noted, the forces can be modified to convert this technique to a manipulation.
PATIENT POSITION	The patient is in a side-lying position facing the therapist with the side to be tested on top.
THERAPIST POSITION	The therapist stands with a diagonal stance facing the front of the patient.
HAND PLACEMENT	Caudal hand: The radial aspect of the index finger is placed between the targeted ribs to be tested.
	Cranial hand: This hand holds and supports the patient's top arm proximal to the elbow.
PROCEDURE	As the therapist palpates the space between the targeted ribs, the patient's shoulder is abducted into end range and overpressure is applied to induce lateral flexion of the thorax to the targeted segment. The therapist attempts to palpate the bucket-handle motion of the superior rib in relation to the adjacent inferior rib.
NOTES	This technique can be easily converted to a rib mobilization technique with holding the inferior of the rib pairs and applying overpressure either through the rib or through the arm. This technique can be converted to an isometric manipulation (Fig 5.30B) with resisting the patient's shoulder into adduction as firm pressure is applied to the lower member of the rib pair. The isometric muscle action theoretically pulls the superior rib of the pair superiorly and applies a stretch to the joints and soft tissues of the targeted rib pair. After a 10-second isometric hold, further passive stretch is applied for 10 seconds. This sequence is repeated three to four times.

▶ Rib Exhalation Passive Accessory Motion Test and Manipulation

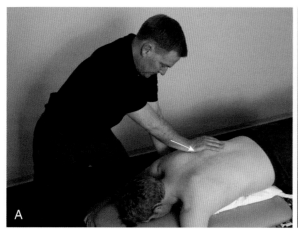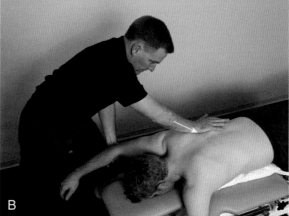

FIG. 5.31 See Videos 5.16 and 5.17. A, Rib exhalation passive accessory motion test. B, Rib exhalation manipulation with use of the upper extremity to provide added leverage.

PURPOSE	The test assesses the mobility and level of reactivity of the costotransverse and costovertebral joints of the targeted rib. If hypomobility is noted, the forces can be modified to convert this technique to a manipulation.
PATIENT POSITION	The patient is prone with a pillow under the chest/trunk and the arm off the side of the table or supported by the armrest on a mobilization table.
THERAPIST POSITION	The therapist stands with a diagonal stance at the side of the targeted rib on the side of the head of the patient.
HAND PLACEMENT	Caudal hand: This hand supports the therapist's own body weight with positioning of the hand along the side of the treatment table.
	Cranial hand: The hypothenar eminence is placed at the superior aspect of the posterior rib angle of the targeted rib.
PROCEDURE	The therapist gradually applies force in an inferior and anterior direction to move the posterior rib angle in an inferior direction. Either a midrange thrust (i.e., spring) force or a gradually intensified force can be used. The amount of passive rib mobility available at the targeted segment and pain provocation are noted. The procedure is repeated from the third to the 12th rib and left versus right is compared.
NOTES	If pain is provoked with this procedure, but not with PA PAIVM tests of the thoracic spine, the more irritable joints at the involved segment are likely rib joints (costotransverse and costovertebral). If pain is provoked with both the thoracic vertebra PAIVM and the rib accessory motion tests, the irritable joints could be either rib or vertebral facet joints or both. This technique can be converted to a mobilization technique by varying the depth and frequency of oscillations. The arm of the side being mobilized can be used to improve the mechanical advantage of the manipulation technique (Fig 5.31B). The therapist can lift the same side arm into end-range forward flexion to assist in taking up the tissue slack above the rib level to be manipulated. Once this position is attained, an isometric shoulder extension force can be resisted as the exhalation rib force is held at the targeted rib. The isometric force can be held 10 seconds and followed by a 10-second stretch with the hand on the rib. This sequence can be repeated for three to four cycles. Caution should be used in forcing the shoulder to the end range of motion if the patient has any signs of shoulder impingement, instability, or pain.

▶ First Rib Accessory Motion (Spring) Test

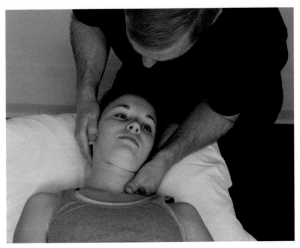

FIG. 5.32 See Video 5.18. First rib accessory motion (spring) test.

PATIENT POSITION	The patient is supine with the head on a pillow.
THERAPIST POSITION	The therapist stands at the head of the patient.
PROCEDURE	The therapist uses the radial aspect of the index finger and metacarpophalangeal joint to palpate the first rib. The first rib is located in the space lateral to the C7 transverse process, posterior to the clavicle and anterior to the scapula. The position of the rib is noted. To spring test the first rib, the therapist side bends the head and neck toward the side tested to place the scalene muscles on slack and then takes up the tissue slack and gives a slight spring to assess the mobility.
NOTES	Any stiffness or tenderness is noted, and right and left sides are compared. This evaluation can also be a pain provocation test. The spring test assesses the mobility of the first costovertebral, costotransverse, and sternocostal joints. Smedmark et al.[95] reported reliability of 0.35 (kappa) with testing first rib accessory motion in 61 subjects with nonspecific neck problems.

⏵ First Rib Depression Manipulation

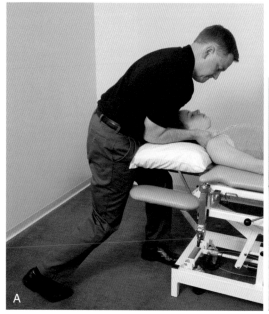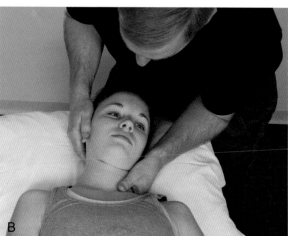

FIG. 5.33 See Video 5.19. A, First rib depression manipulation with demonstration of the therapist body and forearm position. B, First rib depression manipulation.

PURPOSE	The purpose is to manipulate (depress) a hypomobile first rib to restore first rib mobility.
PATIENT POSITION	The patient is supine with the head on a pillow.
THERAPIST POSITION	The therapist stands with a diagonal stance at the head of the patient toward the side to be manipulated.
HAND PLACEMENT	Left hand: The radial or volar aspect of the index finger metacarpophalangeal joint manipulates the left first rib.
	Right hand: The radial or volar aspect of the index finger metacarpophalangeal joint manipulates the right first rib.
PROCEDURE	The radial or volar aspect of the index finger metacarpophalangeal joint of the right hand palpates the right first rib. The first rib is located in the space lateral to the C7 transverse process, posterior to the clavicle and anterior to the scapula. The therapist side bends and rotates the head and neck slightly toward the right and takes up the slack and oscillates the first rib. The manipulation is coordinated with the patient's breathing, with progressive oscillation into greater depression with each oscillation. The procedure is repeated through three breathing cycles. On completion of the manipulation, the mobility of the right first rib is retested.
	The therapist manipulates the left first rib by repeating the procedure with the radial or volar aspect of the index finger metacarpophalangeal joint of the left hand to contact the left first rib. On completion of the manipulation, the mobility of the first rib is retested.
NOTES	Indication for use of this technique is elevation and mobility deficits of the first rib. During the performance of this technique, the manipulating hand is reinforced with bracing the elbow with the ipsilateral hip. The direction of the manipulating force should be toward the patient's umbilicus. An elevated and hypomobile first rib is commonly associated with signs and symptoms characteristic of TOS.

▶ First Rib Posterior Glide Manipulation in Supine

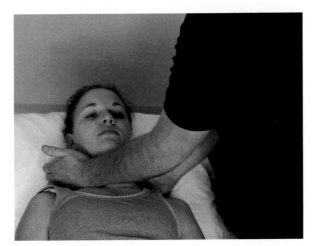

FIG. 5.34 See Video 5.20. First rib posterior glide manipulation in supine.

PURPOSE	The purpose is manipulation of a hypomobile first rib and restoration of first rib and T1–T2 rotation mobility.
PATIENT POSITION	The patient is supine with the head on a pillow.
THERAPIST POSITION	The therapist stands on the opposite side to be manipulated.
HAND PLACEMENT	Left hand: The ulnar aspect of the left hand on the anterior aspect of the right first rib just superior and posterior to the clavicle to manipulate the right first rib.
	Right hand: The pad of the long finger is placed at the left lateral aspect of the T2 spinous process to block T2 rotation.
PROCEDURE	The ulnar aspect of the fifth metacarpal of the left hand provides an anteroposterior force into the first rib as the right hand blocks T2. The therapist takes up the slack and oscillates the first rib. The manipulation is coordinated with the patient's breathing, with progressive oscillation into slightly greater posterior glide with each oscillation. The procedure is repeated through approximately three breathing cycles. On completion of the manipulation, the mobility of the right first rib is retested.
NOTES	Indication for use of this technique is decreased mobility of the first rib and limited rotation of the T1–T2 spinal segment. Ipsilateral pain and limited motion at the cervicothoracic junction during cervical rotation AROM testing is also an indication for this technique. Supine cervical rotation AROM can be used as a pretest and posttest for this manipulation.

SCAPULOTHORACIC SOFT TISSUE TECHNIQUES

Scapular Passive Mobility Assessment and Mobilization

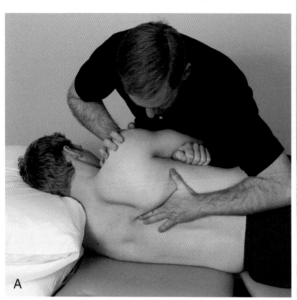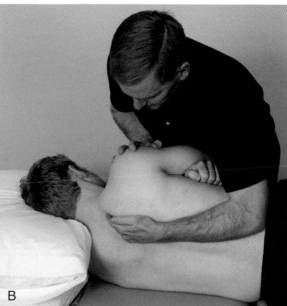

FIG. 5.35 A, Scapular passive mobility assessment and mobilization. B, Parascapular soft tissue mobilization, bordering the scapula.

PURPOSE	The purpose of this test is to assess and treat muscular and connective tissue restrictions of the parascapular tissues.
PATIENT POSITION	The patient is in a side-lying position facing the therapist with the targeted scapula on top.
THERAPIST POSITION	The therapist stands in front of the patient very close to edge of the table.
HAND PLACEMENT	Caudal hand: The web space is positioned at the edge of the inferior angle of the scapula.
	Cranial hand: The hand is placed across the anterior aspect of the patient's shoulder.
PROCEDURE	The therapist gradually applies an anteroposterior force of the shoulder girdle complex with the cranial hand as the caudal hand presses anterior and superior to slide the hand under the inferior angle of the scapula. Once the caudal hand is positioned under the inferior angle of the scapula, the pads of the fingers and thumb can be pressed into the thorax to lift the anterior aspect of the scapula away from the thorax with the dorsal aspect of the caudal hand.
PROCEDURE MODIFICATION	If restricted soft tissue mobility or muscle guarding is noted, soft tissue mobilization techniques (such as the "bordering the scapula" technique shown in Fig. 5.35B) may be needed before performance of this technique to allow further mobilization of the scapular tissues. The "bordering the scapula" soft tissue mobilization technique is performed by rhythmically gliding the caudal hand along the medial border of the scapula as the cranial hand presses the shoulder girdle into a retracted position. The soft tissue mobilization is repeated multiple times until the muscle tone in the region begins to relax.

Pectoralis Minor Muscle Length Test and Stretch

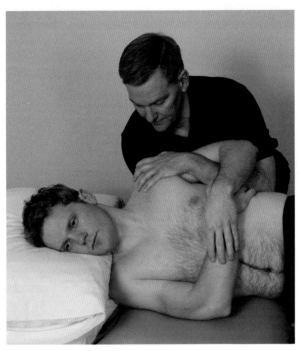

FIG. 5.36 Pectoralis minor muscle length test and stretch.

PURPOSE	This test assesses and treats muscle length restrictions of the pectoralis minor muscle.
PATIENT POSITION	The patient is side-lying and facing away from the therapist with the targeted pectoralis minor muscle on top.
THERAPIST POSITION	The therapist stands behind the patient very close to edge of the table.
HAND PLACEMENT	Caudal hand: The forearm is placed under the patient's top arm, and the hand is positioned at the anterior aspect of the shoulder.
	Cranial hand: The hand is placed on the posterior aspect of the scapula.
PROCEDURE	The therapist gradually applies a posterior force with the caudal hand and creates a force couple with the cranial hand to move the scapula into retraction.
NOTES	Normal muscle length of the pectoralis minor muscle should allow full passive shoulder girdle retraction motion with this passive motion test. If restricted soft tissue mobility or muscle guarding is noted, soft tissue mobilization techniques may be needed to allow further mobilization of the pectoralis tissues with this technique. A hold-relax stretch technique can be used to stretch the pectoralis minor muscle by asking the patient to press the shoulder forward into protraction as the therapist resists for a 10-second hold. This is followed by a 10-second stretch into further retraction. The sequence is repeated three to four times.

THORACIC SPINE MANIPULATION

▶ Central Posteroanterior (Backward-Bending) Manipulation in Prone

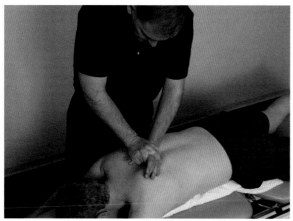

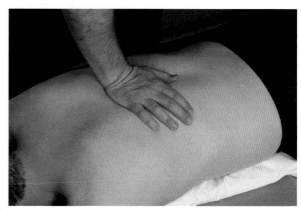

▶ **FIG. 5.37** See Video 5.21. Central posteroanterior backward-bending mobilization: two-handed technique.

▶ **FIG. 5.38** See Video 5.22. Central posteroanterior backward-bending mobilization: alternative one-handed technique.

PURPOSE	The purpose of this technique is to manipulate a specific thoracic segment (T3–T4 through T12–L1) into backward bending.
PATIENT POSITION	The patient lies prone with a pillow under the thorax with the arms along the side of the body, hanging off the edge of the table, or supported on the arm rests of the mobilization table. A pillow can be placed under the lower legs for comfort.
THERAPIST POSITION	The therapist stands at the side of the patient.
HAND PLACEMENT	Left hand: This hand is placed on the patient's back so that the ulnar border of the hand just distal to the pisiform is in contact with the spinous process of the vertebrae to be mobilized. The shoulders are directly over the patient. The left wrist is fully extended with the forearm midway between supination/pronation.
	Right hand: The left hand is reinforced with the right hand so that the second and third digits of the right hand envelop the second metacarpal phalangeal joint of the left hand. The elbows are allowed to slightly flex.
PROCEDURE	The therapist takes up the slack and induces PA force at the specified segment. The manipulation is coordinated with the patient's breathing, with progressive oscillations into slightly greater backward bending with each oscillation. The procedure is repeated through approximately three breathing cycles. On completion of the manipulation, PA PAIVM is retested. The depth and frequency of the forces can be modified to perform graded oscillations I to IV or a thrust manipulation with this technique.
NOTES	Indication for use of this manipulation technique is decreased backward bending (central PA PAIVM motion) at a specific thoracic segment (T3–T4 through T12–L1) or pain provocation with PAIVM motion testing. The force should be perpendicular to the angle of the contour of the region of the spine being manipulated.
PROCEDURE MODIFICATION	This technique could also be done as a one-handed technique with the cranial hand contacting the spinous process with the hypothenar eminence, the elbow flexed, and the forearm perpendicular with the angle of the contour of the surface of the spine (Fig 5.38). The caudal hand rests at the edge of the table to support the therapist's upper body weight as the therapist leans over the patient.

⏵ Thoracic Posteroanterior Forward-Bending Manipulation in Prone

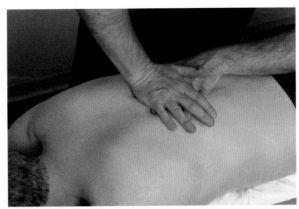

FIG. 5.39 See Video 5.23. Thoracic posteroanterior forward-bending manipulation in prone.

PURPOSE	This technique is used to manipulate a specific thoracic segment (T3–T4 through T12–L1) into forward bending.
PATIENT POSITION	The patient is prone with a pillow under the chest/trunk.
THERAPIST POSITION	The therapist stands with a diagonal stance next to the patient.
HAND PLACEMENT	Caudal hand: The second and third digits are used as dummy fingers, with the pads of the second and third fingers placed on the transverse processes of the specified vertebra.
	Cranial hand: The palmar aspect of the fifth metacarpal is placed over the dummy fingers.
PROCEDURE	The manipulation is coordinated with the patient's breathing, with progressive oscillations into slightly more forward bending with each repetition. As the patient inhales, the therapist holds against the expansion of the thorax. As the patient exhales, more force is applied to take up the tissue slack and mobilize the spinal segment. The procedure is repeated through approximately three breathing cycles. On completion of the manipulation, forward bending is retested. This manipulation can be used for segments T3–T4 through T11–T12. The depth and frequency of the forces can be modified to perform graded oscillations I to IV or a thrust manipulation with this technique.
NOTES	Indication for use of this technique is decreased forward bending of a specific thoracic segment (T3–T4 through T12–L1). The forearm of the arm that applies the force should be perpendicular to the surface contour of the region of the spine to be manipulated. The transverse processes usually are not palpable, but the dummy fingers should feel a firmness as the fingers sink into the soft tissue. Also the transverse processes of one thoracic vertebra are located lateral to the spinous process of the superior vertebra.

Thoracic Posteroanterior Forward-Bending Manipulation in Prone—cont'd

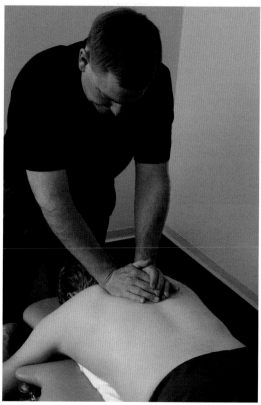

▶ **FIG. 5.40** See Video 5.24. Posteroanterior forward-bending manipulation: alternative two-handed technique.

PROCEDURE MODIFICATION

With the patient lying prone over a pillow, the therapist can stand at the head of the table and position both hypothenar eminences at the transverse processes of the same vertebra (Fig 5.40). As the therapist keeps both elbows straight, a gradual application of PA pressure can be applied to the targeted thoracic vertebra with a force that is perpendicular to the contour of the spine being manipulated. The depth and frequency of the forces can be modified to perform graded oscillations I to IV or a thrust manipulation with this technique. This technique can also be used as a PAIVM test.

▶ Thoracic Rotation Manipulation in Prone

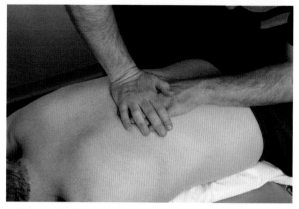

FIG. 5.41 See Video 5.25. Thoracic rotation manipulation in prone for right rotation.

Thoracic Rotation Manipulation in Prone—cont'd

PURPOSE

This technique is used to manipulate a specific thoracic segment (T3–T4 through T12–L1) into rotation.

PATIENT POSITION

The patient is prone with a pillow under the chest/trunk.

THERAPIST POSITION

The therapist stands with a diagonal stance next to the patient.

HAND PLACEMENT

Caudal hand: The second and third digits are used as dummy fingers, and the pads of the second and third digits are placed on the transverse processes of specified adjacent vertebrae.

Cranial hand: The volar aspect of the fifth metacarpal is placed over the dummy fingers.

PROCEDURE

The cranial hand is used to take up the slack and oscillate the T3–T4 segment. The manipulation is coordinated with the patient's breathing, with progressive oscillation into deeper PA pressure and creation of slightly more rotation with each oscillation. As the patient inhales, the therapist holds down the force against the rising thorax; as the patient exhales, the force is deepened further. The procedure is repeated through approximately three breathing cycles. On completion of the manipulation, rotation is retested. A thrust manipulation can also be used at midrange for PIVM testing or end range for treatment effects. Use of a progressive oscillation first is advisable to attain an end-range position before application of the thrust manipulation.

NOTES

The indication for use of this technique is decreased rotation of a specific thoracic segment (T3–T4 through T12–L1). The forearm of the arm that applies the force should be perpendicular to the contour surface of the region of the spine being treated. The transverse processes usually are not palpable, but the dummy fingers should feel a firmness as the fingers sink into the soft tissue. Also the transverse processes of one thoracic vertebra are located lateral to the spinous process of the superior vertebra. This technique follows the *rule of the lower finger*, which states that the direction of the rotation is the same as the side of the lower finger (e.g., if the lower finger is on the right side, right rotation is being induced).

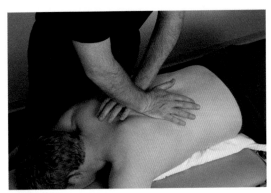

FIG. 5.42 See Video 5.26. Posteroanterior two-handed rotation manipulation in prone for left rotation.

PROCEDURE MODIFICATION

With the patient in prone-lying position over a pillow, the therapist contacts the adjacent transverse processes of the targeted spinal segment with the hypothenar eminences of each hand (Fig 5.42). The therapist is positioned with elbows extended and shoulders placed directly over the targeted segment. PA force can be applied, and the depth and frequency of the forces can be modified to perform a progressive oscillation, graded oscillations II or III, or a thrust manipulation with this technique. Often helpful is combination of the manipulation with the patient's breathing cycle with application of PA force against the chest expansion and further force applied as the breath is released. Osteoporosis is a contraindication for this technique and all manipulation techniques performed in the prone position.

▶ Thoracic Side-Bending Manipulation in Prone

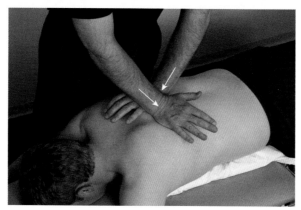

FIG. 5.43 See Video 5.27. Thoracic posteroanterior two-handed side bending manipulation in prone for left side bending.

PURPOSE	The technique is used to manipulate a specific thoracic segment (T3–T4 through T11–T12) into side-bending (lateral flexion) direction.
PATIENT POSITION	The patient is prone with a pillow under the patient's chest.
THERAPIST POSITION	The therapist stands with a diagonal athletic stance next to the patient.
HAND PLACEMENT	Caudal hand: The hand contacts the transverse process of the vertebra with the hypothenar eminence. Cranial hand: This hand contacts the opposite side transverse process of the same vertebrae with the hypothenar eminence and with the arms crossed.
PROCEDURE	The therapist takes up the tissue slack with a PA force to reach a barrier. Once PA force slack is taken up, the ulnar aspects of hands are rotated toward each other to twist the skin for the purpose of taking up more tissue slack to reach a firm barrier. The cranial hand is directed into a caudal direction and the caudal hand is directed into a cranial direction to create a side bending/gliding force. The body weight of the shoulders/thorax is shifted into a downward direction to add a PA thrust. The therapist should consider combining the technique with breathing to first provide a progressive oscillation before providing the thrust.
NOTES	Osteoporosis is a contraindication. Most of the force is into an anteroposterior direction at the targeted vertebra. Because of the natural angle of the forearms in this position, frontal plane cranial- and caudal-directed forces create a slight side bending motion at the targeted spinal segment.

▶ Thoracic Rotation Manipulation in Supine

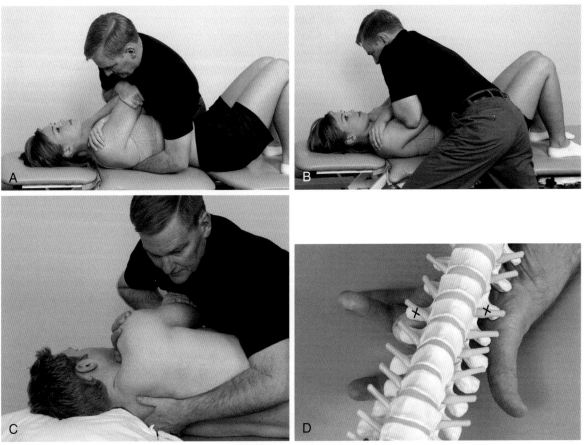

FIG. 5.44 See Video 5.28. A, Thoracic supine rotation manipulation in supine with arms folded. B, Therapist body position for thoracic supine rotation manipulation. C, Roll patient to position hand for thoracic supine rotation manipulation. D, Hand placement on spine model for thoracic supine rotation manipulation.

PURPOSE	The purpose of this technique is to manipulate a specific thoracic segment (T3–T4 through T11–T12) into rotation.
PATIENT POSITION	The patient is supine.
THERAPIST POSITION	The therapist stands next to the patient.
HAND PLACEMENT	Caudal hand: The thenar eminence is placed on the transverse process of the caudal member of the spinal segment, and the dorsal aspect of the middle phalanx of the third digit is placed on the transverse process of the cranial member of the segment.
	Cranial hand: The hand and forearm are used to maneuver the patient's upper body, head, neck, and upper extremities.

Thoracic Rotation Manipulation in Supine—cont'd

PROCEDURE

The patient's arms are folded across the chest. The arm closest to the therapist should be crossed first and underneath the opposite arm. The therapist stands on the patient's left side and uses the cranial hand to reach under the patient's shoulders and support the upper body or places the therapist's forearms over the patient's elbows. The cranial hand is used to roll the patient slightly toward the left side, and the index finger of the caudal hand is used to palpate the specified segment. Once the segment is located, both the distal interphalangeal and proximal interphalangeal joints of the long finger of the caudal hand are flexed. The dorsal aspect of the middle phalanx of the third digit is placed on the left transverse process of the cranial member of the segment. The thenar eminence of the caudal hand is placed on the right transverse process of the caudal member of the segment. The patient is gently rolled back into the supine position onto the caudal hand, and the chest is used to apply force through the patient's forearms to take up the slack and oscillate or thrust the segment.

The manipulation is coordinated with the patient's breathing, with progressive oscillation into slightly more rotation each repetition. The procedure is repeated through approximately three breathing cycles. Once all the tissue slack is taken up, a short-amplitude high-velocity thrust can be imparted. On completion of the manipulation, right rotation is retested.

Additional tissue tension can be created by side bending the patient's thoracic spine superior to the level to be manipulated in the opposite direction of the rotation followed by dropping the same side shoulder girdle (of the direction of rotation) toward the table just before application of the manipulation forces. Skin slack can be taken up by pulling the hand contact slightly inferior just before imparting the thrust.

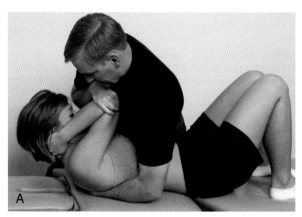

FIG. 5.45 See Video 5.29. A, Thoracic manipulation in supine—hands behind the head variation.

PROCEDURE MODIFICATION: THORACIC ROTATION MANIPULATION IN SUPINE: HANDS BEHIND THE HEAD VARIATION

Another variation can be made with this technique to flex the spine superior to the level to be manipulated to add further tissue tension above the level to be manipulated (Fig 5.45A). Changing the patient's hand position to interlock fingers behind the patient's head/neck can facilitate the addition of flexion to this technique.

Thoracic Rotation Manipulation in Supine—cont'd

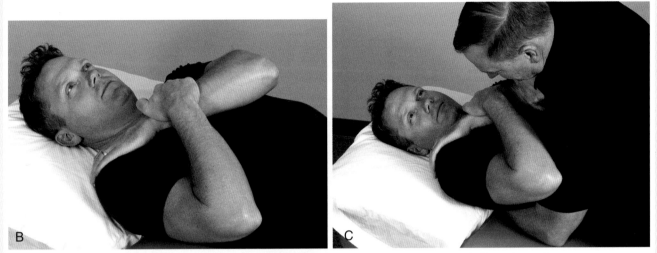

FIG. 5.45, cont'd B, Alternate patient arm position to protect the right shoulder. C, Thoracic manipulation in supine—modification to protect the right shoulder.

PRECEDURE MODIFICATION: THORACIC ROTATION MANIPULATION IN SUPINE: SHOULDER PROTECTION VARIATION	To protect a painful or recent postsurgical shoulder, the patient can grasp the forearm of the unaffected upper extremity with the hand of the affected upper extremity (Fig. 5.45B and C) The anteroposterior force will be directed from the therapist through the unaffected upper extremity to avoid loading the painful shoulder.
NOTES	Indication for use of this technique is decreased rotation of a specific thoracic segment (T3–T4 through T11–T12). The procedure can be performed with the cranial hand used to contact the segment (with the same contact points described previously). This modification prevents the therapist from reaching around the patient to perform the technique. The long finger of the caudal hand (or cranial hand if the modified technique is used) is flexed around a towel or pillowcase to protect the joints from hyperflexion (Box 5.6) (Fig. 5.46). The procedure can also be performed with the patient's arms folded across a pillow to create a barrier between the therapist and patient for patient comfort. This technique follows the rule of the lower finger, which states that the direction of the rotation is the same as the side of the lower finger (e.g., if the lower finger is on the right side, right rotation is being induced). This technique is commonly used to induce a high-velocity thrust manipulation or as a progressive oscillation.

Thoracic Rotation Manipulation in Supine—cont'd

BOX 5.6   Variations of Hand Positions and Use of a Towel to Protect the Joints of the Hand for the Supine Thoracic Manipulation Techniques

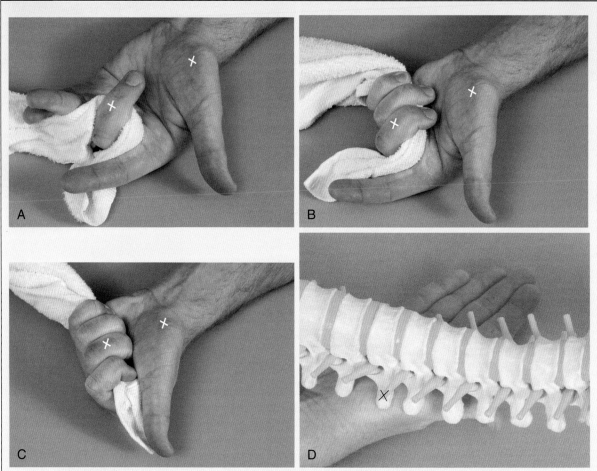

FIG. 5.46 A, Hand position with a flexed third digit and use of a towel to protect joints of third digit for the supine thoracic manipulation techniques. B, "Pistol grip" hand position and use of a towel to protect the joints of the hand for the supine thoracic manipulation techniques. C, Fist grip hand positions and use of a towel to protect the joints of hand for the supine thoracic manipulation techniques. D, The thenar eminence can be used to contact one transverse process with the rest of the hand flat on the table to reduce the stresses on the finger joints and induce rotation via posteroanterior force through one transverse process.

Rib Posteroanterior Manipulation in Supine

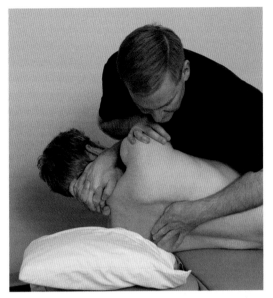

FIG. 5.47 Rib posteroanterior manipulation in supine.

PROCEDURE
MODIFICATION

The supine thoracic manipulation technique can be modified to manipulate a rib by placing the thumb on the posterior aspect of the rib just lateral to the transverse process. The force application is combined with breathing as a progressive oscillation or thrust is applied.

▶ Upper Thoracic Rotation Manipulation in Prone

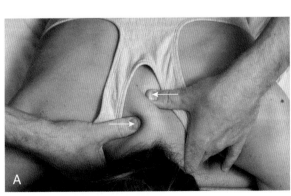

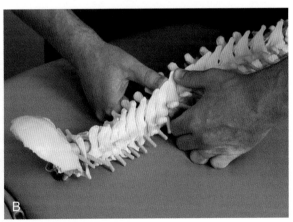

FIG. 5.48 See Video 5.30. A, Upper thoracic rotation manipulation in prone for right rotation. B, Finger placement for prone upper thoracic right rotation manipulation.

Upper Thoracic Rotation Manipulation in Prone—cont'd

PURPOSE	The purpose is manipulation of a specific thoracic segment (C7–T1 through T3–T4) into rotation.
PATIENT POSITION	The patient is prone with a pillow under the chest/trunk and the neck in a neutral position.
THERAPIST POSITION	The therapist stands with a diagonal athletic stance next to the patient.
HAND PLACEMENT	Right hand: The pad of the thumb is used to contact the lateral aspect of the spinous process of one member of the segment. Left hand: The pad of the thumb is used to contact the lateral aspect of the spinous process of the other member of the segment.
PROCEDURE	The therapist stands on the patient's side and uses the pad of the thumb of the left hand to contact the left lateral aspect of the spinous process of the caudal member of the segment. The pad of the thumb of the right hand is used to contact the right lateral aspect of the spinous process of the cranial member of the segment. The therapist manipulates into right rotation by pushing each member of the segment toward the opposite side by using the thumbs to apply an equal and opposite force through the spinous processes. On completion of the manipulation, right rotation is retested. Manipulation into left rotation is accomplished with repeating the procedure with the left thumb contacting the left lateral aspect of the spinous process of the cranial member of the segment and the right thumb contacting the right lateral aspect of the spinous process of the caudal member of the segment. On completion of the manipulation, left rotation is retested.
NOTES	Indication for use of this technique is decreased rotation of a specific thoracic segment (C7–T1 through T3–T4). A flexed index finger can be used to reinforce and support the thumb during the performance of this technique. The therapist should avoid applying the force to the tips of the spinous processes because this is usually uncomfortable to the patient. Grade III oscillations are usually used with this technique. This technique follows the *rule of the upper thumb*, which states that the direction of the rotation is the same as the side of the upper thumb (e.g., if the upper thumb is on the right side, right rotation is being induced).

▶ Upper Thoracic Rotation Mobilization With Movement

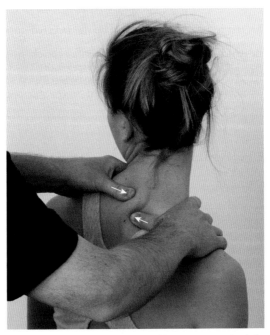

FIG. 5.49 See Video 5.31. Mobilization with movement for left rotation.

PROCEDURE MODIFICATION	The upper thoracic rotation mobilization technique can be followed up with a mobilization with movement in which the same contact and force are used on an upright patient. As the patient actively rotates the neck into the direction of the manipulation, the therapist applies overpressure through the spinous processes at the targeted segment.

▶ Upper Thoracic Gap Manipulation With Facet Locking

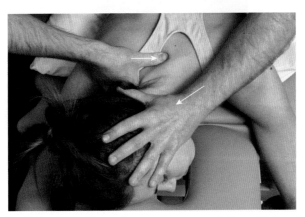

FIG. 5.50 See Video 5.32. Upper thoracic gap manipulation with facet locking.

Upper Thoracic Gap Manipulation With Facet Locking—cont'd

PURPOSE	This test is used to gap/manipulate the targeted upper thoracic facet joint.
PATIENT POSITION	The patient is prone with a pillow under the chest.
HAND PLACEMENT	Right hand: The thumb contacts the lateral aspect of the spinous process of the inferior member of the targeted segment on the side opposite the joint to be manipulated.
	Left hand: The palm is placed across the posterior lateral aspect of the patient's occiput.
PROCEDURE	The therapist uses the left hand to passively side bend the patient's neck away from the targeted facet joint and then rotates the neck toward the targeted facet joint to take up the slack of the cervical and upper thoracic spine down to, but not including, the targeted segment. The therapist presses superiorly with the left hand along the angle of the neck/head and presses laterally with the right thumb across the spinous process with equal forces. Once the slack is taken up, an oscillatory or a thrust force may be imparted.
NOTES	This technique is most effective if the positioning allows maximum tension to the targeted facet joint. The therapist should verbally monitor the patient throughout the technique because the prone position hides facial expressions.

▶ Upper Thoracic Gapping Manipulation in Sitting

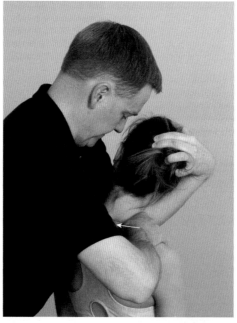

FIG. 5.51 See Video 5.33. Upper thoracic gapping manipulation in sitting.

PROCEDURE MODIFICATION	The same facet locking can be used with the patient in the seated position. A cradle hold of the patient's head with the therapist's arm can facilitate the technique. The forces are the same, with lateral force with the thumb across the spinous process combined with a lifting/distraction force imparted with the therapist's other arm/hand on the patient's head.
	This advanced technique is most commonly used as a thrust technique.

▶ Upper Thoracic Press/Kneading Manipulation in Sitting

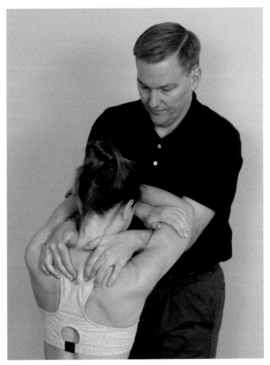

FIG. 5.52 See Video 5.34. Upper thoracic press/kneading manipulation in sitting.

PURPOSE	The technique is used to manipulate a specific thoracic segment (T1–T2 through T4–T5).
PATIENT POSITION	The patient sits on a treatment table with his or her feet flat on the floor with the arms folded and the head resting on the forearms.
THERAPIST POSITION	The therapist stands with a diagonal athletic stance directly in front of the patient.
HAND PLACEMENT	The therapist's arms are placed under the patient's forearms to support the weight of the patient's head, neck, and shoulders. The pads of digits two and three of both hands are placed at the targeted upper thoracic transverse processes.
PROCEDURE	The therapist presses the fingers into the targeted thoracic vertebrae while shifting the weight backward to lean away from the patient and lifting the patient's head/neck/upper thorax from flexion into extension.
NOTES	This technique can be used as a general soft tissue technique or made more specific to target a spinal segment. Firm support of the patient's arms/head/neck and convincing the patient to relax into the rhythmic motions of the mobilization are important. The therapist can modify his force application into asymmetric or diagonal directions to induce lateral flexion and rotation motions at the targeted upper thoracic segments. For instance, the patient's head and neck gliding motion could be angled toward the patient's left as the therapist presses more firmly on the patient's right transverse process to facilitate left rotation at the targeted spinal segment.

⦿ Upper Thorax Posteroanterior Mobilization

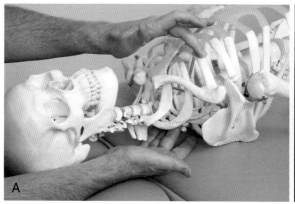 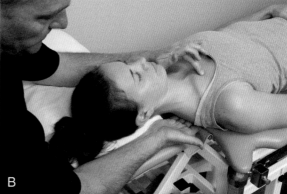

FIG. 5.53 See Video 5.35. A, Upper thorax posteroanterior mobilization finger placement on a skeletal model. B, Upper thorax posteroanterior mobilization.

PURPOSE	The technique is used to manipulate a specific thoracic segment (T1–T2 through T4–T5) and the corresponding ribs at the targeted segment.
PATIENT POSITION	The patient is in the supine position with head/neck supported on a pillow.
THERAPIST POSITION	The therapist stands or sits at the head of the treatment table.
HAND PLACEMENT	The therapist positions the tips of the second and third digits of the right at the targeted right transverse process and posterior angle of the rib with the posterior aspect of the hand resting flat on the table and positions the tips of the second and third digits of the left hand at the anterior aspect of the corresponding rib just lateral to the right edge of sternum.
PROCEDURE	The therapist presses the fingers into the targeted thoracic vertebrae and rib to move the segment forward as the top hand monitors anterior movement of the rib. The anterior hand can alternately press the targeted rib posteriorly to create a reciprocal PA and anteroposterior movement of the motion segment.
NOTES	The location and direction of the forces used with this technique should be localized to mobilize through the location and direction of greatest resistance to passive movement in the upper thorax.

▶ Upper Thorax Isometric Posteroanterior Mobilization

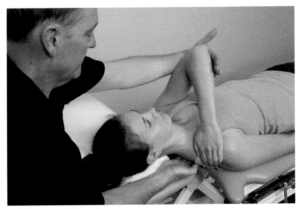

FIG. 5.54 See Video 5.36. Upper thorax isometric posteroanterior mobilization.

PURPOSE	The technique is used to manipulate a specific thoracic segment (T1–T2 through T4–T5) and the corresponding ribs at the targeted segment.
PATIENT POSITION	The patient is in the supine position with head/neck supported on a pillow and left arm (opposite side to be treated) is positioned in a horizontally adducted position with the left hand holding the patient's right shoulder.
THERAPIST POSITION	The therapist stands or sits at the head of the treatment table.
HAND PLACEMENT	The therapist positions the tips of the right second and third digits at the targeted right transverse process and posterior angle of the rib with the hand resting flat on the table. The left hand is positioned under the medial aspect of the patient's elbow.
PROCEDURE	The therapist presses the fingers into the targeted thoracic vertebrae and rib to move the segment forward and simultaneously asks the patient to match a moderate level of pressure applied at the medial aspect of the left elbow. The therapist applies a force to lift the patient's elbow off her chest, and the patient isometrically matches the force. The isometric force is held for 10 seconds and can be repeated three to five times.
NOTES	The location and direction of the forces used with this technique should be localized to mobilize through the location and direction of greatest resistance to the PA passive movement in the upper thorax. The isometric force through the opposite shoulder facilitates the passive rotation motion applied to the upper thoracic segment.

Variation: Upper Thorax Isometric Posteroanterior Mobilization

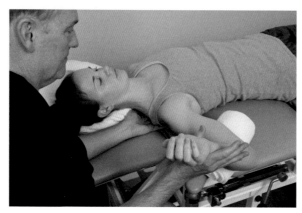

FIG. 5.55 Variation: upper thorax isometric posteroanterior mobilization with isometric shoulder external rotation.

PROCEDURE MODIFICATION   This technique can be modified to include isometric resistance of shoulder external rotation on the same side shoulder as the side of the PA mobilization force application.

Upper Thoracic Lift Manipulation

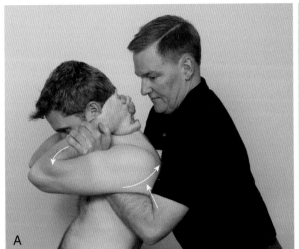
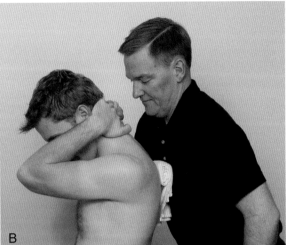

FIG. 5.56 See Video 5.37. A, Upper thoracic lift manipulation. B, Towel placement for upper thoracic lift manipulation technique.

PURPOSE	The technique is used to manipulate a specific thoracic segment (T1–T2 through T4–T5).
PATIENT POSITION	The patient sits on a treatment table with the fingers interlocked behind the neck.
THERAPIST POSITION	The therapist stands with a diagonal athletic stance behind the patient, and the chest is placed against a rolled hand towel against the targeted spinal segment.
HAND PLACEMENT	The hands are used to grasp the patient's forearms in each hand.
PROCEDURE	The patient's neck and upper thoracic spine are fully flexed to the targeted spinal level, and the patient is asked to squeeze the elbows together into a horizontal adduction motion as the therapist lifts the patient in a superior and posterior direction into the counterforce of the rolled towel and the therapist's chest.
NOTES	This technique is often combined with deep breathing with the manipulative thrust applied as the patient exhales. Because minimal compressive loading forces are used on the thorax and rib cage, this technique is thought to be safe for patients who may have suspected weakened skeletal structure (such as osteopenia).

▶ Mid-Thoracic Lift Manipulation

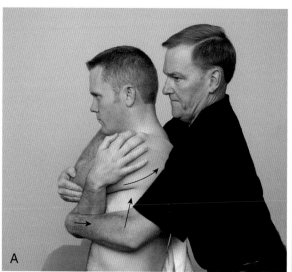
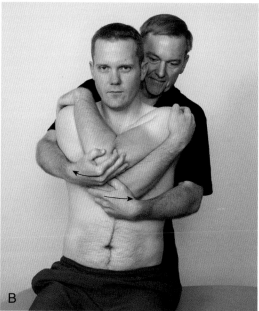

FIG. 5.57 See Video 5.38. A, Mid-thoracic lift manipulation. B, Mid-thoracic lift manipulation anterior view to demonstrate hand placements.

PURPOSE	This technique is used to manipulate a specific thoracic segment (T3–T4 through T10–T11).
PATIENT POSITION	The patient sits on a treatment table with the arms folded across the chest and the hands grasping each opposite shoulder girdle. The arm on the side to be targeted with the manipulation should be positioned superior to the other arm.
THERAPIST POSITION	The therapist stands with a diagonal athletic stance behind the patient, and the chest is placed against a rolled hand towel at the targeted spinal segment.
HAND PLACEMENT	The patient's elbows are grasped in each opposite hand so that the left hand grasps the right elbow and right hand grasps the left elbow (Fig 5.57).
PROCEDURE	The patient's arms are pulled into further adduction as the upper thoracic spine is extended to the targeted spinal level, and the therapist lifts and squeezes the patient in a superior and posterior direction into the counterforce of the rolled towel and the therapist's chest.
NOTES	This technique is often combined with deep breathing with the manipulative thrust applied as the patient exhales. Because minimal compressive loading forces are used on the thorax and rib cage, this technique is thought to be safe for patients who may have suspected weakened skeletal structure (such as osteopenia).

CASE STUDIES AND PROBLEM SOLVING

The following patient case reports can be used by the student to develop problem-solving skills by considering the information provided in the patient history and tests and measures and developing appropriate evaluations, goals, and plans of care. Students should also consider the following questions:

1. What additional historical/subjective information would you like to have?
2. What additional diagnostic tests should be ordered, if any?
3. What additional tests and measures would be helpful in making the diagnosis?
4. What impairment-based classification does the patient most likely fit? What other impairment-based classifications did you consider?
5. What are the primary impairments that should be addressed?
6. What treatment techniques that you learned in this textbook will you use to address these impairments?
7. How do you plan to progress and modify the interventions as the patient progresses?

Mrs. Thoracic Kyphosis

History

An 83-year-old woman has a 2-year history of progressively increasing intensity lumbar and thoracic pain (Fig. 5.58). The patient needs a walker for ambulation but states that her thoracic area pain is worse with lifting the walker. The patient is very limited functionally and needs assistance for all self-care activities because of pain provocation with all functional mobility, especially attempting to roll over and lie supine.

What diagnostic tests should be done on this patient before beginning treatment?

Tests and Measures

1. Observation: The patient is a frail-looking woman with moderately increased thoracic kyphosis who tends to use the upper extremities to support the trunk in sitting.
2. Gait: The patient's gait is slow and laborious with a grimace each time she lifts the walker.
3. Functional mobility: The patient is unable to tolerate supine or prone positions because of pain.
4. Thoracolumbar AROM: The patient has limited thoracolumbar AROM in all planes because of pain, with patient demonstrating approximately 20% to 25% of expected AROM in all planes of motion.

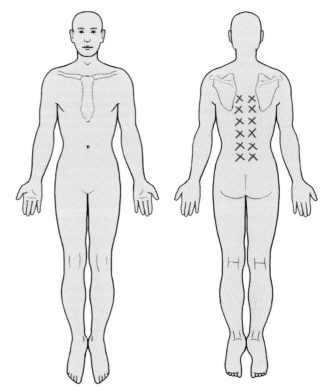

FIG. 5.58 Body chart for Mrs. Thoracic Kyphosis.

5. Palpation: Patient is tender and guarded at the mid-thoracic and lower lumbar paraspinal muscles.
6. Strength: Grossly fair strength is noted throughout trunk and extremities, with poor strength in lower and middle trapezius.
7. Balance: Patient has good static balance and fair dynamic balance.

Evaluation

Diagnosis
Problem list
Goals
Treatment plan/intervention

Mrs. P. Neck

History

A 35-year-old acute care nurse has tightness and discomfort in the mid-thoracic spine and mid-cervical area that is provoked with prolonged sitting and work activities (Fig. 5.59). Symptoms started 24 days before the initial evaluation after the nurse transferred a heavy patient. The Fear-Avoidance Beliefs Questionnaire (FABQ) physical activity subscale score was 11.

Tests and Measures

1. Structural examination: Results indicate mild forward head posture with diminished (flattened) upper thoracic kyphosis.
2. Cervical AROM in standing: Patient displays 75% in all planes of motion with mid-cervical pain reported at the end range of each motion.
3. Cervical extension: Extension is 25 degrees.
4. Thoracic AROM: Testing indicates 60% backward bending, 85% forward bending, 80% bilateral rotation and side bending with ipsilateral mid-thoracic pain reported with bilateral rotation.
5. PIVM testing: Hypomobility and mild reactivity noted with PA testing T3–T4 and T5–T6 segments with bilateral rotation and forward-bending PAIVM testing; downglide PIVM hypomobility noted at C2–C3 and C6–C7 bilaterally.
6. Shoulder screen: Patients has active shoulder forward flexion and abduction full range of motion and is pain free.
7. Muscle length: No limitations noted.
8. Strength: Lower and middle trapezius are 4–/5; deep neck flexors are 3+/5.
9. Neurologic screen: Neurologic tests are negative.
10. Palpation: Patient is tender and guarded at bilateral mid-thoracic and mid-cervical paraspinal muscles.

Evaluation

Diagnosis
Problem list
Goals
Treatment plan/intervention

Mr. Stiff Thorax

History

A 50-year-old college professor has tightness and discomfort in the mid-thoracic spine that is provoked with taking a deep breath and with prolonged sitting (Fig. 5.60).

Tests and Measures

1. Structural examination results: Examination indicates moderate forward head posture with protracted scapulae.
2. Cervical AROM in standing: Patient displays AROM of 85% in all planes of motion and is pain free.
3. Thoracic AROM: Patient ROM is 25% backward bending, 85% forward bending, 50% bilateral rotation and side bending with ipsilateral mid-thoracic pain reported with bilateral rotation.

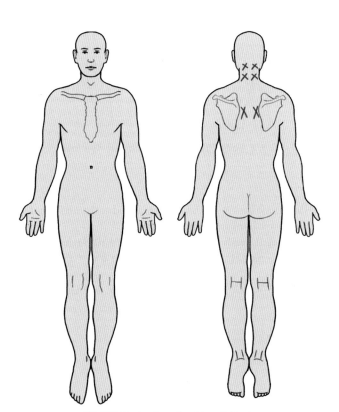

FIG. 5.59 Body chart for Mrs. P. Neck.

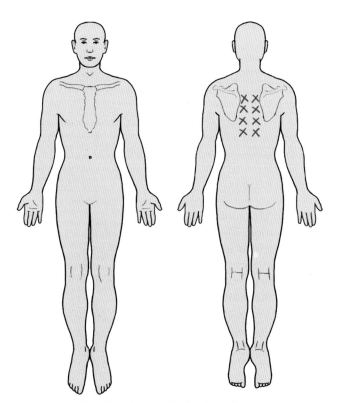

FIG. 5.60 Body chart for Mr. Stiff Thorax.

4. PIVM testing: Hypomobility and moderate reactivity are noted with PA testing T4–T5 and T5–T6 segments with bilateral rotation and forward-bending PAIVM testing.

5. Shoulder screen: Active shoulder forward flexion and abduction are 145 degrees bilaterally with a mild symptom of mid-thoracic tightness at end range of motion.

6. Muscle length: Patient has moderately tight right levator scapula and minimally tight bilateral pectoralis major and minor.

7. Strength: Lower and middle trapezius are 4-/5; deep neck flexors are 3+/5.

8. Neurologic screen: Neurologic tests are negative.

9. Palpation: Patient is tender and guarded at bilateral mid-thoracic paraspinal muscles.

Evaluation

Diagnosis
Problem list
Goals
Treatment plan/intervention

Ms. Tina O. Smith

History

A 45-year-old female nurse with a 6-month history of gradually worsening pain and tension focused at the right cervicothoracic junction and paresthesia into the ulnar aspect of the right hand and forearm (Fig. 5.61).

Tests and Measures

1. Structural examination: Patient displays moderate forward head posture with protracted scapulae.

2. Cervical AROM in standing: Tests indicate 75% cervical AROM in all planes of motion with myofascial tightness noted with bilaterally side bending; upper thoracic mobility is 25% of expected range of motion.

3. Right shoulder screen: AROM is 170 degrees flexion and abduction with arm pain at end range.

4. PROM: Patients displays 170 flexion and abduction with arm pain at end range.

5. Tissue tension signs: Strength is normal and pain free with isometric resistance.

6. Accessory motion tests: Results are normal for right shoulder.

7. Nerve tension tests: Positive right upper limb nerve tension test (ULNT) 1 at –25 degrees elbow extension with provocation of right hand/forearm pain/paresthesia at the ulnar aspect of the hand/forearm.

8. Muscle length: Mildly tight right levator scapula and moderately tight bilateral pectoralis major and minor are noted.

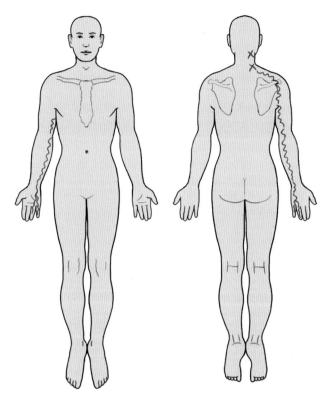

FIG. 5.61 Body chart for Ms. Tina O. Smith.

9. Strength: Tests indicate strength is 3+/5 bilateral lower trapezius, middle trapezius, and serratus anterior; 3/5 deep neck flexor muscles.

10. Spurling test: Test is negative for provocation of right arm pain.

11. Distraction test: Test indicates decreased neck pain but no effect on arm symptoms.

12. Neurologic screen: Neurologic tests results are normal.

13. Palpation: Patient is tender and guarded at the muscle/soft tissues of the right cervicothoracic junction and supraclavicular region.

14. PIVM tests: Mobility deficits are noted at C7–T1, T3–T4, and T4–T5 left and right rotation.

15. Accessory motion testing: Hypomobility is noted with depression of the right first rib.

16. Special tests: Patient has positive test results for right arm symptom reproduction, including Roos test, Adson's maneuver, and hyperabduction test (at 60 degrees abduction), but no vascular signs noted.

Evaluation

Diagnosis
Problem list
Goals
Treatment plan/intervention

REFERENCES

1. Briggs AM, Bragge P, Smith AJ, et al. Prevalence and associated factors for thoracic spine pain in theadult working population: a literature review. *J Occup Health*. 2009;51:177-192.
2. Leboeuf-Yde C, Nielsen J, Kyvik KO, et al. Pain in the lumbar, thoracic or cervical regions: do age or gender matter? A population-based study of 34,902 Danish twins 20e71 years of age. *BMC Musculoskel Disord*. 2009;10:39.
3. Roquelaure Y, Bodin J, Ha C, et al. Incidence and risk factors for thoracic spine pain in the working population: the French Pays de la Loire study. *Arthritis Care Res (Hoboken)*. 2014;66(11):1695-1702.
4. Neumann DA. *Kinesiology of the Musculoskeletal System*, ed 3. St. Louis: Elsevier; 2017.
5. Panjabi MM, Koichiro T, Goel V, et al. Thoracic human vertebrae, quantitative three-dimensional anatomy. *Spine*. 1991;16(8):888-901.
6. Geelhoed MA, McGaugh J, Brewer PA, et al. A new model to facilitate palpation of the level of the transverse processes of the thoracic spine. *J Orthop Sports Phys Ther*. 2006;36(11):876-881.
7. Edmondston S, Waller R, Vallin P, et al. Thoracic spine extension mobility in young adults: Influence of subject position and spinal curvature. *J Orthop Sports Phys Ther*. 2011;41(4):266-273.
8. Sizer PS, Brismee JM, Cook C. Coupling behavior of the thoracic spine: a systematic review of the literature. *J Manipulative Physiol Ther*. 2007;30(5):390-399.
9. National Health and Medical Research Council. Acute thoracic spinal pain. In: *Australian Acute Musculoskeletal Pain Guidelines: Evidence-Based Management of Acute Musculoskeletal Pain*. Brisbane: Australian Academic Press; 2003.
10. April C, Dwyer A, Bogduk N. Cervical zygapophyseal joint pain patterns II: a clinical evaluation. *Spine*. 1990;15:458-461.
11. Dwyer A, Aprill C, Bogduk N. Cervical zygapophyseal joint pain patterns I: a study in normal volunteers. *Spine*. 1990;15:453-457.
12. Fukui S, Ohseto K, Shiotani M, et al. Referred pain distribution of the cervical zygapophyseal joints and cervical dorsal rami. *Pain*. 1996;68:79-83.
13. Hockaday JM, Whitty CWM. Patterns of referred pain in the normal subject. *Brain*. 1967;90:481-495.
14. Schellhas KP, Pollei SR. Thoracic discography: a safe and reliable technique. *Spine*. 1994;19:2103-2109.
15. Wainner RS, Fritz JM, Irrgang JJ, et al. Reliability and diagnostic accuracy of the clinical examination and patient self-report measures for cervical radiculopathy. *Spine*. 2003;28(1):52-62.
16. Johnell O, Kanis JA. An estimate of the worldwide prevalence and disability associated with osteoporotic fractures. *Osteoporos Int*. 2006;17:1726-1733.
17. Kanis JA, Oden A, Johnell O, et al. The burden of osteoporotic fractures: a method for setting intervention thresholds. *Osteoporos Int*. 2001;12:417-427.
18. NICE. *Osteoporosis: Assessing the Risk of Fragility Fracture (CG146)*, 2012. Updated February 2017. Available at http://nice.org.uk/guidance. Assessed January 04, 2020.
19. Santavirta S, Konttinene YT, Heliovaara M, et al. Determinants of osteoporotic thoracic vertebral fracture: screening of 57,000 Finnish women and men. *Acta Orthop Scand*. 1992;63:198-202.
20. Melton LJ, Kan SH, Frye MA, et al. Epidemiology of vertebral fractures in women. *Am J Epidemiol*. 1989;129:1000-1011.

21. Patel U, Skingle S, Campbell GA, et al. Clinical profile of acute vertebral compression fractures in osteoporosis. *Br J Rheumatol*. 1991;30:418-421.
22. Hauag C, Ross PD, Wasnich RW. Vertebral fractures and other predictors of back pain among older women. *J Bone Mineral Res*. 1994;11:1026-1032.
23. Cooper C. The crippling consequences of fractures and their impact on quality of life. *Am J Med*. 1997;103(2A):12S-19S.
24. Ettinger B, Black DM, Nevitt MC, et al. Contribution of vertebral deformities to chronic back pain and disability. *J Bone Mineral Res*. 1992;7:449-456.
25. Goodman CC, Fuller KS, Boissonnault W. *Pathology: Implications for the Physical Therapist*, ed 2. Philadelphia: Saunders; 2017.
26. National Osteoporosis Foundation. *Having a bone density test (website)*. Available at www.Nof.org/articles/743. Accessed January 4, 2014.
27. Roman M, Brown C, Richardson W, et al. The development of a clinical decision making algorithm for detection of osteoporotic vertebral compression fracture and wedge deformity. *J Man Manipulative Ther*. 2010;18:45-50.
28. Bennell K, Larsen J. Osteoporosis. In: Boyling JD, Jull GA, editors. *Grieve's Modern Manual Therapy: the Vertebral Column*, ed 3. Edinburgh: Churchill Livingstone; 2005.
29. Zehnacker CH, Bemis-Dougherty A. Effect of weighted exercises on bone mineral density in post menopausal women: a systematic review. *J Geriatr Phys Ther*. 2007;30(2):79-88.
30. Howe TE, Shea B, Dawson LJ, et al. Exercise for preventing and treating osteoporosis in postmenopausal women. *Cochrane Database Syst Rev*. 2011;6(7):CD000333.
31. Heneghan NR, Baker G, Thomas K, et al. What is the effect of prolonged sitting and physical activity on thoracic spine mobility? An observational study of young adults in a UK university setting. *BMJ Open*. 2018;8:e019371.
32. Schiller L. Effectiveness of spinal manipulative therapy in the treatment of mechanical thoracic spine pain: a pilot randomized clinical trial. *J Manipulative Physiol Ther*. 2001;24(6):394-401.
33. Kelly JL, Whitney SL. The use of nonthrust manipulation in an adolescent for the treatment of thoracic and rib dysfunction: a case report. *J Orthop Sports Phys Ther*. 2006;36(11):887-892.
34. Maitland GD. *Vertebral Manipulation*, ed 5. Oxford: Butterworth Heinemann; 1986.
35. Conroy JL, Schneiders AG. The T4 syndrome. *Man Ther*. 2005;10:292-296.
36. Evans P. The T4 syndrome. *J Manipulative Physiol Ther*. 1995;18(1):34-37.
37. Bogduk N. Innervation and pain patterns of the thoracic spine. In: Grant R, editor: *Physical Therapy of the Cervical and Thoracic Spines*, ed 3. Edinburgh: Churchill Livingstone; 2002.
38. Hartstein AJ, Lievre AJ, Grimes JK, et al. Immediate effects of thoracic spine thrust manipulation on neurodynamic mobility. *J Manipulative Physiol Ther*. 2018;41:332-341.
39. Jowsey P, Perry J. Sympathetic nervous system effects in the hands following a grade III postero-anterior rotary mobilization technique applied to T4: A randomized, placebo-controlled trial. *Man Ther*. 2010;15(3):248-253.
40. Zusman M. Forebrain-mediated sensitization of central pain pathways: "non-specific" pain and a new image for MT. *Man Ther*. 2002;7(2):80-88.

41. Sterling M, Jull G, Wright A. Cervical mobilization: concurrent effects on pain, sympathetic nervous system activity and motor activity. *Man Ther.* 2001;6(2):72-81.

42. Vincenzino B, Collins D, Benson H, et al. An investigation of the interrelationship between manipulative therapy-induced hypoalgesia and sympathoexcitation. *J Manipulative Physiol Ther.* 1998; 21(7):448-453.

43. Karas S, Pannone A. T4 syndrome: a scoping review of the literature. *J Manipulative Physiol Ther.* 2017;40(2):118-125.

44. Cleland JA, Childs JD, Fritz JM, et al. Development of a clinical prediction rule for guiding treatment of a subgroup of patients with neck pain: use of thoracic spine manipulation, exercise, and patient education. *Phys Ther.* 2007;87(1):9-23.

45. Wainner RS, Whitman JM, Cleland JA, et al. Regional interdependence: a musculoskeletal examination model whose time has come. *J Orthop Sports Phys Ther.* 2007;37(11):658-660.

46. Sueki DG, Cleland JA, Wainner RS. A regional interdependence model of musculo-skeletal dysfunction: research, mechanisms, and clinical implications. *J Man Manip Ther.* 2013;21(2): 90-102.

47. Bialosky JE, Bishop MD, George SZ. Regional interdependence: a musculoskeletal examination model whose time has come. *J Orthop Sports Phys Ther.* 2008;38(3):159-160.

48. McDevitt A, Young J, Mintken P, et al. Regional interdependence and manual therapy directed at the thoracic spine. *J Man Manip Ther.* 2015;23(3):139-146.

49. Sueki DG, Chaconas EJ. The effect of thoracic manipulation on shoulder pain: a regional interdependence model. *Phys Ther Rev.* 2011;16(5):399-408.

50. Cleland JA, Mintken PE, Carpenter K, et al. Examination of a clinical prediction rule to identify patients with neck pain likely to benefit from thoracic spine thrust manipulation and a general cervical ROM exercise: multi-center randomized clinical trial. *Phys Ther.* 2010;90(9):1239-1250.

51. Cleland JA, Glynn P, Whitman JM, et al. Short-term effects of thrust versus nonthrust mobilization/manipulation directed at the thoracic spine in patients with neck pain: a randomized clinical trial. *Phys Ther.* 2007;87:431-440.

52. Gonzalez-Iglesias J: Fernandez-de-las-Penas C, Cleland JA. Thoracic spine manipulation for the management of patients with neck pain: a randomized clinical trial. *J Orthop Sports Phys Ther.* 2009;39:20-27.

53. Casanova-Mendez A, Oliva-Pascual-Vaca A, Rodriguez-Blanco C, et al. Comparative short-term effects of two thoracic spinal manipulation techniques in subjects with chronic mechanical neck pain: a randomized controlled trial. *Man Ther.* 2014;19(4): 331-337.

54. Karas S, Olson Hunt MJ, Temes B, et al. The effect of direction specific thoracic spine manipulation on the cervical spine: a randomized controlled trial. *J Man Manip Ther.* 2018;26(1):3-10.

55. Karas S, Olson Hunt MJ. A randomized clinical trial to compare the immediate effects of seated thoracic manipulation and targeted spine thoracic manipulation on cervical spine flexion range of motion and pain. *J Man Manip Ther.* 2014;22(2):108-114.

56. Cross KM, Kuenze C, Grindstaff T, et al. Thoracic spine thrust manipulation improves pain, range of motion, and self-reported function in patients with mechanical neck pain: a systematic review. *J Orthop Sports Phys Ther.* 2011;41(9):633-642.

57. Young JL, Walker D, Snyder S, et al. Thoracic manipulation versus mobilization in patients with mechanical neck pain: a systematic review. *J Man Manip Ther.* 2014;22(3):141-153.

58. Puentedura EJ, Landers MR, Cleland JA, et al. Thoracic spine thrust manipulation versus cervical spine thrust manipulation in patients with acute neck pain: a randomized clinical trial. *J Orthop Sports Phys Ther.* 2011;41(4):208-220.

59. Masaracchio M, Cleland J, Hellman M, et al. Short-term combined effects of thoracic spine thrust manipulation and cervical spine nonthrust manipulation in individuals with mechanical neck pain: a randomized clinical trial. *J Orthop Sports Phys Ther.* 2013;43(3):118-127.

60. Olson KA, Gilette J. Videofluoroscopic evaluation of spine motion during shoulder elevation: a pilot study [abstract]. *J Man Manipulative Ther.* 1998;6(4):206.

61. Stewart SG, Jull GA, Ng JKF, et al. An initial analysis of thoracic spine movement during unilateral arm elevation. *J Man Manipulative Ther.* 1995;3(1):15-20.

62. Crawford HJ, Jull GA. The influence of thoracic posture and movement on range of arm elevation. *Physiother Theory Pract.* 1993;9:143-148.

63. Edmondston S, Ferbuson A, Ippersiel P, et al. Clinical and radiographic investigation of thoracic spine extension motion during bilateral arm elevation. *J Orthop Sports Phys Ther.* 2012;42(10):861-869.

64. Boyles RE, Ritland BM, Miracle BM, et al. The short-term effects of thoracic spine thrust manipulation on patients with shoulder impingement syndrome. *Man Ther.* 2009;14:375-380.

65. Bergman GJD, Winters JC, Groenier KH, et al. Manipulative therapy in addition to usual medical care for patients with shoulder dysfunction and pain: a randomized, controlled trial. *Ann Intern Med.* 2004;141:432-439.

66. Muth S, Barbe MR, Lauer R, et al. The effects of thoracic spine manipulation in subjects with signs of rotator cuff tendinopathy. *J Orthop Sports Phys Ther.* 2012;42:1005-1016.

67. Peek AL, Miller C, Heneghan NR. Thoracic manual therapy in the management of non-specific shoulder pain: a systematic review. *J Man Manip Ther.* 2015;23(4):176-187.

68. Mintken PE, Cleland JA, Carpenter KJ, et al. Some factors predict successful short-term outcomes in individuals with shoulder pain receiving cervicothoracic manipulation: a single-arm trial. *Phys Ther.* 2010;90:26-42.

69. Mintken PE, McDevitt AW, Michener LA, et al. Examination of the validity of a clinical prediction rule to identify patients with shoulder pain likely to benefit from cervicothoracic manipulation. *J Orthop Sports Phys Ther.* 2017;47(4):252-260.

70. Mintken PE, McDevitt AW, Cleland JA, et al. Cervicothoracic manual therapy plus exercise therapy versus exercise therapy alone in the management of individuals with shoulder pain: a multicenter randomized controlled trial. *J Orthop Sports Phys Ther.* 2016;46:617-628.

71. Shambaugh P. Changes in electrical activity in muscles resulting from chiropractic adjustment: a pilot study. *J Manipulative Physiol Ther.* 1987;10:300-304.

72. Zafereo J, Wang-Price S, Roddey T, et al. Regional manual therapy and motor control exercises for chronic low back pain: a randomized clinical trial. *J Man Manip Ther.* 2018;26(4):193-202.

73. de Oliveira RF, Liebano RE, Costa Lda C, et al. Immediate effects of region-specific and non–region-specific spinal manipulative therapy in patients with chronic low back pain: a randomized controlled trial. *Phys Ther.* 2013;93:748-756.

74. Fisher LR, Alvar BA, Maher SF, et al. Short-term effects of thoracic spine thrust manipulation, exercise, and education in individuals with low back pain: a randomized controlled trial. *J Orthop Sports Phys Ther.* 2020;50(1):24-32.

75. Whitman JM, Flynn TW, Childs JD, et al. A comparison between two physical therapy treatment programs for patients with lumbar spinal stenosis. *Spine*. 2006;31(22):2541-2549.

76. Oda I, Abumi K, Cunningham BW, et al. An in vitro human cadaveric study investigating the biomechanical properties of the thoracic spine. *Spine*. 2002;27(3):E64-E70.

77. Lee DG. Rotational instability of the mid-thoracic spine: assessment and management. *Man Ther*. 1996;1(5):234-241.

78. Pratt NE. Neurovascular entrapment in the regions of the shoulder and posterior triangle of the neck. *Phys Ther*. 1986;66:1894-1900.

79. Watson LA, Pizzari T, Balster S. Thoracic outlet syndrome part 1: clinical manifestations, differentiation, and treatment pathways. *Man Ther*. 2009;14:586-595.

80. Coletta JM, Murray JD, Reeves R, et al. Vascular thoracic outlet syndrome: successful outcomes with multimodal therapy. *Cardiovasc Surg*. 2001;9(1):11-15.

81. Sanders RJ, Hammond SL, Rao NM. Diagnosis of thoracic outlet syndrome. *J Vasc Surg*. 2007;46:601-604.

82. Estilaei SK, Byl NN. Magnetic resonance angiography for diagnosing arterial thoracic outlet syndrome. *J Hand Ther*. 2006;19:410-420.

83. Edgelow P. Neurovascular consequences of cumulative trauma disorders affecting the thoracic outlet: a patient centered treatment approach. In: Donatelli R, editor. *Physical Therapy of the Shoulder*. New York: Churchill Livingstone; 2004:205–238.

84. Ide J, Kataoka Y, Yamaga M, et al. Compression and stretching of the brachial plexus in thoracic outlet syndrome: correlation between neuroradiographic findings and symptoms and signs produced by provocation manoeuvers. *J Hand Surg Br*. 2003;28(3):218-223.

85. Wright IS. The neurovascular syndrome produced by hyperabduction of the arms. *Am Heart J*. 1945;29(1):1-19.

86. Rayan GM, Jensen C. Thoracic outlet syndrome: Provocative examination maneuvers in a typical population. *J Shoulder Elbow Surg*. 1995;4:113-117.

87. Nord KM, Kapoor P, Fisher J, et al. False positive rate of thoracic outlet syndrome diagnostic maneuvers. *Electromyogr Clin Neurophysiol*. 2008;48(2):67-74.

88. Singh D. Arterial complications of thoracic outlet syndrome. *Surg Pract*. 2006;10:52-56.

89. Athanassiadi K, Kalavrouziotis G, Karydakis K, et al. Treatment of thoracic outlet syndrome: long-term results. *World J Surg*. 2001;25(5):553-557.

90. Gillard J, Pérez-Cousin M, Hachulla E, et al. Diagnosing thoracic outlet syndrome: contribution of provocative tests, ultrasonography, electrophysiology, and helical computed tomography in 48 patients. *Joint Bone Spine*. 2001;68:416-424.

91. Lindgren KA. Conservative treatment of thoracic outlet syndrome: A 2 year follow up. *Arch Phys Med Rehab*. 1997;78:373-378.

92. Watson LA, Pizzari T, Balster S. Thoracic outlet syndrome part 1: clinical manifestations, differentiation, and treatment pathways. *Man Ther*. 2010;15:305-314.

93. Brantigan CO, Roos DB. Diagnosing thoracic outlet syndrome. *Hand Clin*. 2004;20:27-36.

94. Christensen HW, Vach W, Vach K, et al. Palpation of the upper thoracic spine: an observer reliability study. *J Manipulative Physiol Ther*. 2002;25(5):285-292.

95. Smedmark V, Wallin M, Arvidsson I. Inter-examiner reliability in assessing passive intervertebral motion of the cervical spine. *Man Ther*. 2000;5(2):97-101.

CHAPTER 6

Examination and Treatment of Cervical Spine Disorders

OVERVIEW

This chapter covers the spinal kinematics of the cervical spine, describes common cervical spine disorders with a diagnostic classification system to guide clinical reasoning and management, and provides a detailed description of manual examination, mobilization/manipulation, and exercise procedures for the cervical spine. Video clips of the majority of the examination and manual therapy procedures are also included.

OBJECTIVES

- Describe the significance and impact of cervical spine disorders.
- Describe cervical spine kinematics.
- Use clinical reasoning to diagnose and classify cervical spine disorders based on signs and symptoms.
- Determine the most effective and perform interventions for cervical spine disorders with emphasis on mobilization/manipulation techniques and therapeutic exercises.
- Demonstrate and interpret cervical spine examination procedures.
- Describe contraindications and precautions for cervical spine mobilization/manipulation.
- Demonstrate mobilization/manipulation techniques of the cervical spine.
- Instruct exercises for cervical spine disorders.
- Incorporate psychologically informed education and management principles for treatment of patients with cervical spine disorders.

▶ *To view videos pertaining to this chapter, please visit the eBook.*

SIGNIFICANCE OF CERVICAL SPINE DISORDERS

Neck pain is reported to be the second most common musculoskeletal disorder that leads to disability and injury claims.[1] The economic burden of neck pain is second only to low back pain in workers' compensation claims in the United States.[2–4] The incidence of neck pain ranges from 3.7% to 25% globally with a mean incidence of 15.95%.[5–6] As much as 50% to 75% of individuals have neck or shoulder pain at least once in their life.[7] The 12-month prevalence of neck pain ranges from 12.1% to 71.5% in the general population and from 27.1% to 47.8% in workers.[8] Out of the 291 conditions studied in the Global Burden of Disease 2010 Study, neck pain ranked fourth highest in terms of disability as measured by years lived with disability and 21st in terms of overall global burden.[9]

The strongest risk factors to develop a first episode of neck pain include high muscular tension, depressed mood, role conflict, and high job demand.[5] Most people with neck pain do not experience a complete resolution of symptoms, with between 50% and 85% of those who experience neck pain reporting neck pain again 1 to 5 years later.[8] Cervical spine–related musculoskeletal disorders account for approximately 25% of the patients seen in outpatient physical therapy in the United States.[10] Societal consequences of neck pain include increase in healthcare expenditure, missed days from work, reduced work productivity, and a rise in insurance costs.[9]

Cervical Spine Kinematics: Functional Anatomy and Mechanics

The cervical spine supports and orients the head in space relative to the thorax to serve the sensory systems.[11] It must therefore have sophisticated mobility and stability mechanisms to meet the demands placed on this region of the musculoskeletal system.[11] The cervical spine is designed for a great deal of mobility and is susceptible to the development of instability impairments. Among male and female subjects of the same age group, female subjects have greater active range of motion (AROM) than male subjects for all AROM except neck flexion.[12] Table 6.1 shows the mean cervical AROM for 20-year-old to 29-year-old men. Cervical AROM tends to decrease with age.

The intervertebral disks of the cervical spine by middle age develop clefts that appear in the posterolateral aspect of the cervical disk and are thought to occur as a result of the shearing forces associated with cervical spine rotation.[13] The disk's gelatinous nucleus pulposis shows evidence of fibrosis by the mid-teens and is replaced with fibrocartilaginous uncovertebral clefts that allow further mobility at the spinal segment.[13] The intervertebral disk is reinforced at the anterolateral aspect by the uncovertebral joints of von Luschka, which allow motion in multiple planes and assist in limiting extreme range of motion (ROM).

TABLE 6.1	Active Range of Motion as Measured With Cervical Range of Motion Device for Men Ages 20 to 29 Years		
MOTION	**MEAN**	**STANDARD DEVIATION**	**RANGE**
Flexion	54.3	8.8	42–68
Extension	76.7	12.8	60–108
Left lateral flexion	41.4	7.1	30–58
Right lateral flexion	44.9	7.2	30–58
Left rotation	69.2	7.0	52–83
Right rotation	69.6	6.0	59–80

Active range of motion (AROM) measurements of cervical spine with cervical range of motion (CROM) instrument showed good intratester and intertester reliability with intraclass correlation coefficients >0.80.
(From Jette A, Delitto A. Physical therapy treatment choices for musculoskeletal impairments, *Phys Ther.* 1997;77(2):145-154.)

The zygapophyseal facet joints of the middle and lower cervical spine (C2–C3 to C7–T1) are angled upward and forward at approximately a 45-degree angle[14] (Figs. 6.1 and 6.2). The motions of forward and backward bending occur parallel with the plane of the facet joints as either a bilateral upslope glide (forward and upward) motion for forward bending or a bilateral

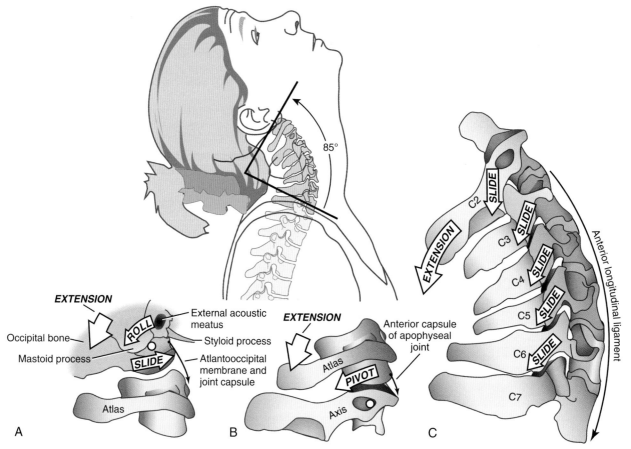

FIG. 6.1 Kinematics of craniocervical extension. A, Atlantooccipital joint. B, Atlantoaxial joint complex. C, Intracervical region (C2–C7). Elongated and taut tissues are indicated with *thin black arrows*. (From Neumann DA. *Kinesiology of the Musculoskeletal System,* ed 3. St Louis: Elsevier; 2017.)

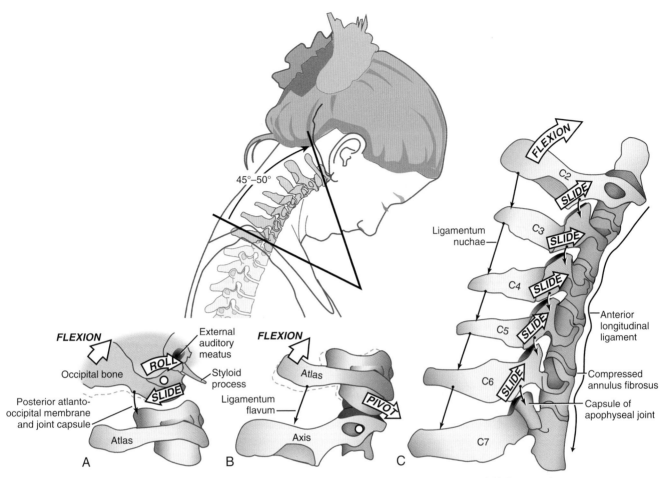

FIG. 6.2 Kinematics of craniocervical flexion. A, Atlantooccipital joint. B, Atlantoaxial joint complex. C, Intracervical region (C2–C7). Note in C that flexion slackens anterior longitudinal ligament and increases space between adjacent laminae and spinous process. Elongated and taut tissues are indicated with *thin black arrows;* slacked tissue is indicated with *wavy black arrow.* (From Neumann DA. *Kinesiology of the Musculoskeletal System,* ed 3. St Louis: Elsevier; 2017.)

downslope glide (backward and downward) motion for backward bending.[15] At the end range of the upslope gliding motion, the cervical vertebrae tilts to create gapping of the posterior aspect of the facet joint with end-range forward bending.[16] The amount of cervical spine segmental motion for sagittal plane motions measured in radiographic and computed tomography (CT) scan studies are described in Table 6.2. The angular plane of the facet joints is important to consider not only in understanding joint mechanics but also in application of passive intervertebral motion (PIVM) testing and joint mobilization/ manipulation technique application. The most effective and most comfortable mobilization/manipulation techniques of the cervical spine for the patient commonly require application of forces parallel with the angle formed by the plane of the facet joints.

The craniovertebral (craniocervical) region is comprised of the atlantooccipital (Occiput–C1) and the atlantoaxial (C1–C2) articulations. The facet joints for C1–C2 are oriented more horizontally than the middle and lower cervical spine facet joints to allow greater mobility and pure translation.[16] The occiput–C1 joints are

TABLE 6.2	Cervical Spine Segmental Flexion-Extension			
SPINAL SEGMENT	**PENNING**	**DVORAK ET AL (SD)**	**PANJABI ET AL.**	**KOTTKE & MUNDALE**
Occiput–C1	30		24	22
C1–C2	30	12	24	11
C2–C3	12	10 (3)		11
C3–C4	18	15 (3)		16
C4–C5	20	19 (4)		18
C5–C6	20	20 (20)		21
C6–C7	15	19 (4)		18

SD, Standard deviation.
(From Dvorak J, Panjabi MM, Novotny JE, et al. In vivo flexion/extension of the normal cervical spine. *J Orthop Res.* 1991;9:828-834; Kottke FJ, Mundale MO. Range of mobility of the cervical spine. *Arch Phys Med Rehabil.* 1959;379-382; Panjabi M, Dvorak J, Duranceau J, et al. Three-dimensional movements of the upper cervical spine. *Spine* 1988;13(7):726-730; Penning L. Normal movement in the cervical spine. *Am J Roentgenol.* 1978;130:317-326.)

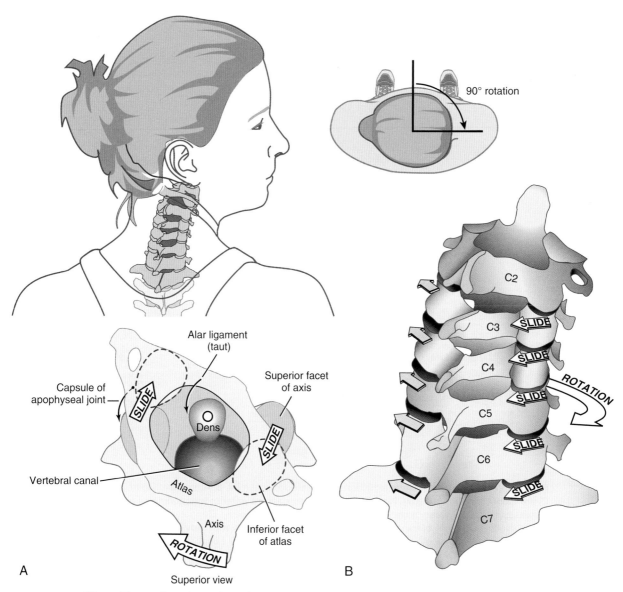

FIG. 6.3 Kinematics of craniocervical axial rotation. A, Atlantoaxial joint complex (C1–C2). B, Intracervical region (C2–C7). (From Neumann DA. *Kinesiology of the Musculoskeletal System*, ed 3. St Louis: Elsevier; 2017.)

formed by a pair of convex-shaped occipital condyles and the concave-shaped superior articular surfaces of the atlas. Therefore the occipital condyles glide in the opposite direction of the motion direction, which follows the convex/concave rule (Figs. 6.1 and 6.2). For instance, the occipital condyles glide posterior with forward bending and glide anterior with backward bending.

Middle and lower cervical rotation and lateral flexion motions are coupled motions from C2–T1, with lateral flexion and rotation occurring toward the same side.[17] The axis of the motion is perpendicular to the angle of the cervical facet joints, with an upslope glide on the contralateral facet joint and a downslope glide on the ipsilateral facet joint (Figs. 6.3 and 6.4).[13] Table 6.3 shows the mean range of rotation motion with the mean amount of coupled lateral flexion at each cervical spine segment measured with biplanar radiographs at the

end range of rotation of middle-aged men.[18] At several cervical spine levels, the standard deviation is greater than the mean of the motion, which indicates a great deal of variability in healthy subjects. However, the means can provide a general idea of the proportion of motion at each segment and the coupling that occurs. Tables 6.4 and 6.5 show findings from multiple studies of the mean segmental motion for cervical rotation and lateral flexion. Although some variability is noted, the C1–C2 segment allows the greatest amount of rotation (~50%). The studies that measured cervical segmental motion consider C6–C7 as the last moving segment with cervical active movements, but clinically, motion is noted in the upper thoracic spinal vertebral segments with cervical active motion. The active and passive mobility of the upper thoracic spinal segments should be evaluated and treated with the cervical

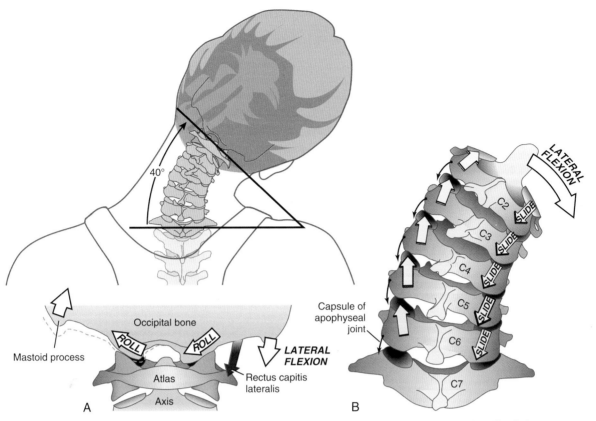

FIG. 6.4 Craniocervical lateral flexion. A, Atlantooccipital joint. B, Intracervical region (C2–C7). (From Neumann DA. *Kinesiology of the Musculoskeletal System,* ed 3. St Louis: Elsevier; 2017.)

TABLE 6.3	Mean Degrees of Rotation in One Direction (Standard Deviation) and Coupled Lateral Flexion (Standard Deviation) as Calculated With Biplanar Radiography in 20 Participants			
LEVELS	**MEAN ROTATION**	**STANDARD DEVIATION**	**MEAN COUPLED LATERAL FLEXION**	**STANDARD DEVIATION**
Occiput–C2	37.5	5.9	–2.4	6.0
C2–C3	3.7	3.2	–1.6	7.7
C3–C4	2.9	2.5	6.2	7.1
C4–C5	2.1	2.9	6.2	7.1
C5–C6	2.7	2.2	4.0	7.9
C6–C7	3.2	1.3	2.7	6.5

Positive degrees of lateral flexion indicate in same direction as rotation.
(From Mimura M, Hideshige M, Tsuneo W, et al. Three-dimensional motion analysis of the cervical spine with special reference to the axial rotation. *Spine.* 1989;14(11):1135-1139.)

TABLE 6.4	Segmental Cervical Rotation (Degrees) in One Direction		
SPINAL SEGMENT	**DUMAS et al. (MEAN [SD])**	**PENNING (MEAN [RANGE])**	**PANJABI et al.**
Occiput–C1	1.4 (2.7)	1.0 (-2–5)	7.2
C1–C2	37.0 (5.8)	40.5 (29–46)	38.9
C2–C3	0.6 (3.4)	3.0 (0–10)	
C3–C4	4.9 (3.7)	6.5 (3–10)	
C4–C5	5.2 (4.2)	6.8 (1–12)	
C5–C6	5.1 (4.5)	6.9 (2–12)	
C6–C7	3.4 (2.7)	5.4 (2–10)	
C7–T1	1.5	2.1 (-2–7)	

SD, Standard deviation.
(From Dumas J, Sainte Rose M, Dreyfus P, et al. Rotation of the cervical spinal column: a computed tomography in vivo study. *Surg Radiol Anat.* 1993;15:333-339; Panjabi M, Dvorak J, Duranceau J, et al. Three-dimensional movements of the upper cervical spine. *Spine* 1988;13(7):726-730; Penning L. Normal movement in the cervical spine. *Am J Roentgenol.* 1978;130:317-326.)

spine. Table 6.6 shows that the upper thoracic spine (T1–T6) provides approximately 25% of the cervical flexion/extension, 10% of the cervical rotation, and 14% of the cervical lateral flexion, which illustrates the importance of manual examination and treatment of thoracic spine mobility deficits in treating cervical spine conditions.[19]

The occiput–C1 and C1–C2 spinal segments allow for fine-tuning of the head position during neck motion and create a distinction between axial cervical rotation and lateral flexion. A relative lateral flexion of the cranium occurs to the contralateral side of the cervical spine rotation, which functions to keep the eyes level with an axial rotation movement of

TABLE 6.5	Cervical Spine Range of Motion: Lateral Flexion in One Direction		
SPINAL SEGMENT	**PENNING**	**WHITE & PANJABI**	**PANJABI et al.**
Occiput–C1	6	7	5.5
C1–C2	6	0	6.7
C2–C3	6	10	
C3–C4	6	11	
C4–C5	6	11	
C5–C6	6	8	
C6–C7	6	7	
C7–T1	6	4	

(From Panjabi M, Dvorak J, Duranceau J, et al. Three-dimensional movements of the upper cervical spine. *Spine* 1988;13(7):726-730; Penning L. Normal movement in the cervical spine. *Am J Roentgenol*. 1978;130:317-326; White A, Panjabi MM. Kinematics of the spine. In: White A, Panjabi MM, editors. *Clinical Biomechanics of the Spine*. Philadelphia: Lippincott; 1978.)

the head.[18] In the process, the atlas glides in the relative opposite direction of the cervical rotation. During cervical lateral flexion, a relative rotation occurs to the opposite side of the lateral flexion at the C1–C2 and occiput–C1 segments to allow the face to remain facing forward in a frontal plane during the lateral flexion.[20]

In the craniovertebral region (occiput–C1, C1–C2), the atlas vertebra may be considered an interposed bearing between the axis vertebra and the occipital condyles that guides and limits the movement between C2 and the occiput.[15] In flexion-extension, the position of the atlas is relatively independent of the actual relationship between the occiput and C2. In any position of the craniocervical region, the posterior atlantal arch may be found somewhere between the occiput and the spinous process of C2 and not necessarily halfway between.[15]

In lateral bending, the atlas has a more rigidly prescribed position[15] because of the shape of the lateral masses of the atlas

as seen in anteroposterior (open-mouth view) radiographic projection. During lateral flexion movement, the odontoid must remain midway between the occipital condyles because of its fixation by the alar ligaments. Thus lateral flexion in the occiput–C1 segment is always combined with lateral flexion in the atlantoaxial segment and vice versa. Also a relative lateral glide of the atlas toward the side of the lateral flexion occurs.[21] Craniovertebral lateral flexion is also facilitated by simultaneous contralateral atlantoaxial rotation as a result of the orientation and function of the alar ligament (Fig. 6.5).[18] The C2 vertebra actually rotates toward the side of craniovertebral lateral flexion in relation to C3, which creates a relative contralateral rotation of C1–C2 spinal segment.[22] The cruciate (transverse portion) ligament also assists in stabilization of the craniovertebral complex, especially to prevent excessive anterior shear of C1 in relation to C2 (Fig. 6.6). If the cruciate ligament is lax or torn, the dens of C2 is no longer held firmly against the anterior arch of C1.

The coupled movement patterns of the cervical spine have been documented with cadaver studies, CT scan, and radiographic studies and can assist in clinical evaluation of movement restrictions.[18,21,23–25] For instance, if cervical spine motion is limited with lateral flexion and rotation to the same side, a middle or lower cervical facet joint restriction is suspected (cervical facet capsular pattern). However, if the most significant limitations in cervical AROM are noted with lateral flexion and rotation to the opposite direction, upper cervical joint restrictions are suspected (i.e., craniovertebral capsular pattern). Jarrett et al.[26] used this finding as part of the criteria to identify craniovertebral motion restrictions and were able to show good reliability (kappa = 0.52) in detection of this type of motion impairment with a cervical range of motion (CROM) device.

Neumann[27] attributes the craniovertebral coupling pattern of contralateral lateral flexion with cervical rotation to the motor control exhibited by the upper cervical muscles that create this side bending motion. Specifically, the rectus capitus lateralis muscle on the left produces left lateral flexion torque to the head via the atlantooccipital joints, and the left obliquus capitis inferior muscle creates left axial rotation of

TABLE 6.6	Mean Angular Displacement in Degrees (Standard Deviation) and Relative Contributions (%) of the Cervical and Thoracic Spine During Active Physiologic Movement of the Neck Measured With Three-Dimensional Electromagnetic Motion Sensors Attached to the Skin at the Head and the T1, T6, and T12 Spinous Processes of 34 Asymptomatic Participants					
SPINAL REGION	**FLEXION**	**EXTENSION**	**LEFT ROTATION**	**RIGHT ROTATION**	**LEFT LATERAL FLEXION**	**RIGHT LATERAL FLEXION**
Cervical Mean (SD)	31.84 (4.54) 67%	27.76 (4.30) 67.7%	60.60 (9.34) 83.9%	61.13 (8.24) 84.8%	25.10 (5.71) 73.1%	27.44 (6.53) 74.9%
Upper thoracic Mean (SD)	11.94 (4.91) 25.1%	9.87 (3.66) 24.1%	7.89 (7.89) 10.9%	7.11 (3.87) 9.9%	4.97 (2.09) 14.5%	4.72 (1.99) 12.9%
Lower thoracic Mean (SD)	3.77 (3.38) 7.9%	3.37 (3.15) 8.2%	3.72 (4.29) 5.2%	3.85 (4.93) 5.3%	4.62 (3.50) 12.4%	4.46 (2.85) 12.2%
Total Mean (SD)	47.55 (8.82)	41.00 (6.70)	72.21 (14.20)	72.09 (12.69)	34.33 (7.63)	36.42 (7.36)

SD, Standard deviation.
(Data from Tsang SMH, Szeto GPY, Lee RYW. Normal kinematics of the neck: the interplay between the cervical and thoracic spines. *Man Ther*. 2013;18:431-437.)

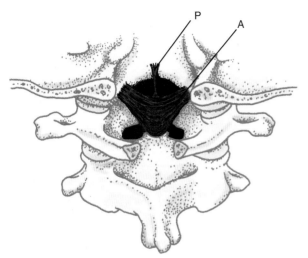

FIG. 6.5 Attachments of alar and apical ligaments. *A,* Alar ligament; *P,* apical ligament. (From Porterfield JA, DeRosa C. *Mechanical Neck Pain.* Philadelphia: Saunders; 1995.)

muscles and provide dynamic stability and neuromuscular control via segmental attachments to cervical vertebrae (Fig. 6.7), and the longus coli and longus capitis (deep neck flexors) provide anterior dynamic stability and neuromuscular control as a result of the position of the muscles anterior to the cervical vertebral bodies[28] (Fig. 6.8). Motor control impairments tend to occur in the neck flexors in patients with chronic neck pain and after whiplash injuries with overactivation of the superficial muscles (anterior scalene and sternocleidomastoid) and underactivation of the deep neck flexors (longus coli and longus capitis).[29] Likewise, the more superficial neck extensor and rotator muscles of the upper cervical spine, such as the splenius capitis muscle, tends to display increased electromyographic (EMG) activity in patients with neck pain with underactivation of the deep neck extensor (multifidus and semispinalis cervicis) muscles of the middle and lower cervical spinal segments[30] (Fig. 6.9). Retraining of the deep neck flexor and extensor muscles is an important component of rehabilitation of many of the cervical spine disorders treated by physical therapists (Figs. 6.7–6.11).

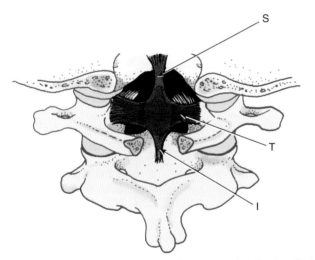

FIG. 6.6 Components of the cruciate ligament. *I,* Inferior band of cruciate ligament; *S,* superior longitudinal band of cruciate ligament; *T,* transverse band of cruciate ligament. (From Porterfield JA, DeRosa C. *Mechanical Neck Pain.* Philadelphia: Saunders; 1995.)

the craniocervical region during right lateral flexion of the cervical spine (Figs. 6.10 and 6.11). The craniovertebral joints must have adequate joint mobility and motor control to smoothly and fully produce these movements. If these active motions are less than full, passive motion assessment of the craniovertebral motion segments assists in differentiation between a motor control deficit and a joint mobility deficit.

Anatomically, the deep neck extensors and deep neck flexors are well suited to control cervical spine segmental movements.[28] The cervical multifidus and the semispinalis cervicis muscles are considered the primary deep neck extensor

Posterior view

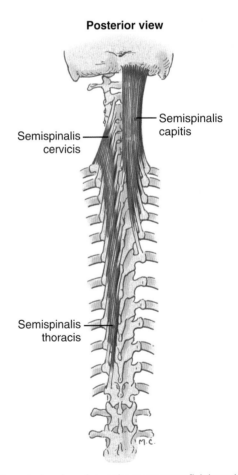

FIG. 6.7 A posterior view shows the more superficial semispinalis within the transversospinal group. For clarity, only the left semispinalis cervicis, left semispinalis thoracis, and right semispinalis capitis are included. (Modified from Luttgens K, Hamilton N. *Kinesiology: Scientific Basis of Human Motion,* ed 9. Madison, WI: Brown and Benchmark; .and Neumann DA. *Kinesiology of the Musculoskeletal System,* ed 3. St Louis: Elsevier; 2017.)

Anterior view

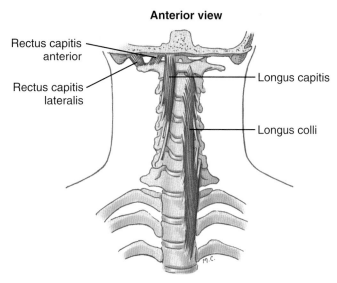

FIG. 6.8 Anterior view of the deep muscles of the neck. The following muscles are shown: right longus capitis, right rectus capitis anterior, right rectus capitis lateralis, and left logus colli. (Modified from Luttgens K, Hamilton N. *Kinesiology: Scientific Basis of Human Motion,* ed 9. Madison, WI: Brown and Benchmark; and Neumann DA. *Kinesiology of the Musculoskeletal System,* ed 3. St Louis: Elsevier; 2017.)

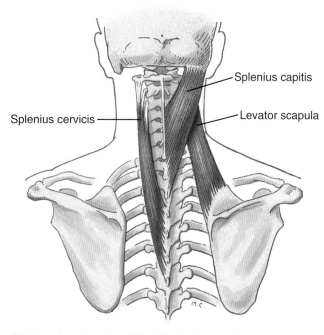

FIG. 6.9 A posterior view of the left splenius cervicis, right splenius capitis, and right levator scapula. (Modified from Luttgens K, Hamilton N. *Kinesiology: Scientific Basis of Human Motion,* ed 9. Madison, WI: Brown and Benchmark; Neumann DA. *Kinesiology of the Musculoskeletal System,* ed 3. St Louis: Elsevier; 2017.)

Posterior view

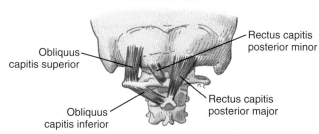

FIG. 6.10 A posterior view of the suboccipital muscles. The left obliquus capitis superior, left obliquus capitis inferior, left rectus capitis posterior minor, and the right rectus capitis posterior major are shown. (Modified from Luttgens K, Hamilton N. *Kinesiology: Scientific Basis of Human Motion,* ed 9. Madison, WI: Brown and Benchmark; Neumann DA. *Kinesiology of the Musculoskeletal System,* ed 3. St Louis: Elsevier; 2017.)

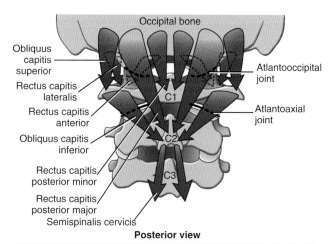

	ATLANTOOCCIPTIAL JOINT			ATLANTOAXIAL JOINT		
MUSCLES	FLEXION	EXTENSION	LATERAL FLEXION	FLEXION	EXTENSION	AXIAL ROTATION*
Rectus capitis anterior	XX	–	X	–	–	–
Rectus capitis lateralis	–	–	XX	–	–	–
Rectus capitis posterior major	–	XXX	XX	–	XXX	XX(IL)
Rectus capitis posterior minor	–	XX	X	–	–	–
Obliquus capitis inferior	–	–	–	–	XX	XXX(IL)
Obliquus capitis superior	–	XXX	XXX	–	–	–

FIG. 6.11 A posterior view depicts the lines of force of muscles relative to the underlying atlantooccipital and atlantoaxial joints. Each of these joints allows two primary degrees of freedom. Note that the attachment of the semispinalis cervicis muscle provides a stable base for the rectus capitis posterior major and the obliquus capitis inferior, two of the larger and more dominant suboccipital muscles. The chart summarizes the actions of the muscles at the atlantooccipital and atlantoaxial joints. A muscle's relative potential to perform a movement is assigned one of three scores: X, minimal; XX, moderate; and XXX, maximum. The *dash* indicates no effective torque production. (From Neumann DA. *Kinesiology of the Musculoskeletal System,* ed 2. St Louis: Mosby; 2010.)

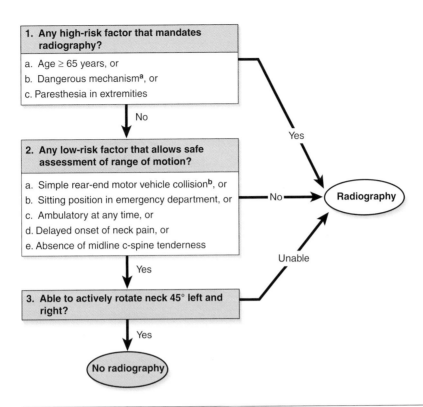

1. Any high-risk factor that mandates radiography?

a. Age ≥ 65 years, or
b. Dangerous mechanism[a], or
c. Paresthesia in extremities

↓ No

2. Any low-risk factor that allows safe assessment of range of motion?

a. Simple rear-end motor vehicle collision[b], or
b. Sitting position in emergency department, or
c. Ambulatory at any time, or
d. Delayed onset of neck pain, or
e. Absence of midline c-spine tenderness

↓ Yes

3. Able to actively rotate neck 45° left and right?

↓ Yes

Radiography ← Yes / No / Unable

No radiography

[a] A dangerous mechanism is considered to be a fall from an elevation ≥3 ft or 5 stairs, an axial load to the head (e.g., diving), a motor vehicle collision at high speed (>100 km/hr), or with rollover or ejection

[b] A simple rear-end motor vehicle collision excludes being pushed into oncoming traffic, being hit by a bus or a large truck, a rollover, and being hit by a high-speed vehicle

FIG. 6.12 The Canadian C-Spine Rule was developed and validated to enhance clinical decision making for determination of when to obtain cervical spine radiographs for patients who have had trauma to their head and neck region.[33] According to a study by Stiell et al., the Canadian C-Spine Rule has a sensitivity of 100% and a specificity of 43%. (Modified from Fernandez de las Penas C. *Neck and Arm Pain Syndromes.* Churchill Livingston: Elsevier; 2011: Stiell IG, Wells GA, Vandemheen KL, et al. The Canadian C-spine rule for radiography in alert and stable trauma patients. *JAMA.* 2001;286(15):1841-1848.)

Diagnosis and Treatment of Cervical Spine Disorders

Cervical spine–related disorders are not a homogeneous group of conditions. Many factors must be considered to arrive at a physical therapy diagnostic classification and to develop a treatment plan of care. Classification systems should adequately define the primary signs and symptoms and guide therapeutic interventions. Once red flags have been screened and the patient, through medical screening procedures, is determined to be an appropriate candidate for physical therapy, further information should be gathered to arrive at a diagnostic classification of the condition.

After a traumatic event, such as a whiplash injury from a motor vehicle accident, the patient should be screened for a vertebral fracture with use of the Canadian C-Spine Rule (Fig. 6.12). If an individual suffers a concussion, examination and treatment of the cervical spine should be incorporated into the management of concussion because there is considerable overlap between the presenting signs and symptoms of whiplash and concussion.[31,32]

The classification system (Table 6.7) used in this textbook is an impairment-based classification of neck disorders commonly treated by physical therapists. The classification terminology developed with the neck pain clinical practice guideline linked to the International Classification of Functioning, Disability, and Health (ICF) from the Academy of Orthopaedic Physical Therapy (AOPT) of the American Physical Therapy Association (APTA) will be incorporated into this chapter and includes the following categories: neck pain with mobility deficits, neck pain with headaches, neck pain with movement coordination impairments, and neck pain with radiating pain.[34,35] Systematic reviews and treatment guidelines conclude that multimodal care, including education, exercise, and manual therapy can benefit patients with neck pain and whiplash-associated disorders (WADs).[35,36]

The AOPT ICF Guideline[35] does not include WAD as a separate classification but includes it in the neck pain with movement coordination impairments classification. For the purpose of this textbook, WAD is separated as a distinct classification because of the special challenges associated with

TABLE 6.7   Classification of Cervical Spine Disorders

CLASSIFICATION	SYMPTOMS	IMPAIRMENTS	INTERVENTIONS
Cervical mobility deficits ICF classification: Neck pain with mobility deficits	• Neck pain • Neck motion limitations • Onset of symptoms is often linked to recent unguarded/awkward movement or position • Associated referred upper extremity pain may be present	• Limited cervical ROM • Neck pain reproduced at end range of active and passive motions • Restricted cervical and thoracic segmental mobility • Neck and neck-related upper extremity pain reproduced with provocation of the involved cervical or upper thoracic segments	• Cervical mobilization/manipulation • Thoracic mobilization/manipulation • Stretching and mobility exercises • Coordination, strengthening, and endurance exercises
Cervical radiculopathy ICF classification: Neck pain with radiating pain	• Neck pain with associated radiating (narrow band of lancinating) pain in the involved upper extremity • Upper extremity paresthesia, numbness, and weakness may be present	• Neck and neck-related radiating pain reproduced with the following: • Spurling A test • ULNT test 1 • Neck and neck-related radiating pain relieved with cervical distraction • May have upper extremity sensory, strength, or reflex deficits associated with involved nerves	• Upper quarter and nerve mobilization procedures • Traction (manual and/or mechanical) • Craniocervical flexion exercises • Postural exercises • Thoracic mobilization/manipulation
Cervical spine clinical instability ICF classification: Neck pain with movement coordination impairments	• Neck pain and associated (referred) upper extremity pain • Remote history of trauma • Symptoms provoked with sustained weight-bearing posture • Symptoms relieved with nonweight-bearing postures	• Hypermobility with loose end feel of cervical motion segments • Strength, endurance, and coordination deficits of deep cervical spine flexor and extensor muscles • Aberrant motion with cervical AROM • Greater cervical AROM in supine (nonweight-bearing) position than in standing (weight-bearing) position • Neck and neck-related upper extremity pain reproduced with provocation of the involved cervical segments	• Coordination, strengthening, and endurance exercises for the neck and postural muscles • Stretching exercises • Mobilization/manipulation above and below hypermobilities • Ergonomic corrections
Whiplash-associated disorders	• High pain and disability scores • Recent history of trauma • Referred symptoms into upper extremity	• Limited/guarded cervical AROM • Poor tolerance to manual examination procedures	• Gentle AROM within patient tolerance • Activity modification to control pain • Relative rest • Physical modalities • Intermittent use of cervical collar • Gentle manual therapy and exercises but avoidance of pain-inducing manual therapy techniques or exercises
Cervicogenic headache ICF classification: Neck pain with headaches	• Noncontinuous unilateral neck pain and associated (referred) headache • Unilateral headache with onset preceded by neck pain • Headache precipitated or aggravated by neck movements or sustained positions	• Headache pain elicited by pressure on posterior neck, especially at one of three upper cervical joints[37] • Limited cervical ROM • Upper cervical (C1–C2) segmental mobility deficits and/or pain noted with the flexion-rotation test • Strength and endurance deficits of the deep neck flexor muscles	• Cervical and thoracic mobilization/manipulation • Strengthening, endurance, and coordination exercises for the neck and postural muscles • Postural education

AROM, Active range of motion; *CROM,* cervical range of motion; *ICF,* International Classification of Functioning, Disability, and Health; *ULNT,* upper limb neurodynamic test; *WAD,* whiplash-associated disorder.
See Tables 6.7 and 6.8 for further classification of whiplash-associated disorders.
(Modified from Childs JD, Cleland JA, Elliott JM, et al. Neck pain: clinical practice guidelines linked to the International Classification of Functioning, Disability, and Health from the Orthopaedic Section of the American Physical Therapy Association. *J Orthop Sports Phys Ther.* 2008;38(9):A1-A34.)

WAD; the depth and breadth of research specific to WAD; and the fact that patients with WAD may present with many signs and symptoms that may not be solely associated with movement coordination impairments. For instance, a longitudinal analysis of 2578 patients with neck pain found that patients with WAD had more self-reported pain and disability and experienced worse outcomes at 1-year than those with nonspecific neck pain.[38]

WHIPLASH-ASSOCIATED DISORDERS

Most people with whiplash injuries from motor vehicle accidents fully recover within a few weeks, but a significant proportion (14%–42%) develop persistent ongoing pain, with 10% reporting constant pain.[39] Ritchie et al.[40] report that 50% of individuals with WAD experience full recovery within 3 months; approximately 25% continue to experience persistent moderate/severe disability, and 25% continue to have mild levels of pain and disability. A metaanalysis found 12 variables to be predictors of poor outcome status at a 6-month or longer follow-up after whiplash, including a high baseline pain intensity (>5.5/10), report of headache at inception, less than postsecondary education, no seat belt in use during the accident, report of low back pain at inception, high Neck Disability Index (NDI) score (>29%), preinjury neck pain, report of neck pain at inception (regardless of intensity), high catastrophizing, female sex, WAD grade 2 or 3, and WAD grade 3 alone.[41] High baseline pain intensity (>5.5/10) and high NDI scores (>29%) are the strongest predictors of poor outcomes, but the impact of multiple risk factors in a single person is not fully understood.[41]

The Quebec Task Force (QTF) classification of WADs was developed to standardize the terminology associated with diag-

TABLE 6.8	Quebec Task Force Classification for Whiplash-Associated Disorders
QUEBEC TASK FORCE CLASSIFICATION GRADE	**CLINICAL PRESENTATION**
0	No symptom of neck pain No physical signs
I	Neck symptom of pain, stiffness, or tenderness only No physical signs
II	Neck symptom Musculoskeletal signs including: • Decreased range of movement • Point tenderness
III	Neck symptom Musculoskeletal signs Neurologic signs including: • Decreased or absent deep tendon reflexes • Muscle weakness • Sensory deficits
IV	Neck symptoms and fracture or dislocation

(From Spitzer W, Skovron M, Salmi L, et al. Scientific monograph of Quebec Task Force on whiplash associated disorders: redefining "whiplash" and its management. *Spine*. 1995;20:1-73.)

TABLE 6.9	Sterling Proposal to Further Subdivide Whiplash-Associated Disorders II

Whiplash associated disorders (WAD) II A	Neck pain
	Motor impairment
	   Decreased range of motion (ROM)
	   Altered muscle recruitment patterns (CCFT)
	Sensory impairment
	   Local cervical mechanical hyperalgia

WAD II B	Neck pain
	Motor impairment
	   Decreased ROM
	   Altered muscle recruitment patterns (CCFT)
	Sensory impairment
	   Local cervical mechanical hyperalgia
	Psychologic impairment
	   Elevated psychologic distress

WAD II C	Neck pain
	Motor impairment
	   Decreased ROM
	   Altered muscle recruitment patterns (CCFT)
	   Increased joint positioning errors
	Sensory impairment
	   Local cervical mechanical hyperalgia
	Generalized sensory hypersensitivity (mechanical, thermal, bilateral upper limb neurodynamic test 1 limitation)
	Some may show sympathetic nervous system disturbances
	Psychologic impairment
	   Elevated psychologic distress
	   Elevated levels of acute posttraumatic stress

(From Sterling M. A proposed new classification system for whiplash associated disorders: implications for assessment and management. *Man Ther.* 2004;9:60-70.)

nosis and management of WAD[42] (Table 6.8). Based on studies that examined the complex clinical features of patients with WAD and tracked the outcomes of these patients, Sterling[43] came to the conclusion that the QTF classification system (Table 6.8) is too simplified and does not adequately classify patients with WAD to guide clinical decision making. In particular, Sterling[43] found that WAD II is the most common classification and should be subdivided further on the basis of specific clinical findings within the classification that alter the treatment approach and potentially predict treatment outcomes. The clinical outcomes of patients within the WAD II classification vary greatly from full recovery at 6 months after injury to reports of continued moderate/severe symptoms.[43]

Sterling[43] has proposed three subclassifications for WAD II based on motor, sensory, and psychologic impairments (Table 6.9). Patients with chronic WAD with moderate/severe ongoing symptoms have been shown to have higher levels of posttraumatic stress and high levels of persistent fear of movement/reinjury. When these factors are identified in a patient with acute WAD, an early psychologic consultation is indicated.[44]

High sensory hyperalgia in the neck is common with most WAD II subclassifications, but the more severe WAD IIC classification also has sensory hyperalgia throughout the body (i.e., generalized). Treatment of this patient population is challenging, and recommendations are to avoid treatments that are

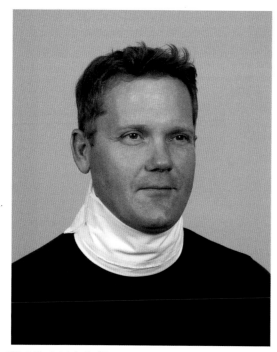

FIG. 6.13 A folded pillowcase wrapped around the neck.

noxious and pain provoking for these patients.[43] Only the most gentle, nonprovocative manual therapy techniques should be used, combined with active movement within the patient's tolerance. Positioning can be helpful; the neck and shoulder girdle muscles can be supported at rest with use of a folded pillowcase wrapped around the patient's neck (Fig. 6.13) and use of pillows to support the arms in sitting when possible. Movement and activity should be encouraged but overstraining the painful structures of the neck should be avoided. Frequent short doses of exercise and activity are encouraged throughout the patient's day. Activities that the patient fears should be gradually introduced as the patient gains ROM and motor control to assist the patient in overcoming fears of movement and activity. Early active exercise within the patient's tolerance has been shown to result in favorable patient outcomes.[45,46]

Motor impairments of patients with WAD can be evaluated with the craniocervical flexion test (CCFT) as described by Jull et al.[47] (Box 6.1). The test assesses precision and control to determine whether a patient can use the deep neck flexor muscles and hold a contraction. The deep neck flexors include the longus colli, longus capitis, and rectus capitis anterior and lateralis; these muscles work with the neck extensor muscles as dynamic stabilizers of the cervical segments. EMG recordings of superficial and deep neck flexor muscles were recorded on 10 control subjects and 10 subjects with chronic neck pain during the CCFT.[29] Subjects with neck pain demonstrated reduced activation of deep neck flexor muscles across all stages of the CCFT with increased activity of the superficial muscles (anterior scalene and sternocleidomastoid muscles).[29] In motor control problems of the neck, a higher level of use of the superficial neck flexors compensates for inadequate contractile

---

BOX 6.1 The Craniocervical Flexion Test (Video 6.1)

1. The starting position:
   a. The testing position is in the crook-lying position with the craniocervical and cervical spine in a midrange neutral position. For the neutral neck position, position with a horizontal face line and a horizontal line bisecting the neck longitudinally.
   b. Layers of towel may be placed under the head to achieve the neutral position. Ensure that the towel is aligned with the base of the occiput and the upper cervical region is free to move.
2. Preparation of the stabilizer (pressure biofeedback unit):
   a. Fold the blue airbag of the stabilizer and clip it together.
   b. Place the stabilizer behind the suboccipital region of the neck.
   c. Inflate the stabilizer to 20 mm Hg.
3. The formal test:
   Stage 1: The craniocervical flexion action:
   a. Explain that the test is assessing the precision and control to determine whether the patient can use the deep neck muscles and hold a contraction.
   b. Explain the movement to the patient and describe the craniocervical flexion as "gently nodding your head as though you were saying yes."
   c. Let the patient practice the movement to ensure that the patient is performing a pure nod but not head retraction or lifting of the head.
   d. Instruct the patient to place the front one-third of the tongue on the roof of the mouth, with the lips together but the teeth slightly separated to relax the jaw.
   e. The movement should be performed gently and slowly.
   f. Turn the dial to the patient.
   g. Ask the patient to slowly nod to target 22 mm Hg and then 24 mm Hg and in turn 26, 28, and 30 mm Hg. The therapist observes the head movement and watches for a pattern of progressively increasing craniocervical flexion with each stage of the test. The therapist does not watch the dial but observes for proper head movements.
   Stage 2: Testing the holding capacity of the deep neck flexors:
   a. Instruct the patient to gently and slowly nod to target 22 mm Hg and attempt to hold the position steadily for 10 seconds with a good quality craniovertebral nodding movement.
   b. If successful at 22 mm Hg pressure, have the patient relax and repeat at each target pressure separately at 2 mm Hg increments up to a maximum of 30 mm Hg.
   c. Once the maximum pressure that the patient can hold steady with a good quality of movement and with minimal superficial muscle activity is determined, use this pressure level to measure endurance capacity (i.e., 10 repetitions of 10-second holds).
4. Normal performance of deep neck flexors:
   a. Normal performance is the achievement of pressure of at least 26 mm Hg with the pressure held steady for 10 seconds with 10 repetitions. Ideal performance is to successfully target and hold 28 to 30 mm Hg. The craniocervical flexion action should be able to be performed without dominant activity in the superficial muscles of the neck.

(From Jull G, Kristjansson E, Dall'Alba P. Impairment in cervical flexors: a comparison of whiplash and insidious onset neck pain patients. *Man Ther.* 2004;9:89-94.)

properties of the deep neck flexor muscles.[47] The intra- and interreliability for the CCFT has been reported as between "fair to good" and "good to excellent" (intraclass correlation coefficient [ICC]: 0.63–0.86).[48] The minimum detectable change of the CCFT of two target levels (4 mm Hg) is less than ideal, but CCFT results have been correlated with measures of disability, such as the NDI, which makes the test clinically relevant.[48]

The airbag biofeedback device can be used as a training tool to recruit deep neck flexor muscles and also can be used to retrain joint position sense of the cervical spine by attempting to reproduce neck positions as visual feedback is provided by the biofeedback device (Fig. 6.14). When the airbag biofeedback device is used as a tool to enhance muscle tonic

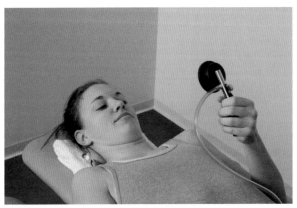

FIG. 6.14 See Video 6.1. Craniocervical flexion test and training program with airbag pressure biofeedback device.

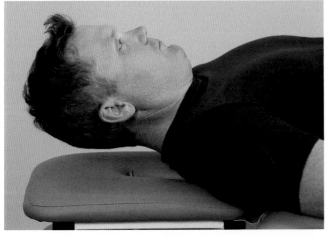

FIG. 6.15 Deep neck flexor muscle endurance test: while maintaining craniovertebral flexion, patient is asked to raise and hold head 2.5 cm off table and the test stops when the individual can no longer hold head up or maintain craniovertebral flexion. Normal performance for individuals without neck pain has been reported as ability to hold the head up in the test position for at least 38 seconds, but subjects with neck pain tested at 24 seconds.[50] This can also be used as a strengthening exercise for anterior neck flexor muscles but would be considered a progression from the craniocervical flexion training program.

endurance, the patient holds the targeted pressure for 10 seconds for up to 10 repetitions.

Another effective means to strengthen the anterior cervical flexor muscles is to have the patient maintain craniocervical neutral in the supine position as the patient lifts the head off the folded towel (or pillow) and repeat for up to three sets of 12 repetitions. This has also been described as an endurance test of the neck flexors (Fig. 6.15). Repeated use of this exercise was shown to be just as effective at training neck flexor muscle strength as the Jull protocol.[49] This exercise might be considered a progression from the isolated craniocervical flexion exercise.

Higher levels of pain and disability, older age, cold hyperalgia, impaired vasoconstriction, and moderate posttraumatic stress symptoms have been shown to be associated with poor outcomes 6 months after whiplash injury.[44] Patients with ongoing moderate/severe symptoms at 2 to 3 years after the initial injury continue to have decreased ROM, increased EMG activity of the superficial neck flexor muscles during the CCFT (an indication of inhibition of the deep neck flexors), sensory hypersensitivity, and elevated levels of psychologic distress compared with individuals with full recovery or milder symptoms.[44] Higher initial NDI scores (>30%), older age, cold hyperalgia, and posttraumatic stress symptoms are predictors of poor outcomes.[44]

In a randomized controlled trial (RCT) of 71 patients with chronic WAD II, a manual physical therapy ($n = 36$) treatment approach addressing specific impairments was compared with a self-management program ($n = 33$).[51] The results demonstrated that manual physical therapy that combined gentle nonpain-inducing manual therapy techniques with deep neck flexor control exercises reduced pain and disability in the chronic WAD patients and restored deep neck flexor control.[51] More than 70% of these patients had sensory hypersensitivity changes at baseline with the mechanical hyperalgesia, measured with pain pressure threshold or cold hyperalgesia.[51] It is believed that sensory hypersensitivity with WAD represents the presence of an augmented central pain processing mechanism.[52] The subgroup of patients with both widespread mechanical and cold hyperalgesia had the least improvement, but patients with mechanical hyperalgesia or cold hyperalgesia alone still demonstrated improvements with the manual physical therapy.[51]

When individuals with moderate/severe symptoms present with a more complex, debilitated pain state and their clinical picture is complicated by the presence of widespread sensory hypersensitivity and psychologic distress, these patients may benefit from early management strategies using a multidisciplinary professional approach that includes physical therapy, psychologic support, and pharmaceutical pain management.[52] In comparison, those with lesser symptoms are not likely to demonstrate such severe impairments, and the clinical management of these patients should consist of strategies addressing impairments, such as limited spinal mobility and altered muscle recruitment patterns with active exercise.[52]

Ritchie et al.[40] analyzed the results of two clinic trials ($n = 91$ and $n = 171$) of patients with WAD to develop a clinical prediction rule (CPR) to determine which patients are most likely to fully recover and which will go on to develop

	Not at all or only one time			Five or more times per week/ almost always
Trouble sleeping	0	1	2	3
Irritability	0	1	2	3
Difficulties concentrating	0	1	2	3
Being overly alert	0	1	2	3
Being easily startled	0	1	2	3

FIG. 6.16 Hyperarousal subscale of the Posttraumatic Diagnostic Scale (PDS). (Modified from Foa EB, Cashman L, Jaycox L, et al. The validation of a self-report measure of posttraumatic stress disorder: the Posttraumatic Diagnostic Scale. *Psychol Assess*. 1997;9:445-451.)

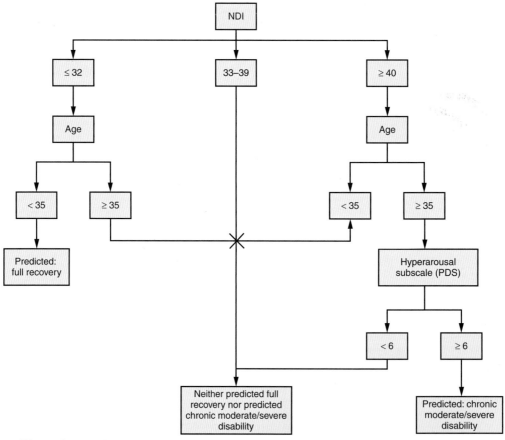

FIG. 6.17 Proposed clinical prediction rule to predict both chronic moderate/severe disability and full recovery following an acute whiplash injury. *NDI*, Neck Disability Index; *PDS*, Posttraumatic Diagnostic Scale. (From Ritchie C, Hendrikz J, Kenardy J, et al. Derivation of a clinical prediction rule to identify both chronic moderate/severe disability and full recovery following whiplash injury. *Pain* 2013;154:2198-2206.)

moderate/severe pain and disability from whiplash injuries. An increased probability of developing chronic moderate/severe disability was predicted in the presence of:
- Older age (>40 years),
- Initially higher levels of disability with NDI of 40% or more, and

- Hyperarousal symptoms (≥6 on hyperarousal subscale of the Posttraumatic Diagnostic Scale [PDS]) with positive predictive value (PPV) = 71%[40,53] (Fig. 6.16).

The probability of full recovery was increased in younger individuals (<35) with initially lower levels of neck disability (NDI <32%) with PPV = 71%[40] (Fig. 6.17).

A validation study of the whiplash CPR was done with a secondary analysis of data from 101 individuals with acute WAD who had previously participated in either a randomized controlled clinical trial or prospective cohort study.[54] Full recovery was defined as NDI score at 6 months of 10% or less, and ongoing moderate/severe disability were defined as an NDI score at 6 months of 30% or greater.[54] The PPV of ongoing moderate/severe pain and disability was 90.9% in the validation cohort, and the PPV of full recovery was 80.0%, which provided external validation of the whiplash CPR to confirm the accuracy and reproducibility of this dual-pathway tool.[54] A group of physical therapists were surveyed and reported that the whiplash CPR was simple, understandable, easy to use, and was an acceptable prognostic tool.[54]

It has been proposed that patients with an acute whiplash injury who are at low risk of ongoing pain and disability (i.e., predicted to fully recover) should receive up to three sessions of guideline-based education and specific neck exercise advise with their healthcare provider.[55] Patients at medium or high risk of developing ongoing pain and disability should be referred to a physical therapist specialist with expertise in whiplash who can conduct a more in-depth physical and psychologic assessment.[55] Based on the results of further assessment, the treatment should consist of primarily education, advice, and specific exercise, or if there are mild to moderate signs of central sensitization or posttraumatic stress, a psychologically-informed approach of physical therapy care that combines specific exercise, gentle manual therapy, and pain science education.[55] If the patient exhibits severe signs of posttraumatic stress or central sensitization, referral to a cognitive behavioral specialist may be indicated. Clinical trials need to be completed to determine if this stratified approach results in better patient outcomes.[55]

Fatty infiltrates of the neck extensor muscles have been noted in subjects following whiplash injury as early as 4 weeks following the injury.[56] The degree of muscle fatty infiltrates increased over time and were significantly higher at 3 and 6 months in the subjects who were moderate/severely disabled (NDI >30%) compared with those who were recovered and mildly disabled.[56] Karlsson et al.[57] reported similar findings with 38% greater fat infiltration of the C4 to C7 cervical multifidus muscle in patients with chronic severe WAD (NDI ≥40%) compared with healthy controls and 45% greater fat infiltration compared with patients with mild/moderate WAD disability (Fig. 6.18).

The initial degree of posttraumatic stress disorder symptoms following whiplash injury has been positively correlated with the severity of pain, disability, and muscle fatty infiltrates at 6 months.[56] Muscle fatty infiltrate values were shown in another study by Elliott et al.[58] to be significantly higher in the group of patients who met the whiplash CPR for severe disability. Elliott et al.[56] have speculated that the whiplash injury may create extreme levels of stress in some patients that can activate various biologic processes, including the release of cortisol by the adrenal glands. Sustained hypercortisolemia can impact overall health status including the degeneration of

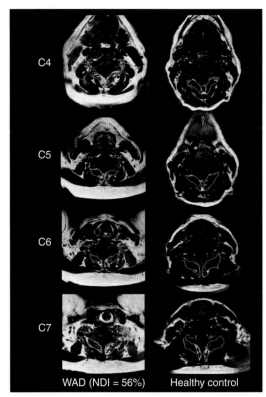

FIG. 6.18 Cross-sections at vertebral levels C4 through C7 of the multifidus muscle, marked on the fat images of (left) a participant with severe disability secondary to WAD and (right) an age- and sex-matched control. *NDI*, Neck Disability Index; *WAD*, whiplash-associated disorder. (From Karlsson A, Leinhard OD, Aslund U, West J, et al. An investigation of fat infiltration of the multifidus muscle in patients with severe neck symptoms associated with chronic whiplash-associated disorder *J Orthop Sports Phys Ther*. 2016;46(10):886-893.)

skeletal muscle.[59] Additional biologic consequences associated with exposure to extreme stress include autonomic reactivity, disturbed sleep, lowered immunity and altered perception of symptoms.[60] Therefore increased levels of neck muscle fatty infiltrates could be related to alterations of the neuroendocrine system in some patients following whiplash, suggesting a neuropsychobiologic link with poor outcomes.[56]

Sterling et al.[61] compared an evidence-based physical therapist guided exercise program (*n* = 55) with the same exercise program combined with stress inoculation training (*n* = 53) for patients with acute WAD. Stress inoculation training is a cognitive behavioral approach that teaches problem-solving and coping strategies to manage stress-related anxiety (i.e., relaxation training, cognitive restructuring, and positive self-statements), provides important information to injured individuals about the impact of stress on their physical and psychologic wellbeing, and focuses on transferring these skills to daily life[61-63] (Table 6.10). The patients in the stress inoculation training combined with exercise intervention group demonstrated superior reduction in disability and psychologic measures of stress, anxiety, and depression after 6 weeks of treatment and at 6- and 12-month follow-up compared with

TABLE 6.10	Description of the Stress Inoculation Training Intervention	
OBJECTIVE(S)	**STRESS INOCULATION TRAINING SESSION**	**CONTENT DESCRIPTION**
A. Identify and understand stress by identifying specific stressors and how these impact on pain, behavior, emotions, physical performance and thoughts	1. Program overview, theories of stress and pain, abdominal breathing exercises	Rationale for stress inoculation training (SIT), introduction to gate control theory, abdominal breathing explanation, demonstration and practice including facilitation of home practice.
B. Develop skills for managing stress through relaxation, problem solving and helpful coping self-statements	2. Muscle relaxation training 3. Problem solving for stressful situations 4. Use of positive coping statements	Rationale, strategy and practice of body scan including cues to initiate and facilitation of home practice. Review body scan experience. Rationale, strategy and practice of problem solving. Review abdominal breathing exercise experience. Generation of a plan for implementation specific to patient's situation and strategies for evaluation. Review problem solving experience. Rationale and identification of helpful and unhelpful self-talk and coping statements. Guided exercise in relation to specific stressful situation.
C. Apply skills in various stressful situations to develop tolerance and confidence	5. Applying SIT to the real world 6. Coping skills maintenance	Review coping statements experience. Review SIT steps from sessions 1 to 4 and provide context for use. Develop plan for managing patient identified stressor. Review SIT plan experience. Introduction to relapse prevention including early warning signs and developing a coping plan. Encourage ongoing development and practice of strategies.

(From Kelly JM, Bunzli S, Ritchie C, et al. Physiotherapist-delivered stress inoculation training for acute whiplash-associated disorders: a qualitative study of perceptions and experiences. *Musculoskelet Sci Pract*. 2018;38:30-36.)

the exercise alone group.[61] The results demonstrate that physical therapists who are trained to combine a cognitive behavioral approach with specific evidence-based exercises can produce positive outcomes for patients with acute WAD and potentially help to prevent progression to chronic WAD. The advantage of physical therapists delivering the cognitive behavioral training over a psychologist is speculated to be that patients who recently sustained a whiplash injury may not see the need for psychologic counseling but are more inclined to seek care from a physical therapist to address the physical effects of the injury.[61] If the physical therapists implement a psychologically informed approach that can aid the patient to cope with stress and anxiety associated with the WAD, the outcomes are enhanced.

Gentle manual therapy techniques, including isometric manipulation, may be helpful to restore limited mobility associated with WAD, but the patient must be monitored closely to ensure that pain is not provoked with the treatment approach. Intermittent use of a cervical collar may be beneficial to provide relative rest through the day. Frequent short doses of exercises (10 repetitions, four to five times per day) with emphasis on training the deep neck flexors, deep neck extensors, and postural scapular muscles can assist in motor retaining, postural correction, and pain inhibition. More vigorous manipulation techniques can be used to the thoracic spine to inhibit neck pain[64–66] and restore thoracic mobility. Gradual progression of an aerobic exercise program, such as walking or biking within the patient's pain tolerance, can also assist in pain management. Specific exercise and gentle manual therapy

should be combined with pain science education and education tailored to the patient's specific needs on topics, such as positioning, posture, ergonomics, stress management, and sleep hygiene to maximize treatment outcomes. The education needs of a patient can be determined through use of questionnaires described in elsewhere in this textbook, such as the Jenkins sleep questionnaire (Box 2.6), the anxiety depression questionnaire (Table 7.4), hyperarousal scale of the PDS (Fig. 6.16), and the central sensitization questionnaire (Fig. 2.7).

CERVICAL SPINE CLINICAL INSTABILITY
ICF Classification: Neck Pain With Movement Coordination Impairments

Clinical instability is defined by Panjabi[67] as the inability of the spine under physiologic loads to maintain its pattern of displacement so that no neurologic damage or irritation, no development of deformity, and no incapacitating pain occur.

The total ROM of a spinal segment may be divided into the neutral zone and the elastic zone.[68,69] Motion that occurs in and around the neutral mid position of the spine is produced against minimal passive resistance (i.e., neutral zone), and motion that occurs near the end range of spinal motion is produced against increased passive resistance (i.e., elastic zone).[67,70] Clinical instability is believed to be a result of increase in the size of the neutral zone and reduction in the passive resistance to motion created in the elastic zone (Fig. 6.19).

Panjabi[67] conceptualized the components of spinal stability into three functionally integrated subsystems of the spinal

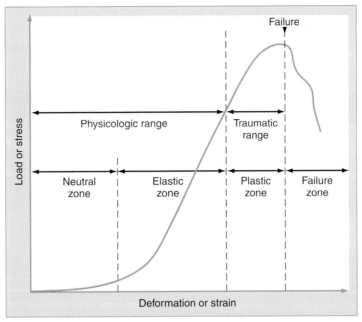

FIG. 6.19 Neutral zone of motion. (Modified from White AA, Panjabi MM. *Clinical Biomechanics of the Spine,* 2nd ed. Philadelphia: Lippincott Williams & Wilkins; 1990: p. 21.)

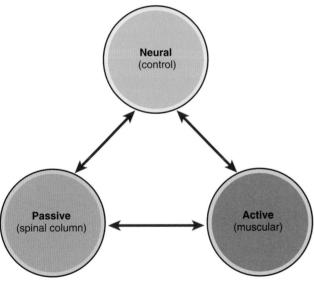

FIG. 6.20 Subsystems of spinal stability.

stabilizing system. According to Panjabi,[67] the stabilizing system of the spine consists of the passive, active, and neural control subsystems (Fig. 6.20).

The passive subsystem consists of the vertebral bodies, facet joints and joint capsules, spinal ligaments, and passive tension from spinal muscles and tendons. The passive subsystem provides significant stabilization of the elastic zone and limits the size of the neutral zone. Also the components of the passive subsystem act as transducers and provide the neural control subsystem with information about vertebral position and motion.

The active subsystem, which consists of spinal muscles and tendons, generates the forces needed to stabilize the spine in response to changing loads. The active subsystem is primarily responsible for controlling the motion that occurs within the neutral zone and contributes to maintaining the size of the neutral zone. The spinal muscles also act as transducers that provide the neural control subsystem with information about the forces generated by each muscle.[71–73]

Through peripheral nerves and the central nervous system, the neural control subsystem receives information from the transducers of the passive and active subsystems about vertebral position, vertebral motion, and forces generated by spinal muscles. With that information, the neural control subsystem determines the requirements for spinal stability and acts on the spinal muscles to produce the required forces.

Clinical spinal instability occurs when the neutral zone increases relative to the total ROM, the stabilizing subsystems are unable to compensate for this increase, and the quality of motion in the neutral zone becomes poorly coordinated and uncontrolled.[67–69] When the condition becomes "clinical," it causes symptoms, and Panjabi would further define clinical spinal instability as a significant decrease in the capacity of the stabilizing system of the spine to maintain the intervertebral neutral zones within physiologic limits, which results in pain and disability.[69] Degeneration and mechanical injury of the spinal stabilization components are some of the potential causes of increases in neutral zone size.[67] Some authors have used the term *functional instability* to describe signs and symptoms associated with clinical instability that can be managed nonsurgically, and use the term *structural instability* for more severe forms of instability that can be documented with medical imaging and likely require surgery if the instability is debilitating, life-threatening, or causes neurologic impairments.[74]

The presence of aberrant motions during active movement has been suggested by several authors to be a key sign of functional or

BOX 6.2   Therapeutic Exercises for Cervical Spine Disorders

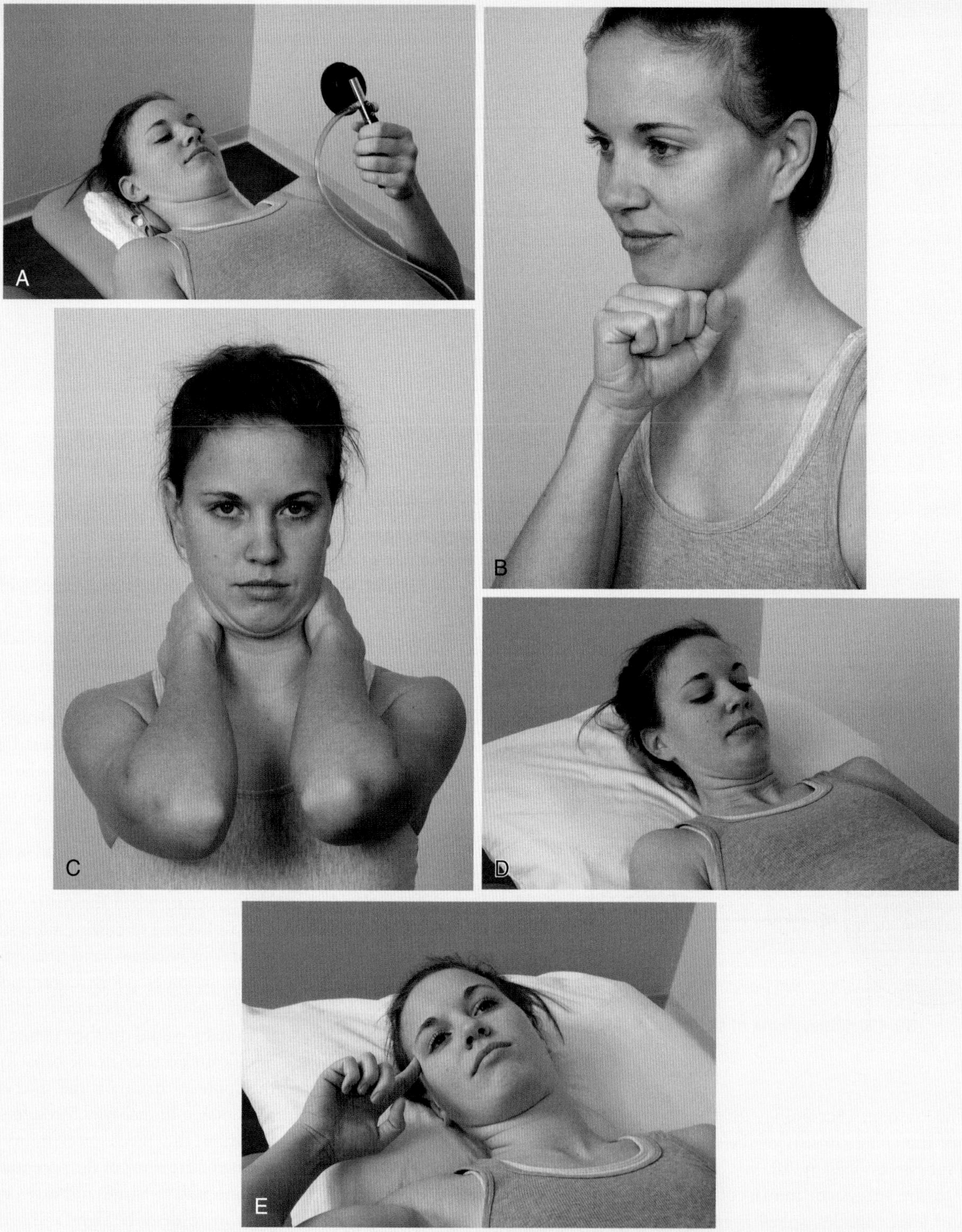

FIG. 6.21   A, Supine craniocervical flexion (nodding). B, Standing isometric craniocervical flexion. C, Standing craniocervical flexion with mid-cervical manual stabilization. D, Supine craniocervical flexion with sustained lift. E, Supine cervical rotation with manual resistance.

BOX 6.2 Therapeutic Exercises for Cervical Spine Disorders—cont'd

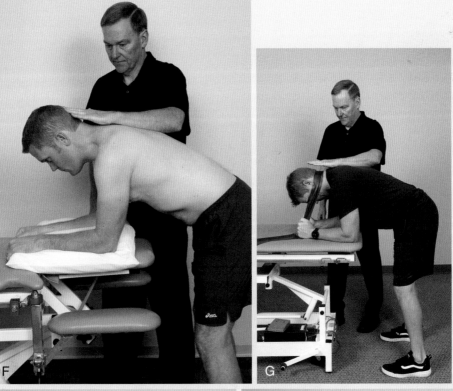
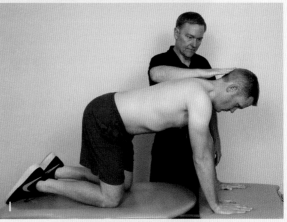
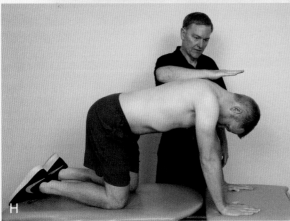

FIG. 6.21, cont'd F, Standing deep neck extensor exercise neutral position. G, Standing deep neck extensor exercise with elastic band resistance. H, Quadruped deep neck extensor exercise flexed position. I, Quadruped deep neck extensor exercise neutral position.

Continued

BOX 6.2   Therapeutic Exercises for Cervical Spine Disorders—cont'd

FIG. 6.21, cont'd J, Supine resistive shoulder D2 flexion. K to M, Cervical rotation active range of motion in semiflexed (three-fingers to sternum) position.

BOX 6.2 Therapeutic Exercises for Cervical Spine Disorders—cont'd

FIG. 6.21, cont'd N, Quadruped deep neck extensor exercise neutral position with elastic band resistance. O, Quadruped deep neck extensor exercise with laser. P, Quadruped deep neck extensor exercise with arm raise and laser. Q, Prone on elbows deep neck extensor exercise in flexed position with elastic resistance. R, Standing resistive shoulder retraction. S, Standing resistive scapular retraction: reciprocal.

Continued

BOX 6.2   Therapeutic Exercises for Cervical Spine Disorders—cont'd

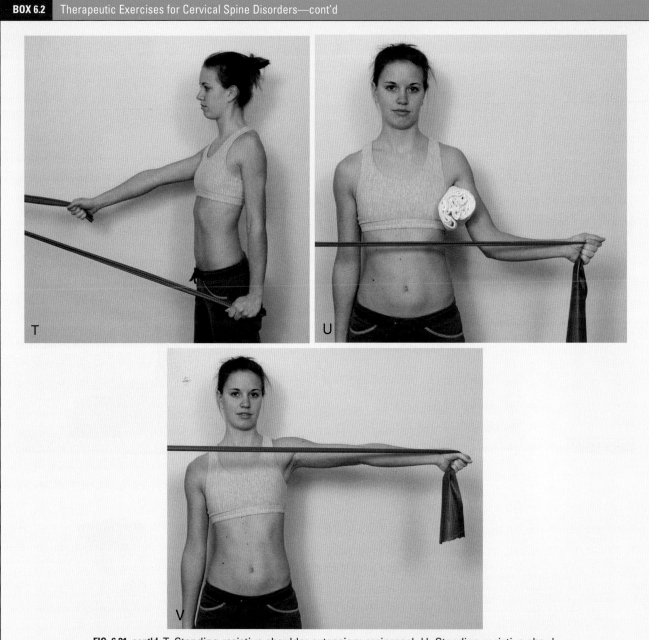

FIG. 6.21, cont'd T, Standing resistive shoulder extension: reciprocal. U, Standing resistive shoulder external rotation. V, Standing resistive shoulder horizontal abduction.

clinical instability,[75,76] and because poor quality of motion is a key aspect of cervical spine functional instability, the term *movement coordination impairments* has been adopted to classify this condition in the ICF clinical practice guidelines.[34,35] Aberrant motions are described as either sudden accelerations or decelerations of movement, such as shaking, juddering, and poor neuromuscular control, or motions that occur outside the intended plane of movement.[37,75] PIVM and joint play test results may reveal hypermobility and decreased passive restraints to motion at the end range of passive spinal segmental motion (i.e., a loose end feel).[77]

Cook et al.[78] used a Delphi survey method to establish consensus among orthopaedic manual physical therapy (OMPT) experts on the signs and symptoms of clinical cervical spine instability and reported the following symptoms as reaching the highest consensus: "intolerance to prolonged static postures"; "fatigue and inability to hold head up"; "better with external support, including hands and collar"; "frequent need for self-manipulation"; "feeling of instability, shaking, or lack of control"; "frequent episodes of acute attacks"; and "sharp pain, possibly with sudden movements."[78] The physical examination findings related to cervical instability that reached highest consensus among the clinical OMPT experts were: "poor coordination/neuromuscular control, including poor recruitment and dissociation of cervical segments with movement"; "abnormal joint play"; "motion that is not smooth throughout ROM, including segmental hinging, pivoting, and fulcruming"; and "aberrant movement."[78]

Objective criteria have been established in the analysis of end-range flexion and extension radiographs for diagnosis of cervical spine structural instability.[75,79–81] However, radiographs do not yield information about the quantity or quality of motion that occurs in the neutral zone (i.e., midrange), which limits the value of radiographs in the diagnosis of cervical spine functional instabilities.[75] Video fluoroscopy shows some promise as a means to analyze the quality of spine motion at midrange, but its use is still experimental for this purpose. PIVM and joint play testing have diagnostic value with assessment of neutral zone size, but the tests have poor interrater reliability and only assess passive motion.[70,82] Because a definitive diagnostic tool for cervical spine functional instability has not been established, cervical functional instability continues to be diagnosed on clinical findings, including history, subjective symptoms, visual analysis of active motion quality, and manual examination methods.[77]

When cervical functional instability does not severely involve or threaten neurologic structures, nonsurgical treatment is indicated. The goal of nonsurgical treatment is to enhance the function of the spinal stabilizing subsystems with emphasis on motor control and to decrease the stresses on the involved spinal segments. With proper training, the subsystems are more capable of compensating for an increase in neutral zone size.[67]

Spinal mobilization/manipulation above and below the region of instability and posture education may decrease stresses on the passive subsystem.[83] Proper posture is believed to reduce the loads placed on spinal segments at end ranges and returns the spine to a biomechanically efficient position.[83]

Spinal mobilization/manipulation can be performed at hypomobile segments above and below the level of instability, which commonly includes the upper thoracic and upper cervical spinal segments.[83] With improved mobility of these segments, spinal movement is thought to be more evenly distributed across several segments and mechanical stresses on the level of clinical instability are thought to be decreased.[83] There will also be positive neurophysiologic effects of the manual therapy techniques which will effect muscle tone and pain in a therapeutic manner.[84] When cervical spine functional instability seems to be the primary impairment, thoracic manipulation techniques may be a viable adjunct to a cervical motor control exercise program.

Neuromuscular control exercises enhance the function of the active subsystem.[67] The cervical multifidus may provide stability via segmental attachments to cervical vertebrae, and the longus coli and longus capitis may provide anterior stability as a result of the position of the muscle anterior to the cervical vertebral bodies (Fig. 6.8). Strengthening the stabilizing muscles of the cervical spine enables these muscles to improve the quality and control of movement that occurs within the neutral zone. Jull et al.[47] identified muscle synergy impairments between the superficial and deep anterior cervical spine muscles in patients with both insidious onset and whiplash neck pain disorders. Compared with a healthy population, both groups of patients excessively activated the sternocleidomastoid muscles when performing an active craniocervical flexion motion in supine. Previous research by Falla[85] showed that when there is overactivation of the sternocleidomastoid measured with a surface EMG, underactivation of the deep anterior neck flexor muscles tends to occur. Falla[85] also showed deficits in the motor control of the deep and superficial cervical flexor muscles in people with chronic neck pain, characterized by a delay in onset of neck muscle contraction associated with movement of the upper limb, cognitive activity, and functional tasks; Falla suggests a rehabilitation program to address retraining to restore the coordination of the deep neck flexor muscles and inhibit the superficial anterior neck muscles.

Falla et al.[86] had 14 women with chronic neck pain complete a program of specific craniocervical flexion exercise training to target the deep neck flexors twice per day for 6 weeks (Fig. 6.21A). After training, the activation of the deep neck flexors increased with the greatest change occurring in patients with the lowest values of deep neck flexor EMG amplitude at baseline.[86] There was a significant relationship between change in pain level with training and change in EMG amplitude for the deep neck flexors during craniocervical flexion.[86] This study provides evidence for the clinical benefits of targeting specific muscle training for the deep neck flexors in patients who demonstrate deficits in the neuromuscular control of these muscles. A systematic review and metaanalysis based on 10 RCTs reports a statistically significant effect size for positive clinical outcomes for reduction of neck pain and improvement in disability using craniocervical flexion motor control exercises compared with other treatments for patients with nonspecific chronic neck pain.[87] The AOPT ICF neck pain clinical practice guideline recommends specific neck and shoulder girdle strengthening and endurance exercises combined with education and manual therapy for treatment of neck pain with movement coordination impairments based on weak to moderate strength of evidence.[35]

The deep neck flexors can also be activated with isometric resistance provided under the patient's chin by the patient's closed fist placed under the chin (Fig. 6.21B, in Box 6.4). This provides a method to isolate the deep neck flexors in a standing or seated position, but this variation of deep neck flexor training has not been tested with quality RCTs.

Anatomically, the deep neck extensors are well suited to control segmental movements with the deep neck flexors.[28] O'Leary[88] used functional magnetic resonance imaging (MRI) to demonstrate that isolated activation of the lower deep neck extensor muscles (multifidus/semispinalis cervicis muscles) in patients with neck pain is obtained more efficiently by performing neck extensor exercises with the craniovertebral region positioned in neutral rather than extension. The neutral position of the cervical spine can be attained in a prone or quadruped position by having the patient's face parallel with the floor (Fig. 6.21I). A standardized method of testing the deep neck extensor muscles has been described using a laser with the patient in the prone position with their head off the head of the table and asking the patient to hold the neutral cervical position for up to 120 seconds[48] (Fig. 6.22). For patients who have difficulty attaining the prone test position, quadruped or prone on elbows positions can be used; and a standing with forearms on a table position could also be used to test and train the deep neck

extensors, but the key is to place the face parallel with the floor to attain a neutral cervical spine position (Fig. 6.21F, G, H, and I). To assess deep neck extensor function with the patient in quadruped, the patient should first be taught to attain the neutral cervical spine position. Next, the patient is instructed to forward bend the cervical spine by bringing the chin toward the chest, stopping at the point of tension, and then is asked to return to the neutral cervical spine position (Fig. 6.21H). The patient should be able to perform at least 10 repetitions with good control. To test the strength and endurance of the deep neck extensor muscles, the patient should be able to hold the quadruped neutral cervical spine position for a minimum of 2 minutes. Training could progress from active movements to include adding elastic band resistance to the neck extension movements (Fig. 6.22G, N, and Q). Holding the head and neck in neutral while performing arm, leg, and other spinal movements in the quadruped position can further train the deep neck extensors, and visual feedback to maintain the neutral neck position can be provided with a laser on the forehead and target on the table (Fig. 6.21O and P).

In patients with neck pain, the splenius capitis muscle tends to display increased EMG activity and the semispinalis cervicis muscle (Fig. 6.9) displays reduced and less defined activation, resulting in a common clinical presentation of increased muscle tone and guarding of the suboccipital muscles and lack of neuromuscular control of the middle and lower cervical spinal segments.[30] Schomacher[30] demonstrated enhanced EMG activation of the deep neck extensor (semispinalis cervicis) muscle relative to the craniocervical extensor (splenius capitis) muscle by placing the thumb and index finger on the vertebral arch of C2 and pushing anteriorly while asking the patient to maximally resist in a seated position. Based on this finding, it is thought that segmental activation of the deep neck extensor muscles can be attained by application of static manual pressure at the vertebral arch just cranial to the targeted portion of the muscle. Further dynamic control of the neck extensor muscles can be obtained by having the patient move into combined cervical extension with rotation repetitively to each side. Manual resistance to cervical rotation can also be applied to cervical rotation in the supine position to activate and train the neuromuscular control of the deep neck rotator muscles (Fig. 6.21E). The deep rotators can also be activated segmentally in sitting or supine with segmental stabilization with one hand and manual resistance of rotation with the other hand as applied with a cervical isometric mobilization technique (Figs. 6.59–6.62). Preliminary data supports that training the deep neck flexors and extensors can result in increased muscle cross section area of both muscle groups and reduction of muscle fatty infiltrations in the cervical multifidus muscles following a 10-week physical therapist guided neuromuscular exercise retraining program.[89] These changes coincided with increased strength and reduction in neck pain disability in five women with chronic whiplash-related neck pain.[89] In a larger RCT of patients with chronic whiplash, a specific neck exercise treatment program supervised by physical therapists for 12 weeks that targeted the deep neck flexor, deep neck extensor, and

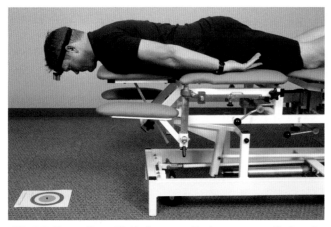

FIG. 6.22 Prone Deep Neck Extensor Endurance test. Patient is positioned prone with legs straight and arms at the side with a laser attached to the head and aimed at a target on the floor (60 cm distance). The patient performs a low cervical extension with the craniocervical region maintained in neutral with the face parallel to the floor and the laser on the target and is asked to hold this position for up to 120 seconds. The test is complete once the laser comes off the center of the target. Means have been reported as 29 seconds for patients with neck pain ($n = 21$) and 49 seconds for normal control subjects ($n = 21$). Reliability for this test has been reported as intraclass correlation coefficient values ranging from 0.75 to 0.90. (From Jorgensen R, Ris I, Falla D, et al. Reliability, construct and discriminate validity of clinical testing in subjects with and without chronic neck pain. *BMC Musculoskelet Disord.* 2014;15:408.)

deep neck rotator muscles demonstrated superior gains with 3- and 6-month follow-ups in neuromuscular neck muscle endurance, reduction in pain after the neck muscle endurance testing, and more satisfaction with treatment than a program of general exercise training.[90] The addition of a behavioral approach to the neck specific exercise program resulted in similar outcomes to the neck specific exercise program alone for this group of patients with chronic WAD.[90] These studies illustrate that neck neuromuscular control can be enhanced with a physical therapists guided training program that specifically targets the deep muscles of the neck.

Upper cervical structural instability with breakdown of the passive structural elements (i.e., bone and ligaments) of the upper cervical spine can be life threatening, is a contraindication for cervical spine manual therapy techniques, and, when suspected, is an indication for further diagnostic testing. The most common causes of upper cervical structural instability are caused by breakdown or damage of the passive stabilizing subsystem that can be caused by rheumatoid arthritis (RA), Down syndrome, or after a traumatic event, such as a motor vehicle accident.[91] Physical therapists must screen for the signs and symptoms associated with upper cervical structural instability, such as bilateral foot and hand dysesthesia, feeling of a lump in the throat, metallic taste in the mouth (cranial nerve VII), arm and leg weakness, and lack of bilateral extremity coordination[92] and could consider incorporating passive mobility and stability tests that target the upper cervical spinal segments as part of the examination (see Alar Ligament Stress Test, Anterior Shear Test, and Sharp-Purser Test). If the history and signs and symptoms are consistent with the red flag signs associated with upper cervical structural instability, radiographs and MRI are indicated to further assess the bony and ligamentous integrity of this spinal region.

When cervical spine instability is seen with severe and progressively worsening neurologic involvement, cervical fusion is the most common surgical intervention.[93] Postsurgical rehabilitation involves a similar approach as treatment of movement coordination impairments with progression of low level neuromuscular control exercises for the deep neck flexor and extensor muscles and parascapular postural muscles.

CERVICAL RADICULOPATHY
ICF Classification: Neck Pain With Radiating Pain

Cervical radiculopathy is a neuropathic pain disorder of the spinal nerve root commonly caused by space-occupying lesions of the cervical neural foramen (such as cervical disk herniation, spondylitic spurs, or cervical osteophytes), resulting in nerve root inflammation or impingement.[94,95] Cervical radiculopathy involves neck pain with associated radiating (narrow band of lancinating) pain in the involved upper extremity. Upper extremity paresthesia, numbness, and weakness may also be present. The most common cause of cervical radiculopathy (in 70%–75% of cases) is foraminal encroachment of the spinal nerve from a combination of factors, including decreased disk

height and degenerative changes of the uncovertebral joints anteriorly and zygapophysial joints posteriorly (i.e., cervical spondylosis).[95] Herniation of the intervertebral disk is responsible for only about 25% of the cases.[95] Other space-occupying lesions, such as tumors, are rarely the cause of cervical radiculopathy.[96]

Cervical radiculopathy must be differentiated from other possible causes of upper extremity pain, which might include thoracic outlet syndrome; referral patterns from cervical and upper thoracic anatomic structures; shoulder girdle impairments, such as a rotator cuff impingement; elbow impairments, such as lateral epicondylitis; and wrist/hand impairments, such as carpal tunnel syndrome. AROM and passive range of motion (PROM) and palpation should be carried out to screen each region of the upper quarter. Depending on the pain pattern, symptom behavior, and response to these initial screening procedures, additional upper extremity special tests and accessory motion testing should also be carried out. The goal of the examination is differentiation of local pain from referred pain and referred pain from true radicular (i.e., lancinating nerve root) pain.

Wainner et al.[97] identified a test item cluster of four clinical examination procedures for identification of patients with cervical radiculopathy that was confirmed and correlated with electrodiagnostic testing if all four test items were positive. The four test items include positive Spurling A test, neck distraction test, upper limb neurodynamic (ULND) test 1, and limited ipsilateral cervical spine rotation AROM of 60 degrees or less.[97]

In the Wainner et al. study,[97] the single best test for screening for cervical radiculopathy was ULND test 1, with a change in probability of the presence of the condition from 23% to 3% when the test results were negative. If the ULND test 1 results are negative, cervical radiculopathy can be essentially ruled out. If three of the four test cluster items are positive, the probability of the condition increases to 65%. If all four variables are present, the probability increases to 90%.[97]

In a systematic review of physical tests to diagnose cervical radiculopathy, Thoomes et al.[98] concludes that when consistent with patient history, clinicians could use a combination of Spurling's (Fig. 6.29), Neck Distraction (Fig. 6.32), and Arm Squeeze (Fig. 6.30) tests to increase the likelihood of a cervical radiculopathy, and the combined results of four negative neurodynamics tests (ULND tests 1, 2a, 2b, and 3 at Fig. 6.34) and an Arm Squeeze test could be used to rule out the disorder. Apelby-Albrecht et al.[99] demonstrated enhanced sensitivity of 0.97 and a specificity of 0.69 with the combined ULND test that is considered positive for radiculopathy when one or more of the four ULND tests were positive and negative for radiculopathy when all four ULND tests are negative. Among the four ULDN individual tests, the specificity was highest in this study with the upper limb neurodynamic test 3 (0.87).[99]

Waldrop[100] used the test item cluster developed by Wainner and colleagues and reported on a case series of six patients who met the diagnostic criteria for cervical radiculopathy. The six patients were treated for a mean of 10 visits (range, 5–18 visits) over an average of 33 days (range, 19–56 days). Four of the six patients had an MRI scan performed that confirmed cervical nerve root encroachment or impingement. Reductions in pain

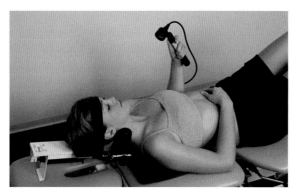

FIG. 6.23 Cervical mechanical traction with portable hydraulic traction device.

BOX 6.3	Clinical Prediction Rule to Determine Which Patients With Cervical Radiculopathy Would Have Positive Response to Cervical Mechanical Traction

- Patient reported peripheralization with lower cervical spine (C4–C7) posteroanterior mobility testing
- Positive shoulder abduction test
- Age >55 years
- Positive upper limb neurodynamic (ULND) test 1
- Positive neck distraction test

(From Raney NH, Peterson EJ, Smith TA et al. Development of a clinical predication rule to identify patients with neck pain likely to benefit from cervical traction and exercise. *Eur Spine J.* 2009;18(3):382-391.)

and disability were reported with all six patients with a treatment approach that included thoracic thrust manipulation techniques, patient education on proper posture, deep neck flexor strengthening exercises, and mechanical cervical traction (Fig. 6.23). Cleland et al.[93] reported on a similar treatment approach that combined manual physical therapy, cervical traction, and specific neck and parascapular muscle exercises to successfully treat a case series of 10 of 11 patients who met the criteria for cervical radiculopathy. Cleland[101] evaluated the clinical findings and interventions used that resulted in successful outcomes in treating 96 patients with cervical radiculopathy and calculated a 71.3% probability of success in patients who received multimodal treatment, including manual therapy, cervical traction, and deep neck flexor muscle strengthening for at least 50% of the visits. The other three factors that positively affected the treatment outcome included younger age (<54 years), dominant arm is not affected, and looking down does not worsen symptoms. The probability of success improved to 90.4% if all four of these factors were present. Young et al.[102] compared one session of a thoracic thrust manipulation in supine with a sham manipulation in the same position for patients with cervical radiculopathy, and the manipulation group demonstrated improved neck pain, disability, cervical ROM, and deep neck flexor endurance immediately after treatment and at a 48- to 72-hour follow-up compared with those treated with sham manipulation. Patients treated with manipulation were also more likely to report at least moderate change in their neck and upper extremity symptoms at 48 to 72 hours following treatment, but the change in upper extremity symptoms did not reach the same level of statistical significance between groups as the improvement in neck pain.[102]

Raney et al.[103] developed a CPR to determine which patients with cervical radiculopathy would have a positive response to cervical mechanical traction based on the results of treatment of 68 patients with neck pain with or without upper extremity symptoms who received cervical traction (60 seconds on/20 seconds off for 15 minutes) and active exercise (supine deep neck flexor strengthening and seated posture) twice a week for 3 weeks. A total of 30 of the 68 patients achieved a Global Rating of Change score of +6 or greater ("a great deal better" or "a very great deal better") on the final physical therapy visit.

The five variables in the CPR are included in Box 6.2. Pretest probability for success was 44%; and if three of five predictors are present, positive likelihood ratio (+LR) is 4.81 with a 79.2% probability of success; if four of five predictors are present, +LR is 23.1 with 94.8% probability of success.[103]

In contrast to the Raney et al. and Cleland et al. studies, Young et al.[104] compared manual therapy, exercise, and intermittent cervical traction (50 seconds on/10 seconds off) for the treatment group to a control treatment group consisting of manual therapy, exercise, and sham traction (5 pounds) twice per week for 4 weeks for both groups. Significant improvements were noted in both groups at the 2- and 4-week follow-up for NDI, numeric pain rating scale, and patient specific functional scale but no significant differences were noted between the two groups in the outcome measures.[104] These studies provide conflicting evidence on the benefits of cervical traction, and the ideal dosage of traction has not been determined, with the majority of the published studies using various protocols of intermittent traction. Continuous cervical traction should also be considered in future research.

Fritz et al.[105] completed a clinical RCT that compared three treatment groups for 86 patients with neck pain with radiating arm pain that included an exercise-only group, an exercise plus mechanical traction group, and an exercise plus over-the-door home traction group. The treatment lasted for 4 weeks, and there was follow-up for 12 months. Lower NDI scores were noted at 6 months in the mechanical traction group compared with the exercise group and over-the-door traction group and at 12 months in the mechanical traction group compared with the exercise group.[105] This study was unable to find a significant difference in treatment outcomes when patients were subgrouped based on the CPR for cervical traction developed by Raney et al.[103] The overall findings of this study demonstrate that patients who have cervical radiculopathy but do not meet the CPR for cervical traction criteria are still likely to have positive outcomes with mechanical traction in addition to an exercise program that targets deep neck flexors and postural muscles. Fritz et al.[105] admit that the study may have been underpowered to fully validate or refute the cervical traction CPR, and the patients in this study were required to have arm symptoms to be enrolled; thus it is possible that the magnitude of the interaction between status on the cervical traction CPR criteria and treatment outcome might have been larger had Fritz et al. enrolled a broader group of patients with neck pain, similar to that included in the study by Raney et al. Romeo et al.[106] completed a systematic review and metaanalysis with five RCTs meeting the inclusion criteria and determined that mechanical traction had a significant effect on pain at short- and intermediate-term and a significant effect on disability at intermediate term. These studies used intermittent mechanical traction with the number of sessions ranging from 7 to 15 and duration of traction treatment ranged from 15 to 50 minutes with the traction force ranging from 5 kg and 9 kg and was incrementally adjusted based on patient tolerance and symptom response.[106] Manual traction also had significant effect on pain at short term based on two studies.[106] The studies included in this review combined traction with other physical therapy interventions, such as manual therapy and exercise, and Romeo et al.[106] concluded that the literature supports the use of cervical traction combined with other physical therapy interventions for the treatment of cervical radiculopathy. The AOPT ICF neck pain clinical practice guideline recommends cervical traction combined with mobilization/manipulation of the cervical and thoracic spine and specific neck exercises for treatment of neck pain with radiating pain based on a moderate strength of evidence.[35]

The use of cervical and thoracic mobilization/manipulation techniques combined with specific exercises targeting the deep neck flexor muscles appears to be beneficial in the treatment of neck pain with radiculopathy. If manual cervical traction provides relief of the symptoms, a trial of cervical mechanical traction would be an appropriate intervention to combine with the manual therapy and exercise. Upper-extremity neural mobilizations with active and passive motion exercises and/or cervical lateral glide mobilizations can also be added to the treatment program. The ULND test positions that reproduce upper-extremity symptoms are used to the point of tension (i.e., "neural glide mobilizations") and performed repeatedly actively or passively as part of the treatment program (Fig. 6.34). In a systematic review of effectiveness of neural mobilizations for neck-related neck and arm pain, neural mobilizations that included a lateral glide mobilization of cervical spine (Fig. 6.48) had a positive effect on pain reduction and positive clinical outcomes.[107] Upper extremity neural mobilizations can also be combined with manual cervical traction. In an RCT involving 42 patients with cervical radiculopathy, Savva et al.[108] reported that neural mobilization with simultaneous intermittent manual cervical traction improved pain, function, disability, grip strength and CROM in the intervention group ($n = 21$) compared with a control group ($n = 21$).

CERVICAL MOBILITY DEFICITS
ICF Classification: Neck Pain With Mobility Deficits

When the primary impairment is mobility deficits of the neck, as noted with AROM/PROM and PIVM testing, and in the absence of radicular arm symptoms, specific spinal manipulation techniques are indicated as the primary intervention. The specific application of technique depends on a number of factors. Skilled manual physical therapists tend to base their clinical judgment of technique selection on multiple factors, including joint mobility and end feel assessment, tissue reactivity, acuity of onset, nature of the symptoms, the patient's emotional state and expectations, and the clinician's manual skill level. Neck pain guidelines recommend a combination of mobilization/manipulation combined with specific neck and shoulder girdle exercises for acute, subacute, and chronic neck pain with mobility deficits based on a moderate strength of evidence.[35,109]

Hoving et al.[110] showed in a RCT that physical therapists with advanced training in specific manipulation skills produced significantly better outcomes in treating patients with neck pain compared with both physical therapists with more general training and general medical practitioners. At the 7-week follow-up examination, the results showed a 68% success rate for the patients treated with specific nonthrust mobilization techniques and specific exercises provided by the physical therapists with advanced training in manual therapy compared with a 51% success rate for the patients treated by the physical therapists with more general training and a 36% success rate for patients treated by a general medical practitioner. Korthals-de Bos et al.[111] published a cost-analysis study based on the Hoving clinical trial and reported that manual physical therapy required fewer treatment sessions for a more favorable outcome, with the cost of the manual physical therapy about one-third the cost of the other two treatment groups. Korthals-de Bos et al.[111] concluded that manual physical therapy was more cost effective for treatment of neck pain than general physical therapy or general practitioner care.

A 2004 Cochrane systematic review of RCTs concluded that thrust manipulation or nonthrust mobilization techniques used with exercise are beneficial for persistent mechanical neck disorders with or without headache.[112] A 2010 Cochrane systematic review attempted to delineate if thrust manipulation or nonthrust mobilization used alone has a therapeutic effect on adults experiencing neck pain.[113] The authors concluded that moderate quality evidence showed cervical thrust manipulation and nonthrust mobilization produced similar effects on pain, function, and patient satisfaction at intermediate-term follow-up and a similar conclusion was reached from a 2015 Cochrane review.[113,114] The authors further conclude that multiple cervical manipulation sessions may provide better pain relief and functional improvement than certain medications at immediate/intermediate/long-term follow-up.[114]

Walker et al.[115] completed an RCT on 94 patients with neck pain (47 each group) that compared manual physical therapy interventions of thrust manipulation, nonthrust mobilization, isometric manipulation, or stretching techniques and a home exercise program of cervical retraction, deep neck flexor strengthening, and cervical rotation ROM exercises with general practitioner care that included postural advice, encouragement to maintain neck motion and daily activities, cervical rotation ROM exercise, prescription medication, and subtherapeutic pulsed ultrasound. The manual physical therapy group demonstrated statistically greater improvement in NDI scores at 3-week, 6-week, and 1-year follow-up periods.[115] Pain reduction was statistically greater for the manual physical therapy group at the 3- and 6-week follow-up periods, but a significant difference between groups was not noted at 1 year.[115]

Walker et al.[115] demonstrated good long-term outcomes combining mobilization/manipulation techniques with exercise. A secondary analysis of this study found no difference in outcomes between patients (23 patients) with neck pain who received thrust manipulation and nonthrust mobilization combined with exercise to those patients (24 patients) who received only nonthrust mobilization with exercise. Both groups demonstrated improvements in pain and disability measures of an equal magnitude, but the authors determined that their sample size might have been too small to demonstrate a difference between the groups.[116] Celenay et al.[117] demonstrated superior results for improving disability, pain intensity at night, CROM, and quality of life by combining cervical and scapular muscle exercises with cervical nonthrust mobilization techniques ($n = 51$) to stabilization exercises alone ($n = 51$) in patients with neck pain.

Dunning et al.[118] demonstrated a greater improvement in pain and disability at a short-term (48-hour) follow-up for patients with neck pain who received a thrust manipulation directed to the C1–C2 and T1–T2 spinal segments ($n = 56$) compared with 30-second bout of nonthrust mobilization techniques directed to the same spinal segments ($n = 51$). In addition, the thrust manipulation group had significantly greater improvement in both passive C1–C2 rotation ROM and motor performance of the deep neck flexor muscles compared with the group that received nonthrust mobilization.[118] However, in a study where a more pragmatic approach was used that allowed the physical therapists to choose the level to be mobilized based on pain and stiffness response to cervicothoracic posteroanterior passive accessory intervertebral movement (PAIVM) testing and to provide longer duration of the nonthrust mobilization techniques based on patient response, the outcomes between cervical nonthrust mobilization ($n = 55$) and cervical thrust manipulation ($n = 44$) for short-term results were the same for pain, disability, and deep neck flexor endurance improvement.[119] In a systematic review and metaanalysis of 13 studies who met the inclusion criteria comparing thrust manipulation with nonthrust mobilization for treatment of low back and neck pain, it was determined that when a pragmatic design was used representing actual clinical practice, patients improved with both techniques with no difference between nonthrust mobilization and thrust manipulation, but when clinicians were prescribed techniques, thrust manipulation showed better outcomes than nonthrust mobilization for pain and disability.[120]

Research data have not been fully developed to identify subgroups of patients who will respond more favorably to various types of manipulation techniques, such as thrust versus nonthrust versus isometric manipulations. These clinical reasoning decisions are based more on clinician experience, the opinions of clinical experts, patient preference, and the comfort level/skill of the practitioner with various techniques. In the Walker et al.[115] study, the physical therapists who provided the manual therapy interventions used an impairment-based clinical decision-making model to determine the location and type of manual therapy interventions, which further supports the effectiveness of an impairment-based approach.

Isometric manipulation procedures can be effective when a high level of reactivity has been identified at the hypomobile joint (e.g., when the patient has pain before engaging the barrier to the passive joint motion and reflexive muscle guarding is noted with the passive motion). In this situation, the patient may not tolerate direct sustained force at the joint and the isometric forces tend to be tolerated more effectively. This type of situation is often found when the patient has a recent sudden onset of sharp localized neck pain that was brought on by a minor incident, such as suddenly looking up to reach for a cup on a high shelf. The active and passive motion is painful and limited with lateral flexion and rotation toward the painful side. A specific area of tenderness with overlying muscle holding is noted at a particular facet joint. Once the segment is isolated, an isometric manipulation can be used to restore motion and enhance neuromuscular control of the targeted segment.

Theoretically, the anatomic cause of this type of sudden onset of neck pain is the result of the entrapment of the facet joint meniscus. With a sudden awkward movement, the meniscus becomes entrapped within the edge of the facet joint, which can cause severe pain with attempts to load or move the involved joint. The entrapment can be released with use of the isometric forces directed to the targeted joint or with a thrust manipulation technique that creates joint distraction or gapping. Often, restoration of joint motion is noted after the intervention. Subsequent treatments can assist in correcting surrounding joint and muscle impairments as needed for full rehabilitation.

A more gradual onset of joint stiffness is characteristic of osteoarthritic joint changes, adaptive shortening of joint connective tissues, or adhesion formation after recovery from trauma to the spinal segment or surrounding soft tissues. Postural stresses are believed to contribute to these impairments. Various degrees of joint hypomobility can be identified throughout the spine and various levels of joint reactivity are noted at the hypomobile spinal segments. The stronger thrust manipulation and nonthrust mobilization techniques tend to be used to target the less reactive joints with mobility deficits. The lighter oscillatory nonthrust techniques tend to be used on joints with higher levels of reactivity and surrounding muscle guarding. There is preliminary evidence, as discussed in more detail in Chapter 3, that specific application of a mobilizing force to a targeted cervical spine segment with a passive segment mobility deficit will result in superior improvements in pain and mobility than mobilization of a segment with normal mobility.[121]

A CPR to identify patients with neck pain who are likely to benefit from thrust joint manipulation to the cervical spine has been developed by Puentedura et al.[122] Box 6.3 outlines the four findings that make up the CPR. Eighty-two patients were included in the data analysis, of whom 32 (39%) achieved a successful outcome as measured with the Global Rating of Change score of + 5, 6, or 7 after one or two treatments of an

BOX 6.4	Clinical Prediction Rule to Identify Patients With Immediate Response to a Cervical High-Velocity Thrust Manipulation

- Symptom duration less than 38 days
- A positive expectation that manipulation will help
- Side-to-side difference in cervical rotation ROM of 10 degrees or greater
- Pain with posteroanterior spring testing of the middle cervical spine

ROM, Range of motion.
(From Puentedura EJ, Cleland JA, Landers MR, et al. Development of a clinical prediction rule to identify patients with neck pain likely to benefit from thrust joint manipulation to the cervical spine. *J Orthop Sports Phys Ther.* 2012;42(7):577-592.)

upslope glide cervical thrust manipulation (Fig. 6.53) to the cervical spine (C3–C7) followed by neck ROM exercises (Fig. 6.21K-M) over a 1-week follow-up time frame. The physical therapist was allowed to use an impairment-based clinical decision-making model to determine the level and direction of the manipulation based on identification of a hypomobile cervical spinal segment. If three or more of the four attributes (+LR 13.5) were present, the probability of experiencing a successful outcome improved from 39% to 90%. This CPR still needs to be validated with follow-up RCTs that should include larger groups of patients and a long-term follow-up. An important lesson from this CPR is that patients with a positive expectation that manipulation will help had better outcomes, which is a reminder that patient expectations and values should always be factored into the clinical reasoning associated with patient management. Likewise, patients with a fear of manipulation, lack of confidence in their treating clinician, and/or a poor expectation that manipulation will help should not receive manipulation. Patients who present in this manner should receive more pain science and cognitive behavioral education with an active exercise-based approach.

Thrust manipulation techniques directed to the thoracic spine have also been shown as an effective means to provide immediate relief of neck pain.[64] Cleland et al.[64] developed a CPR to identify patients with neck pain who will most likely benefit from thoracic spine thrust manipulation for relief of neck pain. In an RCT of 140 patients with neck pain designed to validate this CPR, two sessions of thoracic thrust manipulation along with three sessions of stretching and strengthening exercises proved to be an effective means to reduce neck pain disability regardless of whether or not the patient fit the CPR. The authors concluded that patients who received thoracic spine thrust manipulation and exercise exhibited significantly greater improvements in disability at both the short- and long-term (6 months) follow-up periods compared with patients who received five sessions of exercise alone.[65] Because the results of the study did not validate this CPR, the CPR should be abandoned as a clinical decision-making tool.

A study by Masaracchio et al.[66] demonstrated that individuals with mechanical neck pain who received both thoracic spine thrust manipulation and cervical spine nonthrust mobilization plus exercise demonstrated better overall short-term (1-week) outcomes compared with individuals receiving only cervical spine nonthrust mobilization plus exercise. Therefore as long as thoracic spine thrust manipulation is not contraindicated, thoracic spine thrust manipulation is a useful adjunct to the treatment for patients with painful cervical spine conditions and should be combined with an exercise program that addresses specific cervical and thoracic mobility and strength impairments. Combining thoracic spine thrust manipulation with other cervical spine manual therapy techniques and specific therapeutic exercises to address the patients' impairments is the best treatment approach for patients with cervical hypomobility.

For patients with neck pain, thoracic and cervical spine manipulation techniques can be used to effectively restore spinal mobility, reduce pain, and reduce disability. Spinal segments that have hypomobility with PIVM testing are targeted for manipulation. The manipulation technique can be modified with variations in depth of force, duration of force, speed of application of force, and use of isometric versus direct forces. High levels of fear-avoidance beliefs with high levels of anxiety over movement seem to influence the potential effectiveness of manipulation procedures.[64,85] Manual therapy can still be used with patients with high levels of fear-avoidance beliefs, but other strategies may be needed to effectively deal with the fear of movement, such as a positive reinforcement for active participation in the rehabilitation process, active exercise programs, and perhaps psychologic counseling.

The Cochrane systematic reviews on treatment of cervical spine disorders states that mobilization/manipulation is most effective if combined with exercise.[112,113] Some variability exists in the literature regarding specifically what type of exercise should be used to create the most effective clinical outcomes. Jull et al.[47] advocate specific strengthening exercises to target the deep neck flexor muscles combined with stretching muscles that tend to tighten, such as the levator scapulae and the upper trapezius, and strengthen the scapular adductor and retractor muscles (Box 6.4). Cleland et al.[64] had the patients in their study follow up the thoracic spine thrust manipulation with a more general CROM exercise involving cervical rotation in a semiflexed position (Fig. 6.21K-M). Others have advocated for a more general strengthening and full-body endurance program for rehabilitation of neck pain disorders.

Use of an impairment-based clinical reasoning approach tends to follow components of all three possible recommendations depending on the findings of the clinical examination and reexamination of patients as they proceed through the rehabilitation process. If weakness is noted in the deep neck flexors, deep neck extensors, or parascapular muscles, specific exercises should be instructed to target the strength and endurance of these muscles (Box 6.2). If tightness is noted in specific muscles of the upper quarter, specific stretching should be integrated into the treatment approach (Figs. 6.40 and 6.41). Self-mobilization techniques for the thoracic spine (see Box 5.2 in Ch. 5) can also be helpful to enhance the patient's home program for pain control and thoracic mobility. As specific impairments are addressed, a general exercise program is recommended that includes endurance training to enhance the patient's tolerance to functional activities and to assist in pain control through the beneficial analgesic effects associated with aerobic exercise.

The ultimate goal of the rehabilitation program is to restore mobility, inhibit pain, and return the patient to full functional activity. In the process, the physical therapist provides the patient with strategies to self-treat and maintain the improvements made in the physical therapy sessions. Early in the rehabilitation process, a good deal of manual therapy procedures are provided and only mild low-level exercises are instructed. As the physical therapy program progresses, less manual therapy is needed, and the exercise program duration and intensity are progressed under the direction of the physical therapist. Once the patient is independent in the exercise program and in self-management principles, further skilled physical therapy is no longer needed.

Specific exercises emphasize cervical spine motor control, thoracic mobility, and scapular muscle strengthening (Box 6.2). The primary goals of the exercise program are to enhance neuromuscular control of the upper quarter, correct posture, and maintain mobility attained with the manual therapy techniques. In addition to the specific strengthening program, most patients benefit from the addition of a low-impact aerobic exercise program with an exercise that interests the patient and can fit into the patient's lifestyle, such as a walking program or use of an elliptical trainer.

CERVICOGENIC HEADACHE
ICF Classification: Neck Pain With Headaches

The International Classification for Headache Disorder, 3rd edition, (ICHD-3) describes diagnostic criteria for three main primary headaches: migraine, tension-type headache, and trigeminal autonomic cephalalgias (cluster headache) (see Table 7.1 and Box 6.5) A wide-ranging list of secondary headaches are also described in the ICHD-3 with cervicogenic headaches (CGHs) included in the subgroup of secondary "headache or facial pain attributed to disorder of the cranium, neck eyes, ears, nose, sinuses, teeth, mouth or other facial or cervical structures."[123]

There is debate in the literature regarding the contribution of cervical musculoskeletal impairments to headache.[124] Although the results of a systematic review suggested that the pathogenesis of migraine headaches is probably not influenced by musculoskeletal impairments,[125] patients with migraines have a high prevalence of neck pain,[126,127] and neck muscle and joint impairments have been hypothesized to act as triggers for migraine attacks.[128] In patients with tension type headache, muscle tenderness and trigger points are consistent findings.[129,130] The interaction between trigeminal and cervical afferents in the trigeminocervical nucleus at the brainstem has been hypothesized to explain why neck pain frequently accompanies headaches.[131,132] CGH by definition is the most likely subgroup of headache to present with musculoskeletal impairments in the neck[133–135] (Box 6.5).

| **BOX 6.5** | Primary Headache Classifications From The International Classification of Headache Disorders, 3rd edition |

Migraine Without Aura
Description: Recurrent headache disorder with attacks lasting 4 to 72 hours. Typical characteristics of headache are unilateral location, pulsating quality, moderate or severe intensity, aggravation by routine physical activity and associated with nausea and/or photophobia and phonophobia.
    Diagnostic criteria
A. At least five attacks fulfilling criteria B–D
B. Headache attacks lasting 4–72 hours (when untreated or unsuccessfully treated)
C. Headache has at least two of the following four characteristics:
    1. Unilateral location
    2. Pulsating quality
    3. Moderate or severe pain intensity
    4. Aggravation by or causing avoidance of routine physical activity
D. During headache at least one of the following:
    1. Nausea and/or vomiting
    2. Photophonia and phonophonia
E. Not better accounted for by another International Classification of Headache Disorders (ICHD)-3 diagnosis

Migraine With Aura
Description: Recurrent attacks, lasting minutes, of unilateral fully reversible visual, sensory or other central nervous system symptoms that usually develop gradually and are usually followed by headache and associated migraine symptoms.
    Diagnostic Criteria
A. At least two attacks fulfilling criteria B and C

B. One or more of the following fully reversible aura symptoms:
    1. Visual
    2. Sensory
    3. Speech and/or language
    4. Motor
    5. Brainstem
    6. Retinal
C. At least three of the following six characteristics:
    1. At least one aura symptom spreads gradually over >5 minutes
    2. Two or more aura symptoms occur in succession
    3. Each individual aura symptom lasts 5–60 minutes
    4. At least one aura symptoms is unilateral
    5. At least one aura symptom is positive
    6. The aura is accompanied, or followed within 60 minutes, by headache
D. Not better accounted for by another ICHD-3 diagnosis

Frequent Episodic Tension-Type Headache
Description: Frequent episodes of headache, typically bilateral, pressing or tightening in quality and of mild to moderate intensity, lasting minutes to days. The pain does not worsen with routine physical activity and is not associated with nausea, although photophobia or phonophobia may be present.
    Diagnostic criteria
A. At least 10 episodes of headache occurring on 1–14 days/month on average for >3 months (>12 and <180 days/year) and fulfilling B–D
B. Lasting 30 minutes to 7 days

| BOX 6.5 | Primary Headache Classifications From The International Classification of Headache Disorders, 3rd edition—cont'd |

C. At least two of the following four characteristics:
1. Bilateral location
2. Pressing or tightening (nonpulsating) quality
3. Mild or moderate intensity
4. Not aggravated by routine physical activity, such as walking or climbing stairs
D. Both of the following:
1. No nausea or vomiting
2. No more than one of photophobia or phonophobia
E. Not better accounted for by another ICHD-3 diagnosis

Chronic Tension-Type Headache
Description: A disorder evolving from frequency episodic tension-type headache, typically bilateral, pressing or tightening in quality and of mild to moderate intensity, lasting hours to days, or unremitting. The pain does not worsen with routine physical activity, buy may be associated with mild nausea, photophobia or phonophobia
Diagnostic criteria:
A. Headache occurring on >15 days/month on average for >3 months (>180 days/year), fulfilling criteria B–D
B. Lasting hours to days, or unremitting
C. At least two of the following four characteristics:
1. Bilateral location
2. Pressing or tightening (nonpulsating) quality
3. Mild or moderate intensity
4. Not aggravated by routine physical activity, such as walking or climbing stairs
D. Both of the following:
1. No more than one of photophobia, phonophobia or mild nausea
2. Neither moderate or severe nausea nor vomiting
E. Not better accounted for by another ICHD-3 diagnosis.

Cluster Headache (Trigeminal Autonomic Cephalalgias [TACs])
Description: Attacks of severe, strictly unilateral pain which is orbital, supraorbital, temporal or in any combination of these sites, lasting 15 to 80 minutes and occurring from once every other day to eight times a day. The pain is associated with ipsilateral conjunctival injection, lacrimation, nasal congestion,

rhinorrhea, forehead and facial sweating, miosis, ptosis and/or eyelid edema, and/or with restlessness or agitation.
Diagnostic criteria
A. At least 5 attacks fulfilling criteria B–D
B. Severe or very severe unilateral orbital, supraorbital and/or temporal pain lasting 15–180 minutes (when untreated)
C. Either or both of the following
1. At least one of the following symptoms or signs, ipsilateral to the headache:
   a. Conjunctival injection and/or lacrimation
   b. Nasal congestion and/or rhinorrhea
   c. Eyelid edema
   d. Forehead and facial sweating
   e. Miosis and/or ptosis
2. A sense of restlessness or agitation
D. Occurring with a frequency between one every other day and eight per day
E. Not better accounted for by another ICHD-3 diagnosis

Cervicogenic Headache
Description: Headache caused by a disorder of the cervical spine and its component bony, disk and /or soft tissue elements, usually by not invariably accompanied by neck pain.
Diagnostic Criteria
A. Any headache fulfilling criterion C
B. Clinical and/or imaging evidence of a disorder or lesion within the cervical spine or soft tissues of the neck, known to be able to cause headache
C. Evidence of causation demonstrated by at least two of the following:
1. Headache has developed in temporal relation to the onset of the cervical disorder or appearance of the lesion
2. Headache has significantly improved or resolved in parallel with improvement in or resolution of the cervical disorder or lesion
3. Cervical range of motion is reduced, and headache is made significantly worse by provocative maneuvers
4. Headache is abolished following diagnostic blockade of a cervical structure or its nerve supply
D. Not better accounted for by another ICHD-3 diagnosis

(From Headache Classification Subcommittee of the International Headache Society. The International Classification of Headache Disorders 3rd edition. *Cephalalgia* 2018;38:1-211.)

It is unknown if neck pain is a consequence or a potential perpetuating factor of tension-type and migraine headaches. Based on a systematic review, examination of neck ROM, the flexion-rotation test (Fig. 6.44), pressure pain threshold, passive spinal joint mobility assessment, palpation for trigger points, and forward head postural assessment have been recommended to detect the presence of cervical spine impairments in patients with migraine headaches.[136] Jull and Hall[132] further advise to consider CROM, joint dysfunction, and motor output assessment for diagnosis of neck musculoskeletal disorders in patients with migraine and tension-type headaches. Based on the results of the examination, it has been suggested that treatment of these musculoskeletal impairments may help reduce the intensity and frequency of migraine and tension-type headaches, but this should be combined with medical management of these headaches; further research is required to fully determine the effectiveness of this approach.[132,136]

CGHs originate from musculoskeletal dysfunction of the cervical spine.[137] The incidence of CGH is estimated to be 14% to 18% of all chronic headaches[138] and appear to affect women four times more than men.[139] Sjaastad et al.[133] outlined diagnostic criteria for CGH, with one of the primary criteria being headache pain elicited by pressure on the posterior neck, especially at one of the three upper cervical joints. CGHs are thought to arise from musculoskeletal impairments in the neck with the unilateral headache commonly accompanied by suboccipital neck pain, dizziness, and lightheadedness.[140] If dizziness or lightheadedness is present, further diagnostic tests may be indicated to rule out cardiovascular, central nervous system, or vestibular causes of the dizziness, such as benign positional paroxysmal vertigo. Features that tend to distinguish CGH from migraine and tension-type headache include side-locked (one-sided) pain, provocation of typical headache by digital pressure on neck muscles and by head movement, and posterior-to-anterior radiation of pain.[123] However, although these may be features of CGH, they are not unique to it, and they do not necessarily define causal relationships. Migraine can also be one sided headache, but often can switch sides during the episode where a CGH will not tend to switch sides during the headache episode (i.e., sidelocked). Migraine features, such as nausea, vomiting and photo/phonophobia may be present with CGH, although to a lesser degree than in migraine and may differentiate some cases from tension-type headache.[123] CGHs tend to start in the neck, and migraine headaches start in the head.[141] Tension-type headaches will often present with myofascial trigger point of the muscles of the head, face, jaw, and neck.[129]

The clinical tests that have been shown to further assist in differentiating patients with CGH from patients with migraine with an aura and controls include, in patients with CGH, less CROM flexion/extension, a significantly higher incidence of dysfunctions of the upper three cervical joints (facet joint hypomobility and tenderness to palpation assessed by manual examination), and muscle length limitations (tightness of upper trapezius, levator scapula, scalenes, and suboccipital extensor muscles). Hall et al.[142] has demonstrated that the flexion-rotation test is an effective method to detect C1–C2 mobility deficits and upper cervical pain provocation that is commonly present in patients with CGH (Fig. 6.44). Zito et al.[137] found that manual examination could discriminate the CGH group from other subjects (migraine with an aura and control subjects combined) with a sensitivity of 0.80. Zito et al.[137] found that not all hypomobile joints were painful, but all painful joints were hypomobile in the patients with CGHs. However, no differences were found among groups in this study for examination results of static posture, pressure pain threshold, mechanosensitivity of neural tissues, and measures of cervical kinesthetic sense. The patients in the CGH group demonstrated poorer performance in the CCFT, but this finding did not reach statistical significance.[137] Jull et al.[135] showed a sensitivity of 100% and specificity of 94.4% to identify patients with CGH from other headache types by clustering restricted cervical movement with manual examination of C0-C3 joint dysfunction and impairment in the craniocervical flexion test. Loss of CROM is a consistent feature of CGH, but not necessarily migraine or tension-type.[135]

Haas et al.[143] demonstrated effectiveness in reducing frequency and intensity of headache symptoms in a group of 256 adults with chronic CGH with providing thrust joint manipulation of the cervical spine compared with a control group who received light massage. In comparing number of visits with thrust joint manipulation, the group who had 18 sessions had enhanced outcomes compared with 0, 6, and 12 treatment sessions over a 6-week time frame.[143] These enhanced results were still evident at 1 year with reduced CGH days by about half.[143] Approximately 40% of the participants receiving cervical thrust manipulation in this study reported mild to moderate side events, such as transient neck soreness or headache following the treatment, but no severe adverse events were reported.[143]

Jull et al.[144] completed an RCT comparing physical therapy interventions for treatment of 200 patients who met the diagnostic criteria for CGH developed by Sjaastad et al.[141] who were randomly placed in one of the four physical therapy treatment groups of manual therapy, exercise therapy, combined manual therapy and exercise, and a control group. Beneficial effects were found for headache frequency and intensity and neck pain and disability for both manual therapy and exercise used alone and in combination at both 7-week and 12-month follow-up.[144] Of the participants receiving combined manual therapy and exercise, 10% more obtained good and excellent results, lending support for the combined use of specific therapeutic exercise and manual therapy to treat patients with CGHs.[144]

The manual therapy procedures employed by the physical therapists participating in the Jull et al. study[144] included both thrust manipulation and nonthrust mobilization techniques to the cervical spine. The therapeutic exercise regimen incorporated use of a pressure biofeedback unit to train the deep neck flexors, the longus capitis and colli, which are believed to be important in supporting the function of the cervical region.[144] In addition, the exercise regimen included training the muscles of the scapula, particularly the lower trapezius and serratus anterior muscles, to hold scapular adduction and retraction postural positions.[144] Postural instruction and training of the deep neck rotator muscles were also included in the exercise regimen.[144] Muscle-lengthening exercises were also incorporated based on the needs of the patient. Patients received eight to 12 treatment sessions with a physical therapist over a 6-week period. The physical therapists were allowed to vary their treatments based on the initial examination and subsequent reexaminations of the patients in the treatment groups.[144] A similar physical therapy treatment approach has shown to be effective in an RCT with patients aged 50 to 75 years with recurrent cervicogenic ($n = 23$), migraine ($n = 6$), tension-type ($n = 2$) and mixed ($n = 2$) headaches that combined 14 sessions of specific nonthrust mobilization with exercise training of the neck and postural muscles with a 9-month follow-up.[145] These studies illustrates the effectiveness of an impairment-based manual physical therapy approach that combines manual therapy and exercise for treatment of patients with CGH. Likewise, a systematic review concluded that a combination of cervical thrust manipulation and nonthrust mobilization combined with cervical and scapular muscle strengthening was most effective for decreasing the symptoms associated with CGHs.[140] Gross et al.[146] concluded in another systematic review based on 27 RCTs that specific strengthening and endurance exercises of the neck, scapulothoracic and shoulder muscles are supported by moderate quality evidence to be beneficial to treat neck pain and CGH. The AOPT ICF neck pain clinical practice guideline recommends specific neck and shoulder girdle exercises combined with cervicothoracic mobilization/manipulation for treatment of CGH based on moderate strength of evidence.[35]

Cervicogenic dizziness commonly occurs with WAD and can also be a component of CGH. The dizziness symptoms are commonly described as "lightheaded," "unsteady," and "off-balance."[147-149] The cause of cervicogenic dizziness is postulated to be resulting from disturbances to the afferent input from the cervical region caused by injury or chemical irritation as a result of inflammation to the dense network of mechanoreceptors located in the upper cervical spine joints and muscle soft tissues that normally supply proprioceptive input.[150] Before a diagnosis of cervicogenic dizziness can be made, central nervous system, vascular, and vestibular causes of dizziness must first be ruled out. Cervicogenic dizziness is commonly associated with neck pain and cervical spine impairments, including upper cervical spine myofascial and joint hypomobility with lower cervical hypermobility and poor neuromuscular control of deep neck flexors and deep neck extensor muscles. In addition, patients may present with any combination of impairments of balance, cervical joint position sense, and eye movement coordination. The cervical torsion test can be used to assist in differentiation between a vestibular and cervical cause of dizziness and should include assessment of the effect on dizziness symptoms with cervical rotation (head on neck), cervical torsion (body/neck on head motion), and en bloc (body with neck/head) motion.[151] See Fig. 6.39 for further details on performance of the cervical torsion test.

Cervical joint position sense error (JPSE) reflects a person's ability to accurately return his head to a predefined target after neck movement and is a major component of proprioception[152] and Box 6.6 (Fig. 6.24) describes the procedure used to measure JPSE. Cervical proprioception is the sense of position of the head or neck in space and describes the complex interaction between afferent and efferent receptors to the monitor the position and movement.[152] In a systematic review of that included 14 studies on cervical joint position sense error, four studies reported that participants with traumatic neck pain had a significantly higher JPSE than healthy controls.[152] Of the eight studies involving people with nontraumatic neck pain, four reported significant differences between the groups, and the JPSE did not vary between traumatic and nontraumatic neck-pain groups.[152] The JPSE is overall higher in neck pain groups of subjects when it is measured as a mean over at least six trials that typically includes cervical rotation left and right, and cervical flexion and/or extension.[152]

Cervicogenic dizziness can also affect vision and balance. The postulated mechanism is related to the mechanoreceptor input from the upper cervical spine muscles having direct access to a reflex center for coordination between vision and neck movement, which also converges in the central cervical nucleus that serves as a pathway to the cerebellum where vestibular, ocular, and proprioceptive information is integrated.[150] This allows the postural control system to quickly receive information about the position and movement of the head in relation to the body and to integrate cervical information with that from the labyrinths and eyes so that different information from the subsystems can be compared and equalized. Cervicogenic dizziness may also be linked to functional impairment of muscles, such as increased fatigability[150] or degenerative changes in the muscles, such as fiber transformation, fatty infiltration, and muscle inhibition or atrophy.[150] In addition, the effects of pain at various levels of the nervous system can change muscle spindle sensitivity and alter the cortical representation and modulation of cervical afferent input.[154] Psychosocial stresses might also alter muscle spindle activity via activation of the sympathetic nervous system.[155]

For rehabilitation of the visual disturbances associated with cervicogenic dizziness, training eye movement coordination with and without neck movements is recommended (Table 6.11).

Standing balance should also be assessed and trained at a level that challenges the patient with activities, such as standing with a narrow base of support, tandem standing, single leg balance, and standing on a foam pad. As the rehabilitation program is progressed, combining joint position sense training or eye movement coordination training with balance training can enhance functional outcomes with patients with deficits in these areas. Examples of tasks and progressions to improve sensorimotor control in neck disorders are provided in Table 6.11.

The treatment of impairments of the cervical spine with manual therapy techniques to address myofascial and joint restrictions and specific exercise training for motor control/strength deficits must be combined with the sensorimotor training in patients who present with cervicogenic dizziness to attain the best clinical outcomes.[156] A systematic review of the effects of manual therapy on the treatment of cervicogenic dizziness found low-level evidence for improvement in symptoms and signs of dizziness after manual therapy treatment.[157] Another RCT that studied 86 subjects with cervicogenic dizziness found significant reduction in cervicogenic dizziness symptoms after two treatment sessions by a physical therapist who used either upper cervical nonthrust mobilization techniques followed by neck ROM exercises or an upper cervical mobilization with movement technique (Fig. 6.66) compared with a placebo laser treatment. These improvements in dizziness symptoms from the nonthrust mobilization interventions were evident immediately after treatment and were still noted at a 12-week follow-up reassessment.[158]

Jull et al.[159] compared neck proprioception training to a craniocervical flexion motor training program in a group of 64 female patients with persistent neck pain and demonstrated that both training approaches improved the impaired cervical JPSE with marginally more benefit gained from proprioceptive training. The results suggest that improved proprioception following intervention with either exercise protocol may occur through an improved quality of cervical afferent input or by addressing input through direct training of relocation sense.[159] Another study[160] demonstrated significant improvement in neck JPSE immediately following a cervical thrust manipulation technique for a group of patients ($n = 36$) with chronic neck pain compared with a sham manipulation control group ($n = 18$). It seems that the best approach is to tailor the treatment approach to address the impairments identified at both the musculoskeletal and sensorimotor levels with a combination of manual therapy for joint and muscle impairments, specific exercises to address neck motor control deficits, and joint position sense, eye, and balance training to address impairments noted in the examination.[154]

BOX 6.6   Cervical Joint Position Sense Testing and Training

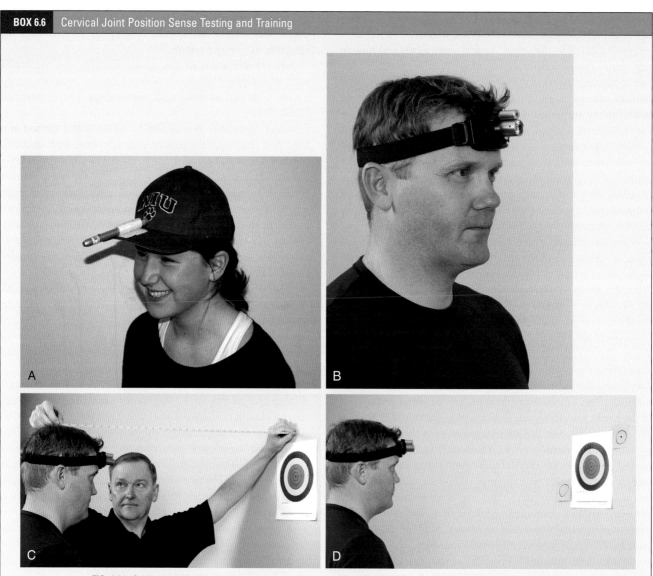

FIG. 6.24 A. Cervical joint position sense error can be measured and documented in a clinical setting by A, securing a laser pointer on a hat or headband or B, purchasing commercially available laser with a head halter, and C, the patient is positioned 90 cm from the top crown of the patient's head to the wall[11]. D, the laser can be used as a training tool for fine control and joint position sense of the cervical joints by using controlled movements along various targeted points in the ROM and by tracing pictorial patterns.

Test Procedure: The patient is asked to attain a natural, neutral rest position looking straight ahead at a blank piece of paper taped on the wall. The neutral position of the laser is marked on the paper. The patient is then asked to close his or her eyes, to fully rotate the neck, and then to return to the neutral start position with eyes closed. A second mark is recorded on the paper where the laser light is positioned. The amount of joint position error is determined by measuring the distance from the second mark to the first mark. This procedure can be repeated for rotation to the opposite direction and for cervical forward and backward bending.

Notes: An angular degree measurement of joint position error can be calculated by the following formula: angle = tan-1

[error distance/90 cm].[150] Therefore an approximately 7-cm error distance would translate to a meaningful error of 4.5 degrees, as long as the subject is sitting 90 cm from the wall.[150] Joint position error of greater than 4.5 degrees (7.1 cm) suggests impairment of relocation accuracy of the head and neck.[150,153] Minimal detectable change for this test has been reported as ranging from 0.44 degrees to 0.63 degrees.[153] After the joint position error is documented, the laser can be used as a training tool for fine control and joint position sense of the cervical joints by using controlled movements along various targeted points in the range of motion and by tracing pictorial patterns[11] (Table 6.11).

TABLE 6.11	Examples of Tasks and Progressions to Improve Sensorimotor Control in Neck Disorders	
AIM	**TASK**	**PROGRESSION**
Cervical position sense	With laser on a hat or headband for feedback, relocate back to neutral head position from head movements with eyes open	Eyes closed, check eyes open Relocate to points in range placed on wall, eyes closed, check eyes open Increase speed Perform in standing Perform on unstable surface
Cervical movement sense	With laser mounted on a hat or headband practice tracing over a pattern placed on the wall, eyes open	Increase speed More difficult and intricate pattern Small finer movements
Eye follow	Sitting in a neutral neck position, keeping the head still and the hands in the laps, move the laser light back and forth across the wall; follow the laser with the eyes only	Sit with neck in relative neck rotated position Eyes up and down, H pattern Increase speed Perform in standing Perform standing on an unstable surface
Gaze stability	Maintain gaze on a dot on the wall as the therapist passively moves the patient's trunk and/or head/neck Maintain gaze on a dot placed on the wall or ceiling as patient actively moves head/neck in all directions	Fix gaze, close eyes, move head and open eyes to check if maintained gaze Change the background of the target, plain, stripes, and checkers Change the focus point to words or a business card Increase speed Increase range of motion (ROM) Progress from lying to sitting to standing Perform on unstable surface
Eye-head coordination	Move eyes to a new focus point and then move the head in the same direction and return to neutral	Actively move head and eyes together same direction Move eyes one direction and the head opposite direction Move eyes and head together when peripheral vision restricted Move eyes, head, neck, and arm with and without vision restricted Rotate eyes, head, neck, and trunk looking as far behind as possible with and without vision restricted Hold a target, keep eyes fixed and move target; head and eyes move together
Balance	Maintain standing balance for 30 seconds	Eyes open, then closed Firm, then soft surface Different stances: comfortable, narrow, tandem, and single limb Walking with head movements—rotation, flexion, and extension—maintaining direction and velocity of gait Performing oculomotor or movement or position sense exercises while balance training

(Modified from Treleaven J. Sensorimotor disturbances in neck disorders affecting postural stability, head and eye movement control—part 2: case studies. *Man Ther.* 2008;13:266-275; Kristjansson E, Treleaven J. Sensorimotor function and dizziness in neck pain: implications for assessment and management. *J Orthop Sports Phys Ther.* 2009;39(5):364-377.)

EXAMINATION TECHNIQUES

SELECTED SPECIAL TESTS FOR CERVICAL SPINE EXAMINATION

 Sharp-Purser Test (Modified)

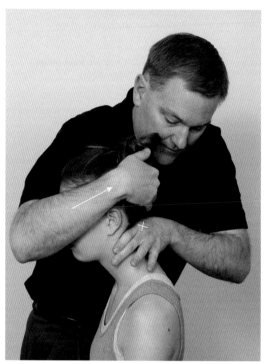

FIG. 6.25 See Video 6.2. Sharp-Purser test with use of forearm and shoulder to glide head.

PURPOSE	This test is used to detect atlantoaxial instability.
PATIENT POSITION	The patient is seated and asked to relax the head in a semiflexed position.
THERAPIST POSITION	The therapist stands at the side of the patient.
HAND PLACEMENT	Cranial hand: The upper arm is placed across the front of the patient's forehead, and the occiput is cupped with the hand.
	Caudal hand: The web space between the index finger and thumb is placed horizontally across the spinous process of C2.
PROCEDURE	The patient's forehead is pressed posteriorly with the cranial arm in a plane parallel with the superior aspect of C2 as the caudal hand provides a stabilizing force at C2. A sliding motion of the head posteriorly in relation to the axis is indicative of atlantoaxial instability. The manual maneuver reduces the atlantoaxial subluxation that occurs with a semiflexed posture in patients with atlantoaxial instability. Perception of excessive posterior glide of the cranium on the stabilized C2 or relief of pain with the manual gliding motion are considered positive findings.

▶ Sharp-Purser Test (Modified)—cont'd

NOTES   A positive Sharp-Purser test has been correlated with atlantoaxial instability in patients with RA at a specificity of 96% and predictive value of 85%.[161] In this study, the results of the Sharp-Purser test were compared with flexion radiograph results and were considered positive for instability if the results measured greater than 4 mm at the interval between the anterior arch of the atlas and the axis.[161] Positive Sharp-Purser test results indicate atlantoaxial instability, which is a contraindication to cervical manipulation techniques that place strain through the craniovertebral region. Atlantoaxial instability is common in RA from weakening of the transverse portion of the cruciate ligament that stabilizes the dens to the anterior arch of the atlas.

In a systematic review, Hutting et al.[162] pooled data from three studies and reported sensitivity ranged from 0.19 to 0.96, and specificity ranged from 0.71 to 1.00. PPVs ranged from 0.11 to 1.00, and negative predictive values ranged from 0.56 to 0.99. Specificity was adequate to rule in instability, but sensitivity was inadequate to rule out instability making the Sharp-Purser test an inadequate screening tool based on the current data.[162]

▶ Alar Ligament Stress Test

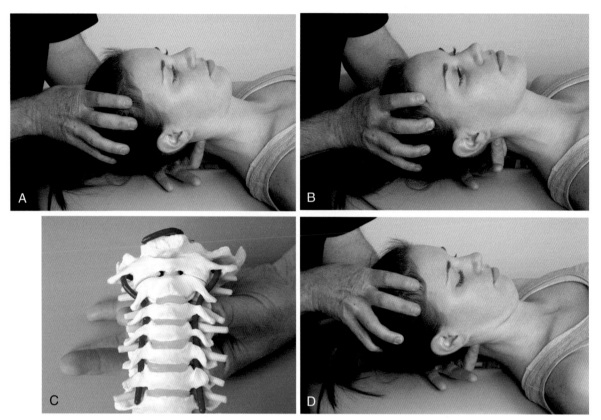

FIG. 6.26 See Video 6.3. A, Alar ligament test performed in neutral position. B, Alar ligament test performed in craniovertebral backward bent position. C, Finger placement on a spine model for the alar ligament test performed in supine. D, Alar ligament test performed in craniovertebral forward bent position.

PURPOSE	The purpose of this test is to determine the stability of the alar ligament and surrounding connective tissues of the craniovertebral region.
PATIENT POSITION	The patient is supine with the head on a pillow and the top of the head even with the edge of the table.
THERAPIST POSITION	The therapist stands at the head of the patient.
HAND PLACEMENT	The therapist firmly stabilizes C2 with the thumb and index finger of the left hand at the spinous process, laminae, and articular pillars of C2 while the right hand is positioned to hold the top of the patient's head.
PROCEDURE	The head and atlas are then side bent around the coronal axis of the atlantoaxial joint. Ipsilateral rotation of the axis is prevented by the stabilization of the C2. The end feel and the amount of motion are assessed. If the alar ligament is intact, little to no side bending can occur, and the end feel should be firm and capsular. The procedure is repeated in a craniovertebral forward bent position and in a craniovertebral backward bent position. Testing should be performed in three planes (neutral, flexion, and extension) to account for variation in alar ligament orientation. For this test to be considered positive for an alar ligament lesion, excessive movement in all three planes of testing should be evident.

Alar Ligament Stress Test: Alternative Technique

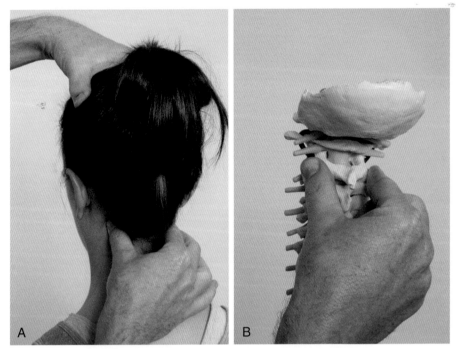

FIG. 6.27 A, Alar ligament test—alternative technique in sitting. B, Finger placement on spine model for alar ligament test performed in sitting.

The alar ligament test can also be performed in a seated position.

NOTES

Signs of instability from an upper cervical ligament stability test may include the following:92 1) increase in motion or empty end feel noted in all three test positions; 2) reproduction of symptoms of instability; 3) production of lateral nystagmus and nausea. The alar ligament stress test has been validated with MRI to demonstrate that strain is applied to the alar ligament with this maneuver.[163] The sitting variation of this test has reported a sensitivity of 80% and a specificity of 76.9% in a small group of patients ($n=7$) with positive MRI confirmed alar ligament lesions.[164]

▶ Anterior Shear Test (Transverse Ligament Stability Test)

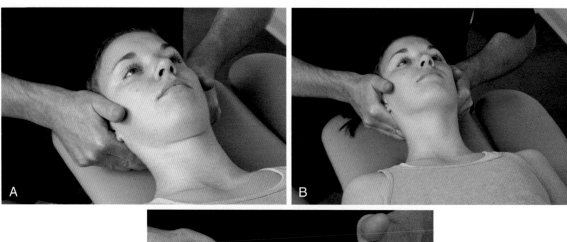

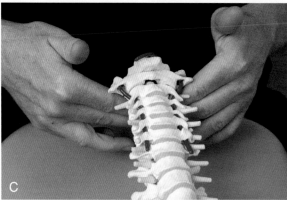

FIG. 6.28 See Video 6.4. A, Anterior shear test start position. B, Anterior shear test end position. C, Anterior shear test finger placement on spine model.

PURPOSE	The purpose of this test is to evaluate the stability of the upper cervical spine ligaments and membranes for signs of instability or reproduction of symptoms (such as headache, dizziness, or lower extremity paresthesia).
PATIENT POSITION	The patient is supine with the head and cervical spine supported in a neutral position on a pillow.
THERAPIST POSITION	The therapist stands at the head of the patient.
HAND PLACEMENT	The therapist supports the occiput in the palms of the hands and the third, fourth, and fifth fingers while the two index fingers are placed in the space between the occiput and the C2 spinous process overlying the neural arch of the atlas.
PROCEDURE	The head and C1 are then lifted (sheared) anteriorly together while the head is maintained in its neutral position and gravity fixes the rest of the neck. The patient is instructed to report any symptoms other than local pain and soreness.
NOTES	Signs of instability from an upper cervical ligament stability test may include the following:[92] (1) increase in motion or empty end feel, (2) reproduction of symptoms of instability, and (3) production of lateral nystagmus and nausea. The sensation of a lump in the throat may also indicate a positive test.
	Mintken et al.[165] described a case of a 23-year-old female with complaints of headaches and lower extremity paresthesia in which the lower extremity paresthesia was provoked with the anterior shear test and then the symptoms were relieved with the Sharp-Purser test. Subsequent radiographs and MRI revealed that the patient had a C2–C3 Klippel-Feil congenital fusion and os odontoideum.[165]

▶ Spurling Test[166]

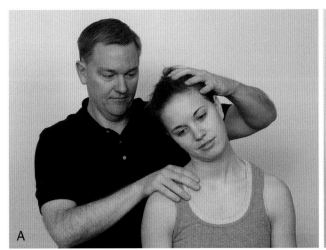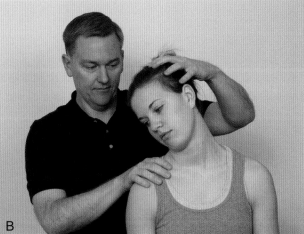

FIG. 6.29 See Video 6.5. A, Spurling test A. B, Spurling test B.

PURPOSE	Results of this pain provocation test are considered positive for cervical nerve root irritation if the patient reports reproduction or intensification of peripheral symptoms with application of the test maneuver.
PATIENT POSITION	The patient is seated in a straight-backed chair. Having the patient face a mirror is also helpful to monitor pain facial expressions during the test.
THERAPIST POSITION	The therapist stands behind the patient.
PROCEDURE	The therapist passively side bends the head toward the symptomatic side and applies compressive overpressure (approximately 7 kg) to the patient's head in the direction of the side bending to perform Spurling test A.
	The procedure for Spurling test B combines cervical extension and rotation with ipsilateral lateral flexion. Application of overpressure for Spurling test B is the same as in Spurling test A.[97]
NOTES	If the patient reports neck or arm symptom reproduction related to the condition at any point during performance of the test, results are considered positive and no further application of force is needed.
	Spurling test B was used on 255 patients who were referred for electrodiagnosis of the upper extremity nerve disorders.[167] Test results were scored positive if symptoms were reported beyond the elbow, and results were correlated with the results of the electrodiagnostic tests. The Spurling test had a sensitivity of 30% and a specificity of 93%, which means that it is not a very useful screening tool but that it is clinically useful to help confirm cervical radiculopathy.[167] Shabet at al[168] reported sensitivity of 95% and specificity of 94% in correlation of imaging findings and Spurling test B in 257 patients.
	Wainner et al.[97] reported kappa of 0.60 (0.32, 0.87) with sensitivity of 0.50, specificity of 0.86, –LR of 0.58 and +LR of 3.5 for correlation with electrophysiologic examination diagnosis of cervical radiculopathy for Spurling test A, and kappa of 0.62 (0.25, 0.99) with sensitivity of 0.50, specificity of 0.74, –LR of 0.67 and +LR of 1.9 for correlation with electrophysiologic examination diagnosis of cervical radiculopathy for Spurling test B.[97] Spurling test A is one of the four findings for the CPR for cervical radiculopathy.[97]

Arm Squeeze Test

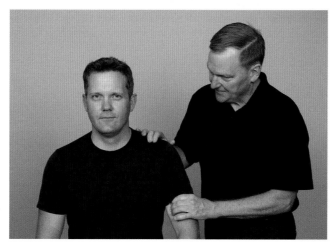

FIG. 6.30 Arm Squeeze Test.

PURPOSE	Test results are positive when the test reproduces arm pain associated with cervical radiculopathy. The test can be used to assist in diagnosis of cervical radiculopathy.
PATIENT POSITION	The patient is standing or sitting with arms relaxed at the side.
THERAPIST POSITION	The therapist stands directly behind and to the side of the patient.
HAND PLACEMENT	One hand rests on the patient's shoulder girdle while the other hand grasps the middle one-third of the patient's upper arm with the thumb at the triceps and fingers 2 to 5 across the biceps.
PROCEDURE	The therapist squeezes the middle one-third of the patient's arm with moderate force (6–8 kg) to provide compression to the skin, subcutaneous and muscle tissues and asks the patient to rate the level of pain (0–10) at the arm associated with the compression. The same level of compression force should then be applied at the acromioclavicular and the anterolateral-subacromial area of the same upper extremity, and the patient is asked to grade the level of pain (0–10) from compression to these two areas.
NOTES	A pain level difference of 3 points or more with compression of the middle one-third of the upper arm compared with the other compression locations is considered a positive test. Gumina et al.[169] reported sensitivity was 0.96; specificity ranged from 0.91 to 1; positive prognostic value ranged from 0.89 to 1; negative prognostic value ranged from 0.81 to 0.99; LRs for an abnormal test result ranged from 10.6 to 48 and LRs for a normal test result ranged from 0.04 to 0.44. The interobserver kappa value was 0.81 and the intraobserver kappa value was 0.87 demonstrating high levels of reliability and diagnostic accuracy for diagnosis of cervical radiculopathy when tested on 1567 patients with neck, arm, and shoulder symptoms and pain-free control subjects.

▶ Shoulder Abduction Test

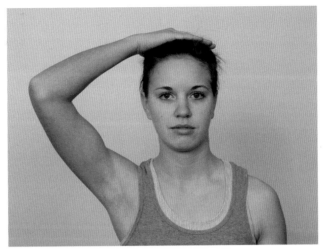

FIG. 6.31 See Video 6.6. Shoulder abduction test.

PURPOSE	If this position alleviates the patient's radicular arm pain, nerve root irritation is suggested as the cause of the arm pain.
PATIENT POSITION	The patient is positioned sitting.
PROCEDURE	The patient is seated and asked to place the hand of the symptomatic extremity on the head. Positive test results occur with reduction or elimination of symptoms.[97] The therapist should ask open-ended questions with this test, such as, "Does this change your symptoms in any way?"
NOTES	Wainner et al.[97] reported a kappa value of 0.20 (0.00, 0.59) with sensitivity of 0.17, specificity of 0.92, –LR of 0.91 and +LR of 2.1 for correlation with electrophysiologic examination diagnosis of cervical radiculopathy.[97] Likewise, Viikari-Juntura[170] reported sensitivity of 0.47, specificity of 0.85, –LR of 0.63 and +LR of 3.03. Therefore this test demonstrates poor reliability and poor diagnostic accuracy. However, there may be a subgroup of patients with cervical radiculopathy who will report relief of radicular symptoms with attaining the arm position associated with this test.

▶ Neck Distraction Test

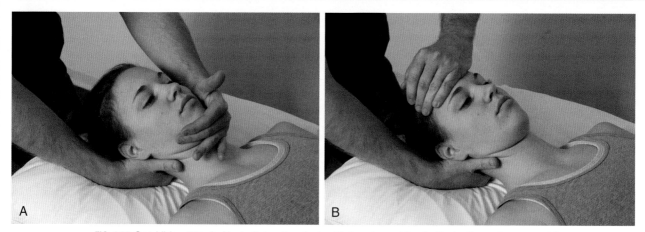

FIG. 6.32 See Video 6.7. A, Neck distraction test with hand on chin. B, Neck distraction test with hand on forehead.

PURPOSE	Test results are positive if the patient reports a reduction of symptoms with application of cervical distraction force. The test is used to assist in diagnosis of cervical radiculopathy.
PATIENT POSITION	The patient is supine with the head resting on a small pillow and the crown of the head even with the top edge of the table.
THERAPIST POSITION	The therapist sits or stands at the head of the treatment table.
HAND PLACEMENT	Dominant hand: The fingers are together with the thumb spread across the occiput to cradle the posterior aspect of the patient's cranium. Nondominant hand: The therapist cups the patient's chin with the fingers or cups the anterior aspect of the patient's forehead.
PROCEDURE	The therapist flexes the patient's neck to a position of comfort by lifting the head off the pillow (20–25 degrees from horizontal) and gradually applies a distraction force up to 14 kg.[97]
NOTES	If this test alleviates symptoms, manual or mechanical cervical traction should be incorporated into the plan of care. The therapist should ask open-ended questions with this test such as, "Does this change your symptoms in any way?" Wainner et al.[97] reported a kappa value of 0.88 (0.64, 1.0) sensitivity of 0.44, specificity of 0.90, –LR of 0.62 and +LR of 4.4 for correlation with electrophysiologic examination diagnosis of cervical radiculopathy.[97] This test is one of the four findings for the CPR to diagnose cervical radiculopathy.[97]

▶ Neck Traction Test

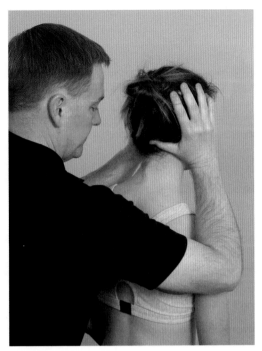

FIG. 6.33 See Video 6.8. Neck traction test.

PURPOSE	Test results are positive if the patient reports a reduction of upper-extremity radicular symptoms with application of cervical distraction force. The test is used to detect signs of cervical radiculopathy.
PATIENT POSITION	The patient sits or stands (preferably facing a mirror).
THERAPIST POSITION	The therapist sits or stands directly behind the patient.
HAND PLACEMENT	The thumbs and thenar eminences of both hands are molded across the inferior aspect of the patient's occiput and the mastoid processes with the forearms placed across the superior aspect of the patient's shoulders.
PROCEDURE	The therapist gradually applies a distraction force by lifting the patient's head superiorly to create cervical traction. Test results are positive if the patient's symptoms are alleviated during the traction.
NOTES	If this test alleviates symptoms, manual or mechanical cervical traction should be incorporated into the plan of care. The therapist should ask open-ended questions with this test such as, "Does this change your symptoms in any way?" Bertilson et al.[171] reported kappa scores of 0.49 if the therapist did not have knowledge of the patient's history and kappa scores of 0.45 if the therapist had knowledge of the patient's history when this test was performed on 100 patients with neck or shoulder problems with or without radiating pain.

Upper Limb Neurodynamic Test 1[172–174]

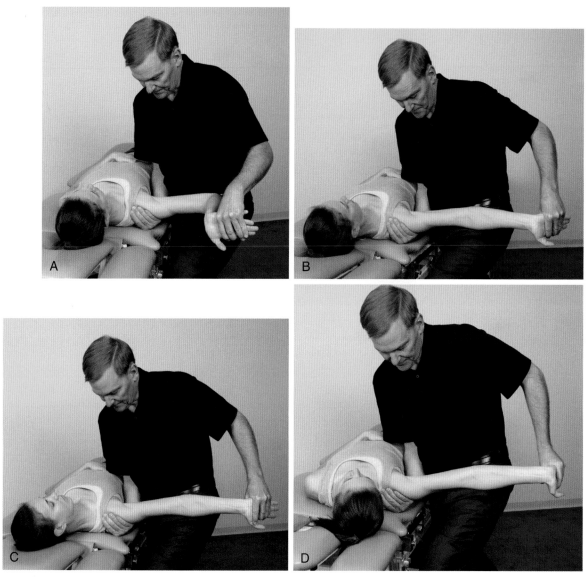

FIG. 6.34 See Video 6.9. A, Upper limb neurodynamic (ULND) test 1, start position. B, ULND test 1, end position. C, ULND test 1, end position with contralateral side flexion. D, ULND test 1, end position with ipsilateral side flexion.

▶ Upper Limb Neurodynamic Test 1—cont'd

PURPOSE

The purpose of this test is to apply tension through the brachial plexus and nerve root sleeves of the cervical spine to determine whether the cause of upper extremity symptoms originates from sensitivity of the cervical nerve roots and surrounding connective tissues. ULND test 1 is designed to focus tension on the median nerve and its corresponding nerve roots.

PATIENT POSITION

The patient lies supine.

THERAPIST POSITION

The therapist stands with a diagonal stance on the side to be tested with the most lateral leg forward and the thigh positioned up against the inferior aspect of the upper arm and the patient's shoulder positioned at 90 to 110 degrees abduction.

HAND PLACEMENT

Left hand: The left hand reaches up and under the posterior aspect of the patient's scapula to place the hand across the posterior and superior aspect of the scapula to depress the shoulder girdle.

Right hand: The therapist's other hand is placed across the palmar surface of the patient's left hand and fingers.

PROCEDURE

The therapist passively depresses the patient's scapula and brings the shoulder to 90 to 110 degrees abduction and 10 degrees horizontal extension and holds this position as the left hand sequentially: (1) extends the wrist and fingers and supinates the patient's forearm, (2) laterally rotates the shoulder, and (3) extends the elbow. The patient is asked to report upper-extremity symptoms throughout the maneuver. Typically, symptoms occur during the final phase of the test with elbow extension. The test results are positive if the patient's symptoms are reproduced with this maneuver and the symptoms can be changed with further structural differentiation.[175] The therapist should note the degree of elbow extension where the symptoms occur. Both sides should be tested, and a difference between sides of greater than 10 degrees may be considered a positive test result.[97]

NOTES

Cervical lateral flexion to the contralateral side can be added as a structural differentiation to further sensitize the neural structures to attempt to elicit positive test results or to generate a positive response sooner in the test sequence. Ipsilateral lateral neck flexion should also be added as a follow-up to a positive test to confirm the findings. If a greater degree of elbow extension is required to elicit positive test results when the neck is placed in ipsilateral lateral flexion, this confirms the positive test findings are from a neural dynamic disorder likely originating from the cervical spine rather than tight upper-extremity muscles. Further tension to the neural system can be added by having a second therapist add a passive straight leg raise on the ipsilateral side before retesting, which applies further tension to dural and neural structures to determine whether loss of central dural extensibility has occurred. Also end ROM sensations of tension, tautness, and tingling may be considered normal, especially if they are at the end of the test range and are present bilaterally. Schmid et al.[176] reported intertester reliability of kappa value of 0.54 with standard error of 0.18. Wainner et al.[97] reported a kappa value of 0.76 (0.51, 1.0). This test is one of the four findings for the CPR for cervical radiculopathy and was the best test in the cluster for ruling out cervical radiculopathy with sensitivity of 0.97, specificity of 0.22, −LR of 0.12 and +LR of 1.3 for correlation with electrophysiologic examination diagnosis of cervical radiculopathy.[97]

▶ Upper Limb Neurodynamic Test 2a[172–174]

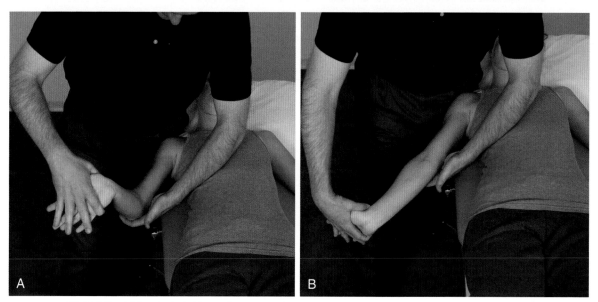

FIG. 6.35 See Video 6.10. A, Upper limb neurodynamic (ULND) test 2a, start position. B, ULND test 2a, end position.

PURPOSE	The test is used to apply tension through the brachial plexus and nerve root sleeves of the cervical spine to determine whether the cause of upper-extremity symptoms originates from irritation of the cervical nerve roots and surrounding connective tissues. ULND test 2a is designed to focus tension on the median nerve and its corresponding nerve roots.
PATIENT POSITION	patient lies supine with the test side shoulder positioned slightly over the edge of the table.
THERAPIST POSITION	The therapist stands with a diagonal stance on the side to be tested with the left hip placed firmly across the superior aspect of the patient's shoulder girdle.
HAND PLACEMENT	Left hand: The left hand supports the patient's upper arm and elbow. Right hand: The therapist's right hand is placed across the palmar surface of the patient's right hand and fingers.
PROCEDURE	The therapist passively depresses the patient's scapula with the hip with the shoulder in 10 degrees abduction and 10 degrees horizontal extension and holds this position as the right hand sequentially: (1) supinates the patient's forearm, (2) laterally rotates the shoulder, (3) extends the wrist and fingers, and (4) extends the elbow. The patient is asked to report upper extremity symptoms throughout the maneuver. Typically, symptoms occur during the final phase of the test with elbow extension. The test results are positive if the patient's symptoms are reproduced with this maneuver and the symptoms can be changed with further structural differentiation.[175] The therapist should note the degree of elbow extension where the symptoms occur. Both sides should be tested, and a difference between sides of greater than 10 degrees may be considered a positive test result.[97]

Upper Limb Neurodynamic Test 2a—cont'd

NOTES   Cervical lateral flexion to the contralateral side can be added as a structural differentiation to further sensitize the neural structures to attempt to elicit positive test results or to generate a positive response sooner in the test sequence. Ipsilateral lateral neck flexion could also be added as a follow-up to a positive test to confirm the findings. If a greater degree of elbow extension is needed to elicit positive test results when the neck is placed in ipsilateral lateral flexion, this confirms that the cause of the positive test findings is from a neural dynamic disorder likely originating from the cervical spine rather than tight upper-extremity muscles. Further sensitization can be added by having a second therapist add a passive straight leg raise on the ipsilateral side before retesting, which applies further tension to dural and neural structures to determine whether a loss of central dural extensibility has occurred. Also end ROM sensations of tension, tautness, and tingling may be considered normal, especially if they are at the end of the test range and are present bilaterally. Schmid et al.[176] reported intertester reliability of kappa value of 0.46 with standard error of 0.18.

▶ Upper Limb Neurodynamic Test 2b[172–174]

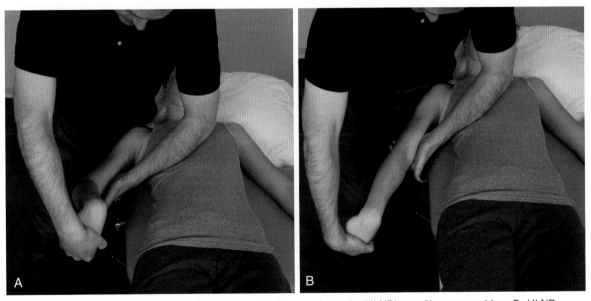

FIG. 6.36 See Video 6.11. A, Upper limb neurodynamic (ULND) test 2b, start position. B, ULND test 2b, end position.

Upper Limb Neurodynamic Test 2b—cont'd

PURPOSE	This test is used to apply tension through the brachial plexus and nerve root sleeves of the cervical spine to determine whether the cause of upper-extremity symptoms originates from irritation of the cervical nerve roots and surrounding connective tissues. In theory, ULND test 2b is designed to focus tension on the radial nerve and its corresponding roots.
PATIENT POSITION	patient lies supine with the test side shoulder positioned slightly over the edge of the table.
THERAPIST POSITION	The therapist stands with a diagonal stance on the side to be tested with the left hip placed firmly across the superior aspect of the patient's shoulder girdle.
HAND PLACEMENT	Left hand: The left hand supports the patient's upper arm and elbow.
	Right hand: The therapist's right hand is placed across the dorsal surface of the patient's right hand and fingers.
PROCEDURE	The therapist passively depresses the patient's scapula and holds this position with the front of the left hip and sequentially introduces: 1) shoulder medial rotation, 2) full elbow extension, and 3) wrist and finger flexion. The patient is asked to report any upper-extremity symptoms throughout the maneuver. Typically, symptoms occur during the final phase of the test with wrist flexion. The therapist can document the test results as positive and note the degree of wrist flexion where the symptoms occurred. Both sides should be tested, and a wrist flexion difference between sides of greater than 10 degrees may be considered a positive test result. The test results are positive if the patient's symptoms are reproduced with this maneuver and the symptoms can be changed with further structural differentiation.[175]
NOTES	Cervical lateral flexion to the contralateral side can be added as a structural differentiation to further sensitize the neural structures to attempt to elicit positive test results or to generate a positive response sooner in the test sequence. Ipsilateral lateral neck flexion could also be added as a follow-up to positive test results to confirm the findings. If a greater degree of wrist flexion is needed to elicit positive test results when the neck is placed in ipsilateral lateral flexion, this helps to confirm that the cause of the positive test findings is a neural tension disorder likely originating from the cervical spine rather than tight forearm muscles. Further sensitization can be added by having a second therapist add a passive straight leg raise on the ipsilateral side before retesting, which applies further tension to dural and neural structures to determine whether a loss of central dural extensibility has occurred. Wainner et al.[97] reported a kappa value of 0.83 (0.65, 1.0) with sensitivity of 0.72, specificity of 0.33, −LR of 0.85 and +LR of 1.1 for correlation for agreement with electrophysiologic examination diagnosis of cervical radiculopathy. Schmid et al.[176] reported intertester reliability of kappa value of 0.44 with standard error of 0.18. Therefore this test has fair to good reliability for reproduction of symptoms, but minimal to no ability to diagnose or rule out cervical radiculopathy as originally described. Manvell et al.[177] measured nerve tension on cadavers during upper limb positioning variations and found that the addition of the following sensitizing maneuvers: 40-degree shoulder abduction, 25-degree shoulder extension, wrist ulnar deviation and thumb flexion to the ULNT2b test places maximum tension on the radial nerve without adding tension to the median or ulnar nerves, which may help to enhance to diagnostic accuracy of this test.

▶ Upper Limb Neurodynamic Test 3[172–174]

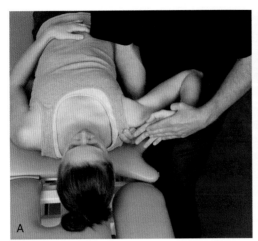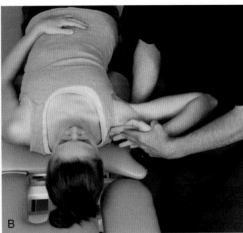

Fig. 6.37 See Video 6.12. A, Upper limb neurodynamic (ULND) test 3, start position. B, ULND test 3, end position.

PURPOSE	This test is used to apply tension through the brachial plexus and nerve root sleeves of the cervical spine to determine whether the cause of upper-extremity symptoms originates from irritation of the cervical nerve roots and surrounding connective tissues. In theory, ULND test 3 is designed to focus tension on the ulna nerve and its corresponding nerve roots.
PATIENT POSITION	The patient lies supine.
THERAPIST POSITION	The therapist stands with a diagonal stance on the side to be tested.
HAND PLACEMENT	Left hand: The therapist's left hand is placed across the palmar surface of the patient's right hand and fingers.
	Right hand: The right hand reaches up and under the posterior aspect of the patient's right scapula to place a hand across the posterior and superior aspect of the shoulder girdle to depress the scapula.
PROCEDURE	The therapist passively depresses the patient's scapula and holds this position as the left hand of the therapist sequentially introduces: (1) shoulder lateral rotation, (2) full elbow flexion, (3) forearm pronation, (4) wrist and finger extension, and (5) shoulder abduction (applied with the thigh of the therapist's front leg). The patient is asked to report any upper-extremity symptoms throughout the maneuver. Typically, symptoms occur during the final phase of the test with shoulder abduction. The test results are positive if the patient's symptoms are reproduced with this maneuver and the symptoms can be changed with further structural differentiation.[175] The therapist should note the degree of shoulder abduction where the symptoms occur. Both sides should be tested, and a difference between sides of greater than 10 degrees may be considered a positive test result.[97]
NOTES	Cervical lateral flexion to the contralateral side can be added as a structural differentiation to further sensitize the neural structures to attempt to elicit positive test results or to generate a positive response sooner in the test sequence. Ipsilateral lateral neck flexion could also be added as a follow-up to positive test results to confirm the findings. If a greater degree of shoulder abduction is needed to elicit positive test results when the neck is placed in ipsilateral lateral flexion, this helps to confirm that the cause of the positive test findings is a neurodynamic disorder likely originating from the cervical spine rather than tight upper-extremity muscles. Further sensitization can be added by having a second therapist add a passive straight leg raise on the ipsilateral side before retesting, which applies further tension to dural and neural structures to determine whether a loss of central dural extensibility has occurred. Schmid et al.[176] reported intertester reliability of kappa value of 0.36 with standard error of 0.18.

▶ Rotation-Extension Vertebral Artery Test

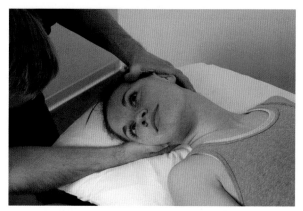

FIG. 6.38 See Video 6.13. Rotation-extension vertebral artery test.

PURPOSE	The purpose of this test is to screen for vertebral artery insufficiency and collateral circulation to the brain.
PATIENT POSITION	The patient is supine with the head on a pillow and the top of the head even with the top edge of the table.
THERAPIST POSITION	The therapist stands at the head of the patient.
HAND PLACEMENT	Left hand: The hand supports the left side of the patient's head with the fingers spread.
	Right hand: The hand supports the right side of the patient's head with the fingers spread.
PROCEDURE	The therapist must instruct the patient to look at the therapist's forehead throughout the procedure, and the therapist must move with the patient to maintain a clear view of the patient's eyes throughout the procedure to assess for nystagmus. The therapist must also continually seek verbal feedback from the patient throughout the test. A delayed response or a report of dizziness, lightheadedness, or nausea is considered positive. As the therapist supports the patient's head, the cervical spine is slowly rotated to the right to the end of available range. The therapist pauses in this position for 3 to 5 seconds to assess the patient's response. If the test results are still negative, the therapist gently adds lateral flexion to the right and extension and holds this position for 5 to 10 seconds. If the test results are negative, the therapist repeats to the opposite side.
NOTES	If the patient has a positive response, the therapist repositions the head to a neutral or slightly flexed position immediately and continues to monitor the patient. The therapist supports the patient's head on one or two pillows and passively positions the patient's legs in a 90/90 position either on a stool or on the therapist's shoulders. The therapist continues to monitor the patient until the positive response completely subsides.
	Cote et al.[178] showed that this test has a sensitivity of approximately 0, which indicates a high likelihood of false-negative results from this commonly performed screening examination procedure.
	In a systematic review that included four studies, Hutting et al.[179] reported sensitivity was low and ranged from 0% to 57%, specificity from 67% to 100%, PPV from 0% to 100%, and negative predictive value from 26% to 96%. The +LR ranged from 0.22 to 83.25 and the −LR from 0.44 to 1.40. The authors concluded that the data on diagnostic accuracy indicate that this premanipulative test is not a valid premanipulative screening procedure.[179] The International Federation of Orthopaedic Manipulative Physical Therapists (IFOMPT) vascular pathology of the neck workgroup does not include this type of testing in the clinical reasoning framework for screening for vascular pathology of the neck before cervical spinal manual therapy treatment.[180]
	See Chapter 3 for more information regarding premanipulation screening.

Cervical Torsion Test (Body on Head Rotation Test)

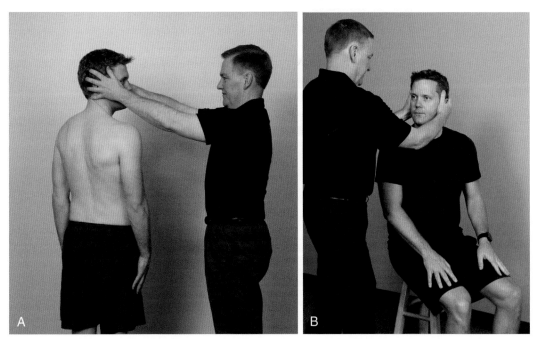

FIG. 6.39 See Video 6.14. A, Cervical torsion test. B, Cervical torsion test sitting on a stool.

PURPOSE	This test screens for a cervical cause for a dizziness symptom (cervicogenic dizziness) while avoiding vestibular activation by avoiding head and inner ear movements. This test should be performed if active cervical rotation causes dizziness.
PATIENT POSITION	The patient stands or sits directly facing the therapist.
THERAPIST POSITION	The therapist stands in front of the patient and holds each side of the patient's head.
PROCEDURE	As the therapist holds the patient's head, the patient is asked to close their eyes and to rotate the body fully toward one side at least 45 degrees and hold that position for 30 seconds as the therapist monitors the patient's response. The procedure is repeated toward the opposite direction.
NOTES	Dizziness caused by active cervical rotation could be resulting from either a vestibular or cervical impairments. The results of this test should be compared with "en bloc" head and neck/trunk rotation (moving head and neck/trunk together), which challenges the vestibular system, but not the cervical. The eyes are closed to avoid visually induced dizziness. If dizziness is noted with cervical rotation and en bloc rotation, but does not occur with the cervical torsion test, the patient may be a candidate for vestibular rehabilitation. If a patient has a positive cervical torsion test and a vascular cause of dizziness has been ruled out, the patient should be treated for cervicogenic dizziness. This test is most commonly performed if the patient has reported dizziness symptoms with testing active or passive cervical rotation movements. This test is best performed with the patient in a seated position. Treleanven et al.[151] reported five of 147 asymptomatic participants reported some symptoms (mild dizziness, visual disturbances, unusual eye movements on opening eyes after the test, motion sickness, or nausea) on one or more of the three test components of this test (rotation, torsion, or en bloc). The specificity when using a positive response to the cervical torsion test (i.e., a negative response to the rotation or en bloc components) was high for the cervical torsion test, 98.64%.[151]

Upper Trapezius Muscle Length Test and Hold/Relax Stretch

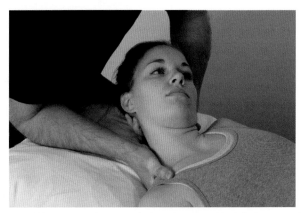

FIG. 6.40 Upper trapezius muscle length test and hold/relax stretch.

PURPOSE	The purpose of this test is to assess the length and stretch the upper trapezius muscle.
PATIENT POSITION	The patient is supine with the head resting on a pillow.
HAND PLACEMENT	Left hand: The left hand cradles the patient's occiput.
	Right hand: The web space and radial aspect of the metacarpal phalange joint are placed firmly across the superior aspect of the first rib and the superior aspect of the scapula.
PROCEDURE	The therapist depresses and holds the right shoulder girdle as the neck is moved into slight forward bending, full contralateral (left) lateral flexion, and ipsilateral (right) rotation. For the stretch, once in the end-range position, the patient is asked to elevate the right shoulder as the therapist holds the shoulder into a depressed position to create an isometric contraction of the upper trapezius. After a 10-second isometric hold, the patient is instructed to relax, and the tissue slack is taken up and held 10 seconds with further shoulder depression or further cervical left side bending, forward bending, or right rotation. This sequence is repeated three to four times and can be followed with instruction in a home stretching program, with the stretch position sustained for 30 to 60 seconds two to three times per day.

Levator Scapula Muscle Length Test and Hold/Relax Stretch

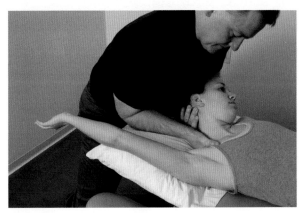

FIG. 6.41 Levator scapula muscle length test and hold/relax stretch.

PURPOSE	The purpose of this test is to assess the length and stretch the levator scapula muscle.
PATIENT POSITION	The patient is supine with the head resting on a pillow with the ipsilateral (right) arm fully flexed.
HAND PLACEMENT	Left hand: The left hand cradles the patient's occiput.
	Right hand: The web space and radial aspect of the metacarpal phalange joint are placed firmly across the superior aspect of the first rib and superior medial angle of the scapula.
PROCEDURE	The therapist depresses and holds the right shoulder girdle as the neck is moved into slight forward bending, full contralateral (left) lateral flexion, and contralateral (left) rotation. For the stretch, once in the end-range position, the patient is asked to elevate the right shoulder as the therapist holds the scapula into a depressed position to create an isometric contraction of the levator scapula. After a 10-second isometric hold, the patient is instructed to relax and the tissue slack is taken up and held 10 seconds with further shoulder depression or further cervical left side bending, forward bending, or left rotation. This sequence is repeated for three to four repetitions and can be followed with instruction in a home stretching program, with the stretch position sustained for 30 to 60 seconds two to three times per day.

PASSIVE INTERVERTEBRAL MOTION TESTING

 Craniovertebral Forward- and Backward-Bending Passive Physiologic Intervertebral Motion Test

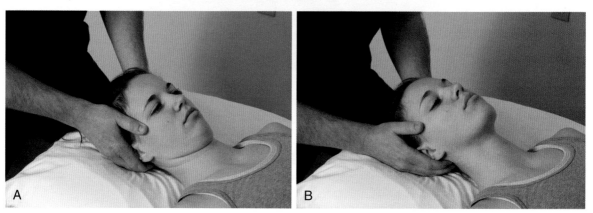

Fig. 6.42 See Video 6.15. A, Craniovertebral forward-bending passive physiologic intervertebral motion (PPIVM) test. B, Craniovertebral backward-bending PPIVM test.

PURPOSE	The purpose of this test is to evaluate the passive forward and backward bending of the cranium (occiput) in relation to C1 and C2.
PATIENT POSITION	The patient is supine with the head on a pillow and the top of the head even with the edge of the table.
THERAPIST POSITION	The therapist stands at the head of the patient.
HAND PLACEMENT	Both hands gently grasp the posterior and lateral aspect of the cranium.
PROCEDURE	Both hands are used to gently isolate craniovertebral backward and forward bending while avoiding full cervical spine movement. Overpressure is applied to assess the end feel and the level of reactivity.
NOTES	The normal amount of craniovertebral forward and backward bending is approximately 10 to 30 degrees of each (Table 6.2). Passive movement restrictions are commonly found with patients with CGH, forward head posture, and mid-cervical instability. The chin tends to deviate toward the side of the craniovertebral restriction with backward bending and away from the side of the restriction with forward bending.

Craniovertebral Side Bending Passive Physiologic Intervertebral Motion Test

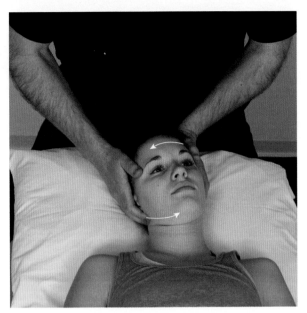

FIG. 6.43 See Video 6.16. Craniovertebral side bending passive physiologic intervertebral motion test.

PURPOSE	This test evaluates the passive side bending of the cranium (occiput) in relation to C1 and C2.
PATIENT POSITION	The patient is supine with the head on a pillow and the top of the head even with the edgethe table.
THERAPIST POSITION	The therapist stands at the head of the patient.
HAND PLACEMENT	Both hands gently grasp the head.
PROCEDURE	Both hands are used to gently side bend the patient's head to the right while avoiding neck movement. The amount of passive side bending available to the right is noted. Overpressure is applied to assess the end feel and the level of reactivity. The procedure is repeated with side bending the head to the left. The amount of motion is noted and compared with the other side. Another variation of this technique is to attempt to palpate movement of transverse process of C1 toward the direction of the side bending motion as passive side bending is induced.
NOTES	The axis of the movement should be through the patient's nose. The normal amount of craniovertebral side bending is approximately 5 to 15 degrees. Passive movement restrictions are commonly found with patients with CGH, forward head posture, and mid-cervical instability. Olsonet al.[181] assessed interrater reliability of craniovertebral side bending in five different positions and found poor interrater (kappa values, −0.03-0.18) and intrarater (kappa values, −0.02-0.14) reliability in all positions. The "Paris physiologic neutral position" with neck flexed approximately 20 degrees proved to be the most reliable position to test craniovertebral side bending.[181] Piva et al.[182] reported kappa values of 0.35 (0.15–0.49) for assessment of mobility asymmetry and 0.35 (0.15–0.55) for pain provocation intertester reliability in 30 patients.

Flexion-Rotation Test (Craniovertebral Rotation Passive Intervertebral Motion Test in Full Cervical Forward Bending)

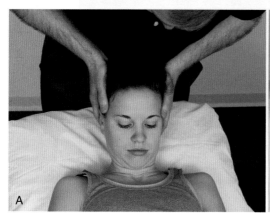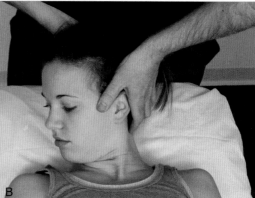

FIG. 6.44 See Video 6.17. A, Start position for the flexion-rotation test. B, End position for the flexion-rotation test.

PURPOSE	The purpose of this test is to evaluate the passive craniovertebral rotation primarily of the C1–C2 segment with the lower cervical spine locked with ligamentous tension.
PATIENT POSITION	The patient is supine with the head on a pillow and the top of the head even with the edge of the table.
THERAPIST POSITION	The therapist stands at the head of the patient.
HAND PLACEMENT	Both hands gently grasp the side of the patient's head.
PROCEDURE	The therapist holds the patient's head and neck in a fully flexed position with the posterior aspect of the cranium supported with the therapist's abdomen. While holding the head and neck in the fully flexed position, the therapist gently rotates the head to end range in one direction and then repeats in the other direction. Left versus right is compared.
NOTES	Asymmetry of movement or pain provocation is noted. Limitations in movement with this test are believed to be the result of stiffness of the C1–C2 spinal segment.

The flexion-rotation test average ROM in healthy individuals is 44 degrees.[183] Ogince et al.[184] demonstrated that highly trained manual therapists using the flexion-rotation test have high sensitivity (0.91) and specificity (0.90) in identifying individuals with CGHs. In clinical practice, the test is deemed positive if there is a 10 degree reduction in the visually estimated range to either side, and this method of test interpretation has been shown to be valid and reliable when compared with goniometry.[183]

Manual examination of the cervical spine was found to be reliable in 60 subjects with CGH with kappa coefficient for interrater reliability of 0.68 for agreement on the most symptomatic segment with PAIVM testing of the upper cervical spine. Examiners identified the C1–C2 segment as the most common symptomatic segment, with 63% of cases positive at this segment.[185] The high frequency of C1–C2 segmental involvement in CGH highlights the importance of examination and treatment procedures for this motion segment.[185] Hall et al.[185] reported a minimal detectable change (MDC) of 7 degrees and intratester reliability of kappa = 0.95 with good consistency in findings over a 2-week time frame in testing patients with CGHs with the flexion-rotation test. In the three studies that examined the flexion-rotation test,[186–188] the sensitivity ranged from 70 to 91.3% and specificity from 70% to 92% with a +LR higher than 5 and a −LR lesser than 0.2, indicating the ability to alter significantly the posttest probability for diagnosis of CGH.[189]

Craniovertebral Rotation Passive Intervertebral Motion Test in Full Cervical Lateral Flexion

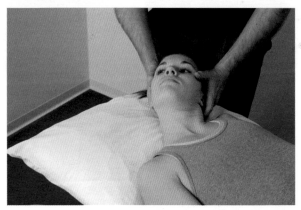

FIG. 6.45 See Video 6.18. Craniovertebral rotation passive intervertebral motion test in full cervical lateral flexion.

PURPOSE	This test evaluates the passive craniovertebral rotation primarily of the C1–C2 segment with the lower cervical spine locked with ligamentous and joint capsular tension.
PATIENT POSITION	The patient is supine with the head on a pillow and the top of the head even with the edge of the table.
THERAPIST POSITION	The therapist stands at the head of the patient.
HAND PLACEMENT	Both hands gently grasp the side of the patient's head.
PROCEDURE	The therapist brings the patient's head and neck to a fully laterally flexed position and then gently rotates the head to the opposite direction of the lateral flexion to the end range in one direction and then repeats in the other direction. Left versus right is compared.
NOTES	Asymmetry of movement or pain provocation is noted. Limitations in movement with this test are believed to be the result of stiffness of the C1–C2 spinal segment.
	Piva et al.[182] reported kappa values of 0.30 (0.17–0.43) for assessment of mobility asymmetry and 0.61 (0.5–0.72) for pain provocation intertester reliability in 30 patients.

▶ Cervical Downglide (Downslope) Passive Intervertebral Motion Test

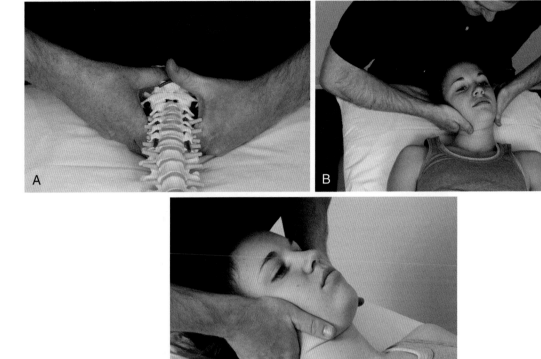

FIG. 6.46 See Video 6.19. A, Hand placement for mid-cervical downglide passive intervertebral motion (PIVM). B, Cervical downglide PIVM (frontal view). Cervical downglide PIVM (frontal view). C, Cervical downglide PIVM (lateral view).

PURPOSE	This test is used to evaluate the passive downglide of cervical segments C2–C3 through C7–T1.
PATIENT POSITION	The patient is supine with the head on a pillow and the top of the head even with the top edge of the table.
THERAPIST POSITION	The therapist stands at the head of the patient.
HAND PLACEMENT	Left hand: The radial border of the metacarpophalangeal joint of the index finger is used to contact the articular pillar of the specified segment, and the fourth and fifth fingers are used to support the patient's head.
	Right hand: The radial border of the metacarpophalangeal joint of the index finger is used to contact the articular pillar of the specified segment, and the fourth and fifth fingers are used to support the patient's head.

Cervical Downglide (Downslope) Passive Intervertebral Motion Test—cont'd

PROCEDURE

Both hands are used to gently grasp the patient's head and neck. The neck is brought into slight flexion (approximately 20 degrees), and the top of the patient's head rests on the therapist's abdomen. The radial border of the metacarpophalangeal joint of the index fingers on both hands is used to contact the articular pillars of C2. The fourth and fifth fingers of both hands are used to support the base of the patient's skull. Right side bending is induced by applying a force (through the contact point of the right hand) that is directed to the left and slightly caudally as the top of the patient's head continues to rest on the stationary therapist's abdomen. The amount of passive downglide available at the segment is noted. Also any swelling or tenderness is noted. Left side bending is induced by applying a force (through the contact point of the left hand) that is directed to the right and slightly caudally as the top of the patient's head continues to rest on the stationary therapist's abdomen. The amount of passive downglide available is noted, as is any swelling or tenderness. The procedure is repeated with assessment of the mobility of the remaining cervical segments. The amount of passive downglide available at each segment and in each direction is noted and compared.

NOTES

This technique can be performed by starting at C2 and proceeding caudally. When the right C2 articular pillar is contacted, the segment being tested is described as a downglide PIVM test of the right C2–C3 facet joint. Counting down from C2 allows for easy location of the cervical vertebrae. The top of the patient's head is supported by the therapist's abdomen and should not move, but rather, the side bending is induced from the passive downgliding motion imparted from the therapist's hand. Also the therapist should be sure that the top of the patient's head is even with the edge of the table and not off the edge of the table. If this procedure induces a pain response at a particular spinal segment, the therapist should slightly readjust the hand placement cephalic or caudal or use the softer volar surface of the hand to induce the force. If the technique continues to cause pain, the cause is likely a reactive facet joint capsule at the level being tested. Smedmark et al.[190] reported a kappa value of 0.43 and a 70% agreement for lateral flexion PIVM between two physical therapists when testing 61 patients with neck pain. Piva et al.[182] reported kappa values ranging from −0.07 to 0.46 for mobility assessment and from 0.29 to 0.76 for pain assessment with this PIVM test, depending on which level was tested, on 30 patients with neck pain.

Cervical Lateral Glide Passive Intervertebral Motion Test

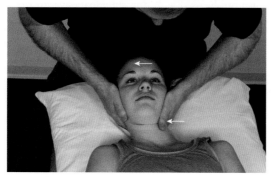

FIG. 6.47 Cervical lateral glide passive intervertebral motion test.

Cervical Lateral Glide Passive Intervertebral Motion Test—cont'd

PURPOSE	This test evaluates the passive lateral glide (joint play) of cervical segments C2–C3 through C7–T1.
PATIENT POSITION	The patient is supine with the head on a pillow and the top of the head even with the topof the table.
THERAPIST POSITION	The therapist stands at the head of the patient.
HAND PLACEMENT	Left hand: The radial border of the metacarpophalangeal joint of the index finger is used to contact the articular pillar of the specified segment, and the fourth and fifth fingers are used to support the patient's head.
	Right hand: The radial border of the metacarpophalangeal joint of the index finger is used to contact the articular pillar of the specified segment, and the fourth and fifth fingers are used to support the patient's head.
PROCEDURE	Both hands are used to gently grasp the patient's head and neck. The neck is brought into slight flexion (approximately 20 degrees), but the top of the patient's head does not rest on the therapist's abdomen. The radial border of the metacarpophalangeal joint of the index fingers on both hands is used to contact the articular pillars of C2. The fourth and fifth fingers on both hands are used to support the base of the patient's skull. Right lateral glide is induced by applying a force (through the contact point of the left hand and with passive head movement) that is directed to the right. The amount of passive lateral glide available at the segment is noted. Also tenderness or pain provocation is noted. Left lateral glide is induced by applying a force (through the contact point of the right hand) that is directed to the left. The cranial cervical spine segments and the head are allowed to move in the same lateral direction. The amount of passive lateral glide available is noted, as is any tenderness or pain provocation, and compared with the right side. The procedure is repeated with assessment of the mobility of the remaining cervical segments. The amount of passive lateral glide available at each segment and in each direction is noted and compared.
NOTES	This technique can be performed by starting at C2 and proceeding caudally, which allows for easy location of the cervical vertebrae (by counting down from C2). If this procedure induces a pain response at a particular spinal segment, the therapist should readjust the hand placement slightly cephalic or caudal or use the softer volar surface of the hand to induce the force. If the technique continues to cause pain, the cause is likely an irritable capsule tissue at the spinal segment being tested. The lateral glide is a general assessment of segmental joint play that tests the mobility of the uncovertebral joints, the facet joints, and neural tissues of the segment. If a restriction is found with the lateral glide PIVM test, graded end-range oscillations (grade III or IV mobilizations) can be used with this same maneuver to free segmental restrictions.
	Fernandez-de-las-Penas et al.[191] compared cervical lateral glide test results with a radiographic assessment of segmental lateral flexion and found a strong correlation between the lateral glide PIVM test with the radiographic assessment in the 25 patients with neck pain assessed in the study.

Lateral Glide Combined With Upper Limb Neurodynamic Test 1 Mobilization

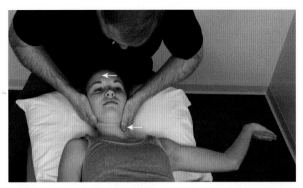

FIG. 6.48 A lateral glide mobilization of the C5–C6 away from the symptomatic upper extremity can be used combined with upper limb neurodynamic test 1 active range of motion to treat cervical radiculopathy. Typically, a sustained lateral glide stretch is used at the mid-cervical spine as the patient moves the elbow in and out of end-range elbow extension for 10 to 15 repetitions.

▶ Cervical Upglide (Upslope) Passive Intervertebral Motion Test

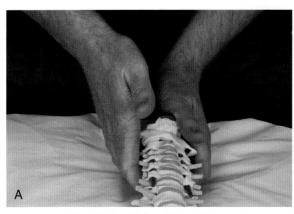
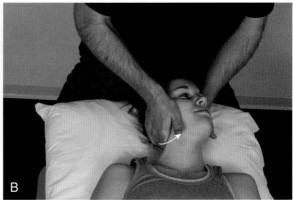

FIG. 6.49 See Video 6.20. A, Finger placement for cervical upglide passive intervertebral motion test. B, Cervical upglide (upslope) passive intervertebral motion test.

PURPOSE	The purpose of this test is to evaluate the passive upglide of cervical segments C2–C3 through T1–T2.
PATIENT POSITION	The patient is supine with the head on a small- to medium-sized soft pillow.
THERAPIST POSITION	The therapist stands at the head of the patient.
HAND PLACEMENT	Right hand: In testing of left rotation, the index finger is hooked around the posterior and lateral aspect of the articular pillar of the superior member of the segment; in testing of right rotation, the right hand is used to support the patient's head.
	Left hand: In testing of left rotation, the left hand is used to support the head; in testing right rotation, the index finger is hooked around the posterior and lateral aspect of the articular pillar of the segment.
PROCEDURE	The index finger of the right hand is used to palpate the right articular pillar of C2. The volar pad of the index finger is hooked posteriorly around the articular pillar and into the lamina. Left rotation is induced by pulling the articular pillar anteriorly cranially 45 degrees and across to the left side. The left hand is used to gently support the head to induce slight right side bending and backward bending and to return the head to midline after the rotation. The amount of passive rotation available at the segment is noted. The procedure is repeated with assessment of the left rotation at the remaining cervical segments. The amount of passive rotation available at each segment is noted and compared. The procedure is repeated with the index finger of the left hand passively rotating each segment to the right. The amount of passive rotation available at each segment and in each direction is noted and compared.
NOTES	This technique can be performed by starting at C2 and proceeding caudally, which allows for easy location of the cervical vertebrae (by counting down from C2). The therapist should ensure that the top of the patient's head is even with the edge of the table and not off the edge of the table.

Cervical Posteroanterior Passive Accessory Motion test

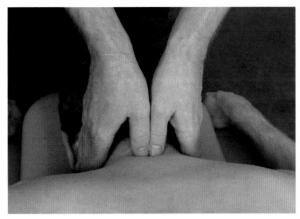

FIG. 6.50 Cervical posteroanterior passive accessory motion test.

PURPOSE	The purpose of this test is to evaluate the passive accessory motion of cervical segments C2–C3 through T1–T2.
PATIENT POSITION	The patient is the prone position with a pillow under the chest and head and neck in a neutral position.
THERAPIST POSITION	The therapist stands at the head of the patient.
HAND PLACEMENT	The tips of both thumbs are positioned over the spinous process of the targeted vertebra.
PROCEDURE	A gentle posterior to anterior force is applied at the targeted vertebra to assess for pain provocation, mobility, and end feel. The force is slowly increased with each repetition up to four to five repetitions.
NOTES	The angle of force can be varied to find the plane of motion that has the most resistance to movement or is most painful. The forces can be varied to turn this assessment into a mobilization for treatment effects. Pain provocation with this maneuver was found to be an important factor in the CPR for effectiveness of cervical spine thrust manipulation.[122] PAIVMs tests C0-C3 were used in two studies for diagnosis of CGH with Kappa values ranging from 0.53 to 0.72[195] and 0.64 to 0.7.[196] Zito et al.[134] studied the values of diagnostic accuracy of the PAIVMs tests C0-C3 obtaining sensitivity values between 59% and 65%, specificity between 78% and 87%, +LR from 2.9 to 4.9 (small shift in probability) and −LR from 0.43 to 0.49 (small shift in probability). Another study[135] showed a sensitivity of 100% and specificity of 94.4% by clustering CROM, manual examination C0-C3 and the craniocervical flexion test for diagnosis of CGH.

⊙ Unilateral Posteroanterior Passive Accessory Motion Test

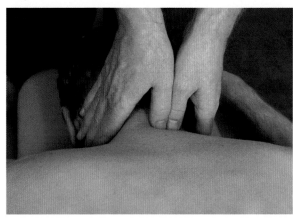

FIG. 6.51 See Video 6.21. Unilateral posteroanterior passive accessory motion test.

PURPOSE	The purpose of this test is to evaluate the passive accessory motion of cervical segments C2–C3 through T1–T2.
PATIENT POSITION	The patient is the prone position with a pillow under the chest and head and neck in a neutral position.
THERAPIST POSITION	The therapist stands at the head of the patient.
HAND PLACEMENT	The tips of both thumbs are positioned over the posterior aspect of the articular pillar of the targeted vertebra.
PROCEDURE	A gentle posteroanterior force is applied at the targeted vertebra to assess for pain provocation, mobility, and end feel. The force is slowly increased with each repetition up to four to five repetitions.
NOTES	The angle of force can be varied to find the plane of motion that has the most resistance to movement or is most painful. The forces can be varied to turn this assessment into a mobilization for treatment effects. PAIVMs tests of C0-C3 were used in two studies for diagnosis of CGH with Kappa values ranging from 0.53 to 0.72[195] and 0.64 to 0.7.[196] Zito et al.[134] studied the values of diagnostic accuracy of the PAIVMs tests of C0-C3 obtaining sensitivity values between 59% and 65%, specificity between 78% and 87%, +LR from 2.9 to 4.9 (small shift in probability) and –LR from 0.43 to 0.49 (small shift in probability). Jull et al.[135] showed a sensitivity of 100% and specificity of 94.4% to identify patients with CGH from other headache types by clustering restricted cervical movement with manual examination of C0-C3 joint dysfunction and impairment in the craniocervical flexion test.

Thoracic Passive Intervertebral Motion Testing and Manipulation

For completion of the cervical spine examination, palpation and PIVM testing must also be completed of the thoracic spine and rib cage. In addition, most patients with cervical spine disorders benefit from manual therapy techniques directed toward correction of thoracic spine dysfunctions. Chapter 5 provides a detailed description of examination and treatment procedures for the thoracic spine.

CERVICAL SPINE MANIPULATION TECHNIQUES

▶ Cervical Spine Downglide (Downslope glide) Manipulation

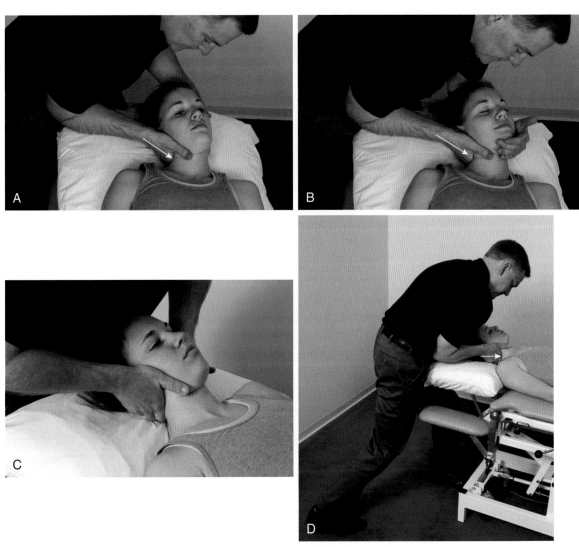

FIG. 6.52 See Video 6.22. A, Cervical spine downglide manipulation (cradle hold). B, Cervical spine downglide manipulation (chin hold). C, Cervical spine downglide manipulation (lateral view). D, Cervical spine downglide manipulation with demonstration of therapist diagonal stance and forearm positioning.

Cervical Spine Downglide (Downslope glide) Manipulation—cont'd

PURPOSE	This technique is used to manipulate a specific cervical segment (C2–C3 through C7–T1) into side bending.
PATIENT POSITION	The patient is supine with the head on a pillow and the top of the head even with the top edge of the table.
THERAPIST POSITION	The therapist stands at the head of the patient.
HAND PLACEMENT	Nonmanipulating hand: This hand supports the patient's head and neck, with fingers draped across the occiput for the cradle hold or the hand wrapped across the chin and forearm across the posterior lateral aspect of the cranium for the chin hold.
	Manipulating hand: The radial border of the metacarpophalangeal joint of the index finger is used to contact the articular pillar of the specified segment.
PROCEDURE	The radial border of the metacarpophalangeal joint of the index finger on the right hand is used to contact the right articular pillar of the specified cervical segment. The left hand supports the patient's head. Side bending of the patient's head slightly to the right is induced by taking up the joint motion in a downslope glide direction. The therapist then shifts the stance to the right and places the elbow at the hip with the forearm aligned with the direction of the force. The patient's neck is moved into rotation to the left down to the targeted spinal level. Further slack can be taken up by side gliding the neck away from the direction of side bending (to the left) and adding cervical distraction. The therapist manipulates into right side bending by applying a force through the contact point of the right hand that is directed to the left and slightly caudally toward the patient's axilla. On completion of the manipulation, right side bending is retested.
	The therapist manipulates into left side bending by side bending the head slightly to the left and applying a force through the contact point of the left hand that is directed to the right and slightly caudally. On completion of the manipulation, left side bending is retested.
NOTES	Indication for use of this technique is decreased side bending (downslope glide) of a specific cervical segment (C2–C3 through C7–T1). Also the top of the patient's head should be even with the edge of the table and not off the edge of the table. If the point of contact is uncomfortable for the patient, the therapist can attempt to adjust the position of the point of contact slightly superiorly or inferiorly or can attempt to use the volar aspect of the index finger metacarpal phalangeal joint to provide a softer point of contact. Once a firm barrier is attained, graded oscillations or a thrust may be used to manipulate the targeted spinal segment.

Cervical Spine Upglide (Upslope glide) Manipulation

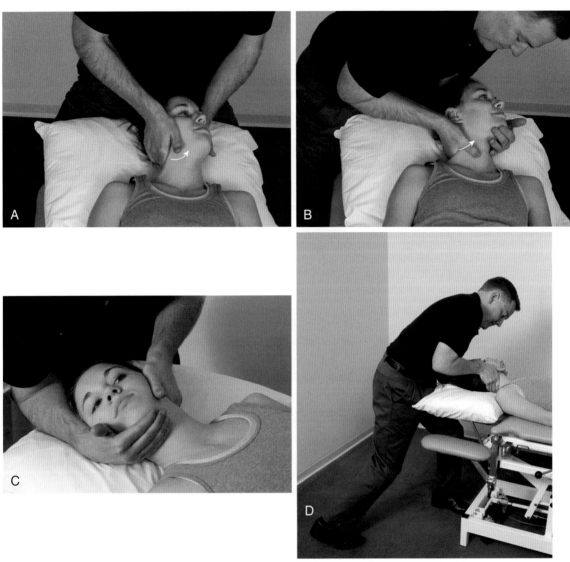

FIG. 6.53 See Video 6.23. A, Mid-cervical spine upglide manipulation (cradle hold). B, Mid-cervical spine upglide manipulation (chin hold). C, Mid-cervical spine upglide manipulation with use of secondary levers. D, Mid-cervical spine upglide manipulation with demonstration of therapist body and forearm position.

Cervical Spine Upglide (Upslope glide) Manipulation—cont'd

PURPOSE	This technique is used to manipulate a specific cervical segment (C2–C3 through C7–T1) into rotation.
PATIENT POSITION	The patient is supine with the head on a pillow.
THERAPIST POSITION	The therapist stands at the head of the patient in a diagonal athletic stance.
HAND PLACEMENT	Left hand: With manipulation into left rotation, the left hand supports the patient's head with fingers draped across the occiput for the cradle hold or the hand wrapped across the chin and forearm across the posterior lateral aspect of the cranium for the chin hold; with manipulation into right rotation, the volar pad of the index finger is hooked around the posterior and lateral aspect of the articular pillar of the segment.
	Right hand: With manipulation into right rotation, the right hand supports the patient's head with fingers draped across the occiput for the cradle hold or the hand wrapped across the chin and forearm across the posterior lateral aspect of the cranium for the chin hold; with manipulation into left rotation, the volar pad of the index finger is hooked around the posterior and lateral aspect of the articular pillar of the segment.
PROCEDURE	The index finger of the right hand palpates the right articular pillar of the specified segment. The index finger hooks posteriorly around the articular pillar and into the lamina. The therapist manipulates into left rotation by lifting the articular pillar anteriorly cranially 45 degrees and across to the left side. The left hand supports the head and provides a counterforce to establish secondary levers of side bending to the right, side glide to the left, extension above the targeted level, and distraction. Once a firm barrier is established, the therapist oscillates or thrusts the targeted facet joint in the left rotation/upslope glide direction (i.e., primary lever). On completion of the manipulation, left rotation is retested. The therapist manipulates into right rotation by repeating the procedure with the left hand to contact the left side of the specified segment. On completion of the manipulation, right rotation is retested. The chin hold of the head creates a broader point of contact for the patient's head and may assist in control of the multiple planes of motion used to create the firm joint barrier, which may assist with patient relaxation during the manipulation.
NOTES	Indication for use of this technique is decreased rotation (upslope glide) of a specific cervical segment (C2–C3 through C7–T1). The patient's head should be kept on the pillow during this technique. Also the top of the patient's head should be even with the edge of the table and not off the edge of the table. The technique can be performed with very small oscillations at the end range (grade IV) or larger oscillations at end-range (III) or midrange (II) or with an end-range, small-amplitude, high-velocity thrust. Measurement with an inclinometer of supine cervical active rotation can be used as an effective premanipulation and postmanipulation ROM test. Use of multiple planes of motion (levers) allows the therapist to create an effective firm manipulative joint barrier without extreme degrees of cervical rotation to take up the tissue slack. This technique builds safety into the technique by avoiding potential strain on the vertebral artery and other cervical soft tissue structures.

▶ Prone Cervical Unilateral Posteroanterior Mobilization

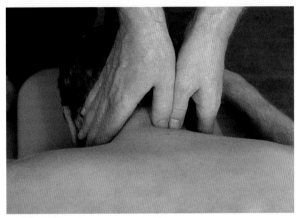

FIG. 6.54 See Video 6.24. Prone cervical unilateral posteroanterior passive accessory interverte-bral motion test and mobilization.

PURPOSE	The technique is used to mobilize a specific cervical or upper thoracic segment (C2–C3 through T3–T4) in a posterior to anterior direction.
PATIENT POSITION	The patient is prone with a pillow under the chest and the forehead resting on a toweland the cervical spine in a neutral position.
THERAPIST POSITION	The therapist stands in a diagonal athletic stance at the head of the patient.
HAND PLACEMENT	The therapist places both thumbs together with fingers in a mid/relaxed position across the posterior lateral aspect of the patient's neck. The tips of both thumbs are placed on the posterior aspect of the targeted articular pillar.
PROCEDURE	The therapist gently applies pressure in an anteroposterior direction in the plane of the facet joint to assess mobility, resistance, end feel, and pain provocation. Gentle oscillations can be used to either inhibit pain (grades I and II) or restore motion (grades III and IV). Slight variations in depth and direction of force can be used to optimize the therapeutic effects of this technique.
NOTES	The forces used in this procedure are very gentle, and the patient should be monitored verbally throughout the procedure to ensure comfort.

Prone Cervical Unilateral Posteroanterior Mobilization: Alternative "Dummy Thumb" Method

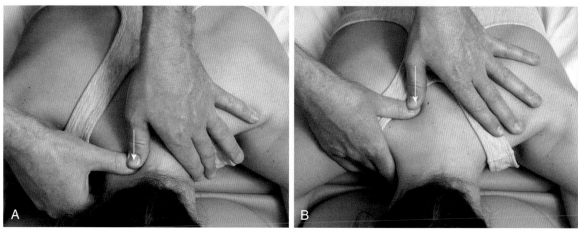

FIG. 6.55 See Videos 6.25 and 6.26. A, Prone cervical unilateral (upglide) posteroanterior passive accessory intervertebral movement (PAIVM) and mobilization with dummy thumb method. B, Prone upper thoracic unilateral (upglide) posteroanterior PAIVM and mobilization with dummy thumb method.

PROCEDURE MODIFICATION	This procedure can be modified by having the therapist stand at the side of the patient with a diagonal stance with the more lateral leg forward and a "dummy thumb" hand placement. The more lateral hand is used as the "dummy thumb" that is placed at the posterior aspect of the articular pillar and the distal pad of the more medial thumb is placed across the top of the "dummy thumb" (on the thumbnail) to provide the manipulative force.
NOTES	This alternative method works well for lower cervical and upper thoracic spinal segments to maintain the force along the plane of the facet joint surfaces, which is 45 degrees in the mid-cervical spine and 30 degrees in the upper thoracic spine.

▶ Suboccipital Release/Inhibitive Distraction

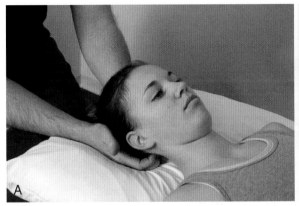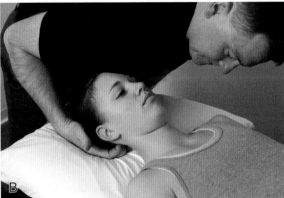

FIG. 6.56 See Video 6.27. A, Suboccipital release/inhibitive distraction B, Suboccipital release/inhibitive distraction with shoulder counterpressure.

PURPOSE	The purpose of this technique is to relax the suboccipital muscles and distract the cranium from C1 to restore craniovertebral mobility.
PATIENT POSITION	The patient is supine with the head on a pillow.
THERAPIST POSITION	The therapist sits at the head of the treatment table.
HAND PLACEMENT	Left hand: This hand contacts the base of the occiput (just caudal to the nuchal line) with the tips of digits 2 to 5.
	Right hand: This hand contacts the base of the occiput (just caudal to the nuchal line) with the tips of digits 2 to 5.
PROCEDURE	The tips of digits 2 to 5 of both hands gently lift the patient's head anteriorly. The dorsum of the hands rest on the pillow. With the tips of the fingers, the therapist gently pulls the head cranially as the patient's suboccipital muscles relax. The therapist continues with this position and takes up tissue slack with distraction as it becomes available. Distraction may continue for up to 5 minutes. Once relaxation of the suboccipital muscles is achieved, the therapist can position the anterior aspect of the shoulder across the patient's forehead to create a firm vice on the head and apply greater suboccipital distraction.
NOTES	Indications for use of this technique are decreased craniovertebral motion or muscle holding of the suboccipital muscles. During the performance of this technique, the forces should be applied to the base of the skull and not to C1. Patient relaxation is the key to the effectiveness of this technique.

⊙ Craniovertebral Distraction With C2 Stabilization

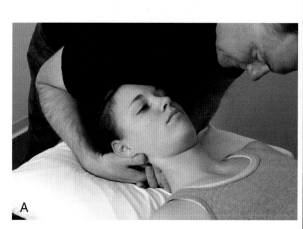

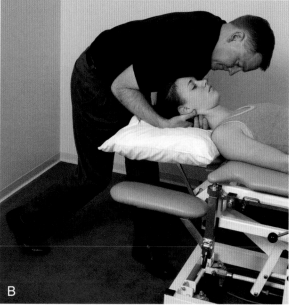

FIG. 6.57 See Video 6.28. A, Craniovertebral distraction with C2 stabilization. B, Craniovertebral distraction with C2 stabilization with demonstration of therapist stance and body position.

PURPOSE	The purpose of this technique is to distract the cranium from C2 to restore craniovertebral mobility.
PATIENT POSITION	The patient is supine with the head on a pillow.
THERAPIST POSITION	The therapist stands at the head of the patient.
HAND PLACEMENT	Left hand: The therapist uses the thumb and index finger to stabilize C2 (through the articular pillar and lamina).
	Right hand: The therapist uses the thumb and index finger to grasp the patient's occiput and the anterior shoulder to create a vice on the patient's forehead.
PROCEDURE	The thumb and index finger of the left hand are used to stabilize C2. The thumb and index finger of the right hand are used to grasp the patient's occiput. The right anterior shoulder is used to create a vice on the patient's forehead. The right hand distracts the cranium. This technique can be performed with a sustained stretch or slow grade III oscillations.

Occipitoatlantal Distraction Manipulation

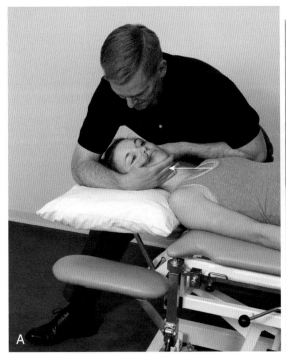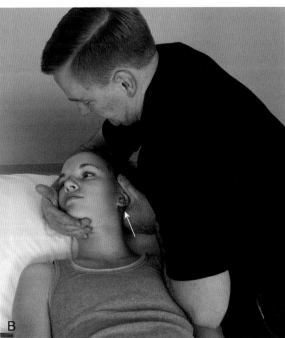

FIG. 6.58 See Video 6.29. A, Occipitoatlantal distraction manipulation with demonstration of therapist body positioning. B, Occipitoatlantal distraction manipulation with demonstration of hand placement and direction of force.

PURPOSE	This technique is used to distract/stretch the occipitoatlantal joint.
PATIENT POSITION	The patient is supine with the head on a pillow and positioned with the head slightly side bent toward and rotated away from the side to be manipulated.
THERAPIST POSITION	The therapist stands at the side of the patient's head with the legs in a lunge position.
HAND PLACEMENT	Left hand: The hand contacts the occiput with the palmar surface of the metacarpophalangeal joint and the forearm is positioned in a sagittal plane.
	Right hand: The hand and forearm support the patient's chin and head.
PROCEDURE	The therapist takes up the slack with a distractive force with the left hand. Next, to create a more effective barrier, the therapist side glides the patient's head and neck toward the side of rotation to further lock the mid-cervical spine. As the position of the head is held firm, the weight is shifted quickly onto the cranial foot with a lunging motion to create a thrust. Most of the force is applied with the left hand into the patient's occiput.

Cervical Spine Isometric Manipulation in Sitting

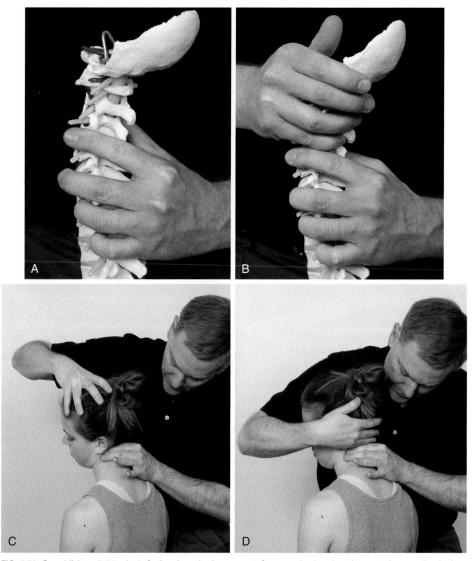

FIG. 6.59 See Video 6.30. A, Inferior hand placement for cervical spine isometric manipulation in sitting. B, Bilateral hand placement for cervical spine isometric manipulation in sitting. C, Cervical spine downglide passive intervertebral motion in sitting. D, Cervical spine isometric manipulation in sitting.

PURPOSE	The purpose of this technique is mobility and neuromuscular control.
PATIENT POSITION	The patient is in a sitting position.
THERAPIST POSITION	The therapist stands to the side of the patient on the opposite side of the joint to be manipulated.
HAND PLACEMENT	Right hand: This hand guides the head movements and applies resistance (with the fifth finger contacting the cranial member of the segment's articular pillar).
	Left hand: The thumb and index finger are used to stabilize the posterolateral aspect (articular pillars) of the caudal member of the segment.

▶ Cervical Spine Isometric Manipulation in Sitting—cont'd

PROCEDURE

The therapist stands on the patient's right side and uses the thumb and index finger of the left hand to palpate and stabilize the posterolateral aspect (articular pillars) of C3. The right hand guides the patient's head into the left posterior quadrant (side bending combined with ipsilateral rotation and backward bending). This procedure is repeated throughout the cervical segments, stabilizing the caudal member of the segment, until the position of the painful entrapment (motion limited by pain/guarding) is located. Once the painful or restricted segment is located, the thumb and index finger of the left hand stabilize the caudal member of the segment. The patient's head is guided into the left posterior quadrant to the point of pain and backed off slightly. The cranial member of the segment is contacted with the volar aspect of the right fifth finger. (The remaining fingers and palm contact the posterolateral aspect of the patient's head.) With the contact points of the right hand, the therapist gently pulls the patient's head out of the left posterior quadrant (into forward bending, side bending, and rotation) while the patient isometrically resists. The position is held for 10 seconds. The head is guided slightly farther into the left posterior quadrant, and the isometric resistance is repeated. The motion is repeated for a total of four to five repetitions. On completion of the technique, the painful segment is reexamined.

If the painful entrapment is located on the patient's right side, the procedure is repeated with the therapist standing on the patient's left side and reversing the roles of the hands.

NOTES

Indication for use of this technique is a Spurling B test result that is positive for neck pain. One should note the placement of the caudal hand of this technique: the thumb and index fingers of the caudal hand should be stabilizing the posterolateral aspect of the caudal vertebral member of the segment.

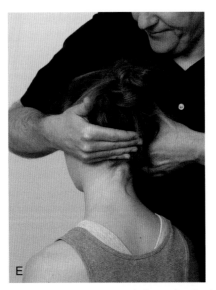

FIG. 6.59, cont'd E, Cervical manual distraction in sitting.

Follow-up of the cervical spine isometric manipulation sitting technique with manual cervical distraction (see Fig. 6.22E). The sitting cervical distraction technique should be combined with deep breathing. The head should be held firmly, with the hands positioned at the patient's mastoid processes, as the patient lets the air out. Manual resistive cervical rotation either in the supine or sitting position is a useful follow-up neuromuscular retraining exercise following this technique.

▶ Cervical Spine Rotation Isometric Manipulation in Supine

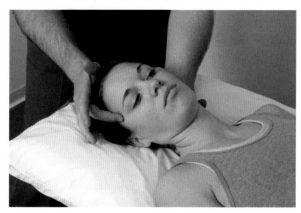

FIG. 6.60 See Video 6.31. Cervical spine rotation isometric manipulation in supine.

PURPOSE	This technique is used to restore (mobilize) the downglide component of cervical rotation mobility and neuromuscular control.
PATIENT POSITION	The patient is supine with the head on a medium-sized pillow.
THERAPIST POSITION	The therapist stands or sits at the head of the treatment table.
HAND PLACEMENT	Right hand: This hand guides the head movements and applies resistance at the patient's temple on the side of the rotation motion that is limited.
	Left hand: The thumb and index or third finger stabilize the posterolateral aspect (articular pillars) of the caudal member of the segment.
PROCEDURE	The thumb and index finger of the left hand palpate and stabilize the posterolateral aspect (articular pillars) of C3. The right hand guides the patient's head into right rotation with slight ipsilateral side bending to the point of resistance or pain. This procedure is repeated throughout the cervical segments, stabilizing the caudal member of the segment, until the position of limited or painful motion is located. Once the painful or restricted segment is located, the thumb and index finger of the left hand are used to stabilize the caudal member of the segment. The patient's head is guided into the right rotated position to the point of pain or resistance and backed off slightly. A light resistance with the pad of the index finger of the right hand is applied at the patient's temple toward left rotation, and the patient is asked to hold against that resistance for 10 seconds. The head is guided slightly farther into the right rotation, and the isometric resistance is repeated. This motion is repeated for a total of four to five repetitions. On completion of the technique, the painful segment is reexamined.
NOTES	Indication for use of this technique is a positive Spurling B test result for neck pain or mid-cervical pain reported on the same side of neck rotation tested in supine or standing. Follow-up of this technique with manual cervical distraction and manual resistive cervical rotation in the supine position is advisable.

▶ Craniovertebral Rotation Isometric Manipulation in Supine

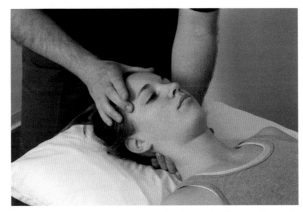

FIG. 6.61 See Video 6.32. Craniovertebral rotation isometric manipulation in supine.

PURPOSE	The purpose of this technique is to restore craniovertebral rotation mobility and neuromuscular control.
PATIENT POSITION	The patient is supine with the head on a medium-sized pillow.
THERAPIST POSITION	The therapist stands or sits at the head of the treatment table.
HAND PLACEMENT	Left hand: The thumb and index or third finger stabilize the posterolateral aspect (articular pillars) of the axis (C2 vertebra).
	Right hand: This hand is spread across the patient's forehead to guide cervical rotation.
PROCEDURE	The thumb and index finger of the left hand palpate and stabilize the posterolateral aspect (articular pillars) of C2. The right hand guides the patient's head into right rotation with slight ipsilateral side bending to the point of resistance or pain, and the patient is asked to hold that position. A light resistance with the pad of the index finger of the right hand is applied at the patient's temple toward left rotation, and the patient is asked to hold against that resistance for 10 seconds. The head is guided farther into the right rotation, and the isometric resistance is repeated. The motion is repeated for a total of four to five repetitions. On completion of the technique, craniovertebral rotation is reexamined.
NOTES	Follow-up of this technique with manual craniovertebral distraction and manual resistive cervical rotation in the supine position is often useful.

⏵ Craniovertebral Side Bending (Lateral Flexion) Isometric Manipulation in Supine

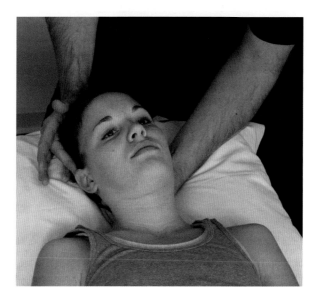

FIG. 6.62 See Video 6.33. Craniovertebral side bending (lateral flexion) isometric manipulation in supine.

PURPOSE	The purpose of this technique is restoration of craniovertebral side bending mobility and neuromuscular control.
PATIENT POSITION	The patient is supine with the head on a medium-sized pillow.
THERAPIST POSITION	The therapist stands or sits at the head of the treatment table.
HAND PLACEMENT	Left hand: The thumb and index or third finger stabilize the posterolateral aspect (articular pillars) of the axis (C2 vertebra).
	Right hand: The hand is spread across the top of the patient's head to guide craniovertebral side bending.
PROCEDURE	The thumb and index finger of the left hand palpate and stabilize the posterolateral aspect (articular pillars) of C2. The right hand guides the patient's head into right craniovertebral side bending (lateral flexion) to the point of resistance or pain, and the patient is asked to hold that position. A light resistance with the pad of the index finger of the right hand is applied just above the patient's right ear, and the patient is asked to hold against the resistance for 10 seconds. The head is guided farther into the right lateral flexion, and the isometric resistance is repeated. The motion is repeated for a total of four to five repetitions. On completion of the technique, passive craniovertebral side bending (lateral flexion) is reexamined.
NOTES	Follow-up of this technique with manual craniovertebral distraction and the active craniocervical flexion exercise is often useful.

Craniovertebral Side Bending (Lateral Press of the Atlas) Mobilization in Supine

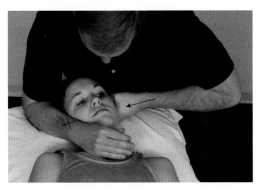

FIG. 6.63 Craniovertebral side bending (lateral press of the atlas) mobilization in supine.

PURPOSE	The purpose of this technique is restoration of craniovertebral side bending.
PATIENT POSITION	The patient is supine with the head on a medium-sized pillow.
THERAPIST POSITION	The therapist stands at the head of the treatment table.
HAND PLACEMENT	Left hand: The palmer surface of the second metacarpal phalangeal joint is placed at the lateral aspect of the atlas transverse process. This is located in the space just anterior to the mastoid process and just posterior to the mandible.
	Right hand: The palmer surface of the forearm is positioned across the lateral aspect of the cranium.
PROCEDURE	As the head is positioned and held at the end range of craniovertebral side bending, a lateral force is applied to the atlas with the left hand along the plane of the occipital condyles into the direction of the side bending positioned cranium. This technique is typically done as a nonthrust technique with a firm, squeezing force applied between the left hand and right forearm. The therapist must monitor the patient closely throughout this technique. The technique should be followed by craniovertebral distraction. On completion of the technique, craniovertebral side bending (lateral flexion) PIVM is reexamined.
NOTES	Because craniovertebral right side bending involves lateral motion of the convexly shaped occipital condyles to the left, there is a relative lateral glide to the right of the atlas. Therefore a mobilization technique that involves pressing the atlas in a lateral direction to the right will tend to improve craniovertebral right side bending. Because craniovertebral right side bending is a component motion of cervical spine left rotation, cervical spine left rotation motion may also improve with following this technique.

Cervical Extension SNAG (Sustained Natural Apophyseal Glides;

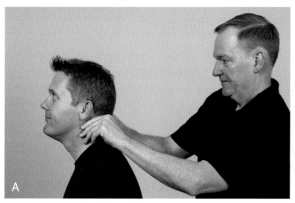
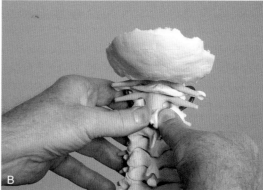

FIG. 6.64 A, Cervical extension SNAG (sustained natural apophyseal glides). B, Cervical extension SNAG hand placement.

PURPOSE	Restore pain free cervical extension and to treat CGHs and cervicogenic dizziness with C2 level SNAG.
PATIENT POSITION	The patient sits on side a treatment table.
THERAPIST POSITION	The therapist stands directly behind the patient.
HAND PLACEMENT	The palmar surface (pad) of distal phalanx of one thumb is placed over the spinous process of the targeted spinous process and the other thumb is placed over the top.
PROCEDURE	The therapist applies an anterior force on the spinous process with both thumbs in the direction parallel with the plane of the facet joints at the targeted level as the patient moves into cervical extension. The direction of force must adapt to the changing position of the neck as the patient moves into extension to assure that the force continues to be parallel with the treatment plane of the facet joints. The anterior thumb pressure is sustained until the patient returns their neck to the starting neutral position. Repeat the SNAG for up to six repetitions.

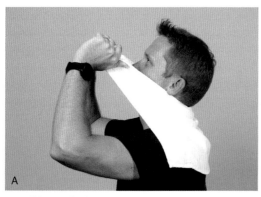
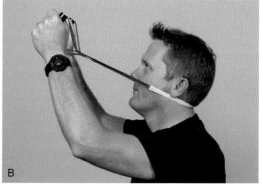

FIG. 6.65 Self- SNAG (sustained natural apophyseal glides) variation. A, Cervical extension SNAG with an edge of a towel. B, Cervical extension SNAG with a mobilization strap.

NOTES	All components of the procedure must be symptom free, and if the patient experiences symptoms, the therapist should readjust the direction of the glide or the point of thumb contact to make the movement pain free (Fig. 6.65).
PROCEDURE MODIFICATION	The cervical extension SNAG can be performed as a self-mobilization technique with use of an edge of a towel or a small mobilization strap placed at the targeted cervical spinous process. The patient must be instructed to sustain the anterior force along the treatment plane that is parallel to the angle of the facet joints of the targeted segment throughout the active neck extension and return to neutral movements. The movements must be symptom free and adjustment of location and direction of force with the strap should be modified until the movement is symptom free.

Cervical Rotation SNAG (Sustained Natural Apophyseal Glides)

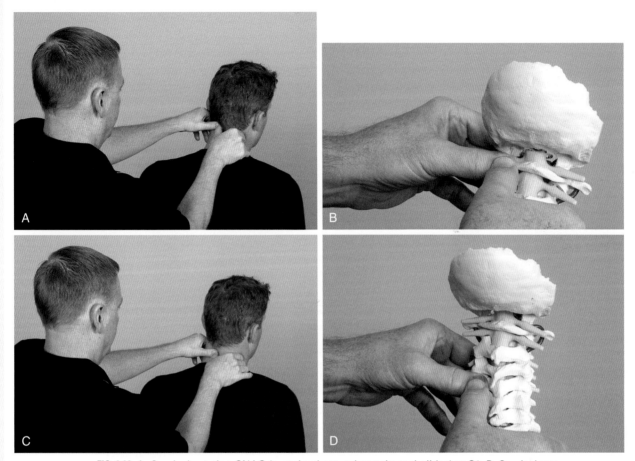

FIG. 6.66 A, Cervical rotation SNAG (sustained natural apophyseal glides) at C1. B, Cervical rotation SNAG at C1 finger placement. C, Cervical rotation SNAG can be modified for mid-cervical spinal levels. D, Cervical rotation SNAG at C4 hand placement.

PURPOSE	Restore pain free cervical extension and to treat CGHs and cervicogenic dizziness with C1 level SNAG.
PATIENT POSITION	The patient sits on side a treatment table.
THERAPIST POSITION	The therapist stands directly behind the patient.
HAND PLACEMENT	The palmar surface (pad) of distal phalanx of one thumb is placed over the posterior aspect of the transverse process/articular pillar of the targeted vertebrae and the pad of the other thumb is placed over the top.
PROCEDURE	The therapist applies an anterior force on the posterior aspect of the transverse process/articular pillar of the targeted vertebrae with both thumbs in the direction parallel with the plane of the facet joint at the targeted level as the patient moves into cervical rotation to the opposite direction of the point of contact. The direction of force must adapt to the changing position of the neck as the patient moves into rotation to assure that the force continues to be parallel with the treatment plane of the facet joints. The anterior thumb pressure is sustained until the patient returns their neck to the starting neutral position. Repeat the SNAG for up to six repetitions for the mid-cervical spine, but only two to five times for the C1 technique.

Cervical Rotation SNAG (Sustained Natural Apophyseal Glides)—cont'd

NOTES　All components of the procedure must be symptom free, and if the patient experiences symptoms, the therapist should readjust the direction of the glide or the point of thumb contact to make the movement pain free (Fig. 6.67).

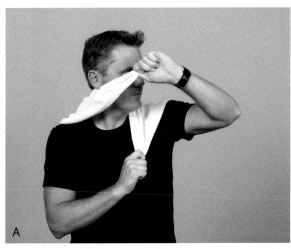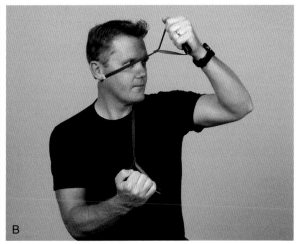

FIG. 6.67 A, Self- SNAG (sustained natural apophyseal glides) variation with a towel edge. B, Self-SNAG variation with a mobilization strap.

PROCEDURE MODIFICATION　The cervical rotation SNAG can be performed as a self-mobilization technique with use of an edge of a towel or a small mobilization strap placed at the targeted cervical vertebrae. The patient must be instructed to sustain the anterior force along the treatment plane that is parallel to the angle of the facet joints of the targeted segment throughout the active neck rotation and return to neutral movements. The movements must be symptom free and adjustment of location and direction of force with the strap should be modified until the movement is symptom free.

The following patient case reports can be used by the student to develop problem-solving skills by considering the information provided in the patient history and tests and measures and developing appropriate evaluations, goals, and plans of care. Students should also consider the following questions:

1. What additional historical/subjective information would you like to have?
2. What additional diagnostic tests should be ordered, if any?
3. What additional tests and measures would be helpful in making the diagnosis?
4. What impairment-based classification does the patient most likely fit? What other impairment-based classifications did you consider?
5. What are the primary impairments that should be addressed?
6. What treatment techniques that you learned in this textbook will you use to address these impairments?
7. How do you plan to progress and modify the interventions as the patient progresses?

9. Neurologic screen: Negative
10. Palpation: Tender and guarded in area of right C2–C3 facet joint and right suboccipital muscles
11. PIVM tests: Hypomobility right C2–C3 upglide and downglide and craniovertebral right side bending

Evaluation

Diagnosis
Problem list
Goals
Treatment plan/intervention

Ms. Head Ache

History

A 32-year-old female secretary has a diagnosis of CGH with pain focused in the right ocular area and the right upper cervical spine (Fig. 6.68).

Tests and Measures

1. Structural examination: Moderate forward head posture with protracted scapulae
2. Cervical AROM: 75% left side bending and left rotation, 50% right side bending and right rotation with provocation of pain, 60% forward bending with deviation to the right
3. Cervical PROM: Overpressure to right rotation increases pain and has a capsular end feel
4. Shoulder AROM and strength: Normal
5. Muscle length: Moderately tight right levator scapula and minimally tight bilateral pectoralis major and minor muscles
6. Strength: 3+/5 bilateral lower trapezius, middle trapezius, and serratus anterior; CCFT 24 mm Hg × 10 s × 5 repetitions maximum
7. Spurling B test: Positive to the right for provocation of neck pain
8. Distraction test: Decreased pain in the head and neck

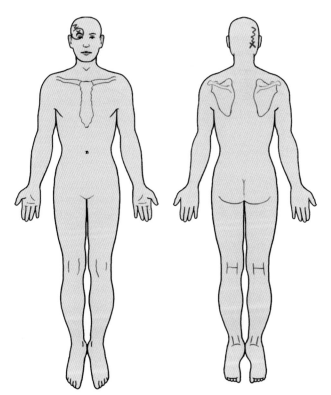

FIG. 6.68 Body chart for Ms. Head Ache.

Ms. Whip Lash

History

A 16-year-old female high school student has a diagnosis of neck pain with pain focused in the left mid-cervical region after a motor vehicle accident caused by a whiplash injury 4 weeks before the initial visit (Fig. 6.69). The patient has been using a rigid cervical collar since the injury.

Tests and Measures

1. Structural examination: Moderate forward head posture with protracted scapulae
2. Cervical AROM in standing: 50% in all planes of motion with provocation of pain at the end of ROMs with poor control noted
3. Cervical AROM in supine: 80% in all planes with less pain reported
4. Cervical PROM: Overpressure to left and right rotation increased pain with a muscle holding end feel
5. Shoulder AROM and strength: Normal
6. Muscle length: Moderately tight right levator scapula and minimally tight bilateral pectoralis major and minor
7. Strength: 3+/5 bilateral lower trapezius, middle trapezius, and serratus anterior; 2/5 longus capitis, longus colli, and cervical multifidus; poor control with craniocervical test and unable to hold contraction for 10 seconds beyond 22 mm Hg

8. Spurling B test: Positive bilaterally for provocation of neck pain
9. Distraction test: Decreased pain in the head and neck
10. Neurologic screen: Negative
11. Palpation: Tender and guarded and inflammation throughout the mid-cervical facet joints and surrounding muscle/soft tissues
12. Ligament stability tests: Alar, anterior shear, and Sharp-Purser tests are negative
13. PIVM tests: Hypomobility T2–T3 and T3–T4 left and right rotation

Evaluation

Diagnosis
Problem list
Goals
Treatment plan/intervention

Mr. Neck A. Armpain

History

A 55-year-old male police officer has a diagnosis of neck and arm pain with the pain focused in the right lateral upper arm, right shoulder, right scapula, and right cervical/thoracic junction (Fig. 6.70).

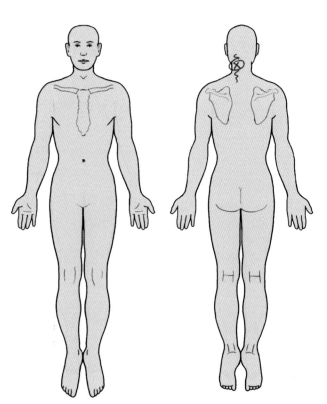

FIG. 6.69 Body chart for Ms. Whip Lash.

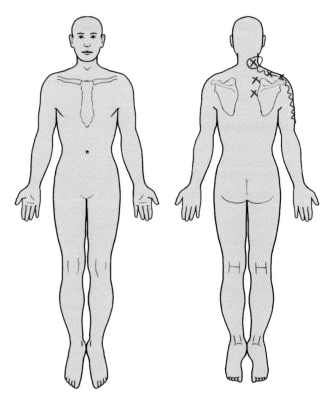

FIG. 6.70 Body chart for Mr. Neck A. Armpain.

Tests and Measures

1. Structural examination: Moderate forward head posture with protracted scapulae; holds the right arm close to the body and supports it with the opposite arm
2. Cervical AROM in standing: 50% in all planes of motion with provocation of pain at the end of ROMs with poor control noted; upper thoracic mobility is 25% of expected ROM
3. Cervical AROM in supine: 45 degrees right rotation, 55 degrees left rotation
4. Cervical PROM: Overpressure to left and right rotation increased pain with a capsular end feel
5. Right shoulder screen:
   - AROM: 120 flexion and 110 abduction with pain arm pain at end range
   - PROM: 120 flexion and 110 abduction with pain arm pain at end range
   - Tissue tension signs: Strength was normal and pain free with resistance
   - Accessory motion tests: Normal for right shoulder
   - Nerve tension tests: Positive ULND test 1 at −60 elbow extension
6. Muscle length: Moderately tight right levator scapula and minimally tight bilateral pectoralis major and minor
7. Strength: 3+/5 bilateral lower trapezius, middle trapezius, and serratus anterior; 3/5 deep neck flexor muscles
8. Spurling A: Positive right for provocation right arm pain
9. Distraction test: Decreased arm pain
10. Neurologic screen: Diminished biceps reflex but normal sensation
11. Palpation: Tender and guarded and inflammation at the right C5–C6 and C6–C7 facet joints and surrounding muscle/soft tissues
12. PIVM tests: Hypomobility T3–T4 and T4–T5 left and right rotation

Evaluation

Diagnosis
Problem list
Goals
Treatment plan/intervention

References

1. Shekelle PG, Markovich M, Louis R. An epidemiologic study of episodes of back pain care. *Spine*. 1995;20:1668-1673.

2. Wright A, Mayer TG, Gatchel RJ. Outcomes of disabling cervical spine disorders in compensation injuries: a prospective comparison to tertiary rehabilitation response for chronic lumbar spinal disorders. *Spine*. 1999;24(2):178-183.

3. Bovin G, Schrader H, Sand T. Neck pain in the general population. *Spine*. 1994;19:1307-1309.

4. Cote P, Cassidy JD, Carroll L. The Saskatchewan Health and Back Pain Survey: the prevalence of neck pain and related disability in Saskatchewan adults. *Spine*. 1998;23:1689-1698.

5. Kim R, Wiest C, Clark K, et al. Identifying risk factors for first-episode neck pain: a systematic Review. *Musculoskelet Sci Pract*. 2018;33:77-83.

6. Lethbridge-Cejku M, Schiller JS, Bernadel L. Summary health statistics for US adults: National Health Interview Survey, 2002. *Vital Health Stat*. 2004;10:1-151.

7. Nygren A, Berglund A, von Koch M. Neck and shoulder pain, an increasing problem: strategies for using insurance material to follow trends. *Scand J Rehabil Med*. 1995;32:107-112.

8. Haldeman S, Carroll L, Cassidy D, et al. The Bone and Joint Decade 2000–2010 Task Force on neck pain and its associated disorders. *Spine*. 2008;33(4S):S5-S7.

9. Hoy D, March L, Woolf A, et al. The global burden of neck pain: estimates from the global burden of disease 2010 study. *Ann Rheum Dis*. 2014;73(7):1309-1315.

10. Jette A, Delitto A. Physical therapy treatment choices for musculoskeletal impairments. *Phys Ther*. 1997;77(2):145-154.

11. Jull G, Sterling M, Falla D, et al. *Whiplash, headache, and neck pain*. London: Churchill Livingstone/Elsevier; 2008.

12. Youdas JW, Garret TR, Suman VJ, et al. Normal range of motion of the cervical spine: an initial goniometric study. *Phys Ther*. 1992;72(11):770-780.

13. Mercer SR, Jull GA. Morphology of the cervical intervertebral disc: implications for McKenzie's model of the disc derangement syndrome. *Man Ther*. 1996;2:76-81.

14. :>Williams PL, Dyson M, Bannister LH, editors. *Gray's anatomy*, ed 37. New York: Churchill Livingstone; 1989.

15. Penning L. Normal movement in the cervical spine. *Am J Roentgenol*. 1978;130:317-326.

16. Dvorak J, Panjabi MM, Novotny JE, et al. In vivo flexion/extension of the normal cervical spine. *J Orthop Res*. 1991;9:828-834.

17. Cook C, Hegedus E, Showalter C, et al. Coupling behavior of the cervical spine: a systematic review of the literature. *J Manipulative Physiol Ther*. 2006;29:570-575.

18. Mimura M, Hideshige M, Tsuneo W, et al. Three-dimensional motion analysis of the cervical spine with special reference to the axial rotation. *Spine*. 1989;14(11):1135-1139.

19. Tsang SMH, Szeto GPY, Lee RYW. Normal kinematics of the neck: the interplay between the cervical and thoracic spines. *Man Ther*. 2013;18:431-437.

20. Ishii T, Mukai Y, Hosono N, et al. Kinematics of the cervical spine in lateral bending: in vivo three-dimensional analysis. *Spine*. 2006;31:155-160.

21. Werne S. Studies in spontaneous atlas dislocation. *Acta Orthop Scand Suppl*. 1957;23:1-150.

22. Ishii T, Mukai Y, Hosono N, et al. Kinematics of the subaxial cervical spine in rotation in vivo three-dimensional analysis. *Spine*. 2004;29:2826-2831.

23. Dumas J, Sainte Rose M, Dreyfus P, et al. Rotation of the cervical spinal column: a computed tomography in vivo study. *Surg Radiol Anat*. 1993;15:333-339.

24. Lysell E. Motion in the cervical spine: an experimental study on autopsy specimens. *Acta Orthop Scand Suppl*. 1969;40(Suppl 123):1-61.

25. Penning L, Wilmink JT. Rotation of the cervical spine: a CT study in normal subjects. *Spine*. 1987;12(8):732-738.

26. Jarrett JL, Olson KA, Bohannon RW. *Reliability in examining craniovertebral sidebending* (Master's thesis). University of St. Augustine for Health Sciences; 2004.

27. Neumann DA. *Kinesiology of the Musculoskeletal System: Foundations for Physical Rehabilitation*, ed 2. St. Louis: Mosby; 2010.

28. Schomacher J, Falla D. Function and structure of the deep cervical extensor muscles in patients with neck pain. *Man Ther*. 2013;18(5):360-366.

29. Falla DL, Jull GA, Hodges PW. Patients with neck pain demonstrate reduced electromyographic activity of the deep cervical flexor muscles during performance of the craniocervical flexion test. *Spine*. 2004;29(19):2108-2114.

30. Schomacher J, Petzke F, Falla D. Localised resistance selectively activates the semispinalis cervicis muscle in patients with neck pain. *Man Ther*. 2012;17(6):544-548.

31. Marshall CM, Vernon H, Leddy JJ, et al. The role of the cervical spine in post-concussion syndrome. *Phys Sportsmed*. 2015;43:274-284.

32. Elkin BS, Elliott JM, Siegmund GP. Whiplash injury or concussion? A possible biomechanical explanation for concussion symptoms in some individuals following a rear-end collision. *J Orthop Sports Phys Ther*. 2016;46(10):874-885.

33. Stiell IG, Wells GA, Vandemheen KL, et al. The Canadian C-spine rule for radiography in alert and stable trauma patients. *JAMA*. 2001;286(15):1841-1848.

34. Childs JD, Cleland JA, Elliott JM, et al. Neck pain: clinical practice guidelines linked to the International Classification of Functioning, Disability, and Health from the Orthopaedic Section of the American Physical Therapy Association. *J Orthop Sports Phys Ther*. 2008;38(9):A1-A34.

35. Blanpied PR, Gross AR, Elliott JM, et al. Neck Pain: Revision 2017, Clinical Practice Guidelines linked to the international classification of functioning, disability and health from the Orthopaedic Section of the American Physical Therapy Association. *J Orthop Sports Phys Ther*. 2017;47(7):A1-A83.

36. Sutton DA, Cote P, Wong JL, et al. In multimodal care effective for the management of patients with whiplash-associated disorders or neck pain and associated disorder? A systematic review by the Ontario Protocol for Traffic Injury Management (OPTIMa) Collaboration. *Spine J*. 2016;16:1541-1565.

37. Paris SV, Loubert PV. *Foundations of clinical orthopaedics*. St Augustine, FL: Institute Press; 1986.

38. Anstey R, Kongsted A, Kamper S, et al. Are people with whiplash-associated neck pain difference from people with nonspecific neck pain? *J Orthop Sports Phys Ther*. 2016;46(10):894-901.

39. Barnsley L, Lord S, Bogduk N. Clinical review: whiplash injury. *Pain*. 1994;58:283-307.

40. Ritchie C, Hendrikz J, Kenardy J, et al. Derivation of a clinical prediction rule to identify both chronic moderate/severe disability and full recovery following whiplash injury. *Pain*. 2013;154:2198-2206.

41. Walton DM, Macdermid JC, Giorgianni AA, et al. Risk factors for persistent problems following acute whiplash injury: Update

of a systematic review and meta-analysis. *J Orthop Sports Phys Ther*. 2013;43(2):31-43.

42. Spitzer W, Skovron M, Salmi L, et al. Scientific monograph of Quebec Task Force on whiplash associated disorders: redefining "whiplash" and its management. *Spine*. 1995;20:1-73.

43. Sterling M. A proposed new classification system for whiplash associated disorders: implications for assessment and management. *Man Ther*. 2004;9:60-70.

44. Sterling M, Jull G, Kenardy J. Physical and psychological factors maintain long-term predictive capacity post-whiplash injury. *Pain*. 2006;122:102-108.

45. McKinnry LA. Early mobilization and outcome in acute sprains of the neck. *Brit Med J*. 1989;299:1006-1008.

46. Rosenfeld M, Bunnarsson R, Borenstein P. Early intervention in whiplash-associated disorders: a comparison of two treatment protocols. *Spine*. 2000;25:1782-1787.

47. Jull G, Kristjansson E, Dall'Alba P. Impairment in cervical flexors: a comparison of whiplash and insidious onset neck pain patients. *Man Ther*. 2004;9:89-94.

48. Jorgensen R, Ris I, Falla D, et al. Reliability, construct and discriminate validity of clinical testing in subjects with and without chronic neck pain. *BMC Musculoskelet Disord*. 2014;15:408.

49. O'Leary S, Jull G, Kim M, et al. Specificity in retraining craniocervical flexor muscle performance. *J Orthop Sports Phys Ther*. 2007;37(1):3-9.

50. Harris KD, Heer DM, Roy TC, et al. Reliability of a measurement of neck flexor muscle endurance. *Phys Ther*. 2005;85:1349-1355.

51. Jull G, Sterling M, Kenardy J, et al. Does the presence of sensory hypersensitivity influence outcomes of physical rehabilitation for chronic whiplash? A preliminary RCT. *Pain*. 2007;129:28-34.

52. Elliott JM, Noteboom JT, Flynn TW, et al. Characterization of acute and chronic whiplash-associated disorders. *J Orthop Sports Phys Ther*. 2009;39(5):312-323.

53. Foa EB, Cashman L, Jaycox L, et al. The validation of a self-report measure of posttraumatic stress disorder: the Posttraumatic Diagnostic Scale. *Psychol Assess*. 1997;9:445-451.

54. Ritchie C, Hendrikz J, Jull G, et al. External validation of a clinical prediction rule to predict full recovery and ongoing moderate/severe disability following acute whiplash injury. *J Orthop Sports Phys Ther*. 2015;45(4):242-250.

55. Rebbeck T, Leaver A, Bandong AN, et al. Implementation of a guideline-based clinical pathway of care to improve health outcomes following whiplash injury (Whiplash ImPaCT): protocol of a randomized, controlled trial. *J Physiother*. 2016;62:111.

56. Elliott J, Pedler A, Kenardy J, et al. The temporal development of fatty infiltrates in the neck muscles following whiplash injury: an association with pain and posttraumatic stress. *PLoS One*. 2011;6(6):e21194.

57. Karlsson A, Leinhard OD, Aslund U, et al. An investigation of fat infiltration of the multifidus muscle in patients with severe neck symptoms associated with chronic whiplash-associated disorder. *J Orthop Sports Phys Ther*. 2016;46(10):886-893.

58. Elliott JM, Courtney M, Rademaker A, et al. The rapid and progressive degeneration of cervical multifidus in whiplash. *Spine*. 2015;40:E694-E700.

59. Paddon-Jones D, Sheffield-Moore M, Cree MG, et al. Atrophy and impaired muscle protein synthesis during prolonged inactivity and stress. *J Clin Endocrinol Metab*. 2006;91:4836-4841.

60. Nemeroff CB, Bremner JD, Foa EB, et al. Posttraumatic stress disorder: a state-of-the-science review. *J Psychiatr Res*. 2006;40:1-21.

61. Sterling M, Smeets R, Keijzers G, et al. Physiotherapist-delivered stress inoculation training integrated with exercise versus physiotherapy exercise alone for acute whiplash-associated disorder (StressModex): a randomized controlled trail of a combined psychological/physical intervention. *Br J Sports Med*. 2019;53:1240-1247.

62. Ritchie C, Kenardy J, Smeets R, et al. StressModEx – Physiotherapist-led inoculation training integrated with exercise for acute whiplash injury: study protocol for a randomized controlled trial. *J Physiother*. 2015;61:157.

63. Kelly JM, Bunzli S, Ritchie C, et al. Physiotherapist-delivered stress inoculation training for acute whiplash-associated disorders: a qualitative study of perceptions and experiences. *Musculoskelet Sci Pract*. 2018;38:30-36.

64. Cleland JA, Childs JD, Fritz JM, et al. Development of a clinical prediction rule for guiding treatment of a subgroup of patients with neck pain: use of thoracic spine manipulation, exercise, and patient education. *Phys Ther*. 2007;87(1):9-23.

65. Cleland JA, Mintken PE, Carpenter K, et al. Examination of a clinical prediction rule to identify patients with neck pain likely to benefit from thoracic spine thrust manipulation and a general cervical range of motion exercise: multi-center randomized clinical trial. *Phys Ther*. 2010;90(9):1239-1250.

66. Masaracchio M, Cleland J, Hellman M, et al. Short-term combined effects of thoracic spine thrust manipulation and cervical spine nonthrust manipulation in individuals with mechanical neck pain: a randomized clinical trial. *J Orthop Sports Phys Ther*. 2013;43(3):118-127.

67. Panjabi MM. The stabilizing system of spine. Part II: neutral zone and instability hypothesis. *J Spinal Disord*. 1992;5(4):390-396.

68. Panjabi MM. The stabilizing system of the spine. Part I: function, dysfunction, adaptation, and enhancement. *J Spinal Disord*. 1992;5(4):383-389.

69. Panjabi MM, Lydon C, Vasavada A, et al. On the understanding of clinical instability. *Spine*. 1994;23:2642-2650.

70. Oxland TR, Panjabi MM. The onset and progression of spinal injury: a demonstration of neutral zone sensitivity. *J Biomechanics*. 1992;25:1165-1172.

71. Hohl M. Normal motions in the upper portion of the cervical spine. *J Bone Joint Surg*. 1978;46A(8):1777-1779.

72. Panjabi MM, Krag MH, Chung TQ. Effects of disc injury on mechanical behavior of the human spine. *Spine*. 1984;9:707-713.

73. White AA III, Johnson RM, Panjabi MM, et al. Biomechanical analysis of clinical instability in the cervical spine. *Clin Orthop Related Res*. 1975;109:85-96.

74. Beazell JR, Mullins M, Grindstaff TL. Lumbar Instability: an evolving and challenging concept. *J Man Manip Ther*. 2010;18(1):9-14.

75. Frymoyer JW, Selby DK. Segmental instability: rationale for treatment. *Spine*. 1985;10:280-286.

76. Ogon M, Bender BR, Hooper DM, et al. A dynamic approach to spinal instability, part I: sensitization of intersegmental motion profiles to motion direction and load condition by instability. *Spine*. 1997;22:2841-2858.

77. Olson KA, Joder D. Cervical spine clinical instability: a resident's case report. *J Orthop Sports Phys Ther*. 2001;31(4):194-206.

78. Cook C, Brismee JM, Fleming R, et al. Identifiers suggestive of clinical cervical spine instability: a Delphi study of physical therapists. *Phys Ther*. 2005;85(9):895-906.

79. Shippel AH, Robinson GK. Radiological and magnetic resonance imaging of cervical spine instability: a case report. *J Manipulative Physiol Ther*. 1987;10:317-322.

80. Jull G, Bogduk N, Marsland A. The accuracy of manual diagnosis for cervical zygapophysial joint pain syndromes. *Med J Aust.* 1988;148:233-236.

81. Pope MH, Frymoyer JW, Krag MH. Diagnosing instability. *Clin Orthop Related Res.* 1992;279:60-67.

82. Herkowitz HN, Rothman RH. Subacute instability of the cervical spine. *Spine.* 1984;9:348-357.

83. Paris SV. Cervical symptoms of forward head posture. *Topics Geriatr Rehabil.* 1990;5(4):11-19.

84. Bialosky JE, Bishop MD, Price DD, et al. The mechanisms of manual therapy in the treatment of musculoskeletal pain: a comprehensive model. *Man Ther.* 2009;14(5):531-538.

85. Falla D. Unraveling the complexity of muscle impairment in chronic neck pain. *Man Ther.* 2004;9:125-133.

86. Falla D, O'Leary SP, Farina D, et al. The change in deep cervical flexor activity after training is associated with the degree of pain reduction in patients with chronic neck pain. *Clin J Pain.* 2012;28(7):628-634.

87. Martin-Gomez C, Sestelo-Diaz R, Carrillo-Sanjuan V, et al. Motor control using cranio-cervical flexion exercises versus other treatments for non-specific chronic neck pain: a systematic review and meta-analysis. *Musculoskelet Sci Pract.* 2019;42:52-59.

88. O'Leary S, Cagnie B, Reeve A, et al. Is there altered activity of the extensor muscles in chronic mechanical neck pain? A functional magnetic resonance imaging study. *Arch Phys Med Rehabil.* 2011;92:929-934.

89. O'leary S, Jull G, Van Wyk L, et al. Morphological changes in the cervical muscles of women with chronic whiplash can be modified with exercise- a pilot study. *Muscle Nerve.* 2015;52(5):772-779.

90. Peterson GE, Ludvigsson MHL, O'Leary SP, et al. The effect of 3 different exercise approaches on neck muscle endurance, kinesiophobia, exercise compliance, and patient satisfaction in chronic whiplash. *J Manipulative Physiol Ther.* 2015;38(7):465-476.

91. Swinkels R, Beeton K, Alltree J. Pathogenesis of upper cervical instability. *Man Ther.* 1996;1:127-132.

92. Rushton A, Rivett D, Carlesso L, et al. *International framework for examination of the cervical region for potential of cervical arterial dysfunction prior to orthopaedic manual physical therapy intervention.* International Federation of Orthopaedic Manipulative Physical Therapists; 2012. Available at www.IFOMPT.org. Accessed September 02, 2013.

93. Torrens M. Adult: cervical spondylosis: part I: pathogenesis, diagnosis, and management options. *Curr Orthop.* 1994;8:255-263.

94. Cleland JA, Whitman JM, Fritz JM, et al. Manual physical therapy, cervical traction, and strengthening exercises in patients with cervical radiculopathy: a case series. *J Orthop Sports Phys Ther.* 2005;35(12):803-811.

95. Radhakrishnan K, Litchy WJ, O'Fallan M, et al. Epidemiology of cervical radiculopathy: a population-based study from Rochester, Minnesota, 1976-1990. *Brain.* 1994;117:325-335.

96. Shelerud RA, Paynter KS. Rarer causes of radiculopathy: spinal tumors, infections, and other unusual causes. *Phys Med Rehabil Clin North Am.* 2002;13:645-696.

97. Wainner RS, Fritz JM, Irrgang JJ, et al. Reliability and diagnostic accuracy of the clinical examination and patient self-report measures for cervical radiculopathy. *Spine.* 2003;28(1):52-62.

98. Thoomes EJ, van Geest S, van der Windt DA, et al. Value of physical tests in diagnosing cervical radiculopathy: a systematic review. *Spine J.* 2018;18(1):179-189.

99. Apelby-Albrecht M, Andersson L, Kleiva IW, et al. Concordance of upper limb neurodynamic tests with medical examination and magnetic resonance imaging in patients with cervical radiculopathy: a diagnostic cohort study. *J Manipulative Physiol Ther.* 2013;36:626-632.

100. Waldrop MA. Diagnosis and treatment of cervical radiculopathy using a clinical prediction rule and a multimodal intervention approach: a case series. *J Orthop Sports Phys Ther.* 2006;36(3):152-159.

101. Cleland JA, Fritz JM, Whitman JM, et al. Predictors of short-term outcome in people with a clinical diagnosis of cervical radiculopathy. *Phys Ther.* 2007;87(12):1619-1632.

102. Young I, Pozzi F, Dunning J, et al. Immediate and short-term effects of thoracic spine manipulation in patients with cervical radiculopathy: a randomized controlled trial. *J Orthop Sports Phys Ther.* 2019;49(5):299-309.

103. Raney NH, Peterson EJ, Smith TA, et al. Development of a clinical predication rule to identify patients with neck pain likely to benefit from cervical traction and exercise. *Eur Spine J.* 2009;18(3):382-391.

104. Young IA, Michener LA, Cleland JA, et al. Manual therapy, exercise, and traction for patients with cervical radiculopathy: a randomized clinical trial. *Phys Ther.* 2009;89(7):632-642.

105. Fritz JM, Thackeray A, Brennan GP, et al. Exercise only, exercise with mechanical traction, or exercise with over-door traction for patients with cervical radiculopathy, with or without consideration of status on a previously described subgrouping rule: a randomized clinical trial. *J Orthop Sports Phys Ther.* 2014;44(2):45-57.

106. Romeo A, Vanti C, Boldrini V, et al. Cervical radiculopathy: effectiveness of adding traction to physical therapy—a systematic review and meta-analysis of randomized controlled trials. *Phys Ther.* 2018;98:231-242.

107. Basson A, Olivier B, Ellis R, et al. The effectiveness of neural mobilization for neuromusculoskeletal conditions: a systematic review and meta-analysis. *J Orthop Sports Phys Ther.* 2017;47(9):593-615.

108. Savva C, Giakas G, Efstrathiou M, et al. Effectiveness of neural mobilization with intermittent traction in the management of cervical radiculopathy: a randomized controlled trial. *Int J Osteopath Med.* 2016;21:19-28.

109. Bier JD, Scholten-Peeters WGM, Staal JB, et al. Clinical practice guideline for physical therapy assessment and treatment in patients with nonspecific neck pain. *Phys Ther.* 2018;98:162-171.

110. Hoving JL, Koes BW, de Vet HCW, et al. Manual therapy, physical therapy, or continued care by a general practitioner for patients with neck pain: a randomized controlled trial. *Ann Intern Med.* 2002;136:713-722.

111. Korthals-de Bos IBC, Hoving JL, van Tulder MW, et al. Cost effectiveness of physiotherapy, manual therapy, and general practitioner care for neck pain: economic evaluation alongside a randomized controlled trial. *Brit Med J.* 2003;326:1-6.

112. Gross AR, Hoving JL, Haines TA, et al. A Cochrane review of manipulation and mobilization for mechanical neck disorders. *Spine.* 2004;29(14):1541-1548.

113. Gross A, Miller J, D'Sylva J, et al. Manipulation or mobilization for neck pain: a Cochrane review. *Man Ther.* 2010;15:315-333.

114. Gross A, Langevin P, Burnie SJ, et al. Manipulation and mobilization for neck pain contrasted against an inactive control or another active treatment. *Cochrane Database Syst Rev.* 2015;(9):CD004249.

115. Walker MJ, Boyles RE, Young BA, et al. The effectiveness of manual physical therapy and exercise for mechanical neck pain: a randomized clinical trial. *Spine.* 2008;33:2371-2378.

116. Boyles RE, Walker MJ, Young BA, et al. The addition of cervical thrust manipulations to a manual physical therapy approach in patients treated for mechanical neck pain: a secondary analysis. *J Orthop Sports Phys Ther*. 2010;40(3):133-140.

117. Celenay ST, Akbayrak T, Kaya DO. A comparison of the effects of stabilization exercises plus manual therapy to those of stabilization exercises alone in patients with nonspecific mechanical neck pain: a randomized controlled trial. *J Orthop Sports Phys Ther*. 2016;46(2):44-55.

118. Dunning JR, Cleland JA, Waldrop MA, et al. Upper cervical and upper thoracic thrust manipulation versus nonthrust mobilization in patients with mechanical neck pain: a multicenter randomized clinical trial. *J Orthop Sports Phys Ther*. 2011;42(1):5-18.

119. Griswold D, Learman K, Kolber MJ, et al. Pragmatically applied cervical and thoracic nonthrust manipulation versus thrust manipulation for patients with mechanical neck pain: A multicenter randomized clinical trial. *J Orthop Sports Phys Ther*. 2018;48(3):137-145.

120. Roenz D, Broccolo J, Brust S, et al. The impact of pragmatic vs prescriptive study designs on the outcomes of low back and neck pain when using mobilization or manipulation techniques: a systematic review and meta-analysis. *J Man Manip Ther*. 2018;26(3):123-135.

121. Tuttle N, Barrett R, Laakso L. Relation between changes in posteroanterior stiffness and active range of movement of the cervical spine following manual therapy treatment. *Spine*. 2008;33(19):E673-E679.

122. Puentedura EJ, Cleland JA, Landers MR, et al. Development of a clinical prediction rule to identify patients with neck pain likely to benefit from thrust joint manipulation to the cervical spine. *J Orthop Sports Phys Ther*. 2012;42(7):577-592.

123. Headache Classification Subcommittee of the International Headache Society. The International Classification of Headache Disorders 3rd edition. *Cephalalgia*. 2018;38:1-211.

124. Luedtke K, Boissonnault W, Caspersen N, et al. International consensus on the most useful physical examination tests used by physiotherapists for patients with headache: a Delphi Study. *Man Ther*. 2016;23:17-24.

125. Robertson BA, Morris ME. The role of cervical dysfunction in migraine: a systematic review. *Cephalalgia*. 2008;28(5):474-483.

126. Ashina S, Bendtsen L, Lyngberg AC, et al. Prevalence of neck pain in migraine and tension-type headache: a population study. *Cephalalgia*. 2015;35(3):211-219.

127. Calhoun AH, Ford S, Millen C, et al. The prevalence of neck pain in migraine. *Headache*. 2010;50:1273-1277.

128. Vincent MB. Headache and neck. *Curr Pain Headache Rep*. 2011;15(4):324-331.

129. Fernández-de-Las-Peñas C, Cuadrado ML, Pareja JA. Myofascial trigger points, neck mobility, and forward head posture in episodic tension-type headache. *Headache*. 2007;47(5):662-672.

130. Abboud J, Marchand AA, Sorra K, et al. Musculoskeletal physical outcome measures in individuals with tension-type headache: a scoping review. *Cephalalgia*. 2013;33(16):1319-1336.

131. Bartsch T. Migraine and the neck: new insights from basic data. *Curr Pain Headache Rep*. 2005;9:191-196.

132. Jull G, Hall T. Cervical musculoskeletal dysfunction in headache: how should it be defined? *Musculoskelet Sci Pract*. 2018;38:148-150.

133. Sjaastad O, Fredriksen TA, Pfaffenrath V. Cervicogenic headache: diagnostic criteria. *Headache*. 1998;38(6):442-445.

134. Zito G, Jull G, Story I. Clinical tests of musculoskeletal dysfunction in the diagnosis of cervicogenic headache. *Man Ther*. 2006;11(2):118-129.

135. Jull G, Amiri M, Bullock-Saxton J, et al. Cervical musculoskeletal impairment in frequent intermittent headache, part 1: subjects with single headaches. *Cephalalgia*. 2007;27(7):793-802.

136. Szikszay TM, Hoenick S, von Korn K, et al. Which examination tests detect differences in cervical musculoskeletal impairments in people with migraine? A systematic review and meta-analysis. *Phys Ther*. 2019;99:549-569.

137. Zito G, Jull G, Story I. Clinical tests of musculoskeletal dysfunction in the diagnosis of cervicogenic headache. *Man Ther*. 2006;11:118-129.

138. Pfaffenrath V, Kaube H. Diagnostics of cervicogenic headache. *Funct Neurol*. 1990;5:159-164.

139. Hagen K, Einarsen C, Zwart JA, et al. The co-occurrence of headache and musculoskeletal symptoms amongst 51050 adults in Norway. *Eur J Neurol*. 2002;9:527-533.

140. Racicki S, Gerwin S, DiClaudio S, et al. Conservative physical therapy management for the treatment of cervicogenic headache: systematic review. *J Man Manipulative Ther*. 2013;21(2):113-124.

141. Sjaastad O, Fredriksen T, Sand T. The localization of the initial pain of attack: a comparison between classic migrane and cervicogenic headache. *Funct Neurol*. 1989;4:73-78.

142. Hall TM, Robinson KW, Fujinawa O, et al. Intertester reliability and diagnostic validity of the cervical flexion-rotation test. *J Manipulative Physiol Ther*. 2008;31:293-300.

143. Haas M, Bronfort G, Evans R, et al. Dose-response and efficacy of spinal manipulation for care of cervicogenic headache: a dual-center randomized controlled trial. Spine J. 2018;18(10):1741-1754.

144. Jull G, Trott P, Potter H, et al. A randomized controlled trial of physiotherapy management for cervicogenic headache. *Spine*. 2002;27:1835-1843.

145. Uthaikhup S, Assapu J, Watcharasaksip K, et al. Effectiveness of physiotherapy for seniors with recurrent headaches associated with neck pain and dysfunction: a randomized controlled trial. *Spine J*. 2017;17:46-55.

146. Gross AR, Paauin JP, Dupont G, et al. Exercises for mechanical neck disorders: a Cochrane review update. *Man Ther*. 2016;24:25-45.

147. Treleaven J, Jull G, Sterling M. Dizziness and unsteadiness following whiplash injury-characteristic features and relationship to cervical joint position error. *J Rehabil Med*. 2003;35:36-43.

148. Loudon JK, Ruhl M, Field E. Ability to reproduce head position after whiplash injury. *Spine*. 1997;22:865-868.

149. Kristtjansson E, Dall'Alba P, Jull G. A study of five cervicocephalic relocation tests in three different subject groups. *Clin Rehabil*. 2003;17:768-774.

150. Kristjansson E, Treleaven J. Sensorimotor function and dizziness in neck pain: implications for assessment and management. *J Orthop Sports Phys Ther*. 2009;39(5):364-377.

151. Treleaven J, Joloud V, Nevo Y, et al. Normative responses to clinical tests for cervicogenic dizziness: clinical cervical torsion test and head-neck differentiation test. *Phys Ther*. 2020;100:192-200.

152. De Vries J, Ischebeck BK, Voogt LP, et al. Joint position sense error in people with neck pain: a systematic review. *Man Ther*. 2015;20:736-744.

153. Dugailly PM, De Santis R, Tits M, et al. Head repositioning accuracy in patients with neck pain and asymptomatic subjects: concurrent validity, influence of motion speed, motion direction and target distance. *Eur Spine J*. 2015;24(12):2885-2891.

154. Treleaven J. Sensorimotor disturbances in neck disorders affecting postural stability, head and eye movement control. *Man Ther.* 2008;13(1):2-11.

155. Passatore M, Roatta S. Influence of sympathetic nervous system on sensorimotor function: whiplash associated disorders (WAD) as a model. *Eur J Appl Physiol.* 2006;98:423-449.

156. Treleaven J. Sensorimotor disturbances in neck disorders affecting postural stability, head and eye movement control—part 2: case studies. *Man Ther.* 2008;13:266-275.

157. Reid SA, Rivett DA. Manual therapy treatment of cervicogenic dizziness: a systematic review. *Man Ther.* 2005;10:4-13.

158. Reid S, Rivett D, Katekar MG, et al. Comparison of Mulligan sustained natural apophyseal glides and maitland mobilizations for treatment of cervicogenic dizziness: a randomized controlled trial. *Phys Ther.* 2014;94(4):466-476.

159. Jull G, Falla D, Treleaven J, et al. Retraining cervical joint position sense: the effect of two exercise regimes. *J Orthop Res.* 2007;25(3):404-412.

160. Garcia-Perez-Juana D, Fernandez-de-las-Penas C, Arias-Buria JL, et al. Changes in cervicocephalis kinesthetic sensibility, widespread pressure pain sensitivity, and neck pain after cervical thrust manipulation in patients with chronic mechanical neck pain: a randomized clinical trial. *J Manipulative Physiol Ther.* 2018;41(7):551-560.

161. Uitvlugt G, Indenbaum S. Clinical assessment of atlantoaxial instability using the sharp-purser test. *Arthritis Rheum.* 1988;31(7):918-922.

162. Hutting N, Scholten-Peeters GGM, Vijverman V, et al. Diagnostic accuracy of upper cervical spine instability tests: a systematic review. *Phys Ther.* 2013;93:1686-1695.

163. Osmotherly PG, Rivett DA, Lindsay JR. Construct validity of clinical tests for alar ligament integrity: an evaluation using magnetic resonance imaging. *Phys Ther.* 2012;92:718-725.

164. Von PH, Maloul R, Hoffman M, et al. Diagnostic accuracy and validity of three manual examination tests to identify alar ligament lesions: results of a blinded case-control study. *J Man Manip Ther.* 2019;27(2):83-91.

165. Mintken PE, Metrick L, Flynn TW. Upper cervical ligament testing in a patient with os odontoideum presenting with headaches. *J Orthop Sports Phys Ther.* 2008;38(8):465-475.

166. Spurling RG, Scoville WB. Lateral rupture of the cervical intervertebral discs: a common cause of shoulder and arm pain. *Surg Gynecol Obstet.* 1944;78:350-358.

167. Tong HC, Haig AJ, Yamakawa K. The Spurling test and cervical radiculopathy. *Spine.* 2002;27(2):156-159.

168. Shabat S, Leitner Y, David R, et al. The correlation between Spurling test and imaging studies in detecting cervical radiculopathy. *J Neuroimaging.* 2012;22:375-378.

169. Gumina S, Carbone S, Albino P, et al. Arm Squeeze Test: a new clinical test to distinguish neck from shoulder pain. *Eur Spine J.* 2013;22:1558-1563.

170. Viikari-Juntura E, Porras M, Laasonen EM. Validity of clinical tests in the diagnosis of root compression in cervical disc disease. *Spine.* 1989;14:253-257.

171. Bertilson B, Grunnesjo M, Strender L. Reliability of clinical tests in the assessment of patients with neck/shoulder problems: impact of history. *Spine.* 2003;28:2222-2231.

172. Butler D, Gifford L. The concepts of adverse mechanical tension in the nervous system: part 1: testing for "dural tension". *Physiotherapy.* 1989;75(11):622-628.

173. Elvey RL. Treatment of arm pain associated with abnormal brachial plexus tension. *Aust J Physiother.* 1986;32:224-229.

174. Butler DS. *Mobilisation of the Nervous System.* Edinburgh: Churchill Livingstone; 1991.

175. Nee RL, Jull GA, Vicenzino B, et al. The validity of upper-limb neurodynamic tests for detecting peripheral neuropathic pain. *J Orthop Sports Phys Ther.* 2012;42(5):413-424.

176. Schmid AB, Brunner F, Luomajoki H, et al. Reliability of clinical tests to evaluate nerve function and mechanosensitivity of the upper limb peripheral nervous system. *BMC Musculoskelet Disord.* 2009;10:11.

177. Manvell JJ, Manvell N, Snodgrass S, et al. Improving the radial nerve neurodynamic test: an observation tension of the radial, median and ulnar nerves during upper limb positioning. *Man Ther.* 2015;20:790-796.

178. Cote P, Kreitz BG, Cassidy JD, et al. The validity of the extension-rotation test as a clinical screening procedure before neck manipulation: a secondary analysis. *J Manipulative Physiol Ther.* 1996;19:159-164.

179. Hutting N, Verhagen AP, Vijverman V, et al. Diagnostic accuracy of premanipulative vertebrobasilar insufficiency tests: a systematic review. *Man Ther.* 2013;18(3):177-182.

180. Rushton A, Carlesso LC, Rivett D, Flynn T, Hing W, Kerry R. International Framework for Examination of the Cervical Region for potential of vascular pathologies of the neck prior to Orthopaedic Manual Therapy intervention. *Man Ther.* 2014;19(3):222-228.

181. Olson K, Paris S, Spohr C, et al. Radiographic assessment and reliability study of the craniovertebral sidebending test. *J Manual Manipulative Ther.* 1998;6(2):87-96.

182. Piva SR, Erhard RE, Childs JD, et al. Inter-rater reliability of passive intervertebral and active movements of the cervical spine. *Man Ther.* 2006;11(4):321-330.

183. Hall T, Chan HT, Christensen L, et al. Efficacy of a C1-C2 self-sustained natural apophyseal glide (SNAG) in the management of cervicogenic headache. *J Orthop Sports Phys Ther.* 2007;37:100-107.

184. Ogince M, Hall T, Robinson K, et al. The diagnostic validity of the cervical flexion-rotation test in C1-C2-related cervicogenic headache. *Man Ther.* 2007;12:256-262.

185. Hall T, Briffa K, Hopper D, et al. Long-term stability and minimal detectable change of the cervical flexion-rotation test. *J Orthop Sports Phys Ther.* 2010;40(4):225-229.

186. Ogince M, Hall T, Robinson K, et al. The diagnostic validity of the cervical flexion-rotation test in C1/2-related cervicogenic headache. *Man Ther.* 2007;12(3):256-262.

187. Hall TM, Robinson KW, Fujinawa O, et al. Intertester reliability and diagnostic validity of the cervical flexion-rotation test. *J Manip Physiol Ther.* 2008;31(4):293-300.

188. Hall T, Briffa K, Hopper D, et al. Comparative analysis and diagnostic accuracy of the cervical flexion-rotation test. *J Headache Pain.* 2010;11:391-397.

189. Rubio-Ochoa J, Benitez-Martinez J, Lluch I, et al. Physical examination tests for screening and diagnosis of cervicogenic headache: a systematic review. *Man Ther.* 2016;21:35-40.

190. Smedmark V, Wallin M, Arvidsson I. Inter-examiner reliability in assessing passive intervertebral motion of the cervical spine. *Man Ther.* 2000;5:97-101.

191. Fernandez-de-las-Penas C, Downey C, Miangolarra-Page JC. Validity of the lateral gliding test as tool for the diagnosis of intervertebral joint dysfunction in the lower cervical spine. *J Manipulative Physiol Ther.* 2005;28(8):610-616.

192. Panjabi M, Dvorak J, Duranceau J, et al. Three-dimensional movements of the upper cervical spine. *Spine*. 1988;13(7):726-730.

193. Kottke FJ, Mundale MO. Range of mobility of the cervical spine. *Arch Phys Med Rehabil*. 1959;379-382.

194. White A, Panjabi MM. Kinematics of the spine. In: White A, Panjabi MM, editors. *Clinical Biomechanics of the Spine*. Philadelphia: Lippincott; 1978.

195. Jull G, Zito G, Trott P, et al. Inter-examiner reliability to detect painful upper cervical joint dysfunction. *Aust J Physiother*. 1997; 43:125-129.

196. Hall T, Briffa K, Hopper D, et al. Reliability of manual examination and frequency of symptomatic cervical motion segment dysfunction in cervicogenic headache. *Man Ther*. 2010;15(6): 542-546.

CHAPTER 7

Examination and Treatment of Temporomandibular Disorders

OVERVIEW

This chapter includes descriptions of the kinematics and functional anatomy of the temporomandibular joint (TMJ) and related structures and the examination, diagnostic classification, and treatment of temporomandibular disorders (TMDs). Video clips of the majority of the examination and manual therapy procedures are also included.

OBJECTIVES

- Describe the functional anatomy and kinematics of the temporomandibular joint (TMJ) disorders.

- Use clinical reasoning to diagnose and identify the classification of TMD based on signs and symptoms and describe the components of each disorder.

- Differentiate TMD from other causes of craniofacial pain.

- Perform a comprehensive examination of the TMJ and related structures.

- Determine the most effective and perform treatment procedures for TMD, including soft tissue mobilization, joint mobilization/manipulation, and exercise instruction.

- Describe the functional and neurophysiologic interrelationships between the TMJ and the cervical spine, and identify why examination and treatment of the cervical spine are important to include with the effective management of TMDs.

- Incorporate psychologically informed education and management principles for treatment of patients with TMDs.

▶ *To view videos pertaining to this chapter, please visit the eBook.*

SIGNIFICANCE OF THE PROBLEM

More than 17 million people in the United States are estimated to have TMDs.[1] The phrase "temporomandibular disorders (TMDs)" is a collective term that describes a number of clinical problems that involve the masticatory musculature, the TMJ and associated structures, or both.[2]

The lifetime incidence rate of TMD is reported to be 34%, with a 2% annual incidence rate.[3] Dworkin and LeResche[3] estimate that 178 lost activity days per 1000 persons per year can be attributed to TMD. Other estimates state that symptoms of TMDs occur in approximately 6% to 12% of the adult population.[4] Although TMJ problems can occur in individuals of any age, they are most common in individuals 18 to 45 years of age and are four to five times more prevalent in women than in men.[5-7] TMD is a musculoskeletal condition

that results in craniofacial pain, functional limitations, and disability.[8] Symptoms associated with TMD can include TMJ pain, decreased jaw motion, joint clicking, headaches, neck pain, facial pain, and pain with chewing.[9] TMDs may be the result of osteoarthritic degeneration, articular disk subluxation, or muscle guarding/myofascial trigger points of the muscles of mastication.[9]

Treatment options for TMD include surgery, injections, medications, intraoral appliances, biofeedback, dry needling, and physical therapy. Outcomes reported with the use of surgery and intraoral appliances in treatment of TMD have been disappointing. A retrospective cohort study revealed that at a 6-month follow-up examination, only 50% of patients who underwent TMJ arthroplasty viewed the outcome as favorable.[10] Intraoral appliances, which are used in theory to create a natural resting position of the mandible to inhibit excessive tension in the muscles of mastication and relieve pain, have been shown to be less effective than a manual physical therapy approach in the management of TMJ articular disk anterior displacement without reduction syndrome.[11] The group that used manual therapy combined with active exercise showed significant reductions in pain and increases in range of motion (ROM), and the group with the soft repositioning splint did not show significant changes in either dependent measure.[11] A systematic review and meta-analysis on the use of manual therapy techniques to treat TMD showed significance for short-term improvement compared with other conservative interventions to increase active range of motion (AROM) of mouth opening and to decrease pain during active mouth opening.[12] Another systematic review showed "promising effects" of manual physical therapy alone or in combination with exercises at the jaw or cervical spine for treatment of TMD.[13] This chapter focuses on the physical therapy diagnosis and management of TMD using an impairment-based manual physical therapy approach that has been supported in the literature.[14–17]

TEMPOROMANDIBULAR KINEMATICS: FUNCTIONAL ANATOMY AND MECHANICS

The TMJ is a synovial articulation between the mandible and the temporal bone of the cranium with an articular disk interposed between the two bony structures. The articular disk divides the joint into an upper and lower compartment. The TMJ is classified as a hinge joint with a moveable socket because of the hinge-like motion of the lower compartment and the gliding movement of the upper compartment.[18] The

articular disk is biconcave, with the thin intermediate portion composed of an avascular and aneural fibrous structure that is well suited for the stresses of the joint surfaces (Fig. 7.1).[19] The anterior and posterior portions of the disk are two to three times thicker than the intermediate portion and have vascular and nerve supplies.[20] The biconcave shape of the disk offers congruency of the articular surfaces and contributes greatly to the stability of the TMJ.

The posterior aspect of the TMJ is referred to as the bilaminar region and is composed of the posterior ligament, which has two heads: the inferior stratum, which attaches the disk to the neck of the mandibular condyle; and the superior stratum, which attaches the disk to the posterior aspect of the temporal bone. The retrodiscal pad is interspersed between the two heads of the posterior ligament and includes highly vascularized and innervated loose connective tissue that attaches to the posterior wall of the capsule[18] (Fig. 7.1). The superior head of the lateral pterygoid muscle attaches to the anterior medial portion of the disk, and additional fibrous capsular tissues attach to the anterior portion of the disk.[18] The lateral and medial collateral ligaments connect the disk to the lateral and medial poles of the condyle to form a bucket-handle configuration, which allows the disk to slide anterior/posterior on the condyle.[19] The fibrous joint capsule envelops the entire joint and is reinforced laterally by the temporomandibular ligament. With hypermobility of the TMJ, the posterior ligament and collateral ligaments tend to lose their ability to stabilize the disk on the mandibular condyle, and the lateral pterygoid tends to pull the disk anterior and medially as the disk dysfunction progresses to cause a disk dislocation.[19]

The innervation of the TMJ is from the auriculotemporal and masseteric branches of the mandibular nerve, and the

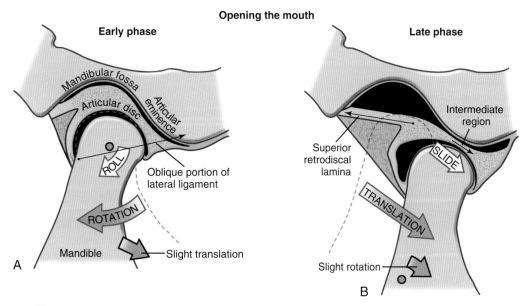

FIG. 7.1 A lateral view of a sagittal plane cross-section through a normal right temporomandibular joint. The mandible is in a position of maximal intercuspation, with the disk in its ideal position relative to the condyle and the temporal bone. (From Neumann DA. *Kinesiology of the Musculoskeletal System: Foundations for Physical Rehabilitation,* ed 3. St Louis: Elsevier; 2017.)

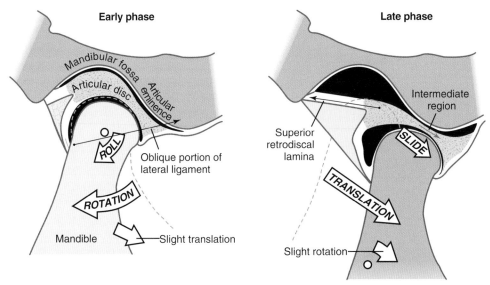

FIG. 7.2 Arthrokinematics of opening mouth: early phase and late phase. (From Neumann DA. *Kinesiology of the Musculoskeletal System: Foundations for Physical Rehabilitation*, ed 3. St Louis: Elsevier; 2017.)

blood supply is from the superficial temporal and maxillary arteries.[18]

The osteokinematics of the mandible include depression (opening), elevation (closing), protrusion, retrusion, and lateral excursion. Mandibular depression is measured as the space between the maxillary and mandibular incisors; normal ROM can vary from 35 mm to 50 mm, depending on the size and shape of the mouth and teeth, with 40 mm of opening typically considered normal ROM.[18,20] Lateral excursion and protrusion motions are approximately 10 mm. A 4:1 ratio of depression to lateral excursion is considered ideal and is an important consideration in restoration of motion to a TMJ with mobility deficits.[19]

Arthrokinematically, mandibular depression begins with the first 25 mm of opening that occurs primarily as a rotational motion (roll-gliding) of the condyle in the inferior joint space (Fig. 7.2). Once the collateral ligaments tauten, the opening continues as primarily a translatory gliding motion in the upper joint space until 35 mm is reached and the posterior and collateral ligaments are taut. Opening greater than 35 mm results from further translation with overrotation and further stretching applied to the posterior and collateral ligaments.[19] The lateral pterygoid, inferior head, provides a protracting force on the condyles and disks; the geniohyoid and digastric muscles produce a depressing and retracting force on the chin; and the mylohyoid muscle pulls downward on the body of the mandible to combine to produce the rotatory and translatory movements of the jaw that occur with mandibular depression[19] (Figs. 7.3 and 7.4).

Elevation of the mandible to close the mouth is initiated by the posterior fibers of the temporalis muscle contracting to retract the condyle of the mandible and clear the articular eminence of the temporalis bone (Fig. 7.5). The temporalis, masseter, and medial pterygoid contract on both sides to elevate the mandible, and the lateral pterygoid (Fig. 7.6) stabilizes

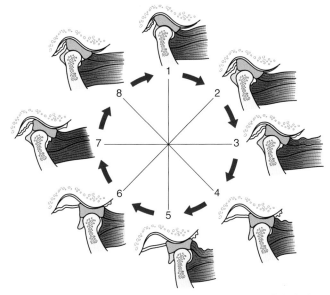

FIG. 7.3 Normal functional movement of condyle and disk during full range of opening and closing. (From Magee DJ. *Orthopedic Physical Assessment*, ed 6. St. Louis: Saunders; 2014.)

the disk/condyle complex against the articular eminence during closing.[18,19]

Protrusion of the mandible is created with symmetrical anterior translation of both condyle/disk complexes on the articular eminence, and the motion occurs at the superior joint space. Protrusion is created by contraction of the inferior head of the lateral pterygoid and holding action of the masseter and medial pterygoid muscles.[19] The lateral pterygoid pulls the condyle and disk forward and down along the articular eminence while the elevator and depressor muscles maintain the mandibular position.[19] Retrusion is the return to rest position from the protrusion position and is created by the contraction

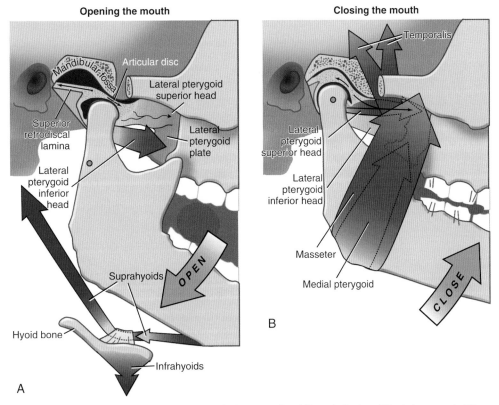

Opening the mouth

Closing the mouth

A

B

FIG. 7.4 The muscle and joint interaction during opening (A) and closing (B) of the mouth. The relative degree of muscle activation is indicated by the different intensities of red. In B, the superior head of the lateral pterygoid muscle is shown eccentrically active. The locations of the axes of rotation (shown as *small green circles* in A and B) are estimates only. (From Neumann DA. *Kinesiology of the Musculoskeletal System: Foundations for Physical Rehabilitation*, ed 3. St Louis: Elsevier; 2017.)

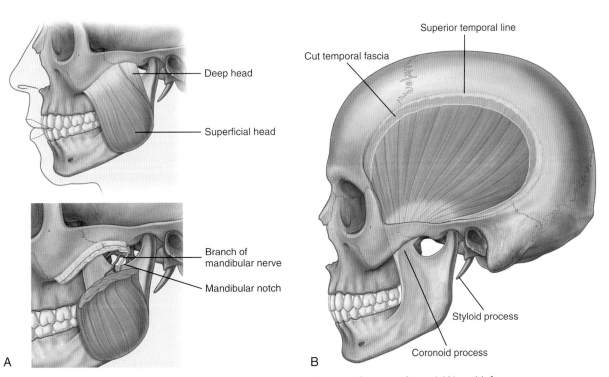

A

B

FIG. 7.5 Illustration highlighting the left masseter (intact and cut specimens) (A) and left temporalis (B) muscles. (From Drake RL, Vogl W, Mitchell AWM. *Gray's Anatomy for Student*. St Louis: Churchill; 2005.)

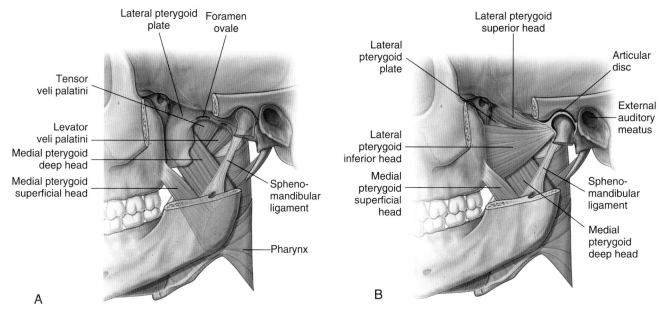

FIG. 7.6 Illustration highlighting the left medial pterygoid (A) and lateral pterygoid (B) muscles. The mandible and zygomatic arch have been cut for better exposure of the pterygoid muscles. (From Drake RL, Vogl W, Mitchell AWM. *Gray's Anatomy for Student.* St Louis: Churchill; 2005.)

of the middle and posterior fibers of both temporalis muscles while the depressors and elevators maintain a slight opening of the mouth.[19]

Lateral excursion occurs when the condyle and disk of the contralateral side are pulled forward, downward, and medially along the articular eminence. The condyle on the ipsilateral side performs minimal rotation around a vertical axis and a slight lateral shift.[19] These motions take place primarily in the upper joint space. Lateral excursion is created by contraction of the lateral pterygoid muscles on the contralateral side of the direction of the motion combined with the ipsilateral side temporalis muscle contracting to hold the rest position of the condyle to prevent the mandible from deviating anteriorly.[19]

Cervical Spine Influence on the Temporomandibular Joint

The cervical spine can influence TMJ function in a variety of ways, and postural interrelationships have been noted through a series of studies. McClean et al.[21] found that occlusional contacts change as the body position is altered on a tilt table. The mandible was consistently in a more retruded position with the participants in supine, and the occlusional contact became more anterior as the participants assumed a more upright position.[21]

Funakoshi et al.[22] measured jaw muscle activity changes associated with head position and found that with cervical forward bending, increased electromyographic (EMG) activity was noted in the bilateral digastric muscles. With cervical backward bending, increased EMG activity was noted in the bilateral temporalis muscles. With cervical rotation and side bending, increased EMG activity was noted in the ipsilateral temporalis, masseter, and digastric muscles. This increased

EMG activity was believed to occur in an attempt to maintain the rest position of the mandible in various head and neck postural positions.[22]

Darling et al.[23] showed that head and neck postural positioning could be improved with 4 weeks of physical therapy and that an increase in the vertical postural position of the mandible occurred as the head and neck postural positioning improved. The vertical postural position is the rest position of the mandible in which the teeth are not occluded, the lips are in light contact, and only a minimal amount of muscular activity occurs to maintain and balance the postural position. In other words, as the patient's head and neck posture improved, the mandible assumed a more relaxed neutral position.

Goldstein et al.[24] found that the vertical distance of mandibular closure from the rest position of the mandible decreased significantly as a maximum forward head posture was assumed in comparison with the same participants in their best "normal" posture. As a result, they also saw a change in trajectory of mandibular occlusion with forward head posture positioning and a change in initial tooth contact.[24] These postural influences on mandibular function have been postulated as causing a "pseudomalocclusion" that could contribute to increased strain on the joint capsule and myofascial structures associated with TMJ function.[25]

Not only can head and neck posture affect TMJ function, but also mandibular rest position change can affect head and neck posture. Daly[26] had 30 participants sit with an 8-mm spacer between the teeth for 1 hour and found that all participants had an altered craniovertebral angle after 1 hour, with 27 participants having a more extended position of the head on the neck and three participants assuming a more flexed position. One hour after removal of the spacer appliance, all participants showed at least partial recovery toward the original head position.[26] These study results reinforce the interdependence of cervical, cranial, and mandibular positioning and function and may assist in explaining why patients occasionally have worse symptoms in the head and neck after initiation of an intraoral appliance therapy.

The cervical spine can also be a source of referred pain to the head and face and must be thoroughly screened as part of the comprehensive examination of a patient with symptoms of head and facial pain. A strong correlation has been demonstrated that the more impairments and pain identified with TMD, the greater the level of observable cervical musculoskeletal impairments.[27] Patients with findings of cervicogenic headache combined with TMD have an even greater number of cervical musculoskeletal impairments, including mobility deficits, pain provocation with examination of the upper cervical spine, and motor control deficits of the deep neck flexors.[28,29] The most likely anatomic sources of referred pain to the head and face include impairments of the suboccipital muscles and the upper cervical and C2–C3 facet joints and entrapment neuropathies of the greater and lesser occipital nerves. The strain associated with suboccipital muscle guarding may impinge on the greater occipital nerve and may result in referred pain into the craniofacial region, most typically into the distribution of the trigeminal nerve.[30] In a study by Aprill et al.,[31] 21 of 34 participants who underwent a nerve block to C1–C2 had complete resolution of headache symptoms. These findings suggest a high prevalence rate of headache and facial pain symptoms referred from the upper cervical spine. Studies have demonstrated improvement in TMD signs and symptoms following manual therapy interventions directed to the cervical spine.[17,32,33] In addition, enhancement of clinical outcomes for management of cervical spine impairments has been demonstrated with manual therapy treatment of TMD impairments in addition to treatment of the cervical musculoskeletal impairments.[29]

Therefore palpation and provocation tests for both the TMJ and upper cervical spine must be completed to differentiate the source of the symptoms. A thorough examination of the cervical and thoracic spine is a necessary component of examination of patients with primary symptoms of headaches and facial pain to differentiate the source of the symptoms and biomechanical factors that could potentially contribute to perpetuation of a TMD. Physical therapy treatment outcomes are enhanced when interventions are concurrently used to address both TMD and cervical impairments.

TEMPOROMANDIBULAR DISORDERS

The International Headache Society[34] classifies headache into three broad categories: (1) primary headache (migraine, tension type, cluster, and other primary); (2) secondary headache caused by another disorder, such as increased intracranial pressure, cranial neoplasm, TMDs, medication reaction, eyes, ears, nose, sinuses, teeth, psychiatric, infection, trauma, and/or cervical; and (3) cranial neuralgias.[35,36] Therefore the International Headache Society classifies TMD as a secondary headache that results from disorders of the TMJ or related structures.

Care must be taken to complete a thorough history and physical examination for patients with orofacial pain to differentiate TMD from a primary or secondary headache versus a systemic problem, such as cardiovascular or rheumatoid disorders[36] (Table 7.1). In addition to the normal physical therapy examination questions as outlined in Chapter 2, the TMJ examination should include completion of the Jaw Functional Limitation Score (JFLS) questionnaire (Table 7.2) and additional TMD history questions (Table 7.3) for identification of whether the facial and jaw pain originates from the TMJ and for determination if the patient has parafunctional oral habits that could be perpetuating the TMD.

The JFLS includes 20 items related to jaw function including mastication, verbal and emotional expression, and vertical

TABLE 7.1	Location, Duration, and Clinical Features of Three Primary Types of Headaches Compared With Cervicogenic Headache		
TYPE OF HEADACHE	**PAIN LOCATION**	**DURATION**	**CLINICAL FEATURES**
Migraine	Unilateral side of head; may shift	4–72 hours	More prevalent in women than men; Nausea, vomiting, throbbing, light-headedness, aura, photophobia, and phonophobia interfere with everyday life
Tension type	Bilateral tight band encircling head at the level of the temples	30 minutes to 7 days	Head and neck pain, muscle tightness, and dull pressure—like tight band
Cluster	Severe unilateral orbital pain	Occurs in cyclical patterns; 15 minutes to 2 hours	More prevalent in men than women; sudden onset, tearing, rhinorrhea, and "alarm clock" headache during morning sleep
Cervicogenic	Occipital to frontal; tends to be unilateral	Variable duration; Headache pain triggered by neck movements or positions	Unilateral headache with onset preceded by neck pain Headache pain elicited by pressure on the posterior neck especially at one of three upper cervical joints

(Modified from Harrison AL, Thorp JN, Ritzline PD. A proposed diagnostic classification of patients with temporomandibular disorders: implications for physical therapists. *J Orthop Sports Phys Ther.* 2014;44(3):182-197; Jull G, Trott P, Potter H, et al. A randomized controlled trial of physiotherapy management for cervicogenic headache. *Spine* 2002;27:1835-1843.)

TABLE 7.2	Jaw Functional Limitation Scale		
For each of the items listed here, indicate the level of limitation during the past month. If the activity was completely avoided because it is too difficult, indicate 10. If you avoid an activity for reasons other than pain or difficulty, then leave the item blank.			
		NO LIMITATION	**SEVERE LIMITATION**
1. Chew tough food*			0 1 2 3 4 5 6 7 8 9 10
2. Chew hard bread			0 1 2 3 4 5 6 7 8 9 10
3. Chew chicken (e.g., prepared in oven)*			0 1 2 3 4 5 6 7 8 9 10
4. Chew crackers			0 1 2 3 4 5 6 7 8 9 10
5. Chew soft food (e.g., macaroni, canned or soft fruits, cooked vegetables, and fish)			0 1 2 3 4 5 6 7 8 9 10
6. Eat soft food requiring no chewing (e.g., mashed potatoes, applesauce, pudding, and pureed food)*			0 1 2 3 4 5 6 7 8 9 10
7. Open wide enough to bite from a whole apple			0 1 2 3 4 5 6 7 8 9 10
8. Open wide enough to bite into a sandwich			0 1 2 3 4 5 6 7 8 9 10
9. Open wide enough to talk			0 1 2 3 4 5 6 7 8 9 10
10. Open wide enough to drink from a cup*			0 1 2 3 4 5 6 7 8 9 10
11. Swallow*			0 1 2 3 4 5 6 7 8 9 10
12. Yawn*			0 1 2 3 4 5 6 7 8 9 10
13. Talk*			0 1 2 3 4 5 6 7 8 9 10
14. Sing			0 1 2 3 4 5 6 7 8 9 10
15. Putting on a happy face			0 1 2 3 4 5 6 7 8 9 10
16. Putting on an angry face			0 1 2 3 4 5 6 7 8 9 10
17. Frown			0 1 2 3 4 5 6 7 8 9 10
18. Kiss			0 1 2 3 4 5 6 7 8 9 10
19. Smile*			0 1 2 3 4 5 6 7 8 9 10
20. Laugh			0 1 2 3 4 5 6 7 8 9 10

Items 1 to 6 represent mastication, items 7 to 10 represent mobility, and items 11 to 20 represent verbal and emotional communication. Items with an asterisk (*) are those used for the Jaw Functional Limitation Score (JFLS-8) (short form). Responses used a 0-to-10 numeric rating scale, with 0 anchored as "no limitation" and 10 anchored as "severe limitation."

(From Ohrbach R, Larsson P, List T. The jaw functional limitation scale: development, reliability, and validity of 8-item and 20-item versions. *J Orofac Pain* 2008;22(3): 219-229.)

jaw opening.[37] Patients are asked to rate each item on a numeric rating scale from 0 (no limitation) to 10 (severe limitation). A shorter version (JFLS-8) of this scale has been developed with use of eight of the selected functional activities for a more global functional limitation score.[37] Both the JFLS-20 and JFLS-8 have been found to have high levels of internal consistency (0.87 for the JFLS-8 and 0.95 for the JFLS-20), reliability, and construct validity.[37,38] The JFLS-20 and JFLS-8 are excellent functional measures for patients with TMD.

Mental health disorders, such as depression or anxiety, or both, are more common in patients with TMD (16%-40%) than in the general population (16%).[39] Physical therapists must screen patients for psychosocial characteristics, such as anxiety and depression, that could be contributing to the orofacial pain. The Four-Item Patient Health Questionnaire (PHQ-4) for Depression and Anxiety is a brief, self-report screen validated for anxiety and depression and is shown to predict functional impairment, healthcare usage, and disability days (Table 7.4). The PHQ-4 has been shown to have good validity and responsiveness.[40] A score of 3 to 5 suggests mild anxiety/depression, 6 to 8 is moderate, and 9 to 12 is severe.[41] Moderate to severe anxiety/depression may be an indication for referral to a behavioral health specialist. In a study with 162 patients with chronic TMD, screening showed that referral was required in 28 (17%) with a probable major depressive disorder and 32 (20%) with a general anxiety disorder.[39]

Central sensitization and depression tend to occur at a higher prevalence in individuals with chronic TMD than the general population.[42,43] Campi et al.[42] assessed 45 women (mean age 37.5 years; 16 with TMD) who were free of headache, fibromyalgia, or other painful conditions. Patients with painful chronic TMD had higher pain sensitivity to vibration

TABLE 7.3	History/Interview Questions for a Temporomandibular Joint Examination

I. Subjective Examination

A. Pain
1. Have you had pain or stiffness in the face, jaw, temple, in front of the ear, or in the ear in the past month?
2. Is there jaw pain with opening, closing, chewing, yawning, talking, singing, or kissing?
3. Ear symptoms of pain, fullness, or ringing?
4. Headaches? If yes, where? _____

B. Function
1. Difficulty opening?
2. Have you ever had your jaw lock or catch so that it would not open all the way? If so, was this limitation in jaw opening severe enough to interfere with your ability to eat?
3. Have you ever noticed clicking, popping, or other sounds in your joint?
4. Have you had any recent changes in occlusion (the way teeth seem to come together)?
5. Have you had any difficulty swallowing?
6. Do you have any parafunctional habits, such as clenching, grinding, nail biting, smoking, pen chewing, or other?
7. In what position do you tend to sleep?   On your back:_____   On your stomach:_____   On your side: Left:_____   Right:_____

and lower pressure pain threshold values in the lateral mandibular condyle, masseter, anterior temporalis, and forearm muscles.[42] Patients with chronic TMD were also more likely to have signs of depression, and the patients with TMD and depression had increased pain sensitivity to pressure and vibration.[42] The presence of hyperalgesia and allodynia among women with a painful chronic TMD provides evidence for the presence of central sensitization.[42]

Lorduy et al.[44] also noted that patients with myalgia TMDs and patients with more than one TMD diagnosis had the most symptoms of central sensitization syndromes and higher reports of pain and pain-related disability than other classifications of the 250 patients studied with acute TMD. A metaanalysis study of case-control and cohort/cross-sectional studies also supports the existence of differences in widespread pressure

pain sensitivity in patients with TMD when compared with asymptomatic subjects, which further supports the increased likelihood that patients with TMD will also be more likely to present with central sensitization than asymptomatic individuals.[45]

The central sensitization inventory questionnaire is a screening tool to help to identify patients with central sensitization syndrome and should be used as part of the examination of patients with TMD. See Chapter 2 for further explanation of central sensitization and the central sensitization inventory (Fig. 2.7). In patients with central sensitization, a psychologically informed approach that includes pain neuroscience education is recommended. Providing explanations of the neurophysiology associated with pain perception and the impact that psychosocial factors, such as stress, anxiety, and depression have on pain perception can help the patient better cope with and manage TMD symptoms. In addition, because central sensitization is associated with hyperalgesia, the therapist must use very gentle, nonprovocative manual forces to effectively incorporate manual therapy interventions in the management of patients with TMD.

Key history questions have been determined to have strong sensitivity and specificity in identification of TMDs as the source of pain.[36,46,47] One initial question is, "Have you had pain or stiffness in the face, jaw, temple, in front of the ear, or in the ear in the past month?" A positive response should be followed with a question about whether the symptoms are altered by jaw activities, such as chewing, talking, singing, yawning, kissing, or moving the jaw.[36,48] Another key question is directed toward identifying the presence of a disk displacement,[46,48] "Have you ever had your jaw lock or catch so that it would not open all the way? If so, was this limitation in jaw opening severe enough to interfere with your ability to eat? Have you ever noticed clicking, popping, or other sounds in your joint?"[48]

An international consortium recently revised the Research Diagnostic Criteria for Temporomandibular Disorders,[46] a classification system based on an integration of impairments and symptoms, that is referred to as the Diagnostic Criteria/ Temporomandibular Disorders (DC/TMD).[36,48] The DC/ TMD criteria describe two axes of focus for examination, with Axis I including the physical examination of body structure/ function impairments in the muscle and joint conditions and

TABLE 7.4	The Four-Item Patient Health Questionnaire for Anxiety and Depression			
OVER THE LAST 2 WEEKS, HOW OFTEN HAVE YOU BEEN BOTHERED BY THE FOLLOWING PROBLEMS?	**NOT AT ALL**	**SEVERAL DAYS**	**MORE THAN HALF THE DAYS**	**NEARLY EVERY DAY**
Feeling nervous, anxious, or on edge	0	1	2	3
Not being able to stop or control worrying	0	1	2	3
Feeling down, depressed, or hopeless	0	1	2	3
Little interest or pleasure in doing things	0	1	2	3

The first two items make up the anxiety subscale, and the last two items make up the depression subscale. Subscale scores of ≥3 are used to screen for depression or anxiety impairments. Composite scores of 3 to 5 suggest mild anxiety/depression, 6 to 8 is moderate, and 9 to 12 is severe.[41]

Axis II focusing on identifying psychosocial characteristics that play a role in the primary complaints.[40] Axis I contains three broad classification groups: group 1, masticatory muscle disorders; group 2, joint disorders related to temporomandibular disk derangements (disk displacement with reduction and disk displacement without reduction); and group 3, joint disorders related to TMJ arthralgia, arthritis, and arthrosis.[36,48]

The classification system presented in this chapter includes the components of the Axis I DC/TMD with supplemental information provided in an attempt to provide a classification system that is comprehensive and useful to guide physical therapist clinical reasoning in management of TMD. Table 7.5

provides a summary of the common signs and symptoms associated with each disorder. Patients may have a combination of TMD classifications, which makes management of this condition challenging.

The TMJ examination should also include a thorough cervical spine and upper thoracic examination as described in Chapters 2, 5, and 6, with particular attention directed toward screening for signs of a cervicogenic headache (Table 7.1).[36,49]

Arthralgia (Capsulitis/Synovitis)

Arthralgia is the term used for TMJ pain caused by capsulitis/synovitis, which is an inflammatory condition of the articular

TABLE 7.5	Signs and Symptoms of Temporomandibular Disorders
TEMPOROMANDIBULAR DISORDER CLASSIFICATION	**SIGNS AND SYMPTOMS**
Arthralgia (capsulitis/synovitis)	Tender to palpation at TMJ lateral condyle or posterior compartment Pain with biting on opposite side Pain with retrusive overpressure Pain with accessory motion testing
Capsular fibrosis	Limited mandibular AROM Limited mobility with TMJ accessory motion tests No joint sounds Deviation of mandible with opening and protrusion toward TMJ with mobility deficits Limited contralateral lateral excursion History of trauma or surgery

Masticatory muscle myalgia (with or without limited opening)	No joint sounds
	Pain with palpation of the muscles of mastication/myalgia
	Parafunctional oral behaviors
	Pain with biting on same side of the facial pain
	Masseter and/or temporalis:
	   Palpation of either reproduces chief complaint
	   Mouth opening painful at end range and may be limited to ≤40 mm (confirming if lateral excursion and protrusion are not painful or limited)
	Lateral pterygoid:
	   Chief complaint is lateral face pain
	   Pain reproduced with resisted protrusion
	   Pain with power stroke or biting on bilateral tongue depressors (confirming if end-range mouth opening does not reproduce complaint)

Hypermobility	Excessive AROM with opening >40 mm Joint sound at end range of opening Hypermobility with accessory motion testing Movement coordination impairments noted with variable S or C curves with opening/closing
Anterior disk displacement with reduction	Reciprocal joint sound with opening and closing (at least one of three repetitions); or opening or closing joint sound during one of three repetitions and a joint sound with one of three lateral excursions or protrusions S curve with opening Full AROM (unless combined with arthralgia/myalgia)
Anterior disk displacement without reduction (with or without limited opening)	History of joint sounds or TMJ locking/catching Limited opening <40 mm if acute with deviation of mandible toward the limited side Normal mandibular motions when chronic No current joint sounds (crepitus may be noted)
Osteoarthritis	TMJ crepitus as noted with stethoscope Pain with TMJ palpation Pain with loading TMJ Radiographic evidence of osteoarthritis

AROM, Active range of motion; *TMJ,* temporomandibular joint.
(Modified from Harrison AL, Thorp JN, Ritzline PD. A proposed diagnostic classification of patients with temporomandibular disorders: implications for physical therapists. *J Orthop Sports Phys Ther.* 2014;44(3):182-197.)

capsule and soft tissues that surround the TMJ, especially the highly vascularized and innervated extracapsular articular tissues. The patient has pain with palpation and loading the TMJ. Pain may also be noted with accessory motion testing. Chewing and biting down with the molars on the contralateral side of the involved TMJ tend to be painful. If capsulitis continues chronically over time, capsular fibrosis could form. Capsulitis can be combined with any of the other common TMJ disorders or can present in isolation.

The cause of capsulitis/synovitis has been explained as microtrauma or macrotrauma.[19] Microtrauma includes low-level repeated stresses and strains on the TMJ and surrounding tissues that may occur with parafunctional habits, such as clenching and grinding the teeth, chewing gum, or chewing on a pencil. Macrotrauma occurs with greater force, such as a blow to the jaw or surgery to the TMJ.

Antiinflammatory treatment, such as iontophoresis, gentle ROM activities, and ice, can often be helpful. In a study by Majwer and Swider,[50] 27 of 32 patients with posttraumatic TMD benefited with decreased pain from the application of dexamethasone ($n = 8$) or lidocaine (Xylocaine) ($n = 24$) through iontophoresis. Schiffman et al.[51] also demonstrated improvements in mandibular range of active motion and reduction in disability after three iontophoresis treatments with dexamethasone or lidocaine compared with a placebo iontophoresis treatment with saline. Reduction of the parafunctional activities through behavior modification may assist as well. Creation of a good environment for proper TMJ function, such as postural correction exercises and treatment of cervical and upper thoracic impairments, can also facilitate the rehabilitation process.

A physical therapy treatment approach was compared with use of splint therapy for a group of patients with signs and symptoms of TMJ arthralgia. Mandibular opening and pain levels improved with both groups, and at a 3-month follow-up, the group of patients who received physical therapy demonstrated a slightly better outcome.[52]

Furto et al.[14] had successful outcomes that included reduction of pain and disability with use of an impairment-based manual physical therapy approach in a case series of 15 patients with TMD as the primary symptom. At a 2-week follow-up examination, the group had received a mean of 4.3 physical therapy treatment sessions. Specific interventions included manual physical therapy techniques, such as intraoral soft tissue mobilization and nonthrust joint mobilization/manipulation to the cervical spine, TMJ, and thoracic spine. Five of the patients also received iontophoresis with dexamethasone to the symptomatic TMJ. Some 80% of the patients received instruction in TMJ proprioception and postural exercises. The mean TMD disability index scores were 32.1% at baseline and 18.3% at the 2-week follow-up examination, an improvement of 13.9% (confidence interval [CI], 8.2%, 19.5%; $P < .05$). Eleven patients (73%) reported they were "somewhat better" to "a very great deal better" on the global rating of change questionnaire, and patient specific functional scale scores improved 3.1 points (CI, 2.3–3.9; $P < .05$).[14] The treatment approach used in this case series is representative of an impairment-based approach in which manual physical therapy and exercise interventions were used to address the specific impairments noted at the cervical spine and craniomandibular region. Iontophoresis was used as an adjunct to reduce the pain and inflammation at the TMJ capsular tissues.

Furto et al.[14] used a TMJ exercise program developed by Rocabado[53] to facilitate dynamic neuromuscular control through the use of repetitive lateral deviation motions with a 0.5-inch piece of rubber tubing placed between the incisors to assist with mobility, proprioception, and pain inhibition. Box 7.1 (Fig. 7.7) provides an illustration of TMJ proprioception exercises. The first (ROM) phase involves AROM lateral excursion while the rubber tubing is rolled between the incisors, with movement away from the side of TMJ pain or hypermobility; the second (bite) phase involves a submaximal biting-down contraction in the lateral excursion position with the bite let off before a return to midline; and the third phase involves biting down on the tube with the lateral excursion motion and with return to midline. In theory, the biting with motion recruits the muscles of mastication to apply a compressive force to the disk to improve the condylar-disk-eminence congruency and TMJ function.[53] Phases 4 to 6 of this program involve a similar progression with mandibular protrusion active motions. Patients are instructed to perform six repetitions every 2 hours. Although limited evidence exists to support the theoretical effect of this treatment approach, the patients in the case series had improvements in function, pain, and disability.[14]

Capsular Fibrosis

Capsular fibrosis is characterized by a mandibular opening of less than 40 mm (commonly <25 mm) because of adhesions that limit extensibility of the TMJ capsule. The mandible deviates toward the side of the restricted TMJ with opening, lateral excursion to the opposite side of the hypomobile joint is limited, and protrusion deviates toward the affected side. Accessory motion testing of the TMJ shows hypomobility. The causes of capsular fibrosis may include a chronic inflammatory condition, trauma, immobilization, or a subluxed articular disk without reduction relationship that places the mandibular head in a posterior and superior position which may block TMJ motion.[19]

When the capsular fibrosis is coupled with arthralgia or myalgia, these conditions need to be addressed as part of the treatment. Cervical spine and postural disorders should also be appropriately addressed if present with TMD. Joint mobilization/manipulation, active and passive mandibular ROM exercises, and sustained TMJ stretching techniques are indicated to restore TMJ mobility. Sustained TMJ stretching can be accomplished with a stack of tongue depressors placed between the molars on the ipsilateral side of the TMJ with mobility deficits (Box 7.2) (Fig. 7.8). The patient is instructed to maintain the stretch for 15 to 20 minutes three times per day. This technique can be combined with a heat modality, such as moist heat or therapeutic ultrasound. TMJ ROM and proprioception

BOX 7.1   Temporomandibular Joint Proprioception/Movement Coordination Exercises With a Rubber Tube

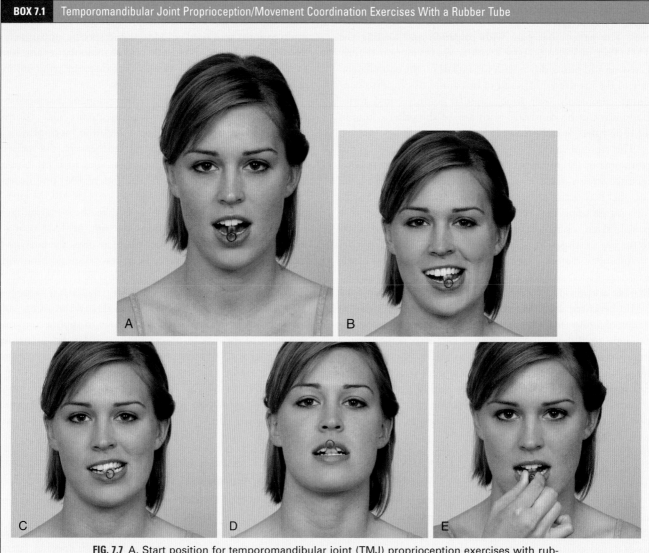

FIG. 7.7 A, Start position for temporomandibular joint (TMJ) proprioception exercises with rubber tube. B, Range-of-motion (ROM) phase (phase 1): perform active lateral deviation away from painful TMJ within pain-free range of motion and without joint sounds. C, Bite phase (phase 2): at end of lateral deviation ROM, patient applies submaximal bite onto tube and holds bite for 5 seconds. Mandible is then returned to midline. This is repeated for five to six repetitions. Next progression (phase 3) is to maintain bite as mandible is returned to midline. D, Phases 4 to 6: protrusion ROM, bite at end range, and bite as return to starting position can be progressed in similar fashion to lateral deviation progression. E, Final progression is to gently pull tube and resist in either protrusion or laterally deviated position.

exercises for opening and lateral excursion should be performed at least five to six times per day.

Masticatory Muscle Myalgia

Masticatory muscle myalgia disorders are most commonly associated with painful guarded muscles of mastication (myalgia) with the presence of taut myofascial bands and trigger points and may progress to include tendonitis, commonly of the temporalis tendon. Palpation of the involved muscles and chewing/biting on the ipsilateral side of the pain provoke the symptoms. Masticatory muscle disorders may be associated

with limited or normal mandibular opening. Okeson[54] recommends activating the inferior portion of the lateral pterygoid through resisted protrusion and the superior portion of the lateral pterygoid through a power stroke (clenching teeth together) to assess masticatory myalgia. The medial pterygoid muscle is also activated with the power stroke but is also stretched with mouth opening unlike the lateral pterygoid muscle.[36] Therefore limited opening associated with masticatory muscle disorders may be caused by myalgia/guarding/tightness of the medial pterygoid, temporalis, and masseter muscles. The lateral pterygoid myalgia could be the source of

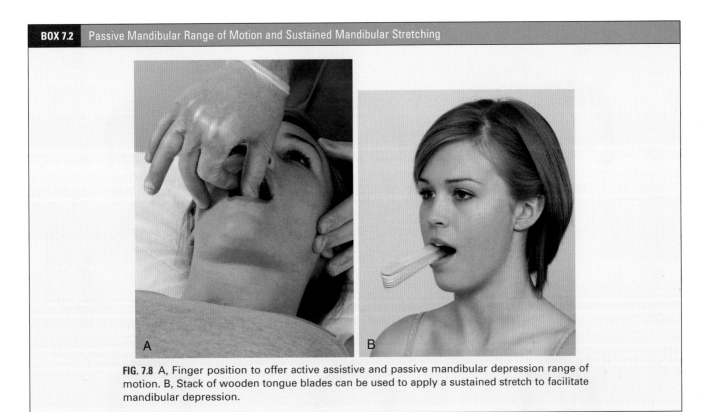

FIG. 7.8 A, Finger position to offer active assistive and passive mandibular depression range of motion. B, Stack of wooden tongue blades can be used to apply a sustained stretch to facilitate mandibular depression.

the muscle pain but still allow full opening. To reduce joint loading while testing the power stroke, the therapist can position tongue depressors between the back molars on each side during clenching, which prevents the joints from compressing during a power stroke (Fig 7.24B). If this maneuver is painful, likely it is caused by masticatory myalgia rather than arthralgia.[36]

TMJ palpation, compression, and accessory motion tests are nonprovocative if the masticatory muscle disorder is present in isolation. Masticatory muscle disorders can occur in isolation or can be combined with other TMJ disorders. The most common cause is parafunctional behaviors that cause irritation and inflammation of the muscles of mastication; most commonly, the closing/clenching muscles are involved, especially the masseter, temporalis, and lateral pterygoid muscles. Parafunctional oral habits (such as gum chewing, chewing on ice, repetitive nonfunctional jaw movements, and frequent leaning of the chin on the palm) have been associated with the presence of TMJ disorders in girls of high school age.[55] Masticatory myalgia may also be associated with stress and anxiety disorders and centrally mediated pain conditions, such as fibromyalgia and chronic pain disorders.[36]

Treatment may include use of heat modalities, such as moist heat, therapeutic ultrasound, or warm water rinses. Instruction in proper tongue/teeth/lip positioning and isometric opening exercises may assist in inhibition of the guarded closing/clenching muscles. The controlled mandibular opening exercise can facilitate muscle relaxation and strengthen the proper tongue function and placement (Box 7.3) (Fig. 7.9). Intraoral and extraoral soft tissue mobilization techniques are

also indicated. The patient can be instructed in self–soft tissue mobilization techniques and educated to limit parafunctional activities. Muscle reeducation and TMJ proprioception exercises can assist to improve masticatory muscle control and function (Box 7.1). Kalamir et al.[56] demonstrated that 30 patients with chronic myofascial pain of the masticatory muscles who received an intraoral soft tissue mobilization technique either alone or combined with education and TMJ exercises demonstrated reduction in pain and improvement in mandibular opening at a 6-month follow-up compared with a control group (Fig. 7.20). In a larger randomized controlled trial, Kalamir et al.[57] demonstrated effective outcomes with use of intraoral myofascial technique after 6 weeks of treatment, and the most effective long-term outcomes at a 1-year follow-up occurred with the group that received both the intraoral myofascial techniques combined with TMJ exercise instruction and education.[57] Myofascial pain of the masticatory muscles can also be effectively treated with dry needling techniques (Fig. 7.10).[58,59]

A study by Oliveira-Campelo et al. demonstrated an increase in pressure pain threshold over latent trigger points of the masseter and temporalis muscles with an increase in maximal active mouth opening immediately after atlantooccipital thrust manipulation or the inhibitive distraction soft tissue technique of the suboccipital muscles, which provides support for a clinical approach that includes manual therapy techniques of the craniovertebral region for treatment of masticatory muscle myalgia.[17]

Von Piekartz and Hall[32] compared manual therapy treatment of the cervical spine with this intervention combined

BOX 7.3   Temporomandibular Joint Movement Coordination Exercises

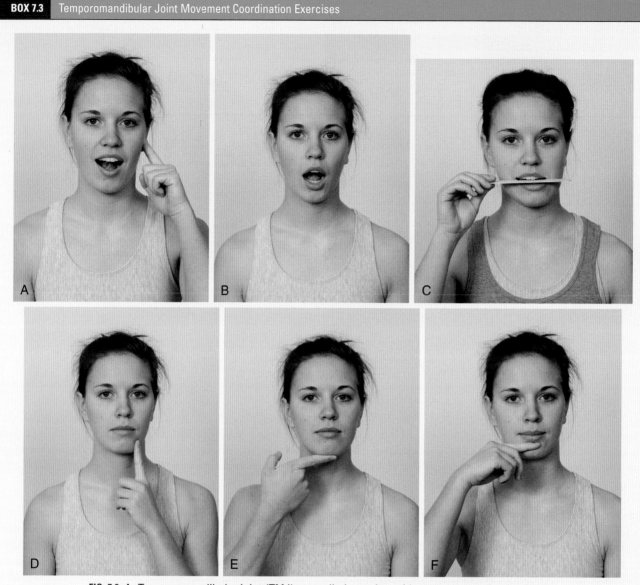

FIG. 7.9 A, Temporomandibular joint (TMJ) controlled opening with tongue up and palpation to isolate spinning of the condyle and limit excessive translation. A, Mirror can be used to assist in retraining symmetric opening. Keeping the tongue up on the roof of the mouth strengthens the tongue and avoids excessive translation of the TMJ. B, TMJ controlled opening with tongue up. C, Lateral excursion active range of motion with tongue blade guidance. D, Mandibular lateral excursion isometric; use only the force of the weight of a finger. E, Mandibular depression isometric; use only the force of the weight of a finger. F, Mandibular protrusion isometric; use only the force of the weight of a finger.

with manual therapy orofacial treatments directed to myofascial trigger points and TMJ restrictions for patients diagnosed with cervicogenic headache. Thirty-eight patients were assessed at baseline, after six treatment sessions (3 months), and at a 6-month follow-up. The outcome criteria were cervical range of movement (including the C1–C2 flexion-rotation test) and manual examination of the upper three cervical vertebrae. The group that received the combined cervical and orofacial treatment showed significant reduction in all aspects

of the cervical impairments after the treatment period and at the 6-month follow-up.

Women with myalgia TMD have been shown to have significantly less upper cervical mobility as measured with the cervical flexion rotation test compared with matched asymptomatic women with the flexion rotation test positive in 90% of the TMD participants versus 5% in the asymptomatic control, which points out a potential common involvement of the upper cervical joints (C1–C2) in women with myalgia

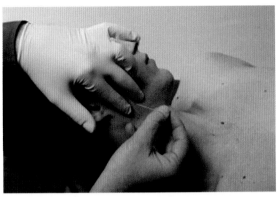

FIG. 7.10 Dry needling of the inferior division of the lateral ptery-goid muscle. (From Dommerholt J, Fernandez-de-las-Peñas C. *Trigger Point Dry Needling: an Evidenced and Clinical Based Approach.* London: Churchill Livingston/Elsevier; 2014.)

TMD.[60] Upper cervical nonthrust mobilization techniques combined with deep neck flexor training has demonstrated significant reduction in orofacial pain and headache impact in a study of 61 women with TMD randomized between an intervention group and control group after 5 weeks of treatment.[61] Positive effects on pressure pain threshold for the muscles of mastication were also noted with the intervention group, but the changes did not reach a clinically meaningful level.[61]

Reynolds et al.[33] demonstrated enhanced outcomes at 1 week and 4 weeks follow-up in comparing high-velocity thrust manipulation of the upper cervical spine to sham manipulation of 50 individuals with myalgia TMD while both groups received standardized behavioral education, soft tissue mobilization, and a home exercise program directed to the TMJ and neck.[33]

These findings support an impairment-based manual physical therapy approach that includes comprehensive treatment of the cervical, TMJ, and muscles of mastication impairments to most effectively treat patients with cervicogenic headache and TMDs.[31,33,60,61]

Hypermobility

Hypermobility of the TMJ is characterized by a mandibular opening greater than 40 mm with an end-range opening click and chin deviation away from the hypermobile joint that clicks. The joint sound in this case is the result of the mandibular condyle snapping across the distal edge of the articular crest. Hypermobility also is noted with accessory motion testing. Neuromuscular control and movement coordination deficits may also be noted with altered trajectory of opening and closing with inconsistent S and Z movement patterns in the absence of midrange joint sounds. Hypermobility of the TMJ may be asymptomatic unless combined with an myalgia or arthralgia condition, and TMJ hypermobility is postulated as being a precursor to articular disk displacement conditions.[19] Treatment is a TMJ movement coordination/stabilization treatment program with an emphasis on multidirectional mandibular

isometric exercises, proprioception exercise, and education to avoid full wide opening (Boxes 7.1 and 7.3). Five to 10 repetitions of each of the TMJ motor control exercises should be performed at least 5 to 6 times per day. The isometric exercises are held 5 to 6 seconds each. Short, frequent doses of exercise can assist in muscle reeducation and pain inhibition. A strategy that is often helpful to avoid end-range stresses on the TMJ is to instruct the patient to maintain the tip of the tongue up on the roof of the mouth with yawning. Cervical spine impairments should also be addressed as part of the rehabilitation program of all TMDs.

Articular Disk Displacement With Reduction

Articular disk displacement with reduction (ADDwR) is considered a progression of the dysfunction of a hypermobile TMJ. As the joint becomes more lax, the posterior ligament and collateral ligaments elongate and are unable to maintain the articular disk in its ideal position in relation to the mandibular condyle throughout the range of mandibular motion. As the mouth closes, the disk tends to slide forward and medial, which produces a joint noise.[19] With mandibular depression, a joint sound occurs as the condyle translates far enough anterior to recapture the disk-condyle relationship to create an opening click. The mandible tends to deviate to the ipsilateral side because of the initial restriction of condyle anterior translation by the anterior medial position of the disk. Once the disk is recaptured, a joint click is produced at the apex of the mandibular deviation and then the mandible moves back toward midline as the opening proceeds. The greater the degree of ligamentous laxity, the later in the range of the motion the joint sound occurs with mandibular depression (Fig. 7.11).[19] The most reliable method to detect

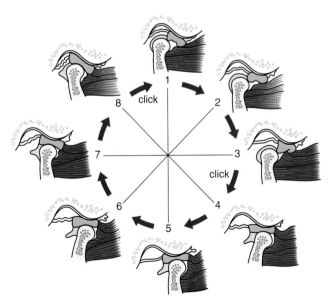

FIG. 7.11 Anterior disk dislocation with reduction. Note joint sound that occurs with opening as disk is reduced and joint sound with closing that occurs as disk dislocates. (From Magee DJ. *Orthopedic Physical Assessment*, ed 6. St. Louis: Saunders; 2014.)

joint sounds is to use a stethoscope (Fig. 7.16). An audible joint sound with opening and closing should be heard on at least one of three repetitions to diagnose articular disk displacement with reduction. The closing joint sound tends to be more muffled than the opening joint sound.[36] The patient could also meet the diagnostic criteria with an opening or a closing joint sound during one of three repetitions when combined with a joint sound with one of three lateral excursion or protrusion mandibular motions.[36]

Treatment is similar to TMJ hypermobility, with an attempt to stabilize the joint and improve the neuromuscular control and movement coordination. If arthralgia or masticatory muscle myalgia is evident, these conditions also need to be addressed. Education on TMJ stress reduction (Box 7.4) combined with an exercise program is used to prevent the condition from progressing to an acute articular disk displacement without reduction (ADDwoR).

The proprioception and movement coordination exercises described in Box 7.1 can be modified first to protrude the mandible to recapture the disk and then to perform the lateral excursion progression of ROM, ROM with the end-range bite, and ROM with the sustained bite. Rocabado[62] theorizes that this exercise regimen can assist in remodeling the disk and re-educating the local TMJ muscles to attempt to correct and stabilize the disk displacement. If the disk displacement is a more chronic condition, TMJ capsular tightness may be evident as a result of the tendency of the mandibular condyle to rest in a more superior, retracted position with the disk displaced.[62] TMJ distraction mobilization techniques may be needed to assist in restoration of normal capsular mobility.

In a randomized clinical trial, Yoda et al.[63] compared an exercise program with an education program for patients with anterior disk displacement with reduction. The results showed that the exercise program group had better outcomes for decreased pain and increased ROM ($P = .0001$).[63] Some 42 patients participated in the study; 61.9% of the exercise group had favorable outcomes (13/21 patients) and 0% of the control (education program) group had favorable results.[62] Success

was measured on the severity of joint sounds or pain with maximal mouth opening. Of the 13 patients with a successful outcome, only three patients' TMJ articular disks (23.1%) were recaptured with reexamination with magnetic resonance imaging (MRI).[63]

Likewise, Nicolakis et al.[16] reported on the outcomes of 30 patients with TMJ anterior disk displacement with reduction who underwent treatment with TMJ and soft tissue mobilization, ROM and isometric exercises, and postural education for an average of nine visits with a physical therapist. Seventy-five percent of the patients had successful outcomes in this case series, with outcome measures that included pain level and mouth opening measurements at the 6-month follow-up examination; 13% had reduction in TMJ sounds.[16] Tuncer et al.[64] compared physical therapy treatment consisting only of a home exercise program for one group of 20 patients with TMD (14 with ADDwR) with a second group of 20 patients with TMD (17 with ADDwR) who received both a home exercise program and soft tissue and TMJ manual therapy interventions three times per week for 4 weeks. At the end of the 4 weeks, the group that received both the exercise program plus the manual therapy demonstrated better outcomes for pain and pain-free mouth opening.[64] These studies support the use of exercise combined with gentle manual therapy techniques for treatment of anterior disk displacement with reduction.

Articular Disk Displacement Without Reduction

ADDwoR is a progression of ADDwR. When the condition is acute, the opening is limited to less than 25 mm with an end-range deviation toward the affected joint, limited contralateral lateral excursion, and deviation of the mandible toward the affected side with protrusion. Because this pattern of limited mandibular AROM is the same as with capsular fibrosis, a history of joint sounds can help to distinguish the likelihood of a disk displacement without reduction. The disk displacement without reduction disorder typically has a history of an opening and closing joint sound, but the joint sounds disappear when the acute limitation in mandibular motion occurs. This condition occurs when the articular disk displaces anterior to the condyle and is unable to be reduced with movement of the mandible. The disk blocks further anterior translation with opening, contralateral lateral excursion, and protrusion (Fig. 7.12). Accessory motions of the affected joint are also limited. When the condition is chronic, the posterior ligament and capsular tissues can be stretched to allow full normal mandibular motion. Yatani et al.[65] reported that 80 of 138 patients (58%) who demonstrated MRI evidence of an anterior disk displacement without reduction presented with normal mandibular opening ROM on clinical examination.

Julsvoll describes a cluster of seven TMD examination procedures for clinical diagnosis of ADDwoR and is considered positive if a threshold of five of the seven tests are positive.[66] The cluster included:

- The dental stick test (Fig. 7.24A)
- The isometric test
- Joint provocation test

BOX 7.4	Temporomandibular Joint Education

- Limit parafunctional activities: Nail biting, gum chewing, and clenching and grinding teeth.
- Tongue position: At rest, the tip of the tongue should be at the ridge of the roof of the mouth with the front one-third of the tongue on the roof of the mouth.
- Teeth position: Teeth should be 2 to 3 mm apart at rest.
- Lips should be lightly together with breathing through the nose.
- Keep the tip of the tongue up on the roof of the mouth when yawning.
- Avoid sleeping in the prone position.
- Do not rest chin in hands.
- Soft diet: Avoid hard, crunchy foods.
- Cut food up into small pieces.
- Warm water rinses.
- Perform postural exercises 5 to 6 times per day.

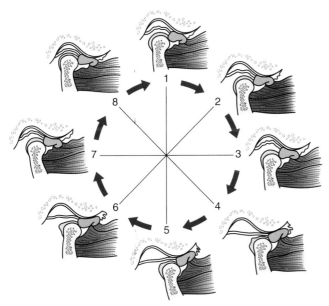

FIG. 7.12 Anterior disk dislocation without reduction. Disk remains dislocated anterior and medial to the condyle, which limits the distance the condyle can translate forward. (From Magee DJ. *Orthopedic Physical Assessment*, ed 6. St. Louis: Saunders; 2014.)

- Joint sound test (crepitus)
- The deviation with mandibular opening test
- The laterotrusion (limited lateral excursion ROM) test
- The joint mobility (reduced anterior glide TMJ accessory motion) test.

Validity of this five-out-of-seven positive cluster was compared with diagnosis of ADDwoR with MRI used as the gold standard, and the authors reported sensitivity 0.71, specificity 0.91, and positive likelihood ratio (+LR) of 7.89, which demonstrates a moderate shift of probability to diagnosis AD-DwoR in a group of patients with chronic TMD.[66] The interrater reliability of this five-of-seven cluster was reported as kappa 0.76 and 0.72 in another paper by the same research group.[67] The dental stick test had the best validity for a single test with sensitivity of 0.71, specificity of 0.77 and +LR of 3.09.[66] The dental stick test also had high reliability with kappa scores 0.88 (0.29–1.0) when tested on this patient population with chronic TMD.[67]

Cleland and Palmer[68] showed a good clinical outcome in a single-case design study of a patient with bilateral ADDwoR that was confirmed with MRI. The treatment approach included TMJ mobilization techniques, cervical spine mobilization/manipulation techniques, postural and neck exercises, and patient education regarding parafunctional habits, soft diet, relaxation techniques, activity modification, and tongue resting position. The patient had a return of normal mouth opening and a reduction in pain and disability measures as a result of the physical therapy approach.[68]

Patients with anterior disk displacement without reduction can make functional and symptomatic improvements with the use of joint mobilization and therapeutic exercise. Over time, the shape of the articular disk tends to change and the likelihood of reducing and maintaining a normal disk condyle relationship is minimal. Some speculation exists that over time the posterior ligament can become more fibrous and function similar to a disk. However, without a properly positioned and functioning disk, the TMJ may be more susceptible to development of osteoarthritic changes. On occasion, the anterior disk displacement begins to reduce again and the joint sounds return as the ROM and function of the mandible improves. In this situation, the rehabilitation program should progress as outlined for an anterior disk displacement with reduction.

Temporomandibular Joint Osteoarthritis

Osteoarthritis of the TMJ is common and may be an added source of pain and limited mandibular motion. Joint crepitus is present with osteoarthritis of the TMJ and is best noted with use of a stethoscope (Fig. 7.16). Radiographs or arthroscopic visualization are needed to confirm the diagnosis. Israel et al.[69] tested 84 participants with symptoms of TMJ pain with auscultation for crepitus with a stethoscope and compared the findings with arthroscopic visualization results to find a sensitivity of 0.70, a specificity of 0.43, a +LR of 1.23, and a negative likelihood ratio (–LR) of 0.70 for detection of osteoarthritis with positive findings of TMJ crepitus. Acceptable levels of sensitivity (0.67) and specificity (0.84) for diagnosis of advanced osteoarthritis were also made with auscultation of TMJ crepitus with a stethoscope when compared with findings noted with a TMJ arthroscopic procedure in 200 patients with TMD.[70]

Nicolakis et al.[15] had successful outcomes in a series of 20 patients with osteoarthritis of the TMJ with improved measures of pain at rest, incisional opening, and function. The interventions included joint mobilization of the TMJ, soft tissue techniques, active and passive TMJ exercises, and postural exercises.[15] Data collected on these patients at a 12-month follow-up examination continued to suggest favorable results for the use of exercise and manual physical therapy in the management of TMD.[16]

Postsurgical Temporomandibular Joint

A variety of surgical procedures are performed to treat TMDs. A detailed surgical report and the surgeon's postsurgical precautions should be obtained. A common example of TMJ surgery is an arthroscopic procedure in which a small scope is used to remove joint adhesions. After TMJ surgery, the patient often has findings similar to the arthralgia (capsulitis/synovitis) classification; therefore interventions to reduce inflammation and restore joint function are indicated. In addition, underlying impairments may be present, such as articular disk, muscle, and postural/cervical spine disorders that need to be addressed as part of the overall treatment plan. Education as outlined in Box 7.4 can assist with management of postsurgical conditions. TMJ ROM exercises also are a vital part of the treatment approach. Joint mobilization techniques and sustained stretching with tongue depressors are indicated if joint mobility restrictions are present and the surgeon has cleared the patient for passive stretching techniques.

TEMPOROMANDIBULAR JOINT EXAMINATION

The following is a detailed description of TMJ examination procedures, including AROM, palpation, provocation tests, and accessory motion tests, which when completed and considered in clusters of positive findings should allow the therapist to properly diagnose/classify the TMD and create a problem list that can be addressed with physical therapy interventions. Assessment of teeth and occlusion should be completed as part of the TMJ examination; obvious malocclusions, such as premature contact, missing teeth, or worn patterns characteristic of bruxism, should be noted and brought to the attention of the patient's dentist (Fig. 7.13).

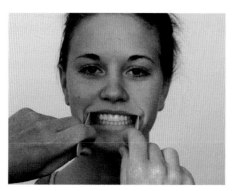

FIG. 7.13 See Video 7.1. Occlusion and teeth assessment. Use two tongue depressors to move the lips and cheeks out of the way to allow inspection of occlusion. Note signs of premature contacts, crossbite, missing teeth, or teeth wear patterns characteristic of bruxism.

TEMPOROMANDIBULAR JOINT ACTIVE RANGE OF MOTION AND MAPPING MOTION

Each mandibular AROM is tested at least three times. With the first trial of AROM, the therapist observes for the quality and ROM. With the subsequent trials, the therapist palpates the TMJ to attempt to identify joint sounds and notes at what point in the ROM the joint sound occurs. If joint sounds are suspected, auscultation of the TMJ with a stethoscope should be completed as the patient opens/closes for three additional cycles (Fig. 7.16). The therapist should note whether the joint sound occurs during opening or closing and whether deviation from midline occurs with the joint sound. These deviations and joint sounds are mapped on the mandibular dynamics chart (Fig. 7.14). With the final trial, a millimeter ruler is used to measure the ROM (Fig. 7.15B).

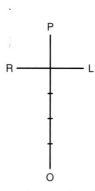

FIG. 7.14 Mandibular dynamics mapping chart: a *line* is drawn to document the path of opening and closing, and an "*x*" is used to mark joints sounds within the range of motion (ROM). A small slash mark is used to mark end of ROM. The therapist should also note whether pain is provoked with each motion and where the pain is focused.

The amount of mandibular depression has been found to be affected by the head and neck position; therefore the patient should be instructed to attain and hold the best natural, comfortable postural position before and throughout the testing of mandibular AROM.[71] The postural position should be reproduced for subsequent reassessments of mandibular AROM to attain a valid measure of the effects of the therapy.

Mandibular Depression

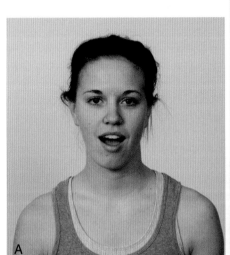
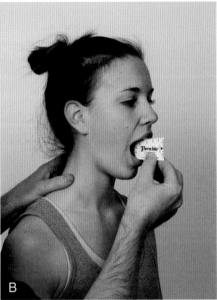
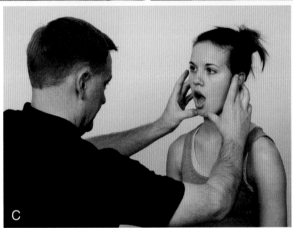

FIG. 7.15 See Videos 7.2 and 7.3. A, Mandibular depression active range of motion (AROM). B, Interincisor measurement of mandibular depression with millimeter ruler. C, Therapist positioning for mapping mandibular dynamics and palpating the mandibular condyles during AROM testing.

PATIENT POSITION	The patient sits or stands with good postural alignment.
THERAPIST POSITION	The therapist stands or sits in front of the patient.
PROCEDURE	Depression refers to opening the mouth in the sagittal plane. The patient is instructed to actively open the mouth as wide as possible. The therapist observes for symmetrical opening. A deviation to either side during opening is noted. (Deviation usually occurs to the side of the TMJ mobility deficit.) The amount of mandibular depression is noted with a millimeter ruler to measure the distance between the maxillary and mandibular central incisors.

Mandibular Depression—cont'd

NOTES

The distance between the incisors at maximal opening should be 35 to 50 mm, and the mandible should track in midline throughout the AROM. Walker et al.[72] used a millimeter ruler to measure the opening on 15 patients with TMD and 15 participants without TMD and reported an interclass correlation coefficient (ICC) for interexaminer reliability of 0.98 for those without TMD and 0.99 for those with TMD. Of the six motions measured (opening, left excursion, right excursion, protrusion, overbite, and overjet) by two therapists in this study, mouth opening (mandibular depression) was the only TMJ ROM measurement to discriminate between participants with and without TMJ disorders (mean, 36.2 ± 6.4 mm versus 43.5 ± 6.1 mm).[72] Interrater reliability for measurement of mouth opening for a group of 40 patients with long-standing TMD has been reported as ICC = 0.97 (0.95–0.98).[67]

The presence of a joint sound should also be noted. Interexaminer reliability for detection of joint sounds has been reported as a kappa value of 0.24 in 79 patients referred to a craniomandibular disorder clinic.[73] The presence of an audible palpable joint click has been correlated with MRI confirmation of an anterior disk displacement with reduction in 146 patients seen at a craniofacial pain clinic with a sensitivity of 0.51, a specificity of 0.83, a +LR of 3.0, and a –LR of 0.59. No clicking with opening has been correlated with an anterior disk displacement without reduction with a sensitivity of 0.77, a specificity of 0.24, a +LR of 1.01, and a –LR of 0.96.[74] Joint sounds of crepitus have been reported in a group of 35 patients with chronic TMD as part of a joint cluster to diagnosis ADDwoR and when compared with MRI, the specificity for joint sound detection with palpation and stethoscope was sensitivity 0.71, specificity 0.77, and +LR 3.09.[66] Reliability by the same research group was reported as kappa 0.94 (0.82–1.0) for joint sounds with opening when testing 40 patients with long standing TMD.[67]

Box 7.5 (Fig. 7.16) provides an illustration of use of a stethoscope to facilitate identification of a TMJ sound with mandibular AROM testing.

BOX 7.5   Auscultation of the Temporomandibular Joint With Stethoscope for Detection of Joint Sounds

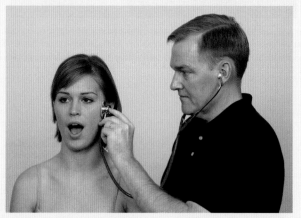

FIG. 7.16 See Video 7.4. Auscultation of the temporomandibular joint with stethoscope for detection of joint sounds.

▶ Mandibular Protrusion

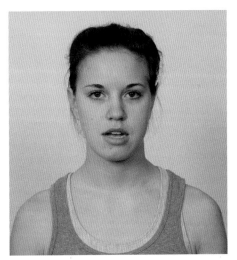

FIG. 7.17 See Video 7.5. Mandibular protrusion active range of motion.

PATIENT POSITION	The patient sits or stands with good postural alignment.
THERAPIST POSITION	The therapist stands or sits in front of the patient.
PROCEDURE	Protrusion refers to the anterior movement of the mandible in the horizontal plane. The patient is instructed to actively protrude the mandible. The therapist observes for symmetrical protrusion. A deviation to either side during protrusion is noted. (Deviation usually occurs toward the side of the TMJ mobility deficit.) The amount of protrusion can be measured with a millimeter ruler to measure the distance between the maxillary and mandibular central incisors.
NOTES	This motion is difficult to measure, but the mandibular incisors should move past the maxillary incisors by several millimeters. Walker et al.[72] used a millimeter ruler to measure protrusion on 15 patients with TMD and 15 participants without TMD and reported an ICC for interexaminer reliability of 0.95 for those without TMD and 0.98 for those with TMD. The presence of a joint sound should also be noted. Interexaminer reliability for detection of joint sounds has been reported as a kappa value of 0.47 in 79 patients referred to a craniomandibular disorder clinic.[73]

▶ Mandibular Lateral Excursion

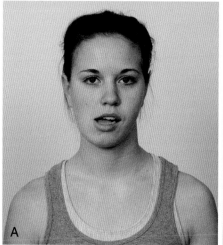 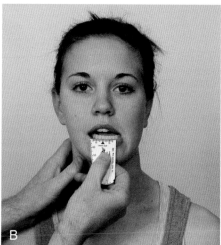

FIG. 7.18 See Videos 7.6 and 7.7. A, Mandibular lateral excursion active range of motion. B, Mandibular lateral excursion measurement with millimeter ruler.

PATIENT POSITION	The patient sits or stands with good postural alignment.
THERAPIST POSITION	The therapist stands or sits in front of the patient.
PROCEDURE	Lateral excursion refers to the mandible moving laterally in the horizontal plane. The patient is instructed to actively move the mandible laterally to the right. A millimeter ruler can be used to measure the amount of lateral excursion by placing the ruler against the bottom lip with the zero lined up with the space between the two central maxillary incisors. The ruler is held against the lip as the patient moves into lateral excursion and the measurement on the ruler in relation to the central maxillary incisor space is taken at end range. A more accurate measurement can be made with marking a vertical line along the maxillary and mandibular central incisors with a marking pencil while in a neutral position and measuring the horizontal distance between the two marks at the end range of lateral excursion left and right.
NOTES	This motion is difficult to measure, but the mandibular canine should move past the maxillary canine by several millimeters. Lateral excursion of 10 mm in each direction is considered a normal ROM. Importantly, the motion should be equal in each direction. Lateral excursion will tend to be limited in the direction away from the TMJ with a mobility deficit. Walker et al.[72] used a millimeter ruler to measure lateral excursion on 15 patients with TMD and 15 participants without TMD and reported an ICC for interexaminer reliability of 0.95 for those without TMD and 0.94 for those with TMD for left lateral excursion and reported an ICC for interexaminer reliability of 0.90 for those without TMD and 0.96 for those with TMD for right lateral excursion. The presence of a joint sound should also be noted. Interexaminer reliability for detection of joint sounds has been reported as a kappa value of 0.50 in 79 patients referred to a craniomandibular disorder clinic.[73]
	In another study of 40 patients with long standing TMD, interexaminer reliability for detection of crepitus with lateral excursion was report as kappa 0.88 and for a click kappa 0.77.

PALPATION

▶ Muscles of Mastication External Palpation

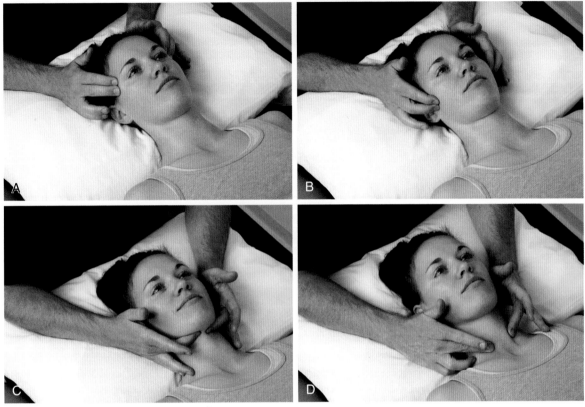

FIG. 7.19 See Video 7.8. A, Palpation of the temporalis. B, Palpation of the masseter. C, Palpation of the suprahyoid muscles. D, Palpation of the infrahyoid muscles.

PATIENT POSITION	The patient is supine with the head on a pillow.
THERAPIST POSITION	The therapist stands at the head of the patient.
PROCEDURE	The therapist uses the pads of the second and third digits to palpate the temporalis, the masseter, the suprahyoid muscles, and the infrahyoid muscles. Swelling, tenderness, trigger points, or excessive tension in the muscles is noted.
NOTES	Cacchiotti et al.[75] examined 41 patients who sought treatment for TMD and 40 healthy participants and graded the results of palpation examination on a 0 to 3 scale, with 0 indicating no response and 3 indicating that the patient pulled the head away in anticipation of palpation and reported significant pain. The results for use of palpation of the muscles of mastication for identification of patients with TMD were sensitivity of 0.76, specificity of 0.90, +LR of 7.6, and −LR of 0.27.

▶ Muscles of Mastication Intraoral Palpation

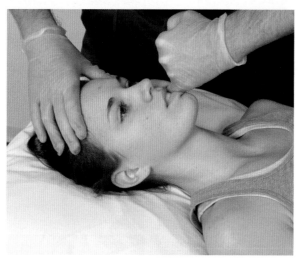

FIG. 7.20 See Video 7.9. Intraoral palpation of muscles of mastication.

PATIENT POSITION	The patient is supine with the head on a pillow.
THERAPIST POSITION	The therapist stands next to the patient.
PROCEDURE	The therapist wears a latex glove and uses the tip of the fifth digit to palpate the upper lateral corner of the patient's mouth between the teeth and cheek. Pain provocation and swelling, tenderness, or excessive tension in the muscles are noted. The therapist palpates and compares both sides.
NOTE	This technique is designed to palpate the lateral pterygoid muscle, but debate exists as to whether the fifth digit can actually reach far enough to palpate this muscle.[76] The tendon of the temporalis is also near this site of palpation, as is the masseter muscle. Dworkin et al.[77] reported a kappa value of 0.90 for intraoral palpation interexaminer reliability in 64 healthy volunteers. This palpation technique can also be used as an intraoral soft tissue mobilization treatment technique by sustaining direct pressure at the trigger points noted in the muscles of mastication for up to 90 seconds until tension and tenderness ease with the sustained pressure. A randomized controlled trial that used this type of intraoral myofascial technique demonstrated effective outcomes with patients with myalgia TMD after 12 treatments sessions over 6 weeks.[57] Superior long-term outcomes (1-year follow-up) were noted when myofascial techniques are combined with a TMD exercise and education program.[57]

▶ Temporomandibular Joint Lateral Pole Palpation

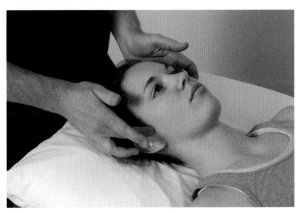

FIG. 7.21 See Video 7.10. Palpation of the lateral condyle.

PATIENT POSITION	The patient is supine with the head on a pillow.
THERAPIST POSITION	The therapist stands at the head of the table.
PROCEDURE	The pad of the third digit is used to palpate the lateral pole of the TMJ just anterior to the ear. Any swelling or tenderness is noted. The therapist palpates the opposite side, noting any swelling or tenderness.
NOTES	Tenderness of the lateral pole is an indication of inflammation of the TMJ capsule or lateral TMJ ligament which is a sign of TMJ arthralgia. de Wiker et al.[78] reported a kappa value of 0.33 for interexaminer reliability for pain provocation with palpation of the lateral pole of the TMJ in 79 patients referred to a TMJ disorder and orofacial pain department. Manfredini et al.[79] reported intraexaminer reliability of kappa of 0.53 for pain provocation for palpation of lateral pole of the TMJ on 61 patients with TMJ pain and correlated pain with palpation with the presence of joint effusion as seen on MRI findings with a sensitivity of 0.83, a specificity of 0.69, a +LR of 2.68, and a −LR of 0.25.

▶ Posterior Compartment Palpation

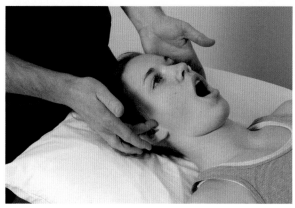

FIG. 7.22 See Video 7.10. Palpation of posterior compartment of temporomandibular joint.

PATIENT POSITION	The patient is supine with the head on a pillow.
THERAPIST POSITION	The therapist stands at the head of the table.
PROCEDURE	The pad of the third digit palpates just posterior to the condyle of the mandible. The patient is instructed to actively open the mouth. The therapist palpates for tenderness or swelling of the posterior compartment during opening of the mouth. The procedure is repeated with assessment of the opposite side. Any differences between right and left sides are noted.
NOTES	Tenderness and swelling of the posterior compartment of the TMJ is an indication of inflammation/irritation of the posterior ligaments and joint capsule of the TMJ which is a sign of TMJ arthralgia. Manfredini et al.[79] reported intraexaminer reliability of kappa of 0.48 for pain provocation with palpation of the posterior compartment of the TMJ in 61 patients with TMJ pain and correlated pain with palpation with presence of joint effusion as seen on MRI findings with a sensitivity of 0.85, a specificity of 0.62, a +LR of 2.24, and –LR of 0.24. Reliability has also been reported for a group of patients with chronic TMD at high levels with kappa 0.81 (0.55–0.95).[67]

PROVOCATION TESTS

▶ Forced Retrusion (Compression) Temporomandibular Joint Provocation Test

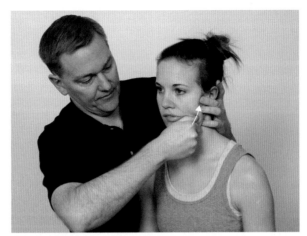

FIG. 7.23 See Video 7.11. Forced retrusion (compression) temporomandibular joint provocation test.

PATIENT POSITION	The patient is in a sitting position.
THERAPIST POSITION	The therapist stands in front and to the side of the patient and on the opposite side of the TMJ to be tested.
PROCEDURE	The thumb and index finger are used to grasp the patient's chin. The opposite hand stabilizes the back of the patient's head. With the patient relaxed and the teeth slightly apart, the therapist applies a pressure directed posteriorly and slightly superiorly. Pain provocation is noted.
NOTES	Test results are considered positive if the test increases or reproduces the patient's symptoms. This test is not specific to either the right or left TMJ, but the force can be directed toward one joint at a time to attempt to isolate each joint. de Wiker et al.[78] reported a kappa value of 0.47 for interexaminer reliability of pain provocation with a TMJ compression test in 79 patients referred to a TMJ disorder and orofacial pain department.

▶ Forced Biting Provocation Test (Dental Stick Test)

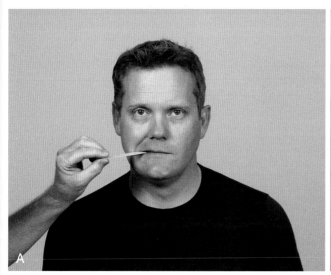
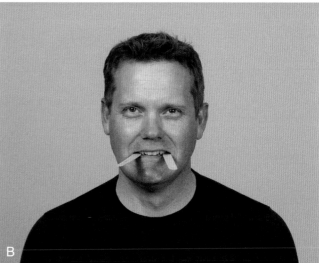

FIG. 7.24 See Video 7.12. A, Forced biting provocation test (Dental stick test). B, Power Stroke Test (Bilateral forced biting test).

PATIENT POSITION	The patient is in a sitting position.
THERAPIST POSITION	The therapist stands in front of the patient.
PROCEDURE	The therapist places gauze, a cotton ball, or a tongue depressor between the patient's back molars. The patient is instructed to firmly bite down. Pain provocation is noted. The test can be modified to include biting on tongue depressors bilaterally (power stroke test). Test results are considered positive if the test increases or reproduces the patient's symptoms.
NOTES	For the dental stick test, if pain is produced in the ipsilateral side, it is likely from muscle/tendon irritation (myalgia) associated with a masticatory muscle disorder; if the pain is reproduced on the contralateral TMJ, it is likely from TMJ arthralgia (capsulitis/synovitis). A confirmatory test can be used by having the patient firmly bite down with tongue depressors placed between both sides of molars. Pain produced by this power stroke maneuver is likely caused by masticatory myalgia rather than TMJ arthralgia because both TMJs are unloaded when the molars are separated.[36] A positive power stroke test combined with pain-free end range mouth opening is most likely indicative of myalgia of the superior lateral pterygoid muscle.
	The dental stick test demonstrated fair validity for a single test with sensitivity of 0.71, specificity of 0.77 and +LR of 3.09 for diagnosis of ADDwoR in a group of patients with chronic TMD.[66] The dental stick test also had high reliability with kappa scores 0.88 (0.29–1.0) when tested on this patient population with chronic TMD.[67]

Muscles of Mastication Isometric Resistive Provocation Tests (Isometric Test)

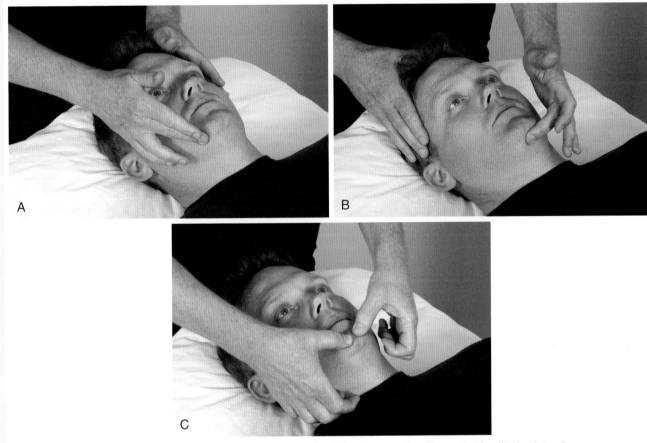

FIG. 7.25 Muscles of Mastication Isometric Resistive Provocation Tests. A, Mandibular lateral excursion. B, Mandibular depression. C, Mandibular protrusion.

PATIENT POSITION	The patient is in a supine position.
THERAPIST POSITION	The therapist stands at the head of the table.
PROCEDURE	The therapist applies a gentle isometric force at the lateral aspect of the chin of the mandible for 10 seconds and asks the patient to hold and meet the resistance. Pain provocation is noted. The test is repeated for contralateral lateral excursion, opening (inferior chin finger placement), and protrusion (anterior chin finger placement). Test results are considered positive if the test increases or reproduces the patient's symptoms.
NOTES	In theory, if pain is produced with isometric resisted protrusion, lateral pterygoid myalgia is likely involved. If there is no pain with isometric resisted lateral excursion or protrusion, the masseter and/or temporalis muscles are likely the primarily involved muscles with signs of myalgia.[36]

ACCESSORY MOTION TESTS AND MOBILIZATIONS

▶ Temporomandibular Joint Distraction Accessory Motion Test and Mobilization

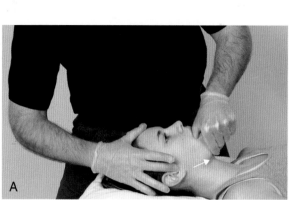
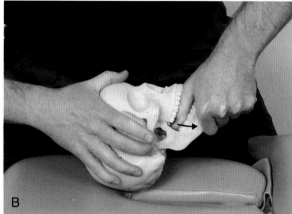

FIG. 7.26 See Video 7.13. A, Temporomandibular joint (TMJ) distraction accessory motion test and mobilization. B, Distraction accessory motion test and mobilization of TMJ with hand placement on a model.

PATIENT POSITION	The patient is supine with the head on a pillow.
THERAPIST POSITION	The therapist stands next the patient on the side opposite the TMJ to be tested or mobilized.
PROCEDURE	The therapist stands on the patient's left side and inserts the left thumb into the patient's mouth. The thumb is placed on top of the patient's right mandibular molars, and digits 2 to 5 are gently folded around the lateral inferior aspect of the mandible (externally). The thumb is used to apply an inferior scooping force against the molars along the ramus of the mandible to distract the joint. The pad of the third digit of the right hand is used to palpate the right TMJ (externally). The amount of motion available at the joint is noted, and the procedure is repeated with assessment of the left side. The therapist stands on the patient's right side and uses the right thumb on the left mandibular molars. Pain provocation and the amount of motion available at the joint are noted and compared with the right side.
	This technique can be turned into a nonthrust mobilization with application of a sustained stretch to the joint or with oscillation of the joint. Thrust manipulation to the TMJ is rarely indicated. A successful outcome can be obtained with gentle nonthrust mobilization techniques.
NOTES	The therapist stands on the side opposite of the joint to be assessed. The therapist should wear a latex glove during this technique. Gentle forces are used to assess and mobilize the joint. The amount of accessory motion of a normally functioning TMJ is very small. Manfredini et al.[79] correlated pain with joint distraction and joint effusion as seen on MRI findings in 61 patients with TMJ pain with a sensitivity of 0.80, a specificity of 0.39, a +LR of 1.31, and a −LR of 0.51; joint play intraexaminer reliability was reported as kappa of 0.20. Lobbezoo-Scholte et al.[73] reported a kappa value of 0.46 for interexaminer reliability for testing of TMJ joint play in 79 randomly selected patients referred to a craniomandibular disorder department.

⊙ Temporomandibular Joint Lateral Glide Accessory Motion Test and Mobilization

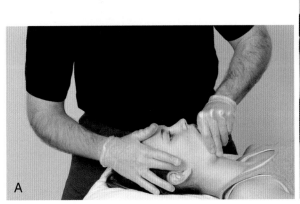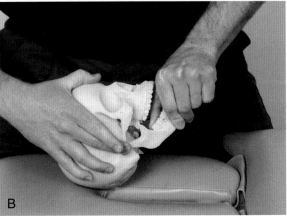

FIG. 7.27 See Video 7.14. A, Temporomandibular joint (TMJ) lateral glide accessory motion test and mobilization. B, TMJ lateral glide accessory motion test and mobilization with hand placement on a model.

PATIENT POSITION	The patient is supine with the head on a pillow.
THERAPIST POSITION	The therapist stands next to the patient on the side opposite the TMJ.
PROCEDURE	The therapist stands on the patient's left side and inserts his left thumb into the patient's mouth. The pad of the thumb is used to contact the medial aspect of the patient's right mandibular molars. The thumb is used to apply a lateral force toward the patient's right side, and the pad of the third digit of the right hand is used to palpate the TMJ (externally). The amount of motion available at the joint is noted, and the procedure is repeated with assessment of the left side. The therapist stands on the patient's right side and uses the right thumb to contact the left mandibular molars. Pain provocation and the amount of motion available at the joint are noted and compared with the other side. This technique can be turned into a nonthrust mobilization with application of a sustained stretch to the joint or with oscillation of the joint.
NOTES	The therapist stands on the side opposite the joint to be assessed and wears a latex glove during this technique. Gentle forces are used to assess and mobilize the joint. The amount of accessory motion of a normally functioning TMJ is very small. Lateral glide is a joint play motion for the TMJ being tested.

▶ Temporomandibular Joint Medial Glide Accessory Motion and Joint Mobilization

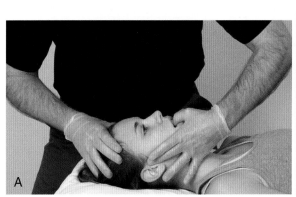
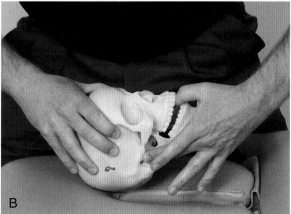

FIG. 7.28 See Video 7.15. A, Temporomandibular joint (TMJ) medial glide accessory motion and joint mobilization. B, TMJ medial glide accessory motion and joint mobilization with hand placement on a model.

PATIENT POSITION	The patient is supine with the head on a pillow.
THERAPIST POSITION	The therapist stands next to the patient on the side opposite of the TMJ.
PROCEDURE	While standing on the patient's left side, the therapist places the left thumb between the patient's maxillary and mandibular incisors. The pads of the second and third digits are used to contact the lateral pole of the right TMJ. The third digit applies a medial force toward the patient's left side. The amount of motion available at the joint is noted, and the procedure is repeated with assessment of the left side. The therapist stands on the patient's right side and uses the pad of the third digit of the right hand to apply a medial force to the lateral pole of the left TMJ. Pain provocation and the amount of motion available at the joint are noted and compared with the other side.
	This technique can be turned into a nonthrust mobilization with application of a sustained stretch to the joint or with oscillation of the joint.
NOTES	The therapist stands on the side opposite of the joint to be assessed and wears a latex glove during this technique. Gentle forces are used to assess and mobilize the joint. The amount of accessory motion of a normally functioning TMJ is very small. Medial glide is a joint play motion for the TMJ being tested.

CASE STUDIES AND PROBLEM SOLVING

The following patient case reports can be used by the student to develop clinical reasoning skills by considering the information provided in the patient history and tests and measures and developing appropriate evaluations, goals, and plans of care. Students should also consider the following questions:

1. What additional historical/subjective information would you like to have?
2. What additional diagnostic tests should be ordered, if any?
3. What additional tests and measures would be helpful in making the diagnosis?
4. What impairment-based classification does the patient most likely fit? What other impairment-based classifications did you consider?
5. What are the primary impairments that should be addressed?
6. What treatment techniques that you learned in this textbook will you use to address these impairments?
7. How do you plan to progress and modify the interventions as the patient progresses?

Ms. TMJ Dysfunction

History
A 23-year-old college student has tightness, discomfort, and clicking in the right TMJ with intermittent occipital headaches (Fig. 7.29). Pain is provoked with stressful situations and with chewing meat and crunchy foods. Central Sensitization Inventory score is 40/100. PHQ-4 for anxiety and depression score is 5. Jenkins Sleep Questionnaire score is 12. JFLS is 60/200.

Tests and Measures
1. Structural examination: Moderate forward head posture with protracted scapulas
2. Cervical AROM in standing: 85% in all planes of motion and pain free except for backward bending, which is 50% and provokes occipital area pain
3. Thoracic AROM: 75% to 85% in all planes of motion and pain free
4. Mandibular dynamics: Opening to 35 mm with midrange deviation to the right and return to midline after midrange of opening joint sound; joint sound also noted at midrange closing; lateral deviation is limited to the left with a joint sound; protrusion also has midrange click

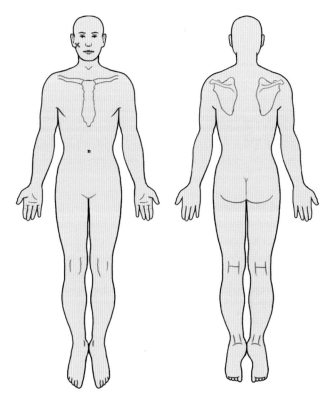

FIG. 7.29 Ms. TMJ Dysfunction Body chart.

5. Passive intervertebral motion (PIVM) testing: Limited craniovertebral forward bending, right side bending, and left rotation; mid-cervical spine PIVM testing reveals hypermobility; upper thoracic slightly restricted at T1–T2 left and right rotation and forward bending
6. Shoulder screen: Full and pain-free bilateral shoulder AROM
7. Muscle length: Mild tightness right levator scapula and minimally tight bilateral pectoralis major and minor
8. Strength: Lower and middle trapezius are 4−/5; deep neck flexors are 3+/5
9. Neurologic screen: Negative
10. Special tests:
    1. Forced biting (dental stick test): Painful right TMJ with biting on left side

2. Retrusive overpressure: Provokes pain on right TMJ
3. Palpation: Tender and guarded right muscles of mastication with internal (intraoral) and external palpation, tender at lateral pole right TMJ, and tender at right C2–C3 facet joint

Evaluation
Diagnosis
Problem list
Goals
Treatment plan/intervention

Mr. Stiff TMJ

History
A 50-year-old construction worker has difficulty opening his mouth after trauma to his jaw from being hit in the jaw during a bar fight 3 months before the initial evaluation. The patient has no history of TMJ sounds. Recent radiographic results were negative for signs of mandibular fracture. The patient complains of right-sided jaw pain and suboccipital headaches (Fig. 7.30). JFLS is 45/200. Central Sensitization Inventory score is 20/100. PHQ-4 for anxiety and depression score is 1. Jenkins Sleep Questionnaire score is 4.

Tests and Measures
1. Structural examination: Mild forward head posture with protracted scapulas
2. Cervical AROM in standing: 85% in all planes of motion and pain free
3. Thoracic AROM: 75% upper thoracic rotation motion and pain free
4. Mandibular dynamics: 20 mm opening with deviation to the right, 5 mm left lateral excursion, 8 mm right lateral excursion, and 4 mm protrusion with deviation to the right; no joint sounds noted
5. TMJ Accessory motion testing: Hypomobility with lateral and medial glide and joint distraction right TMJ
6. PIVM testing: Slight hypomobility craniovertebral forward bending and right side bending; hypomobility T1–T2 left and right rotation
7. Shoulder screen: Active shoulder ROM full and pain free with normal strength

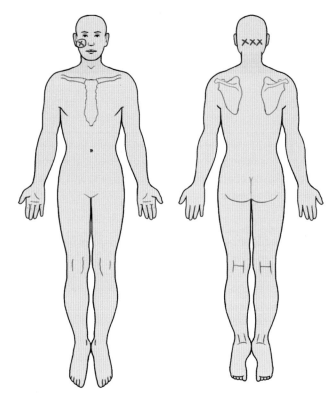

FIG. 7.30 Mr. Stiff TMJ Body chart.

8. Muscle length: No limitations noted
9. Strength: Lower and middle trapezius are 4−/5; deep neck flexors are 3+/5
10. Neurologic screen: Negative
11. Special tests:
    1. Forced biting (dental stick test): Negative
    2. Retrusive overpressure: Negative
    3. Palpation: Tender and guarded right muscles of mastication internally (intraoral) and externally and tender at right lateral mandibular condyle

Evaluation
Diagnosis
Problem list
Goals
Treatment plan/intervention

REFERENCES

1. Dodson TB. Epidemiology of temporomandibular disorders. In: Fonseca RJ, editor. *Oral and Maxillofacial Surgery: Temporomandibular Disorders*, vol. 4. Philadelphia: Saunders; 2000.

2. LeResche L. Epidemiology of temporomandibular disorders: Implications for the investigation of etiologic factors. *Crit Rev Oral Biol Med*. 1997;8:291-305.

3. Dworkin SF, LeResche L. Temporomandibular disorder pain: epidemiologic data. *Am Pain Soc Bull*. 1993;12-13.

4. Lipton JA, Ship JA, Larach,Äê Robinson D. Estimated prevalence and distribution of reported orofacial pain in the United States. *J Am Dent Assoc*. 1993;124:115-121.

5. Helkimo M. Epidemiological surveys of dysfunction of the masticatory system. In: Zarb G, Carlsson G, editors. *Temporomandibular Joint Dysfunction*. St. Louis: Mosby; 1979.

6. Von Korff M, Dworkin SF, Le Resche L, et al. An epidemiologic comparison of pain complaints. *Pain*. 1988;32:173-183.

7. Warren MP, Fried JL. Temporomandibular disorders and hormones in women. *Cells Tissues Organs*. 2001;169:187-192.

8. Merskey H, Bogduk N. *Classification of Chronic Pain*. Seattle: IASP Press; 1994.

9. Kraus SL. *Clinics in Physical Therapy: Temporomandibular Joint Disorders*. New York: Churchill Livingstone; 1994.

10. Godden DRP, Robertson JM. The value of patient feedback in the audit of TMJ arthroscopy. *Br Dent J*. 2000;188:37.

11. Carmeli E, Sheklow S, Bloomenfeld I. Comparative study of repositioning splint therapy and passive manual range of motion techniques for anterior displaced temporomandibular discs with unstable excursive reduction. *Physiotherapy*. 2001;87:26-36.

12. Rodrigues Martins W, Castro Blaszyk J, Furlan de Oliveira MA, et al. Efficacy of musculoskeletal manual approach in the treatment of temporomandibular joint disorder: a systematic review with meta-analysis. *Man Ther*. 2016;21:10-17.

13. Armijo-Olivo S, Pitance L, Neto F, et al. Effectiveness of manual therapy and therapeutic exercise for TMD: systematic review and meta-analysis. *Phy Ther*. 2016;96(1):9-25.

14. Furto ES, Cleland JA, Whitman JM, et al. Manual physical therapy interventions and exercise for patients with temporomandibular disorders. *J Craniomandib Dis*. 2006;24(4):283-291.

15. Nicolakis P, Burak EC, Kollmitzer J, et al. An investigation of the effectiveness of exercise and manual therapy in treating symptoms of TMJ osteoarthritis. *Cranio*. 2001;19:26-32.

16. Nicolakis P, Erdogmus B, Kopf A, et al. Effectiveness of exercise therapy in patients with internal derangement of the temporomandibular joint. *J Oral Rehabil*. 2002;29:362-368.

17. Oliveira-Campelo NM, Rugens-Rebelatto J, Marin-Vallejo FJ, et al. The immediate effects of atlanto-occipital joint manipulation and suboccipital muscle inhibition technique on active mouth opening and pressure pain sensitivity over latent myofascial trigger points in the masticatory muscles. *J Orthop Sports Phys Ther*. 2010;40(5):310-317.

18. Williams PL, Warwick R. *Gray's Anatomy*, ed 37. London: Churchill Livingstone 1989.

19. Rocabado M, Inglarsh A. *Musculoskeletal Approach to Maxillofacial Pain*. Philadelphia: Lippincott; 1991.

20. Neumann DA. *Kinesiology of the Musculoskeletal System: Foundations for Physical Rehabilitation*, ed 3. St. Louis: Elsevier; 2017.

21. McClean LF, Brenman HS, Friedman MG. Effects of changing body position on dental occlusion. *J Dent Res*. 1973;52(5):1041-1045.

22. Funakoshi M, Fujita N, Takehana S. Relations between occlusal interference and jay muscle activities in response to changes in head position. *J Dent Res*. 1976;55(4):686-690.

23. Darling DW, Kraus S, Glasheen-Wray MB. Relationship of head posture and the rest position of the mandible. *J Prosth Dent*. 1984;52(1):111-115.

24. Goldstein DF, Krauss S, Williams WB, et al. Influence of cervical posture on mandibular movement. *J Prosth Dent*. 1984;52(3):421-426.

25. Krauss SL. *TMJ Disorders: Management of the Craniomandibular Complex*. New York: Churchill Livingstone; 1998.

26. Daly P. Postural response of the head to bite opening in adult males. *Am J Orthodont*. 1982;82:157-160.

27. Piekartz von H, Pudelko A, Danzeisen M, et al. Do subjects with acute/subacute temporomandibular disorder have associated cervical impairments: a cross sectional study. *Man Ther*. 2016;26:208-215.

28. Armijo-Olivo S, Silvestre R, Fuentes J, et al. Electromyographic activity of the cervical flexor muscles in patients with temporomandibular disorders while performing the craniocervical flexion test: a cross-sectional study. *Phys Ther*. 2011;91(8):1184-1197.

29. Piekartz von H, Hall T. Orofacial manual therapy improves cervical movement impairment associated with headache and features of temporomandibular dysfunction: a randomized controlled trial. *Man Ther*. 2013;18(4):345-350.

30. Packard RC. The relationship of neck injury and post-traumatic headache. *Curr Pain Headache Rep*. 2002;6:301-307.

31. Aprill C, Axinn M, Bogduk N. Occipital headaches stemming from the lateral atlanto-axial (C1-C2) joint. *Cephalalgia*. 2002;22:15-22.

32. Von Piekartz H, Hall T. Orofacial manual therapy improves cervical movement associated with headache and features of temporomandibular dysfunction: a randomized controlled trial. *Man Ther*. 2013;18:345-350.

33. Reynolds B, Puentedura EJ, Kolber MJ, et al. Effectiveness of cervical spine high velocity low amplitude thrust added to behavioral education, soft tissue mobilization, and exercise in individuals with temporomandibular disorder with myalgia: a randomized clinical trial. *J Orthop Sports Phys Ther*. 2020;1-40.

34. International Headache Society. The international classification of headache disorders 2nd edition. *Cephalalgia*. 2004;24(Suppl 1):9-160.

35. Olesen J. The International Classification of headache disorders 2nd edition (ICHD-2) and the 10th International Classification of Diseases, neurological adaptation (ICD10NA) classification of headache disorders. In: Olesen J, editor. *The Classification and Diagnosis of Headache Disorder*. Oxford: Oxford University Press; 2005:12-19.

36. Harrison AL, Thorp JN, Ritzline PD. A proposed diagnostic classification of patients with temporomandibular disorders: implications for physical therapists. *J Orthop Sports Phys Ther*. 2014;44(3):182-197.

37. Ohrbach R, Larsson P, List T. The jaw functional limitation scale: development, reliability, and validity of 8-item and 20-item versions. *J Orofac Pain*. 2008;22(3):219-229.

38. Ohrbach R, Grandger C, List T, et al. Preliminary development and validation of the jaw functional limitation scale. *Community Dent Oral Epidemiol*. 2008;36:228-236.

39. Yeung E, Abou-Foul A, Matcham F, et al. Integration of mental health screening in the management of patients with temporomandibular disorders. *Br J Oral Maxillofac Surg*. 2017;55: 594-599.

40. Ohrbach R, Turner JA, Sherman JJ, et al. The research diagnostic criteria for temporomandibular disorders. IV: evaluation of psychometric properties of the Axis II measures. *J Orofac Pain*. 2010; 24:48-62.

41. Kroenke K, Spitzer RL, Williams JB, et al. An ultra-brief screening scale for anxiety and depression: the PHQ-4. *Psychosomatics*. 2009;50:613-621.

42. Campi LB, Jordani PC, Tenan HL, et al. Painful temporomandibular disorders and central sensitization: implications for management—a pilot study. *Int J Oral Maxillofac Surg*. 2017;46:104-110.

43. Woolf CJ. Central sensitization: implications for the diagnosis and treatment of pain. *Pain*. 2011;152:S2-S15.

44. Lorduy KM, Liegey-Dougall A, Haggard R, et al. The prevalence of comorbid symptoms of central sensitization syndrome among three different groups of temporomandibular disorder patients. *Pain Pract*. 2013;13(8):604-613.

45. La Touche R, Paris-Alemany A, Hidalgo-Perez A, et al. Evidence for central sensitization in patients with temporomandibular disorders: a systematic review and meta-analysis of observational studies. *Pain Pract*. 2018;18(3):388-409.

46. Dworkin SF, LeResche L. Research diagnostic criteria for temporomandibular disorders: review, criteria, examinations and specifications, critique. *J Craniomandib Disord*. 1992;6:301-355.

47. Gonzalez YM, Schiffman E, Gordon SM, et al. Development of a brief and effective temporomandibular disorder pain screening questionnaire: reliability and validity. *J Am Dent Assoc*. 2011;142: 1183-1191.

48. Schiffman EL, Ohrbach R, Truelove EL, et al. The Research Diagnostic Criteria for Temporomandibular Disorders. V: methods used to establish and validate revised Axis I diagnostic algorithms. *J Orofac Pain*. 2010;24:63-78.

49. Jull G, Trott P, Potter H, et al. A randomized controlled trial of physiotherapy management for cervicogenic headache. *Spine*. 2002;27:1835-1843.

50. Majwer K, Swider M. Results of treatment with iontophoresis of posttraumatic changes of temporomandibular joints with an apparatus of own design. *Protet Stomatol*. 1989;39:172-176.

51. Schiffman EL, Braun BL, Lindgren BR. Temporomandibular joint iontophoresis: a double-blind randomized clinical trial. *J Orofac Pain*. 1996;10(2):157-165.

52. Ismail F, Demling A, Hebling K, et al. Short-term efficacy of physical therapy compared to splint therapy in treatment of arthrogenous. *J Oral Rehab*. 2007;34(11):807-813.

53. Rocabado M. *Intermediate Craniofacial: Course Manual*. Tucson, AZ: International Fundamental Orthopedic Rocabado Center; 2003.

54. Okeson JP. *Management of Temporomandibular Disorders and Occlusion*, ed 7. St. Louis: Mosby Elsevier; 2013.

55. Gavish A, Halachmi M, Winocur E, et al. Oral habits and their association with signs and symptoms of temporomandibular disorders in adolescent girls. *J Oral Rehabil*. 2000;27:22-32.

56. Kalamir A, Pollard H, Vitiello A, et al. Intra-oral myofascial therapy for chronic myogenous temporomandibular disorders: a randomized, controlled pilot study. *J Man Manipulative Ther*. 2010;18(3):139-146.

57. Kalamir A, Bonella R, Graham P, et al. Intraoral myofascial therapy for chronic myogenous temporomandibular disorder: a

58. Smith P, Mosscrop D, Davies S, et al. The efficacy of acupuncture in the treatment of temporomandibular joint myofascial pain: a randomized controlled trial. *J Dentistry*. 2007;35(3):259-267.

59. Dommerholt J, Fernandez-de-las-Penas C. *Trigger Point Dry Needling: an Evidenced and Clinical Based Approach*. Edinburgh: Churchill Livingston/Elsevier; 2013.

60. Greenbaum T, Dvir Z, Reiter S, et al. Cervical flexion-rotation test and physiological range of motion – a comparative study of patients with myogenic temporomandibular disorder versus healthy subjects. *Musculoskelet Sci Pract*. 2017;27:7-13.

61. Calixtre LB, Oliveira AB, de Sena Rosa LR, et al. Effectiveness of mobilisation of the upper cervical region and craniocervical flexor training on orofacial pain, mandibular function and headache in women with TMD. A randomised, controlled trial. *J Oral Rehabil*. 2019;46:109-119.

62. Rocabado M. *Keynote Address*. St. Louis: AAOMPT annual conference; 2007.

63. Yoda T, Sakamoto I, Imai H, et al. A randomized controlled trial of therapeutic exercise for clicking due to disk anterior displacement with reduction in the temporomandibular joint. *Cranio*. 2003;21:10-16.

64. Tuncer AG, Ergun N, Tuncer AH, et al. Effectiveness of manual therapy and home physical therapy in patients with temporomandibular disorders: a randomized controlled trial. *J Bodyw Mov Ther*. 2013;17:302-308.

65. Yatani H, Suzuki K, Kuboki T, et al. The validity of clinical examination for diagnosing anterior disk displacement without reduction. *Oral Surg Oral Med Oral Pathol Oral Radiol Endod*. 1998;85:654-660.

66. Julsvoll EH, Vollestad NK, Robinson HS. Validation of clinical tests for patients with long-lasting painful temporomandibular disorders with anterior disc displacement without reduction. *Man Ther*. 2016;21:109-119.

67. Julsoll EH, Vollestad NK, Opseth G, Robinson HS. Inter-tester reliability of selected clinical tests for long-standing termporomandibular disorders. *J Man Manipulative Ther*. 2017;25(4): 182-189.

68. Cleland J, Palmer J. Effectiveness of manual physical therapy, therapeutic exercise, and patient education on bilateral disc displacement without reduction of the temporomandibular joint: a single-case design. *J Orthop Sports Phys Ther*. 2004;34: 535-548.

69. Israel H, Diamond B, Saed-Nejad F, et al. Osteoarthritis and synovitis as major pathoses of the temporomandibular joint: comparison of the clinical diagnosis with arthroscopic morphology. *J Oral Maxillofac Surg*. 1998;56:1023-1028.

70. Holmlund AB, Axelsson S. Temporomandibular arthropathy: correlation between clinical signs and symptoms and arthroscopic findings. *Int J Oral Maxillofac Surg*. 1996;25:178-181.

71. Higbie EJ, Seidel-Cobb D, Taylor LF, et al. Effect of head position on vertical mandibular opening. *J Orthop Sports Phys Ther*. 1999;29(2):127-130.

72. Walker N, Bohannon RW, Cameron D. Discriminant validity of temporomandibular joint range of motion measurements obtained with a ruler. *J Orthop Sports Phys Ther*. 2000;30:484-492.

73. Lobbezoo-Scholte AM, de Wijer A, Steenks MH, et al. Interexaminer reliability of six orthopaedic tests in diagnostic subgroups of craniomandibular disorders. *J Oral Rehabil*. 1994;21: 273-285.

74. Orsini MR, Kuboki T, Terada S, et al. Clinical predictability of temporomandibular joint disc displacement. *J Dent Res*. 1999; 78:650-660.

75. Cacchiotti DA, Plesh O, Bianchi P, et al. Signs and symptoms in samples with and without temporomandibular disorders. *J Craniomandib Disord*. 1991;5:167-172.

76. Johnstone J. The feasibility of palpating the lateral pterygoid muscle. *J Prosth Dent*. 1980;44(3):318-323.

77. Dworkin SF, LeResche L, DeRouen T, et al. Assessing clinical signs of temporomandibular disorders: reliability of clinical examiners. *J Prosthet Dent*. 1990;63:574-579.

78. de Wiker A, Lobbezoo-Scholte AM, Steenks MH, et al. Reliability of clinical findings in temporomandibular disorders. *J Orofac Pain*. 1995;9:181-191.

79. Manfredini D, Tognini F, Zampa V, et al. Predictive value of clinical findings for temporomandibular joint effusion. *Oral Surg Oral Med Oral Pathol Oral Radiol Endod*. 2003;96: 521-526.

INDEX

Note: Page numbers followed by *"b," "f,"* and *"t"* indicate boxes, figures, and tables, respectively.